Liver Metastasis: Biology and Clinical Management

Cancer Metastasis – Biology and Treatment

VOLUME 16

Liver Metastasis: Biology and Clinical Management

Edited by

Pnina Brodt

Division of Surgical Research, Royal Victoria Hospital, McGill University Health Centre, Montreal, QC, Canada

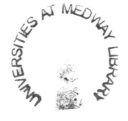

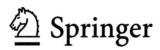 Springer

Editor
Pnina Brodt
Division of Surgical Research
Royal Victoria Hospital
McGill University Health Centre
H3A 1A1 Montreal, QC
Canada
pnina.brodt@mcgill.ca

ISSN 1568-2102
ISBN 978-94-007-0291-2   e-ISBN 978-94-007-0292-9
DOI 10.1007/978-94-007-0292-9
Springer Dordrecht Heidelberg London New York

Library of Congress Control Number: 2011921120

Printed on acid-free paper

Springer is part of Springer Science+Business Media (www.springer.com)

This book is dedicated to all the scientists who devote their lives to the study of disease for the betterment of human health.

Acknowledgement

The editor acknowledges with gratitude the hard work and dedication of all the authors who contributed excellent chapters to this book. Their knowledge and insights were an inspiration.

Contents

Contributors

Pnina Brodt Division of Surgical Research, Royal Victoria Hospital, McGill University Health Center, Montreal, QC, Canada, H3A 1A1, pnina.brodt@mcgill.ca

Miguel N. Burnier Jr. Department of Ophthalmology, McGill University Health Center, McGill University, Montreal, QC, Canada, miguel.burnier@mcgill.ca

Ann F. Chambers London Regional Cancer Program, London, ON, Canada; Department of Oncology and Department of Medical Biophysics, University of Western Ontario, London, ON, Canada, ann.chambers@Lhsc.on.ca

Sean P. Cleary Hepatobiliary and Pancreatic Surgical Oncology and Transplantation, Division of General Surgery, University Health Network-10EN212 Toronto General Hospital, Toronto, ON, Canada, sean.cleary@uhn.on.ca

Christina M. Edwards Division of Surgical Oncology, Department of Surgery, Vanderbilt University Medical Center, Nashville, TN, USA, christina.edwards@vanderbilt.edu

Khaled Elgadi Hepatobiliary and Pancreatic Surgical Oncology and Transplantation, Division of General Surgery, University Health Network-10EN212 Toronto General Hospital, Toronto, ON, Canada, elgadik@gmail.com

Mohamed El Khodary Department of Radiology, McGill University Health Center, Montreal, QC, Canada, mohamed.khodary@gmail.com

Lorenzo Ferri The LD McLean Surgical Research Laboratories, Division of Surgical Research, Department of Surgery, The Montreal General Hospital, McGill University, Montreal, QC, Canada; Division of Thoracic Surgery, Department of Surgery, The Montreal General Hospital, McGill University, Montreal, QC, Canada, lorenzo.ferri@muhc.mcgill.ca

Bruno F. Fernandes Department of Ophthalmology, McGill University Health Center, McGill University, Montreal, QC, Canada, bruno.mtl@gmail.com

Adrian M. Fox University Health Network, University of Toronto, Toronto, ON, Canada, adrian.fox@uhn.on.ca

Steven Gallinger University Health Network, University of Toronto, Toronto, ON, Canada, sgallingen@rogers.com

Jacques Huot Le Centre de recherche en cancérologie de l'Université Laval et le Centre de recherche du CHUQ, L'Hôtel-Dieu de Québec, Québec, QC, Canada, Jacques.Huot@phc.ulaval.ca

Thorsten Jung Department of Tumor Cell Biology, University Hospital of Surgery, Heidelberg, Germany, schunges@gmx.de

Otto Kollmar Department of General, Visceral, Vascular and Pediatric Surgery, University of Saarland, Homburg/Saar, Germany; Institute for Clinical and Experimental Surgery, University of Saarland, Homburg/Saar, Germany, otto.kollmar@uks.eu

Shun Li Department of Medicine, McGill University, Montreal, QC, Canada, shun.li@mail.mcgill.ca

Lance A. Liotta Center for Applied Proteomics and Molecular Medicine, George Mason University, Manassas, VA, USA, lliotta@gmu.edu

Michael D. Menger Institute for Clinical and Experimental Surgery, University of Saarland, Homburg/Saar, Germany, michael.menger@uks.eu

Nipun B. Merchant Division of Surgical Oncology, Department of Surgery, Vanderbilt University Medical Center, Nashville, TN, USA, nipun.merchant@vanderbilt.edu

Laurent Milot Department of Medical Imaging, Sunnybrook Health Sciences Centre, Toronto, ON, Canada, laurent.milot@sunnybrook.ca

Carol-Anne Moulton University Health Network, University of Toronto, Toronto, ON, Canada, carol-anne.moulton@uhn.on.ca

Alexander A. Parikh Division of Surgical Oncology, Vanderbilt University Medical Center, Nashville, TN, USA, alexander.parikh@vanderbilt.edu

Emanuel F. Petricoin Center for Applied Proteomics and Molecular Medicine, George Mason University, Manassas, VA, USA, epetrico@gmu.edu

Mariaelena Pierobon Center for Applied Proteomics and Molecular Medicine, George Mason University, Manassas, VA, USA, mpierobo@gmu.edu

Nicolas Porquet Le Centre de recherche en cancérologie de l'Université Laval et le Centre de recherche du CHUQ, L'Hôtel-Dieu de Québec, Québec, QC, Canada, nicolas.porquet@unice.fr

Trevor Reichman Hepatobiliary and Pancreatic Surgical Oncology and Transplantation, Division of General Surgery, University Health

Network-10EN212 Toronto General Hospital, Toronto, ON, Canada,
trevor.reichman@uhn.on.ca

Caroline Reinhold Department of Radiology, McGill University Health Center,
Montreal, QC, Canada, caroline.reinhold@muhc.mcgill.ca

Martin K. Schilling Department of General, Visceral, Vascular and Pediatric
Surgery, University of Saarland, Homburg/Saar, Germany,
martin.schilling@uks.eu

Peter M. Siegel Goodman Cancer Research Centre, McGill University, Montréal,
QC, Canada; Departments of Biochemistry and Medicine, McGill University,
Montréal, QC, Canada, peter.siegel@mcgill.ca

Alessandra Silvestri Center for Applied Proteomics and Molecular Medicine,
George Mason University, Manassas, VA, USA; CRO-IRCCS, National Cancer
Institute, Aviano, Italy, asilvestri@cro.it

J. Joshua Smith Division of Surgical Oncology, Department of Surgery,
Vanderbilt University Medical Center, Nashville, TN, USA,
josh.smith@vanderbilt.edu

Jonathan Spicer The LD McLean Surgical Research Laboratories, Division of
Surgical Research, Department of Surgery, McGill University Health Center,
Montreal, QC, Canada, jonathan.spicer@mail.mcgill.ca

Sébastien Tabariès Goodman Cancer Research Centre, McGill University,
Montréal, QC, Canada, H3A 1A3; Department of Medicine, McGill University,
Montréal, QC, Canada, H3A 1A3, sebastien.tabaries@mail.mcgill.ca

Jason L. Townson London Regional Cancer Program, London, ON, Canada;
Department of Medical Biophysics, University of Western Ontario, London, ON,
Canada, jtownson@umm.edu

Fernando Vidal-Vanaclocha Institute of Applied Molecular Medicine (IMMA),
CEU-San Pablo University School of Medicine, Madrid, Spain,
fernando.vidalvanaclocha@ceu.es

Shoshana Yakar Division of Endocrinology, Diabetes and Bone Disease, Mount
Sinai School of Medicine, New York, NY, USA, shoshana.yakar@mssm.edu

Margot Zöller Department of Tumor Cell Biology, University Hospital of
Surgery, Heidelberg, Germany; German Cancer Research Centre, Heidelberg,
Germany, margot.zoeller@uni-heidelberg.de

Chapter 1
Introduction

Pnina Brodt

The liver is a common site of metastasis from several of the most prevalent human malignancies, in particular cancers of the gastrointestinal tract such as colorectal (CRC), neuroendocrine, pancreatic, esophageal and gastric carcinomas. Over 50% of CRC patients will present with liver metastases either at the time of diagnosis or after resection of the primary tumor [1]. Although advances in surgery, chemotherapy and targeted biologic therapies have progressively and significantly improved the prognosis of patients with hepatic metastases in the past 15 years, a large proportion of these patients still die of their disease, with the 5 year survival rate ranging from 23 to 45% [2–7]. To improve these dismal statistics, a better understanding of the biology of liver metastasis is essential. This is particularly true for early events that precede, and are required for the successful colonization of the liver, because their blockade may offer a therapeutic window for the prevention of metastasis.

The tumor microenvironment plays an active role in the progression of malignant disease both at the primary site and at sites of metastases. The tumor microenvironment consists of the tumor-associated stroma that includes cells such as resident fibroblasts, adipocytes, blood and lymph vessel-lining endothelial cells and pericytes, extracellular matrix (ECM) proteins produced by these cells, as well as resident and infiltrating host inflammatory and immune cells. These cell populations may have distinct organ-specific properties and molecular profiles that affect their interaction with the metastatic cells. The malignant cells can communicate with these organ-specific microenvironments through soluble mediators such as chemokines, cytokines and growth factors, through cell-cell and cell-ECM contact, mediated by receptors and counter receptors that can themselves evolve as the tumor progresses, and through the activity of proteolytic enzymes that remodel tissue barriers around the expanding tumors and contribute to neovascularization, tumor migration and invasion [8, 9]. In addition, the host innate and acquired immune

P. Brodt (✉)
Departments of Surgery and Medicine, McGill University and the McGill University Health Center, Montreal, QC, Canada
e-mail: pnina.brodt@mcgill.ca

P. Brodt (ed.), *Liver Metastasis: Biology and Clinical Management*, Cancer
Metastasis – Biology and Treatment 16, DOI 10.1007/978-94-007-0292-9_1,
© Springer Science+Business Media B.V. 2011

responses also contribute significantly to tumor progression at the primary and metastatic sites [10–12].

The phenomenon of preferential homing of metastatic cells (site-specific metastasis) has been recognized for decades but its molecular basis, particularly as it pertains to liver metastasis has only recently become better understood. As predicted by the "seed and soil" hypothesis, first postulated by Paget [13, 14], the ability of tumor cells to grow in a secondary site depends on a complementarity between tumor cell properties and the unique microenvironment of the target organ. This also includes the reciprocal communication between invading tumor cells and the unique stroma of the target organ.

The architecture and cellular composition of the liver, the largest gland of the body, is unique. As a bi-functional gland, it is the site of bile production and synthesis of many plasma proteins and endocrine factors and has a well-developed machinery for biosynthesis and metabolic functions. In addition, the liver also plays a major role as a "bio-sieve" detoxifying and excreting into the bile endogenous waste products and removing microbial contaminants, toxins and reactive oxygen intermediates from visceral blood en route to the systemic circulation. To carry out these functions, the liver receives in addition to arterial blood, venous blood draining from visceral organs. In fact, the portal vein draining the blood from the GI tract accounts for 70% of the liver blood supply [15]. This unique feature provides circulating metastatic cells with two vascular routes and ports of entry into the liver. In addition, tumor cells entering the liver encounter a unique population of host cells that includes unique sinusoidal cells specialized in the filtration of plasma, the hepatocytes constituting the major cellular component of this organ and perivascular mesenchymal cells such as fibroblasts and perisinusoidal hepatic stellate cells. Other distinct characteristics of the liver include a parenchymal cell heterogeneity that amplifies its functional capabilities and tissue regenerating potential and distinct innate and adoptive immune defense mechanisms that generate a physiological immune tolerance in this organ. These specialized features of the liver have major consequences for the process of metastasis and their understanding is therefore essential for better insight into the early cellular and molecular events in liver metastasis. An extensive discussion on the unique architectural and physiological properties of the liver is provided to the reader in Chapter 2 of this book. A three dimensional graphic web-based teaching tool known as the *Virtual Liver Project* developed by the authors of Chapter 12 can also be found at: http://pie.med.utoronto.ca/VLiver/index.htm.

Tumor cells or tumor cell clusters that enter the hepatic microvasculature normally arrest in the terminal portal venules and hepatic sinusoids, and their first point of contact is therefore with the sinusoidal endothelial cells. The events that follow tumor cell entry into the sinusoids vary greatly depending on the tumor cell properties and their fate may follow several different scenarios. The tumor cells may be immediately destroyed by physical factors such as deformation-associated trauma and mechanical stress, transient ischemia/reperfusion due to vessel obstruction or local resistance mechanisms. Once in the extravascular space they may enter a state of dormancy as solitary cells and never produce a metastasis, they may initiate a short-lived process of proliferation that is aborted before a metastasis is established or they may actively proliferate to form macrometastases. The chapters included in Part I of this book provide insight into the cellular/molecular mechanisms that determine which of these scenarios prevails. They have been organized in an order that reflects the sequence of events occurring upon tumor entry into the liver. Chapters 2 and 3 by Dr. Vidal-Vanaclocha provide an overview of the liver architecture and its unique cellular/molecular composition (Chapter 2) and against this background a detailed review of the body of knowledge on the different types of hepatic metastases and the diverse interactions between the tumor and its microenvironment that impact metastases formation (Chapter 3). The role of the cancer initiating cell and its unique markers in the process of liver metastasis of colorectal cancer is reviewed by Dr. Zoller and associates in Chapter 4 and the role of chemokines and chemokine receptors in tumor and host cell recruitment into the liver is discussed by Dr. Schilling and associates in Chapter 5.

The first point of contact between metastatic cancer cells and the hepatic microenvironment is the sinusoidal endothelium. This interaction is affected the various factors including the releases of chemotactic and inflammatory mediators by tumor and host cells and also involves host innate immune cells residing in the sinusoids such as Kupffer cells. In turn, the tumor-endothelial cell interaction is an important limiting step in the metastatic process as it can determine whether tumor cells are eliminated or proceed to extravasate and ultimately, form micrometastases. This early step in the metastatic process is reviewed in two of the chapters namely, Chapter 6 on the role of inflammation in the early stages of liver metastasis contributed by Dr. Spicer et al. and Chapter 7 that focuses on signal transduction mechanisms initiated by tumor-endothelial cell interactions, contributed by Drs. Porquet and Huot.

Tumor cells extravasate from the sinusoidal vessels into the space of Disse separating the endothelial and parenchymal compartments where hepatic stellate cells also reside. There they may begin a process of proliferation or migrate further into preferred sites of growth, in response to local chemotactic or growth factors, to form macrometastases. Alternatively, they may enter a state of dormancy as solitary cells or as small microscopic foci and either fail to produce a metastasis or resume proliferation years later in response to local factors that are yet to be identified. The mechanisms underlying tumor cell dormancy and recurrence in the liver and their implications for the clinical management of metastatic disease are reviewed by Drs. Townson and Chambers in Chapter 8, while the role of liver-derived growth factors such as IGF-I in paracrine stimulation of tumor cell growth is reviewed in Chapter 9 by Li et al. Finally, in Chapter 10, Drs. Tabariès and Siegel provide a detailed overview of the cellular and molecular factors that underlie liver metastasis of breast cancer cells, highlighting the contribution of the molecular profiles of the tumor cells and the role of the microenvironment, including pre- and pro-metastatic niches, in the establishment of metastases. Although all of these chapters focus on biological aspects of the metastatic process, the translational/clinical implications are underscored.

The chapters in Part II of the book provide critical overviews on major aspects of the clinical management of hepatic metastases. In Chapter 11 Dr. El Khodary and associates provide a comprehensive and timely description of the imaging modalities presently available for hepatic metastases, the progress of the technology in the past few decades, the advantages and limitations of the different modalities and the context for selecting the appropriate imaging technology. Surgical and chemotherapeutic treatment approaches to the management of colorectal cancer metastases are critically reviewed by Dr. Fox and associates in Chapter 12, while the management of hepatic metastases from non GI origin, with emphasis on the surgical option, is discussed by Dr. Elgadi et al. in Chapter 13. In Chapter 14, Dr. Silvestri and associates eloquently make the case for the use of proteomic porfiling of tumor tissue as a tool for individualization of anti-metastatic therapy and in Chapter 15, the use of targeted biological therapeutics is discussed by Dr. Edwards et al., with emphasis on the accumulated clinical experience with anti-angiogenic drugs for treatment of metastases. The book concludes with a review by Drs. Fernandes and Burnier (Chapter 16) on mechanisms underlying the systemic dissemination and metastasis of uveal melanoma – a prototype of site-specific liver metastasis. The studies reviewed in this chapter reveal that common molecular mechanisms and mediators may be involved in liver metastasis from diverse tumor types, suggesting that a universal "liver-metastasis signature" may eventually emerge.

A common thread that can be found in many of the chapters dealing with the clinical management of hepatic metastasis is the critical importance of the multidisciplinary team in decision making and individualization of disease management. The authors (Chapter 12) recommend that this team should ideally be composed of all the health care providers that deliver care to the patient, including representation from diagnostic radiology, medical oncology, surgery, radiation oncology, pathology, diagnostic radiology, palliative care, nursing staff and social work. It is argued that the involvement of such a team ensures that the patient care recommendations are arrived at through consensus decision making and reflect closely the various parameters that could affect outcome.

In closing, it has not been the objective of this book to provide an exhaustive review of the multiple and complex factors that play a role in the development of hepatic metastases or the various treatment options available to cancer patients that develop inoperable hepatic tumors. An all-inclusive review of this complex disease is clearly beyond the scope of any single volume. Instead, this volume focuses on specific aspects of the process of hepatic metastasis, in particular tumor cell communication with the hepatic microenvironment, as well as on various clinical parameters that have come to light in recent years and whose understanding is essential for better and more individualized design of treatment protocols. In this age of personalized medicine, it is hoped that the information in this book will provide the clinician with additional decision-making tools, contribute to new approaches for patient stratification and improve the management of metastatic disease to the liver.

Acknowledgement   The author wishes to thank the McGill University Health Center Foundation and the Stewart family for the Stewart Fellowship in Research in Haematology and Oncology.

References

1. Alberts SR, Wagman LD (2008) Chemotherapy for colorectal cancer liver metastases. Oncologist 13:1063–1073
2. Selzner M et al (2000) Liver metastases from breast cancer: long-term survival after curative resection. Surgery 127:383–389

3. Lubrano J et al (2008) Liver resection for breast cancer metastasis: does it improve survival? Surg Today 38:293–299

4. Ercolani G et al (2005) The role of liver resections for noncolorectal, nonneuroendocrine metastases: experience with 142 observed cases. Ann Surg Oncol 12:459–466

5. Goldberg RM et al (2007) The continuum of care: a paradigm for the management of metastatic colorectal cancer. Oncologist 12:38–50

6. Jaeck D, Pessaux P (2008) Bilobar colorectal liver metastases: treatment options. Surg Oncol Clin N Am 17:553–568, ix

7. Benoist S, Nordlinger B (2009) The role of preoperative chemotherapy in patients with resectable colorectal liver metastases. Ann Surg Oncol 16:2385–2390

8. Brooks SA et al (2009) Molecular interactions in cancer cell metastasis. Acta Histochem 112:3–25

9. Steeg PS (2006) Tumor metastasis: mechanistic insights and clinical challenges. Nat Med 12:895–904

10. Bissell MJ, Kenny PA, Radisky DC (2005) Microenvironmental regulators of tissue structure and function also regulate tumor induction and progression: the role of extracellular matrix and its degrading enzymes. Cold Spring Harb Symp Quant Biol 70:1–14

11. Robinson SC, Coussens LM (2005) Soluble mediators of inflammation during tumor development. Adv Cancer Res 93:159–187

12. Coussens L, Werb Z (2002) Inflammation and cancer. Nature 420:860–867

13. Paget S (1989) The distribution of secondary growths in cancer of the breast. Cancer Metastasis Rev 8:98–101

14. Fidler IJ (2003) The pathogenesis of cancer metastasis: the 'seed and soil' hypothesis revisited. Nat Rev Cancer 3:453–458

15. Greenway CV, Stark RD (1971) Hepatic vascular bed. Physiol Rev 51:23–65

Part I
Biology

Chapter 2
Architectural and Functional Aspects of the Liver with Implications for Cancer Metastasis

Fernando Vidal-Vanaclocha

Abstract The complex functions of the liver in biosynthesis, metabolism, clearance, and host defense are tightly dependent on its specialized microcirculation and parenchymal/non-parenchymal cell heterogeneity. The same architectural and functional aspects of the liver that guarantee hepatic homeostasis are also determinants of the malignant behavior of cancer cells through the various stages of the metastatic process. First, the functional heterogeneity of the hepatic microcirculation at the lobular level and its unique sinusoidal cell composition influence the trafficking, retention of, and damage to circulating cancer cells reaching the liver through the portal vein or hepatic artery. Second, the perivascular hepatic mesenchymal cells including fibroblasts from perilobular portal tract and perisinusoidal hepatic stellate cells become "tumor-activated myofibroblasts" providing a unique stromal support for metastatic cell growth and tumor angiogenesis. Third, the phenotypic heterogeneity of the hepatic parenchymal cell compartment represents an additional bio-resource for tumor-associated stromal cells and autocrine growth factors through epithelial to mesenchymal transition and fourth, the status of the hepatic regional immunity, including the innate immune response and immunosuppression of the adaptive response also contribute to cancer cell survival and growth. Therefore, the aim of this chapter is to summarize the current state of knowledge on these four aspects of hepatic tissue biology. Taken together, these liver-unique elements constitute a functional microenvironment representing the specific biological background encountered by metastatic cancer cells entering the liver. It has become clear in recent years that functional diversity in this biological background may affect cancer patients susceptibility to hepatic metastasis This raises the possibility that hepatic microenvironment-specific biomarkers could be identified that will provide prognostic tools for metastasis risk prediction and the prevention, surgical management and anti-tumor drug selection for liver metastasis.

F. Vidal-Vanaclocha (✉)
Institute of Applied Molecular Medicine (IMMA), CEU-San Pablo University School of Medicine,
Urb. Montepríncipe, Boadilla del Monte, 28668 Madrid, Spain
e-mail: fernando.vidalvanaclocha@ceu.es

P. Brodt (ed.), *Liver Metastasis: Biology and Clinical Management*, Cancer
Metastasis – Biology and Treatment 16, DOI 10.1007/978-94-007-0292-9_2,
© Springer Science+Business Media B.V. 2011

Keywords Liver sinusoidal cells · Hepatocytes · Microcirculation · Liver immunity · Hepatic fibrogenesis

Abbreviations

SMA	α-smooth muscle actin
COX	cyclooxygenase
HSE	hepatic sinusoidal endothelium
HSEC	hepatic sinusoidal endothelial cell(s)
HSC	hepatic stellate cells
PTF	portal tract fibroblast
LAL	liver-associated lymphocyte
ManR	mannose receptor
NK	natural killer
IL	interleukin
ICAM-1	intercellular adhesion molecule-1
IFNγ	interferon gamma
MHC	major histocompatibility complex
NK	natural killer cells
TNFα	tumor necrosis factor alpha
VCAM-1	vascular cell adhesion molecule-1
PTF	portal tract fibroblast
GFAP	Glial fibrillary acidic protein
TLR	toll-like receptor

Contents

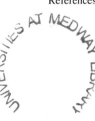

2.1 Introduction

The liver is the largest solid organ and resides beneath the diaphragm between the digestive tract and the lower abdominal organs. The main function of the liver is to maintain the body's metabolic homeostasis through processing of dietary amino acids, carbohydrates, lipids, and vitamins. As a bi-functional gland, it is the site of bile production and the synthesis of many plasma proteins and endocrine factors. As a "bio-protection" platform, the liver contributes to detoxification and excretion into bile of endogenous waste products and pollutants, and to the removal of microbes and toxins in visceral blood en route to the systemic circulation. Hepatic disorders therefore can have far-reaching clinical consequences.

To accomplish these diverse tasks, the liver functions as a "way station" between the splanchnic and systemic circulation, with dual inputs for its blood supply. The portal vein delivers three quarters of the afferent blood volume to the liver and carries a venous drainage originating from the majority of the intra-abdominal viscera that is poor in oxygen but rich in nutrients, bacterial-degradation products and absorbed toxic substances. The hepatic artery delivers approximately one quarter of the total blood output from the heart, and carries well-oxygenated blood to the liver, although most of the hepatic cells are in hypoxia even under normo-oxygenated conditions. These major vessels enter the liver through the *hilum* (*porta hepatis*) and immediately begin to arborize, ensheathed in connective tissue stroma.

According to traditional anatomy, the human liver is divided into four lobes (right, left, quadrate and caudate). These are supplied by right and left branches of the portal vein and hepatic artery, while their bile secretion drains into the right and left hepatic ducts emerging from the liver through the hepatic duct proper. The right lobe is further subdivided in its inferior-posterior surfaces into two smaller lobes, the quadrate and caudate lobes. However, the conventional division of the liver into these lobes is a topographic classification that does not correspond to the functional division of the liver that is defined by the distribution of the right and left portal vein systems. The watershed between these two vascular beds corresponds to a plane that passes superiorly through the left side of the sulcus of the inferior vena cava to the middle of the gallbladder fossa inferiorly. The quadrate lobe and the greater part of the caudate lobe on the posterior aspect of the liver belong functionally to the left hemiliver. Of greater significance to the surgeon is the functional organization of the liver into eight segments, numbered 1–8, the caudate lobe being segment 1 and the remainder, 2–8, moving roughly from left to right across the liver (see Fig. 2.1). Each segment has its own independent vascular and biliary pedicle and venous drainage. This functional anatomic arrangement facilitates limited segmental resections of the liver as is sometimes performed for partial hepatectomy.

The entire liver is covered by the Glisson's capsule, a thin connective tissue layer, which is beneath the single layer of peritoneal mesothelial cells. Seventy percent of the hepatic cellular content (or 80% of the liver volume) is composed of parenchymal cells of endodermal origin. These include hepatocytes, cholangiocytes and their progenitor cells that together provide the glandular, metabolic

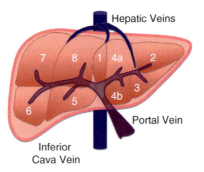

Fig. 2.1 A schematic representation of the segmental anatomy of the liver based on the functional approach of Couinaud. The liver has been divided into eight functionally independent segments. Each segment has its own vascular inflow, outflow and biliary drainage. In the center of each segment there is a branch of the portal vein, hepatic artery and bile duct. In the periphery of each segment there is vascular outflow through the hepatic veins. Because of this division into self-contained units, each segment can be resected without damaging the remaining segments. The portal vein divides the liver into upper and lower segments, while the right hepatic vein divides the right lobe into anterior and posterior segments, the middle hepatic vein divides the liver into right and left lobes and the left hepatic vein divides the left lobe into medial and lateral parts. In a frontal view of the liver, segments 6 and 7 are not visible because they are located more posteriorly, and the right border of the liver is formed by segments 5 and 8. Segment 1 (caudate lobe) is also located posteriorly, not being visible in a frontal view, and often has direct connections to the inferior vena cava through hepatic veins that are separate from the main hepatic vein. Segment 4 is sometimes divided into segments 4a and 4b

and detoxifying needs of the body. The remaining cells consist of a broad family of non-parenchymal cell lineages of mesenchymal and hematopoietic origin, including sinusoidal wall-lining cells, liver-associated lymphocytes and other hepatotropic leukocytes, and connective tissue cells. These specialized cell populations provide the liver with non-glandular capabilities that have systemic relevance such as blood cell filtration, molecular scavenger activities and inflammatory and immune responses. In addition, non-parenchymal cells are also involved in the local control of the liver microcirculation, extracellular matrix composition and liver tissue renewal and regeneration. These unique architectural and functional features are differentiated in the adult liver to perform functions required inside and outside the liver. However, as reviewed in Chapter 3, these organ-specific features also endow the liver with a functional microenvironment that may provide prometastatic cues to circulating cancer cells. Among these architectural/functional aspects of the liver are the following:

(A) The dual, slow and tortuous character of the hepatic microcirculation [1] that provides the hepatic "territory" with a great accessibility and efficient filtration and recognition capabilities for circulating cells, microbes and soluble molecules. This is due to the anastomotic arrangement of networking capillaries within the hepatic tissue and to the special role that organ-specific subtypes of endothelial cells, macrophages and pericytes play in blood flow control [2] (see Section 2.3). These unique hemodynamic features not only provide access to the liver but may also facilitate the mechanical arrest of cancer cell emboli carried in the blood from tumors located in other organs.

Another feature of the hepatic biology that is relevant at the microvascular phase of hepatic metastasis is the rich profile of surface molecules provided to disseminating cancer cells by fenestrated hepatic sinusoidal endothelium cells (HSECs) and organ-specific macrophages i.e. Kupffer cells lining the hepatic capillaries (see Sections 2.5.1 and 2.5.2). Major molecules on the surface of these hepatic scavenger cells include diverse terminal oligosaccharide moieties [3], cell adhesion proteins [4], endocytic receptors [5] and toll-like receptors (TLRs) [6], normally involved in the recognition of pathogen-associated molecular patterns and endogenous TLR ligands termed "damage-associated molecular patterns". More importantly, most of these surface molecules are regulated by inflammatory cytokines and account for the efficient hepatic uptake and clearance of circulating gut-derived nutrients, toxins, microbes, waste molecules, aged cells, and even cancer cells.

(B) The liver contains heterogeneous populations of endoderm-derived parenchyma cells [7] i.e. hepatocytes and cholangiocytes and mesenchymal non-parenchymal cells [8] (see Sections 2.4 and 2.5). These cell populations coordinately behave to establish the functional tissue structure supporting the glandular and metabolic functions of the liver. At the same time, this functional coordination serves to restore hepatic microarchitecture during physiological renewal and regeneration in response to a variety of pathophysiological circumstances [9]. This powerful tissue-reconstitution machinery can also be co-opted during the development of hepatic metastases. In fact, the same hepatic parenchymal and non-parenchymal cells can also contribute to intratumoral stroma and blood vessel generation in response to tumor-derived factors (see Chapter 3), providing a favorable milieu for the survival and growth of disseminating cancer cells.

(C) Perivascular hepatic mesenchymal cells including fibroblasts from perilobular portal tract and perisinusoidal hepatic stellate cells (see Section 2.5.4) become activated myofibroblasts in response to liver insults of viral, metabolic, toxic and tumoral origin [10–12]. These activated mesenchymal cells are the major source of extracellular matrix during liver injury and secrete all the components of the hepatic scar. In addition they also have proangiogenic [13] and parenchymal cell-stimulating activities, contributing to hepatic regeneration [14, 15]. However, when this stromal reaction is induced by tumor-derived factors, it provides a unique stromal cell support for cancer cell invasion and growth and for the induction of tumor angiogenesis with resulting prometastatic effects (see Chapter 3 for a more extensive discussion).

(D) The liver contains specialized subpopulations of the host defense system including resident macrophages, dendritic cells, mast cells, cytotoxic natural killer (NK) cells and T lymphocytes (see Section 2.5.3). These provide potent innate and adaptive immune responses [16]. However, the same defense machinery can also be the source of immune regulatory mediators such as

IL-10, prostanoids, soluble ICAM-1 and TGFβ that induce a regional immune suppression intended to limit the damage to the liver parenchyma that can be caused by prolonged exposure to inflammatory and immune factors [17]. While this local immune suppression can provide a favorable milieu for liver transplantation [18] and increases oral tolerance [19], it may also contribute to the occurrence of autoimmunity, infectious diseases and cancer metastasis in this organ [20]. Not surprisingly, therefore, the hepatic microenvironment can be relatively tolerant to invading microorganisms such as malaria sporozoites [21] and fungi [22] and is also favorable to the development of hepatic metastases (see Chapter 3).

It appears therefore that in addition to specific features of the hepatic microcirculation that facilitate the intrahepatic lodgment of circulating cancer cells the microenvironment and mechanisms that support key hepatic functions such as blood clearance, molecular scavenging, hepatic regeneration, wound healing, and immunity may also play a role in the retention or destruction of circulating cancer cells and ultimately may facilitate the ability of some tumor cells to develop metastases (see Chapter 3).

On this basis, this chapter summarizes those architectural and functional attributes of the hepatic tissue that may be relevant for metastasis. Specific attention has been paid to the hepatic microcirculation, the lobular organization of hepatic parenchymal and sinusoidal (non-parenchymal) cells into functional compartments, the origin and myofibroblastic transdifferentiation of parenchymal and non-parenchymal cells and the regional immunity of the liver. Moreover, because a large percentage of hepatic metastases occur in aging individuals, the structure and function of the aged liver [23, 24] are also discussed.

2.2 Tissue Architecture and Heterogeneity of the Hepatic Lobules

Within the interior of the liver, the Glisson's capsule connective tissue subdivides the parenchymal tissue into small polyhedral units known as the hepatic lobules [25]. At the same time, this connective tissue provides an internal supporting framework for the hepatic parenchyma, and ensheathes inter and perilobular portal venules, hepatic arterioles, biliary ducts, as well as lymphatic vessels and a network of nerve fibers – sympathetic and parasympathetic – that overlap with the perilobular microvasculature. Hepatic lobules are polyhedral prisms of liver tissue, the boundaries of which are demarcated by connective tissue septa. When cut in cross sections, the lobules have a hexagonal shape, and at the angles of the hexagons are typically visible the perilobular connective tissue ensheathing hepatic portal/arterial venules and bile ductules (portal triads). In the center of the hexagonal lobule a central vein is usually visible (the centrilobular vein). The smallest portal venules and hepatic arterioles provide the hepatic lobules with blood that drains through centrilobular veins into

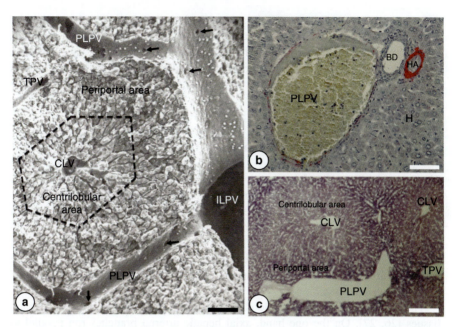

Fig. 2.2 The structure of the hepatic lobule. (**a**) Scanning electron microscopy image of the hepatic lobule. The hepatic lobule has the form of a polyhedral prism that has been sectioned horizontally in this image. Portal tracts situated at the border of the lobule, contain interlobular, perilobular and terminal portal veins (ILPV, PLPV, TPV), perilobular hepatic arteries, lymphatic vessels, nerve fibers and bile ducts (not visible). TPV around the lobule are connected to sinusoids through occasional gates serving the intralobular access of blood (*arrows*). Hepatic parenchymal cells i.e. hepatocytes (H) are organized in plates radially-arranged around the centrilobular vein (CLV) located in the center of the hepatic lobule. Sinusoids (S) provide a microvasculature interspersed among the hepatocytes within the hepatic lobules. They form an anastomotic network in the periportal area, while they are straight in the centrilobular area around the central vein. Blood passes through openings in the TPV into sinusoids and circulates among hepatocytes to be collected by the CLV. There, blood continues to the interlobular veins and, then, into collecting veins draining finally into the hepatic veins leaving the liver through the suprahepatic vein (not shown). Bar: 50 μm. (**b**) Portal space in the corner of a hepatic lobule. It contains the portal triad including a perilobular portal vein (PLPV) surrounded by a thin layer of smooth muscle cells expressing αSMA (in *red*), a small hepatic artery (HA) also stained with anti-αSMA antibodies (in *red*) and a bile duct (BD) without αSMA-expressing cells. Bar: 30 μm. (**c**) Histochemical reaction for succinate dehydrogenase of hepatocytes in a frozen hepatic tissue section. Limits among hepatic lobules are easily seen due to higher enzymatic activity (*dark stained*) of hepatocytes around perilobular portal veins (PLPV) compared to hepatocytes around centrilobular veins (CLV). Bar: 60 μm

hepatic veins leaving the liver (Fig. 2.2). Special capillaries termed hepatic sinusoids drive the blood from the perilobular areas into the center of the hepatic lobule. Both bile secretion and lymphatic fluid flow in the opposite direction from inside the lobules outwardly, draining in a network of hepatic bile ducts and lymphatic venules around the hepatic lobules.

The parenchymal cells of the organ – i.e., the glandular epithelial cells termed hepatocytes – are arranged as single-layered plates, arranged between sinusoids that radiate from the centrilobular vein – axis of the hepatic lobule – to the perilobular vessels. The complex microarchitecture formed by the hepatocytes and sinusoids ensures optimal exchange of metabolites between blood and hepatocytes. However, a limiting plate of hepatocytes surrounding the circumference of the lobules forms a nearly continuous wall in the interior of the lobule, which is connected to hepatocyte plates at the periphery of the lobules.

2.3 The Hepatic Microcirculation

The first-order branches of the portal vein distribution system arise from the terminal branches of the intrahepatic conducting system. These give rise to second-order vessels of approximately 70 μm in diameter that correspond to the terminal portal vein branches seen in portal tracts. Third-order vessels arise from these and correspond to the septal or interlobular branches. In turn, these vessels are branched into special capillaries along the hexagonal lobule before draining into the hepatic vein. These vessels exhibit a classical sinusoidal appearance, lack a connective tissue sheath and have no basement membrane.

The hepatic artery provides blood to both intralobular and portal tract hepatic tissues [26, 27]. On the one hand, axial hepatic arterial branches run parallel to the conducting portal veins and terminate in terminal portal venules and sinusoids, thereby supplying blood to the intralobular parenchyma. On the other hand, axial arteries also give rise to peribiliary branches that supply the accompanying bile ducts and connective tissue at the portal tract interstitium. These arterioles form the peribiliary plexus consisting of efferent and afferent capillaries with a basement membrane that wraps around bile ducts. Small channels from the peribiliary plexus drain into the sinusoids or portal venules. Thus, complex anastomoses exist between the axial arteries and peribiliary arterioles.

Therefore, the hepatic microcirculation is comprised of several anatomically and functionally distinct segments: hepatic arteries and their portal tract capillaries, terminal portal veins, sinusoids, and centrilobular or hepatic veins (Fig. 2.2). The portal vein branches into perilobular portal veins, interlobular veins and terminal portal venules, which feed into the hepatic sinusoids. The hepatic arterioles, derived from the hepatic artery, also feed into sinusoids, which in turn connect afferent portal venules and hepatic arterioles to centrilobular hepatic venules, located at a distance of approximately 0.5–0.8 mm. There are approximately one billion sinusoids in the human liver, forming a rich capillary network that promotes an efficient and prolonged blood-liver cell interaction along hepatic lobules [28]. This peculiar organ-specific vascularity facilitates molecular exchanges between blood and liver cells, and provides an extensive endothelial surface area for interactions with leukocytes and soluble waste macromolecules.

Hepatic sinusoids extend from portal to centrilobular venules and wind through regions having a wide variety of structural and microenvironmental characteristics. The first such region – called hepatic lobule periportal region – is where the highest percentage of hepatic tissue volume is occupied by sinusoids. This is also the location where sinusoids are smallest in diameter and form a network with frequent

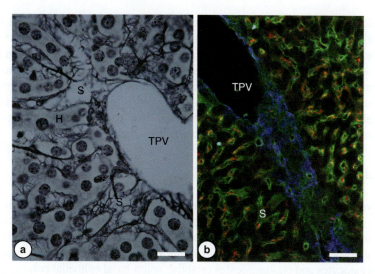

Fig. 2.3 The connective tissue stroma of the liver. (**a**) Histochemical reticulin staining of the hepatic tissue according to the Gordon-Sweets silver impregnation technique. A reticulin-stained fibrilar matrix network supporting the rich microvasculature of terminal portal veins (TPV) and sinusoids is shown. Bar: 20 μm. (**b**) Confocal microscopy of a terminal portal vein (TPV). In *blue* are stained αSMA-expressing cells located around the PV. In *green* are immunohistochemically stained ICAM-1-expressing HSECs and in *red* are stained ManR-expressing Kupffer cells and HSECs. Bar: 40 μm

anastomoses (Fig. 2.3). The second region provides a transition to the most distal region, the centrilobular region, where the sinusoidal segments are somewhat wider and converge straight into the centrilobular venules [28]. Together with intralobular zone-related structural differences, during the passage of blood through the sinusoids, decreasing periportal-to-centrilobular gradients of metabolic substrates and hormones (e.g. glucagon, adrenaline and cortisol) are generated, while at the same time the gradients of other products and mediators (e.g. bile acids, ammonia, IGF-I, NGF, TGFβ, VEGF) increase. This sublobular compartmentalization of signal output becomes even more complex because the output of sympathetic, parasympathetic and other nerves may also be different along the sinusoidal pathway [29].

The *hepatic acinus*, as described by Rappaport [30], is comprised of a three-dimensional arrangement of a small subgroup of liver cells nourished by a microvascular axis including a terminal portal venule and a hepatic arteriole. These vascular components together with the bile ductule comprise the *portal triad*. Liver cells are grouped around sinusoids that drain into terminal hepatic venules corresponding to centrilobular veins. Rappaport's model holds that blood flows from the portal triad at the center of the functional unit to the peripheral cells around the centrilobular veins. Beginning at a centralized portal triad, portal venous and arterial blood flows in an unidirectional fashion to the peripheral centrilobular vein. This flow initiates the formation of absorptive and metabolic gradients for most solutes. Cells in Rappaport's zone 1 receive blood with the highest concentration of oxygen and solutes. While zone 3 hepatocytes receive blood that has been modified by the absorption and secretion of hepatocytes in zones 1 and 2 [30]. Although these zones are referred to as distinct entities, there are no clear-cut boundaries between them. One contemporary trend describes populations of hepatocytes as either proximal or distal to a particular fixed point of origin, such as the terminal portal venule or the centrilobular vein. As a result of this topography, the functional activities of the liver cells, vary along the sinusoidal pathway and are widely distributed among the periportal and centrilobular subpopulations of these cells [31, 32].

2.4 Liver Parenchymal Cells

The liver consists of two types of endodermally-derived epithelial cells, the hepatocytes and cholangiocytes that differentiate from hepatoblasts. Hepatocytes are liver parenchymal cells providing numerous metabolic functions, such as glycogenesis, gluconeogenesis, urea and lipid synthesis [33]. To achieve these functions, both hepatocytes and cholangiocytes establish apico-basal epithelial polarity during liver organogenesis. Interestingly, these cells have different types of polarity; the basal surface of hepatocytes faces the space of Disse and the apical surface forms the bile canalicular space between neighboring cells. In contrast, the basal surface of cholangiocytes is associated with basement membrane while the apical surface forms a microvilli-enriched luminal space connected with bile secretion.

2.4.1 The Hepatocytes

Hepatocytes constitute 60–65% of the total cells in the liver and approximately 80% of the organ volume. In three dimensions, hepatocytes are arranged in plates that anastomose with each other. Parenchymal cells are polygonal in shape and are in contact with the sinusoids (the sinusoidal face with microvilli) and neighboring hepatocytes (Fig. 2.4). Microvilli from the sinusoidal face of the hepatocytes extend into this space, increasing the surface area of hepatocytes available for uptake of plasma molecules. Between abutting hepatocytes are *bile canaliculi*, which are channels 1–2 μm in diameter, formed by grooves in the plasma membranes of the adjacent cells and delineated from the vascular space by tight junctions. Numerous microvilli extend into these intercellular spaces that constitute the outermost reaches of the biliary tree. Hepatocellular actin and myosin microfilaments surrounding the *canaliculus* help propel secreted biliary fluid along the *canaliculi*. These channels drain into the canals of Hering in the periportal region. These canals are trough-like extensions of biliary epithelium into the periportal parenchyma, abutting with hepatocytes to form efficient channels for draining bile [34]. Biliary fluid is conveyed through their lumen to bile ductules, which traverse the portal connective tissue to empty into the terminal bile ducts within the portal tracts.

Hepatocytes contain large, usually spherical nuclei of varying sizes. In fetal and newborn liver, hepatocytes are chiefly mononuclear and diploid, while in adult liver they may exhibit both polyploid nuclei and multinucleated cells. Hepatocyte

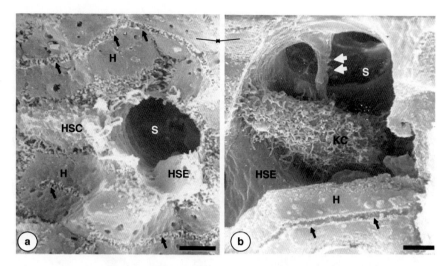

Fig. 2.4 Cells of the hepatic sinusoid. (**a**) This scanning electron microscopic image shows a cross section of a 9- μm in diameter hepatic sinusoid (S) lined by the fenestrated sinusoidal endothelium (HSE) and surrounded by hepatocytes (H) with bile canaliculi (*arrows*). HSC-hepatic stellate cell. Bar: 5 μm. (**b**) Shown is an intrasinusoidal Kupffer cell (KC) occupying the sinusoidal lumen (S) and connected to the endothelial wall by filopodia and a long cytoplasmic extension (*white arrows*). Bile canaliculi (*black arrows*) are shown on the exocrine face of a hepatocyte. Bar: 5 μm. Reproduced with permission from [163]

function (e.g. gene expression profile and biochemical activities), however, is not uniform. Rather, hepatocytes perform different roles depending on their position coordinates within the hepatic lobule (Fig. 2.5a, b). For example, the mitochondria of periportal hepatocytes have greater mean volumes than mitochondria in the centrilobular hepatocytes [35]. Periportal and centrilobular cells receive different signals from the blood because substrates including oxygen and hormones are degraded and modified and new metabolic products and mediators are formed during the passage of blood through the liver. Oxygen tension, which decreases by approximately 50% from periportal to centrilobular regions, has been considered a key regulator for zonal gene expression in hepatocytes. Gradients of metabolic substrates, hormones such as adrenalin, insulin, and cortisol and extracellular matrix are also thought to be important regulators of these zonally-determined phenotypic variations. In addition, the transcriptional rate, the abundance of mRNA and the enzymatic activity of the cells are increased under arterial as compared to venous oxygen. Thus, hepatocytes around the afferent vessels (periportal) differ from those around the efferent vessels (centrilobular) in their contents of key enzymes and therefore have different metabolic capacities. Periportal cells produce glucose via glycogenolysis and gluconeogenesis and the centrilobular cells utilize glucose for glycogen synthesis and glycolysis [31]. Periportal hepatocytes are also enriched in enzymes associated with amino acid degradation and the production of urea. Xenobiotic metabolism, lipogenesis and glutamine synthase activity occur predominantly in the centrilobular hepatocytes. Therefore, the heterogeneous distribution

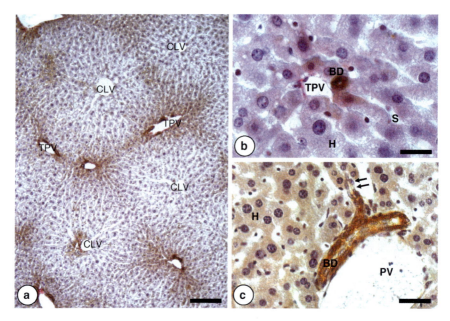

Fig. 2.5 The parenchymal cells of the liver. (**a**) Parenchymal cell heterogeneity across the hepatic lobule, as evidenced by immunohistochemical staining of nerve growth factor-expressing hepatocytes is shown. CLV-centrilobular vein. Bar: 100 μm. Reproduced with permission from [163]. (**b**) A periportal area from the image in (**a**) shows a terminal portal venule (TPV), a bile ductule (BD) with high nerve growth factor (NGF)-expressing cubic epithelium of cholangiocytes and some low-NGF expressing hepatocytes (H) and sinusoids (S). Bar: 20 μm. (**c**) Shown is another portal tract from the image in (**a**). Note the bile ductule of high NGF-expressing cholangiocytes and the Hering canal (*arrows*) connecting a bile ductule to bile canaliculi from hepatocytes. Bar: 20 μm

of enzymes along the sinusoids within the liver lobule results in phenotypic variations of hepatocytes located between the portal and the centrilobular veins. The zonal distribution of the metabolic activity of these cells is an efficient "division of labor" occurring under physiological conditions in the hepatic tissue. In turn, this microenvironment-associated hepatocyte heterogeneity within the hepatic lobule has also implications for liver regeneration, inflammation, fibrogenesis and aging, and also affects hepatocyte susceptibility to inflammatory and infectious agents and cancer. Not surprisingly, the deleterious effects of drugs or toxins, such as carbon tetrachloride on the liver show zonal specificity due to the regional differences in gene expression and the microenvironment [32].

2.4.2 The Cholangiocytes

Cholangiocytes line intrahepatic bile ducts (Fig. 2.5b, c) that serve to secrete the bile produced by hepatocytes into the intestine [36]. Cholangiocytes have primary cilia extending from the apical plasma membrane into the bile duct lumen. These cilia are ideally positioned to detect changes in bile flow, composition, and osmolarity. The bile is an aqueous solution of organic and inorganic compounds initially secreted by hepatocytes (primary bile) and subsequently modified by cholangiocytes (ductal bile) through secretory and absorptive processes. Cholangiocytes modify the fluidity and alkalinity of primary bile by adding ions, primarily Cl− and HCO by absorbing bile salts, glucose, and amino acids and by the passive movement of water into or out of the bile duct lumen in response to osmotic gradients. Cholangiocyte cilia express proteins such as polycystin-1, polycystin-2, fibrocystin, TRPV4, P2Y12 and AC6 that account for ciliary mechano-, osmo-, and chemo-sensory functions [37]. A disturbance of these processes by mutations in genes encoding ciliary-associated proteins results in liver diseases. Abnormalities in ciliary structure and functions are responsible for cholangiopathies. These include, but are not limited to, cystic and fibrotic liver diseases associated with mutations in genes encoding polycystin-1, polycystin-2, and fibrocystin. Cholangiocytes are also the target of both acquired and inherited liver diseases such as polycystic liver disease that occurs in combination with autosomal dominant and autosomal recessive polycystic kidney disease [38].

2.4.3 The Oval Cells

Small portal zone cells with a high nuclear/cytoplasmic ratio and an ovoid nucleus, first observed in rat liver, have become known as "oval cells" [39]. These cells proliferate extensively and, upon migration into the lobule, differentiate into hepatocytes. The term "oval cell" is widely used to describe a heterogeneous population of intermediate hepatobiliary progenitor cells that arise in different species and as a result of different insults. Within the oval cell pool, there are proliferative cells that are derived from liver resident oval cell precursors. These cells are likely bi-potential in that they can differentiate into hepatocytes or bile duct epithelium. Multiple studies support the concept that liver stem cells reside within the biliary tree and are a subset of ductal cells. The most likely origin of the precursors of oval cells in adult tissue is the canal of Hering [40]. The oval cells may in fact be bi-potential, transitional cell types capable of replication that are derived from normally quiescent true stem cells that reside in the biliary tree [41–42]. Cellular markers that will help to identify these various cell types and their inter-relationships are becoming available [43] and it seems likely that future descriptions of hepatic cell populations will include surface marker designations.

2.4.4 Liver Parenchymal Cell Renewal and Tissue Regeneration

Under physiological conditions, hepatocyte replacement occurs relatively slowly and the average life span of adult hepatocytes ranges from 200 to 300 days [44]. A number of different hypotheses have been proposed to explain hepatocyte turnover. According to the "streaming" liver model [45], normal liver turnover would be similar to intestinal regeneration, with young hepatocytes originating in the portal zone and then migrating toward the central vein. Differential gene expression by periportal and centrilobular hepatocytes may arise during the hepatocyte maturation process representing a typical lineage progression [46]. However, the gene expression pattern in hepatocytes is also affected by the direction of blood flow and the lobular zonation and may be modulated by metabolite-induced gene regulation. Although the contribution of stem cells to normal liver turnover in adult animals cannot be ruled out, current evidence suggests that liver maintenance is achieved mainly by hepatocyte and bile duct epithelial cell division [47].

On the other hand, one of the defining features of hepatic parenchymal cells is their capacity to maintain a constant size of the liver despite injury. Moreover, mammals can survive surgical removal of up to 75% of the total liver mass. Within 1 week after liver resection, the total number of liver cells is restored. Although the precise molecular signals involved in the maintenance of liver size are not completely known, it is clear that the liver balances regeneration with overgrowth. The regenerative response after partial hepatectomy is mediated by a number of factors, the most important of which are hepatocyte growth factor (HGF) [48], IL-6, TNFα, TGFα, and EGF. Non-peptide hormones including triiodothyronine [49] and norepinephrine [50] can also stimulate hepatocyte replication in vivo. Much less is known about the signals that stop liver regeneration once the appropriate liver mass is restored. Although the endocrine or paracrine factors that sense overall liver size are unclear, several intercellular signals have been identified. For example, some evidence suggests that TGFβ1 is important in the termination of liver regeneration [51].

Again, both mature hepatic parenchymal cells and facultative stem cells mediate liver maintenance and growth [52]. It has been proposed [53] that the liver has three types of cells in the hepatic parenchymal lineage that respond to injury or carcinogenesis: (1) the mature hepatocyte that responds to partial hepatectomy, centrilobular injury induced by agents such as carbon tetrachloride, and dimethylnitrosamine hepatocarcinogenesis; (2) the ductular "bipolar" hepatic progenitor cell that responds to centrilobular injury when the proliferation of hepatocytes is inhibited, and to N-2-acetylaminofluorene hepatocarcinogenesis; and (3) the putative periductular hepatic stem cell that responds to periportal injury induced by agents such as allyl alcohol and to choline-deficiency models of hepatocarcinogenesis. Hepatocytes are numerous, respond rapidly by one or two cell cycles, but can only give rise to other hepatocytes. The ductular progenitor cells are less numerous, may undergo more cell divisions than hepatocytes and can give rise to cholangiocytes or hepatocytes. Periductular hepatic stem cells are rare in the liver, have an extensive proliferative capacity and may be multipotent, but their full potential has yet to be defined. There is evidence that the periductular stem cells are of extrahepatic (bone marrow) origin because recent data have shown that hepatocytes may express genetic markers of donor hematopoietic cells after bone marrow transplantation [52].

2.5 The Non-parenchymal Cells of the Liver

Multiple types of non-parenchymal cells complement the hepatocyte populations in mediating the liver's capacity as the major metabolic, endocrine, exocrine, and host defense organ of the body. They are a heterogeneous population accounting for 6.3% of the total tissue volume and including: sinusoidal lining cells (endothelial cells and Kupffer cells) and perisinusoidal stellate cells (formerly Ito cells or fat-storing cells); hepatic connective tissue cells forming perilobular stroma; large vessel-type endothelial cells and liver-associated lymphocytes and granulocytes. Consistent with hepatic tissue architecture, these cell lineages also constitute highly diversified cell populations for which a characteristic intrahepatic topography can be seen.

2.5.1 Hepatic Endothelial Cells

Comparison of the phenotypes of hepatic vein-lining and sinusoid-lining endothelial cells (EC) reveals differences of a structural, biochemical, metabolic and immunologic nature. In general, the vein-type EC phenotype involves a continuous endothelium with marginal folds and underlying basement membrane, high expression of *Ulex europaeus* agglutinin I-binding sites and factor VIII-related antigen, the presence of Weible-Palade bodies and the absence of a receptor-mediated endocytic mechanism. In contrast, the sinusoid-lining endothelium (HSE) is fenestrated with discontinuous underlying extracellular matrix, bristle-coated micropinocytic vesicles, several immunocompetent surface antigens, and a well-developed receptor-mediated endocytic apparatus (Fig. 2.6a).

HSECs line the wall of the hepatic sinusoid and separate the sinusoidal blood from hepatocytes. They are specialized endothelial cells that play important roles in liver physiology and disease. HSECs have several features that distinguish them from other endothelial cells. Morphologically, they are characterized by the presence of open *fenestrae* [54] arranged in sieve plates [55] and lack an organized basement membrane. Functionally, HSECs act as scavengers [5] eliminating soluble waste macromolecules or immune complexes from portal venous blood, they are critical for inducing $CD8^+$ T cell tolerance [20, 56] and synthesize and release Factor VIII, a critical co-factor in the intrinsic coagulation pathway [57].

The HSEC fenestrations (Fig. 2.6b) are pores of approximately 50–150 nm in diameter that are grouped in clusters of 20–100 fenestrations known as liver sieve plates [55]. These fenestrations lack a diaphragm and underlying basal lamina, and represent approximately 5–10% of the sinusoidal surface, although a zonal gradient exists with slightly larger fenestrations in the periportal sinusoids and greater porosity in sinusoidal segments around centrilobular veins [58].

The space of Disse (or perisinusoidal space), named after the German anatomist Joseph Disse (1852–1912), is the space between HSECs and hepatocytes that contains the blood plasma. It is thought that this space serves to channel plasma towards the space of Mall (the space between the stroma of the portal tract and the outermost hepatocytes in the hepatic lobule), in turn draining plasma into the true lymphatics coursing through the portal tract [59]. HSEC *fenestrae* act as a bidirectional venue for the transendothelial transport of solutes, and metabolic substrates between the liver sinusoidal blood and the hepatocytes. They have been shown to be responsive

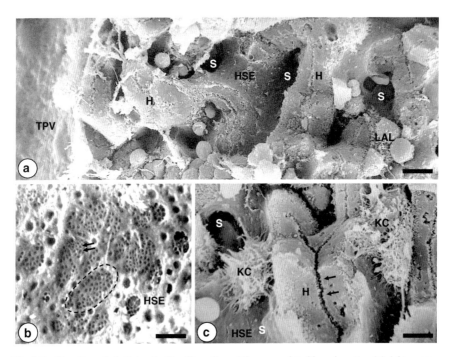

Fig. 2.6 Hepatic endothelial cells, Kupffer cells and liver-associated lymphocytes. (**a**) A low magnification scanning electron microscopic image of the hepatic tissue is shown. The terminal portal vein (TPV) with a non-fenestrated endothelium is on the left. Hepatocytes (H) and a labyrinth of sinusoids (S) in an alternating pattern are shown. Some liver-associated lymphocytes (LAL) are located intrasinusoidally and interact with Kupffer cells (KC). Bar: 10 μm. (**b**) High-power image of the fenestrated surface of the hepatic sinusoidal endothelium. Under physiological conditions, endothelial fenestrae (*arrows*) are transcellular structures of 100–150 nm in diameter that cluster to form highly filtrating microdomains termed sieve plates (encircled with a *broken line*). Bar: 1 μm. Reproduced with permission from [163]. (**c**) Shown are activated Kupffer cells (KC) within the sinusoidal lumen of two sinusoids (S) around a hepatocyte (H) with its bile canaliculi (*arrows*). Bar: 6 μm

in functional processes such as lipoprotein metabolism [60], blood flow regulation [61] and hepatocyte gene transfer [62]. However, fenestration of the endothelium may be obliterated in liver disease, leading to decreased uptake by hepatocytes of nutrients and waste products [63]. Defenestration occurs during the earliest stage of the metastatic process [64], in the pathogenesis of cirrhosis and in chronic alcohol abuse, resulting in alcoholism-associated hyperlipoproteinemia [63]. Absence of HSEC *fenestrae* is associated with capillarization, defined as the formation of an organized basement membrane in the space of Disse with characteristic changes in the HSEC phenotype that lead to HSC activation and transdifferentiation into myofibroblasts (see below). Interestingly, the HSEC phenotype can be maintained by hepatocyte and HSC-derived vascular endothelial growth factor (VEGF). VEGF in turn, stimulates HSECs to produce nitric oxide (NO) – a factor essential for maintenance of differentiated HSECs [65]. In HSEC capillarization that precedes cirrhosis, paracrine production of VEGF is markedly decreased, VEGF-mediated

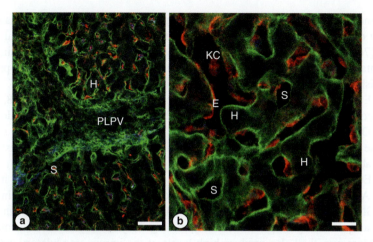

Fig. 2.7 Immunohistochemistry of hepatic vessels and cells. Shown in (**a**) is a confocal microscopy image of a perilobular portal vein (PLPV) and periportal segments of hepatic sinusoids immunostained with anti-ICAM antibodies (*green*). Note that ManR-expressing HSECs and Kupffer cells (in *red*) are located in sinusoids but not in the portal vein. Bar: 50 μm. (**b**) A higher magnification view of the image in (**a**) shows ManR expression on HSECs (E) and some Kupffer cells (KC) lining the network of sinusoids (S) around the hepatocytes (H). Bar: 10 μm

stimulation of NO is lost and only basal NO production persists [66]. In *in vitro* studies, specific matrix molecules (such as collagen I, collagen IV and fibronectin) and short-range soluble signals emanating from hepatocyte-fibroblast cocultures were able to prolong survival and the expression of HSEC markers [67].

HSECs also play a scavenger role in collaboration with Kupffer cells (Fig. 2.7a, b). Major components of the connective tissue, as well as other potential hazardous products are eliminated from the blood rapidly and almost exclusively by HSECs, via receptor-mediated endocytosis [68]. Five different endocytic receptors of HSECs have been described namely, the collagen alpha-chain receptor, the hyaluronan receptor, the IgG Fc receptor, the mannose receptor, and the scavenger receptor [5, 8, 68]. The collagen alpha-chain receptor function has so far only been described in HSECs and shows specificity for free alpha-chains of types I, II, III, IV, V, XI collagen, but not native triple helical collagen [69–71]. The hyaluronan receptor is responsible for the clearance of circulating hyaluronic acid, but also of chondroitin sulphate, dermatan sulphate, and some ligands of the scavenger receptor [72]. The Fc receptor is displayed on both Kupffer cells and HSECs and has been shown to mediate the elimination of circulating IgG immune complexes in the liver. However, of the known Fc-γ receptors, only IIb2 is able to mediate endocytosis of immune complexes and only IIb2 is expressed in HSECs [73]. The mannose receptor (ManR) recognizes the terminal non-reducing sugar residue of the oligosaccharide (fucose, mannose or *N*-acetyl-glucosamine) moiety of glycoproteins [68, 74]. Studies with ManR-deficient knockout mice showed that the clearance of denatured collagen is ManR-mediated [75]. This receptor uses a different binding domain to take up blood-borne collagen alpha chains [74]. Using the same knockout mice model it has been reported that HSEC ManR mediates the import of blood-borne lysosomal enzymes for re-use in the endo/lysosomal apparatus [76]. Furthermore, ManR is also involved in antigen uptake, processing and presentation to T cells by HSECs [77] and it has been suggested that this process diminishes the local immune response of the liver [78].

HSECs are also secretory cells and can release IL-1, TNFα, IL-6, IL-18, IFNγ and eicosanoids, particularly PGI2, PGE2 and TXA2 [64, 79], as well as endothelin and NO [80–82]. Thus, along with Kupffer cells, the HSEC participates in host defense mechanisms and the regulation of sinusoidal blood flow and fenestration permeability in the liver.

HSECs also express high levels of cell surface adhesion molecules including ICAM-1, VCAM-1, liver/lymph node-specific ICAM-3-grabbing, non-integrin (L-SIGN) and vascular adhesion protein-1 (VAP-1) [4, 77, 83], suggesting that they can potentially trap CD4/CD8-expressing T lymphocytes in the sinusoids [17]. Moreover, they also produce high levels of the immunomodulatory cytokine TFG-β [84] and soluble ICAM-1 [85]. Furthermore, galectin-1 – a beta-galactoside binding lectin that is specifically expressed on HSECs is known to bind to, and induce apoptosis in activated T cells [17]. These observations indicate that HSECs may potentially participate in the induction of T cell apoptosis in the liver (see Section 2.5.3). Some of these properties are, however, shared with Kupffer cells and it is therefore difficult to clearly distinguish between the contributions of macrophages and endothelial cells to these processes in the hepatic sinusoids. Moreover, as this sinusoid-lining endothelial cell phenotype exists in a dynamic state, some of the most characteristic features can disappear, while other characteristics generally associated with either vein-type endothelial cells or Kupffer cells, can, under certain circumstances, be accentuated [64]. Thus, during the development of certain chronic liver diseases, such as cirrhosis, HSECs can undergo transformation to a vein-type endothelium with the characteristic appearance of Weible-Palade bodies and factor VIII-related antigen, loss of scavenger capacity and fenestrations and the formation of a true basement membrane [86–88]. Alternatively, under various experimental conditions involving macrophage damage or depletion, HSECs can become phagocytic [64]. Therefore, HSECs can show some phenotypic plasticity and acquire properties characteristic of the large-vessel-type hepatic endothelium that they encounter at sites of terminal portal vein-sinusoidal connections, on one hand, and of intrasinusoidal macrophages, or Kupffer cells, with which they functionally cooperate as reticuloendothelial cells, on the other. Indeed, Kupffer cells and HSECs together are the source of a variety of beneficial, vasoactive or toxic mediators which are thought to be involved in host defense mechanisms, as well as some disease processes in the liver. They also represent the most powerful scavenger system of the body [68]. Indeed, most of the harmful, soluble or insoluble macromolecules entering the body from the gut are transported to the liver via the portal vein and eliminated through uptake by these cells.

2.5.2 The Hepatic Macrophages

Resident hepatic macrophages, known as Kupffer cells (Figs. 2.4b and 2.6c), play a major role in clearance of particulate material and endotoxin from the blood, and in immune response modulation through antigen sequestration by phagocytosis, clearance of immune complexes and the release of IL-1β, IL-18, IL-6, TNFα and IFNγ [89–91]. They account for about 10% of the liver cell population and about 80–90% of the total population of fixed tissue macrophages in the entire body [92]. They are anchored to the luminal surface of HSECs via long and multiple cytoplasmic processes, without forming junctional complexes. Kupffer cells possess migratory capacity and continuously patrol the sinusoids. They are highly variable in their shape, although they are mainly stellate and adopt a Y-shaped morphology when located at sinusoid branching sites [93]. Kupffer cells are heterogeneous [94–96] but endogenous peroxidase is considered a general cytochemical marker for the identification of Kupffer cells in the adult liver [97, 98]. They are found in all regions of the liver but appear to be slightly larger and more concentrated in the periportal region of hepatic lobules. Here, they also have greater phagocytic capacity and higher lysosomal enzyme activities than Kupffer cells in the centrilobular regions. This functional variability may be due to greater concentrations of potential immunogenic material in the region of afferent blood flow [94–96].

Like other organ-specific macrophages, Kupffer cells have a high phagocytic potential and can endocytose bacteria and cellular debris after trauma [90]. In the liver, these macrophages can also phagocytose aged erythrocytes and play a role in iron metabolism by accumulating ferritin and hemosiderin [90, 93]. In the case of acute hemolysis, Kupffer cells can also support intrasinusoidal hematopoietic activity in the adult liver [97]. Kupffer cells are also a key cellular component of hepatic regeneration [98–100] and the innate immune system, and have been implicated in both immunogenic and tolerogenic immune reactions [84, 100–104]. They eliminate pathogens including bacteria and parasites and may directly kill some cancer cells [103, 105] by receptor-mediated phagocytosis or the release of TNFα, reactive oxygen metabolites, NO or proteinases. They express markers distinguishing them from extrahepatic macrophages such as major histocompatibility complex class II molecules, ICAM-1, as well as low levels of CD80 and CD86. As professional, antigen-presenting cells they can also promote adaptive immune responses by processing and presenting antigens via MHC class I and II [104]. In addition, in cases of pathogenic infection or tissue damage, the release of cytokines and chemokines from activated macrophages recruits other cells of the immune system to sites of inflammation and tissue repair.

There is ongoing controversy regarding the origin of Kupffer cells and the mechanism that maintains homeostasis of the Kupffer cell population over time. The traditional view is that tissue macrophages are not self-renewing and are replenished from bone marrow-derived monocytes [106–108]. In contrast, it has been argued that Kupffer cells are a self-renewing population and divide as mature cells or originate from local intrahepatic progenitors [99, 109, 110]. This issue assumes practical importance in clinical situations such as myeloid diseases treated with bone marrow allografts and also during liver transplantation. In both scenarios, large, self-renewing antigen presenting cell populations that are not readily replaced from bone marrow sources are likely to affect the specificity of the immune responses generated. Using multi-parameter flow cytometry of isolated, hepatic leukocytes, two distinct Kupffer cell populations have been identified within the liver [111]. This analysis revealed a predominance of bone marrow-derived Kupffer cells that rapidly replaced resident Kupffer cells after irradiation and bone marrow reconstitution. However, *in situ* analysis by immunohistology revealed a large population of residual, non-bone marrow-derived Kupffer cells that do not rapidly turn over and are completely lost upon various cell isolation protocols [111]. While both the bone marrow-derived and the residual non-bone marrow-derived Kupffer cells share a similar morphology and phagocytic capabilities, only the bone marrow-derived Kupffer cells were shown to be engaged in inflammatory responses [111]. The different biological functions of these two Kupffer cell subpopulations provide a possible explanation for the dichotomy in the immunogenic and tolerogenic responses within the liver.

2.5.3 Liver-Associated Lymphocytes and Hepatic Immunity

The liver is the largest source of lymph in the body, contributing up to 50% of the thoracic duct flow. More lymphocytes migrate through the liver via the lymph than any other non-lymphoid organ. The liver receives gut-derived nutrients, but also toxins and antigens, as well as spleen-derived molecules and cells that are delivered through the splenic vein drainage into the portal vein. This unique location allows many molecules and cells to transit through the liver continuously exposing it to antigens and cells of the immune system. Historically, the focus on the critical metabolic functions of the liver has eclipsed an appreciation of its role as an immune organ. However pioneering morphological studies in the late 20th century that revealed the presence of liver-specific lymphoid cells [112, 113], have drawn attention to the important immuno-regulatory function of the liver and its potential role in systemic and local innate immunity. Intrahepatic lymphocytes are distinct both in phenotype and function from their counterparts in any other organ and in peripheral blood.

2.5.3.1 Subtypes of Hepatic Lymphocytes

The liver contains specific resident lymphocyte subsets called liver-associated lymphocytes [114] (Fig. 2.6a). They include both conventional CD4$^+$ and CD8$^+$ $\alpha\beta$T cell receptor (TCR)$^+$ T cells, B cells and natural killer (NK) cells as well as nonconventional lymphoid cells such as natural killer T (NKT) cells, gamma delta TCR$^+$ T cells and CD4$^-$ CD8$^-$ T cells [17]. Many hepatic T cells express an intermediate TCR level and the great majority of them either co-express NK cell markers (NK T cells) or are apoptotic peripheral T cells. The proportions of activated (CD69$^+$)

and memory (CD45RB low$^+$) lymphocytes are much higher than in the peripheral blood, while naive (CD62L high) and resting T cells, as well as B lymphocytes are underrepresented in the liver as compared to the peripheral blood. The discovery of major populations of lymphoid cells in the liver that differ phenotypically, functionally, and even perhaps developmentally, from populations in other regions has been key to the evolving perception of the liver as a regulatory lymphoid organ [17, 20].

Innate lymphocytes, including both NK and NK T cells are unusually abundant in the liver [115, 116]. Up to 50% of intrahepatic lymphocytes in a normal mouse liver express intermediate levels of the T-cell receptor and NK T cell markers. In vivo imaging revealed that NK T cells patrol hepatic sinusoids and are arrested upon specific recognition of a cognate ligand, α-galactosyl-ceramide that is presented in a CD1-restricted fashion [104]. Most CD4$^+$ NK T cells can readily secrete both Th2 and Th1 cytokines upon stimulation under CD1-restriction. These innate immune cells play a key role in the local defense to pathogens in the liver, but the mechanisms involved remain unclear. In addition, the liver is a preferential site of T-cell apoptosis, acting as a graveyard for activated CD8$^+$ T cells [84, 117–119], as was demonstrated in a number of systems, including transplantation, transgenic models of peripheral tolerance and hepatitis C infection [18, 20].

2.5.3.2 The Dendritic Cells of the Liver

The liver dendritic cells are another important myeloid component of the hepatic immune-microenvironment. They are usually found in the portal triad and the centrilobular veins. Upon antigen capture at the sinusoidal area or the portal tract, these cells can migrate through the HSECs and into the space of Disse and travel toward the celiac lymph nodes while maintaining an immature state [121–124]. HSECs, Kupffer cells, and HSCs are all capable of secreting IL-10 and TGFβ during their activation by a variety of insults that cause inflammation. In response to the increase in local TGFβ concentrations, hepatocytes secrete IL-10 to further promote a tolerogenic microenvironment [20, 125]. Exposure of the dendritic cells to high levels of IL-10 and TGFβ has been shown to reduce the expression of co-stimulatory molecules such as CD80, CD86 and B7 family members, leading to the development of regulatory dendritic cells [78]. In turn, the dendritic cells can prime naïve T cells to differentiate into Th2, Th0 or T-regulatory lymphocytes.

2.5.3.3 Portal Tract-Associated Lymphoid Tissue

Although most T cell activation occurs within the lymph nodes, evidence of T cell proliferation can also be detected in the portal tract-associated lymphoid tissue [123, 124]. After the hepatic dendritic cells process captured antigens, they can migrate to the draining lymph nodes; remain in the site of infection (granuloma) or associate with neighboring B or T cells to form a portal tract-associated lymphoid site. Portal tract-associated lymphoid foci are very similar to the classical lymphoid follicles. These areas are near the portal triad and are the site of dendritic cell interaction with immunoreactive B or T cells. Formation of portal tract-associated lymphoid tissue may allow the hepatic dendritic cells to interact with corresponding T cells without entering the regional lymph nodes. The center of the portal tract-associated lymphoid tissue is composed of B cell follicles populated by antigen loaded follicular dendritic cells. Interspersed among these B cell follicles are the CD4+ T cells. As the large vessel-type endothelium of the portal tract-associated lymphoid tissue is able to secrete CCL21, cells expressing the CCR7 receptor, such as mature dendritic cells and naïve T cells, are readily recruited into this area. Surrounding the B and T cells are the macrophages. Formation of portal tract-associated lymphoid tissue may be indicative of liver inflammation because patients with primary sclerosing cholangitis have multiple portal tract-associated lymphoid tissue formation within their portal area [124].

2.5.3.4 Hepatic Immune Tolerance

The liver possesses a unique ability to induce immune tolerance. Administration of antigens via the portal, rather than the systemic venous system was shown to suppress delayed-type-hypersensitivity and antibody production upon subsequent challenge (the Chase – Sulzberger effect) [126]. In agreement with these experiments, the surgical introduction of a mesenteric-caval shunt, that "short-circuits" the liver, has been shown to impair induction of oral tolerance, suggesting that the intestinal venous drainage through the liver plays a role in the induction of oral tolerance [127]. Liver-tolerized lymphocytes can re-circulate back to mucosa-associated lymphoid tissue in the gut and once there maintain their non-responsiveness. The tolerogenic properties of the liver have also been illustrated in models of transplantation. Moreover, although HSECs and Kupffer cells can efficiently capture antigens and process those for major histocompatibility complex class II presentation, they can perform these functions in the context of immunosuppressive cytokines and/or inhibitory cell surface ligands. Therefore, hepatic immune responses to antigens often result in tolerance. Important human pathogens (including hepatitis C virus and the malaria parasite) and cancer cells exploit the liver's immunosuppressive environment, subvert immunity, and establish persistent infection or cancer metastasis. It is possible, therefore, that the liver plays an active role in the development of specific non-responsiveness to metastatic cancer cells [85].

Induction of antigen-specific tolerance in CD8+ T cells has been attributed to hepatic cell populations that can function as antigen-presenting cells. It is accepted that the initial antigen-specific stimulation of naïve CD8+ T cells in the liver determines their subsequent functional capacity, i.e. tolerance, whereas extrahepatic priming of T cells in the secondary lymphatic tissue leads to the development of T cell immunity that upon antigen-recognition in the liver can develop into autoimmunity [125]. Therefore, a better understanding of the molecular mechanisms regulating the hepatic immune response will further our knowledge on the pathophysiological principles of persistent viral infections of the liver. It will also allow the development of immune tolerance-stimulating drugs for the treatment of autoimmune diseases and of reagents that can stimulate immune reactivity during persistent hepatic viral infection or cancer metastasis.

2.5.4 Hepatic Connective Tissue Cells and Hepatic Fibrogenesis

Two major hepatic connective tissue cell types are recognized in the liver. First, the portal tract fibroblasts (PTFs) that support the hepatic lobule structure and Glisson's capsule, the intrahepatic distribution of blood and lymphatic vessels and the bile duct tree. Second, the perisinusoidal hepatic stellate cells that are located exclusively around sinusoids to participate in the metabolic functions of the liver and can support morpho-dynamic aspects of these specialized capillaries and HSEC differentiation. In addition, both PTFs and HSCs contribute to hepatic fibrogenesis, angiogenesis, regeneration and immune response.

2.5.4.1 The Portal Tract Fibroblasts

Early reports by Popper et al. described mesenchymal cells that were not related to sinusoidal structures and later noted that fibroblast-like cells and matrix deposits were present in the region immediately surrounding proliferating bile ducts in biliary cirrhosis [128, 129]. It has been appreciated for many years that biliary cirrhosis is distinct from the more rapidly progressing non-biliary cirrhosis. As it became clear that the bile duct epithelia are the primary site of injury in chronic cholangiopathies such as primary biliary cirrhosis, and that fibrosis originates in the periductular region in these diseases, the portal localization of portal tract fibroblasts, as opposed to the more distant HSCs, identified them as potential candidates for mediators of biliary fibrosis. Indeed, a model whereby PTFs were first responders in biliary fibrosis, later to be supplanted by HSCs, was proposed [130]. The most commonly used designations for portal region fibroblasts are accordingly, the peribiliary fibrogenic cells, periductular fibroblasts and portal/periportal mesenchymal cells [131–133] (Fig. 2.8).

The expression of elastin, fibulin-2, ecto-ATPase nucleoside triphosphate diphosphohydrolase-2, IL-6, P100, 2-macroglobulin, and neuronal proteins (including neuronal cell adhesion marker and synaptophysin) and the absence of lipid droplets and GFAP have been used to differentiate PTFs from HSCs [134–136]. PTFs appear to be the major elastin-expressing cells (in addition to vascular smooth muscle cells) in the liver, and some investigators have shown that elastin deposition increases as PTFs proliferate and fibrosis progresses [137, 138]. However, p75 neurotrophin receptor-expressing mesenchymal cells in the mouse fetal liver include precursors that can differentiate into distinct parenchymal and portal cell subpopulations, presumably reflecting HSCs and PTFs. Moreover, lineage-tracing analyses using mouse embryos expressing a LacZ reporter gene under the control of the mesodermal marker MesP1 demonstrated a mesodermal origin for HSCs and perivascular mesenchymal cells (desmin$^+$, p75$^+$, αSMA$^+$), as well as a population of submesothelial cells [139–142]. The perivascular mesenchymal cells described may be PTF precursors, suggesting that HSCs and portal tract fibroblasts have a common precursor in the embryo [142].

The recent interest in PTFs has resulted in part from data showing that liver myofibroblasts causing fibrosis are heterogeneous and not always derived from

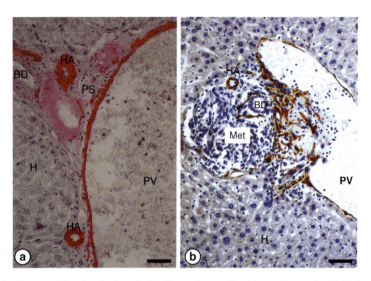

Fig. 2.8 Immunohistochemical analysis of portal tract fibroblasts. Shown in (**a**) is the portal space (PS) of a normal liver containing portal tract fibroblasts (*light basophilic staining*), hepatic arterioles (HA), and a bile duct (BD). Hepatocytes (H) are around the portal area. Bar: 30 μm. Shown in (**b**) is a portal area containing a portal vein-invading micrometastasis (Met) of the murine C26 colorectal carcinoma. Note that some portal vein-associated smooth muscle cells and portal tract fibroblasts are now being recruited into the tumor tissue and express αSMA (cells stained in *brown*). Bar: 100 μm

HSCs. Not surprisingly, portal tract fibroblasts play an important role in liver scar formation, especially in biliary fibrosis [143]. TGFβ, widely appreciated as one of the most important mediators of liver fibrosis, is also required for PTF differentiation. This is in contrast to cultured HSCs that express αSMA independently of TGFβ [144, 145], but is consistent with the model of Gabbiani and colleagues [146] whereby TGFβ, as well as mechanical tension are required for differentiation of myofibroblasts in all tissues. PDGF also enhances PTF proliferation in culture but decreases αSMA expression [144]. PDGF is of particular interest given that it is expressed by cultured bile duct segments from bile duct ligation-treated rats, suggesting a possible mechanism for fibrosis after bile duct ligation. In fact, there is a direct correlation between the intensity of the ductular reaction and the severity of fibrosis in human liver disease of various etiologies, including hepatitis C and nonalcoholic fatty liver disease [147–149].

The PTFs also express the Notch ligand Jagged1, suggesting that these cells may regulate the commitment of hepatoblasts to a biliary lineage [149]. Moreover, cytokines and chemokines, in particular IL-6 and monocyte chemotactic protein-1 (MCP-1), are emerging as important mediators of cell-cell communication between cholangiocytes and PTFs. IL-6 is expressed specifically by cholangiocytes in biliary, as opposed to other forms of fibrosis [150], and PTFs express the IL-6 co-receptor glycoprotein 130 [151]. These cells appears to communicate via a paracrine loop in which IL-6 potently down-regulates nucleoside triphosphate diphosphohydrolase-2

(NTPD2) in PTFs, without altering their myofibroblastic differentiation while in turn NTPD2 regulates G protein-coupled P2Y receptors for extracellular ATP and other nucleotides, which mediate cholangiocyte proliferation [152]. Cholangiocytes are also the liver cells expressing MCP-1 messenger RNA in chronic hepatitis [153] and they signal to PTF through MCP-1 release, up-regulating PTF proliferation, myofibroblastic differentiation and procollagen-1 mRNA expression, while down-regulating NTPD2 expression [155–157].

It has been reported that PTFs are contributing to the stroma and angiogenesis of portal-type hepatic metastases (see Chapter 3) (Fig. 2.8b). Our knowledge of PTFs, however, lags far behind that of the prometastatic effects of HSCs [12, 13]. A better understanding of the differences between HSCs and PTFs with regard to their molecular regulation and relative contribution to hepatic metastasis is needed. This may have implications for the development of anti-metastatic therapies tailored to distinct hepatic metastases containing PTF-derived tumor stroma.

2.5.4.2 The Perisinusoidal Stellate Cells

Hepatic stellate cells (HSCs) are a resident mesenchymal cell type located in the subendothelial space of Disse, interposed between the sinusoidal endothelium and hepatocytes [158]. Under normal physiological conditions HSCs store fat or fat-soluble vitamins [159]. However, these cells can undergo a transdifferentiation into myofibroblasts by a variety of insults that cause inflammation. This results in the production and accumulation of collagen in the space of Disse leading to cirrhosis [160]. While recent studies have identified some heterogeneity in the fibrogenic cells of the liver [133–136], strong evidence implicates HSCs as the key source of extracellular matrix protein production, associated with their activation into myofibroblast-like cells [161].

HSC activation refers to the transition from a quiescent vitamin A-rich cell to one that is proliferative, fibrogenic and contractile with a reduced vitamin A content. HSC activation begins within minutes of liver injury and involves a coordinated induction of genes encoding both regulatory and structural proteins (for review, see reference [10]). Activated HSCs are the major source of extracellular matrix production in liver injury and secrete all components of the hepatic scar. In a model of HSC activation, it has been defined as a two-stage process consisting of initiation followed by perpetuation [162]. Initiation refers to early changes in gene expression and phenotype that render the cells responsive to other cytokines and stimuli, while perpetuation results from the effects of these stimuli in maintaining the activated phenotype and generating fibrosis. Many of the key features of perpetuation include induction of cytokines and their receptors, proliferation, fibrogenesis, contractility and degradation of the normal subendothelial matrix of the liver. Regulators of HSC activation that are particularly relevant during viral infection and alcohol-induced chronic liver disease include oxidative stress and acetaldehyde, but the mechanisms underlying their effects are only partially characterized.

Normal HSCs secrete apolipoprotein E and numerous prostaglandins that contribute to hepatic metabolism and inflammation, as well as to neural cell-mediated vasoregulation. They are also an important source of cytokines in the liver. They secrete HGF, nerve growth factor, stromal-derived growth factor-1, pleiotrophin, epimorphin and EGF, contributing to hepatocyte proliferation and autocrine HSC activation. In addition, they also secrete insulin-like growth factor I and II, PDGF and acidic fibroblast growth factor – all mitogenic cytokines for HSCs. They also produce M-CSF, PAF and MCP-1 that regulate neutrophil and macrophage accumulation and play a role in amplifying the inflammatory and fibrogenic response during liver injury. An increasing number of chemokines has also been ascribed to HSCs, including cytokine-induced neutrophil chemoattractant, RANTES, C-X-C chemokine ligand-1, and macrophage inflammatory protein-2. HSCs also contribute to the acute phase response by secreting IL-6, while are also able to downregulate immune responses and fibrogenesis through the production of IL-10. In addition, HSCs also express several adhesion molecules including ICAM-1, VCAM-1, and neural cell adhesion molecule, contributing to lymphocyte adherence to activated HSCs and thereby modulating the recruitment of inflammatory cells during liver injury. Moreover, in response to injury HSCs secrete latent TGFβ1 that in turn exerts potent fibrogenic effects in an autocrine and paracrine manner and activin, a structurally-related member of the TGFβ family that modulates the effects of TGFβ1 on angiogenesis. Finally, HSCs are a major source and target of endothelin-1 during liver injury. Endothelin-1 has a prominent contractile effect on HSCs and myofibroblasts that may contribute to portal hypertension in the cirrhotic liver. However, HSCs also produce nitric oxide, a physiological antagonist of ET-1 that may play a role in the maintenance of microcirculation during liver injury (for review, see reference [161]).

As discussed at greater length in Chapter 3, normal HSCs can become transdifferentiated myofibroblasts in the tumor microenvironment. More importantly, HSC-derived myofibroblasts are actively recruited into hepatic metastases from its earliest avascular stage. Within the tumor microenvironment, these cells proliferate and secrete several factors that contribute to the regulation of metastatic cell behavior and angiogenesis. Therefore, hepatic myofibroblasts are a key stromal component during hepatic metastases formation, although the mechanisms involved in their activation and recruitment during the initiation of the metastatic process remain to be fully elucidated.

2.6 Conclusion

Over the past few decades, there has been an increasing appreciation of the critical role that the target organ microenvironment plays in the progression of metastasis. While only three decades ago, there was little understanding of how cancer metastasis develops to a life-threatening disease in the liver, and tumorigenesis was thought to be a cell-autonomous process, governed mainly by altered genes of immune-resistant cancer cells, it is now well accepted that cancer cell entering the liver engage in a bidirectional interaction with the local microenvironment that affects both their own behavior and that of the hepatic cells.

The liver contributes to the body's homeostasis through its well-developed and organ-specific machinery for biosynthesis, metabolism, clearance of circulating molecules and host defense. As a bi-functional gland, it is the site of bile production and the synthesis of many plasma proteins and endocrine factors. As a "bio-protection" platform, it contributes to detoxification and excretion into the bile of endogenous waste products and polluting xenobiotics as well as the removal of microbes, toxins and reactive oxygen intermediates in visceral blood en route to the systemic circulation.

To accomplish these diverse functions, the liver receives not just arterial blood, but also blood draining from most intra-peritoneal organs including the spleen. Among the unique functional attributes of the liver are: (1) its specialized microcirculation within organ lobes, segments and lobules, containing unique populations of sinusoidal cells and perivascular mesenchymal cells such as fibroblasts and perisinusoidal hepatic stellate cells; (2) its remarkable parenchymal cell heterogeneity, amplifying its functional capabilities and tissue regenerating potential; and (3) its innate and adoptive immune defense mechanisms generating a physiological immune tolerance.

As our understanding of the biology of specific compartments and cells of the liver has increased, it has become clear that the same molecular mechanisms that guarantee hepatic homeostasis may also influence the behavior of cancer cells during the various stages of the metastatic process. Moreover, the functional diversity in the microenvironment of the liver, representing the biological background encountered by metastatic cancer cells entering the liver may affect cancer patients' susceptibility to hepatic metastasis. This raises the possibility that in patients with malignant tumors, liver-specific biomarkers could be identified that will provide prognostic and therapeutic tools for patient stratification and the personalization of anti-metastatic therapy.

References

1. McCuskey RS (1994) The hepatic microvascular system. In: Arias IM, Boyer JL, Fausto N, Jakoby WB, Schachter D, Shafritz DA (eds) The liver: biology and pathobiology. Raven Press, New York, NY, pp 1089–1106
2. Oda M, Han JY, Yokomori H (2000) Local regulators of hepatic sinusoidal microcirculation: recent advances. Clin Hemorheol Microcirc 23:85–94
3. Barberá-Guillem E, Rocha M, Alvarez A et al (1991) Differences in the lectin-binding patterns of the periportal and perivenous endothelial domains in the liver sinusoids. Hepatology 14:131–139
4. Scoazec JY, Feldmann G (1994) The cell adhesion molecules of hepatic sinusoidal endothelial cells. J Hepatol 20:296–300
5. Seternes T, Sorensen K, Smedsrod B (2002) Scavenger endothelial cells of vertebrates: a nonperipheral leukocyte system for high-capacity elimination of waste macromolecules. Proc Natl Acad Sci USA 99:7594–7597
6. Seki E, Brenner DA (2008) Toll-like receptors and adaptor molecules in liver disease: update. Hepatology 48:322–335
7. Fausto N (2004) Liver regeneration and repair: hepatocytes, progenitor cells, and stem cells. Hepatology 39:1477–1487

8. Smedsrød B, Le Couteur D, Ikejima K et al (2009) Hepatic sinusoidal cells in health and disease: update from the 14th International Symposium. Liver Int 29:490–501
9. Malik R, Selden C, Hodgson H (2002) The role of non-parenchymal cells in liver growth. Sem Cell Dev Biol 13:425–431
10. Friedman SL (1999) The virtuosity of hepatic stellate cells. Gastroenterology 117: 1244–1246
11. Ramadori G, Saile B (2004) Portal tract fibrogenesis in the liver. Lab Invest 84:153–159
12. Olaso E, Santisteban A, Bidaurrazaga J et al (1997) Tumor-dependent activation of rodent hepatic stellate cells during experimental melanoma metastasis. Hepatology 26:634–642
13. Olaso E, Salado C, Egilegor E et al (2003) Proangiogenic role of tumor-activated hepatic stellate cells in experimental melanoma metastasis. Hepatology 37:674–685
14. Libbrecht L, Cassiman D, Desmet V et al (2002) The correlation between portal myofibroblasts and development of intrahepatic bile ducts and arterial branches in human liver. Liver 22:252–258
15. Asai K, Tamakawa S, Yamamoto M et al (2006) Activated hepatic stellate cells overexpress p75NTR after partial hepatectomy and undergo apoptosis on nerve growth factor stimulation. Liver Int 26:595–603
16. Li Z, Diehl AM (2003) Innate immunity in the liver. Curr Opin Gastroenterol 19:565–571
17. Parker GA, Picut CA (2005) Liver immunobiology. Toxicol Pathol 33:52–62
18. Starzl TE, Murase N, Abu-Elmagd K et al (2003) Tolerogenic immunosuppression for organ transplantation. Lancet 361:1502–1510
19. Safadi R, Alvarez CE, Ohta M et al (2005) Enhanced oral tolerance in transgenic mice with hepatocyte secretion of IL-10. J Immunol 175:3577–3583
20. Kern M, Popov A, Kurts C et al (2010) Taking off the brakes: T cell immunity in the liver. Trends Immunol 31:311–317
21. Frevert U, Engelmann S, Zougbédé S et al (2005) Intravital Observation of *Plasmodium berghei* sporozoite infection of the liver. PLoS Biol 3:1034–1046
22. Anttila VJ, Elonen E, Nordling S et al (1997) Hepatosplenic candidiasis in patients with acute leukemia: incidence and prognostic implications. Clin Infect Dis 24:375–380
23. Schmucker DL (2005) Age-related changes in liver structure and function: implications for disease? Exp Gerontol 40:650–659
24. Le Couteur DG, Warren A, Cogger VC et al (2008) Old age and the hepatic sinusoid. Anat Rec 291:672–683
25. Kiernan F (1883) The anatomy and physiology of the liver. Trans R Soc Lond 123:711–770
26. Ekataksin W, Wake K (1997) New concepts in biliary and vascular anatomy of the liver. In: Boyer JL, Ockner RK (eds) Progress in liver diseases. WB Saunders, Philadelphia, PA, pp 1–30
27. Takasaki S, Hano H (2001) Three-dimensional observations of the human hepatic artery (Arterial system in the liver). J Hepatol 34:455–466
28. McCuskey RS (2000) Morphological mechanisms for regulating blood flow through hepatic sinusoids. Liver 20:3–7
29. McCuskey RS (1996) Distribution of intrahepatic nerves: an overview. In: Shimazu T (ed) Liver innervation. John Libbey, London, pp 17–22
30. Rappaport AM (1973) The microcirculatory hepatic unit. Microvasc Res 6:218–228
31. Jungermann K, Katz N (1989) Functional specialization of different hepatocyte populations. Physiol Rev 69:708–764
32. Gumucio JJ (1989) Hepatocellular heterogeneity: the coming of age. Hepatology 9: 154–160
33. Jungermann K (1988) Metabolic zonation of liver parenchyma. Semin Liver Dis 8:329–341
34. Crawford JM (2002) Development of the intrahepatic biliary tree. Semin Liver Dis 22: 213–226
35. Blouin A, Bolender RP, Weibel ER (1977) Distribution of organelles and membranes between hepatocytes and non hepatocytes in the rat liver parenchyma. A stereological study. J Cell Biol 72:441–455

36. Fitz JG (2002) Current concepts in developmental, physiologic, and pathophysiologic aspects of cholangiocyte biology. Semin Liver Dis 22:211–212
37. Masyuk AI, Masyuk TV, LaRusso NF (2008) Cholangiocyte primary cilia in liver health and disease. Dev Dyn 237:2007–2012
38. Masyuk T, LaRusso N (2006) Polycystic liver disease: new insights into disease pathogenesis. Hepatology 43:906–908.
39. Shinozuka H, Lombardi B, Sell S et al (1978) Early histological and functional alterations of ethionine liver carcinogenesis in rats fed a choline-deficient diet. Cancer Res 38:1092–1098
40. Theise ND, Saxena R, Portmann BC et al (1999) The canals of Hering and hepatic stem cells in humans. Hepatology 30:1425–1433
41. Wang X, Foster M, Al-Dhalimy M et al (2003) The origin and liver repopulating capacity of murine oval cells. Proc Natl Acad Sci USA 100:11881–11888
42. Alison MR, Golding M, Sarraf CE et al (1996) Liver damage in the rat induces hepatocyte stem cells from biliary epithelial cells. Gastroenterology 110:1182–1190
43. Dorrell C, Erker L, Lanxon-Cookson KM et al (2008) Surface markers for the murine oval cell response. Hepatology 48:1282–1291
44. Bucher NLR, Malt RA (1971) Regeneration of liver and kidney. Little Brown, Boston, MA
45. Zajicek G, Oren R, Weinreb M Jr (1985) The streaming liver. Liver 5:293–300
46. Ponder KP (1996) Analysis of liver development, regeneration, and carcinogenesis by genetic marking studies. FASEB J 10:673–682
47. Fellous TG, Islam S, Tadrous PJ et al (2009) Locating the stem cell niche and tracing hepatocyte lineages in human liver. Hepatology 49:1655–1663
48. Lindroos PM, Zarnegar R, Michalopoulos GK (1991) Hepatocyte growth factor (hepatopoietin A) rapidly increases in plasma before DNA synthesis and liver regeneration stimulated by partial hepatectomy and carbon tetrachloride administration. Hepatology 13:743–750
49. Short J, Klein K, Kibert L et al (1980) Involvement of the Iodothyronine in liver and hepatoma cell proliferation in the rat. Cancer Res 40:2417–2422
50. Cruise JL (1991) Alpha 1-adrenergic receptors in liver regeneration. Dig Dis Sci 36:485–488
51. Jirtle RL, Carr BI, Scott CD (1991) Modulation of insulin-like growth factor-II/mannose 6-phosphate receptors and transforming growth factor-beta 1 during liver regeneration. J Biol Chem 266:22444–22450
52. Duncan AW, Dorrell C, Grompe M (2009) Stem cells and liver regeneration. Gastroenterology 137:466–481
53. Sell S (2001) Heterogeneity and plasticity of hepatocyte lineage cells. Hepatology 33:738–750
54. Wisse E (1970) An electron microscopic study of the fenestrated endothelial lining of rat liver sinusoids. J Ultrastruct Res 31:125–150
55. Wisse E, De Zanger RB, Charels K et al (1985) The liver sieve: considerations concerning the structure and function of endothelial fenestrae, the sinusoidal wall and the space of Disse. Hepatology 5:683–692
56. Limmer A, Ohl J, Kurts C et al (2000) Efficient presentation of exogenous antigen by liver endothelial cells to CD8 T cells results in antigen-specific T-cell tolerance. Nat Med 6:1348–1354
57. Do H, Healey JF, Waller EK et al (1999) Expression of factor VIII by murine liver sinusoidal endothelial cells. J Biol Chem 274:19587–19592
58. Vidal-Vanaclocha F, Barbera-Guillem E (1985) Fenestration patterns in endothelial cells of rat liver sinusoids. J Ultrastruct Res 90:115–123
59. Trutmann M, Sasse D (1994) The lymphatics of the liver. Anat Embryol (Berl) 190:201–209
60. Fraser R, Dobbs BR, Rogers GWT (1995) Lipoproteins and the liver sieve: the role of the fenestrated sinusoidal endothelium in lipoproteína metabolism, atherosclerosis, and cirrhosis. Hepatology 21:863–874
61. Oda M, Yokomori H, Han JY (2006) Regulatory mechanisms of hepatic microcirculatory hemodynamics: hepatic arterial system. Clin Hemorheol Microcirc 34:11–26

62. Snoeys J, Lievens J, Wisse E et al (2007) Species differences in transgene DNA uptake in hepatocytes after adenoviral transfer correlate with the size of endothelial fenestrae. Gene Ther 14:1–9

63. Braet F, Wisse E (2002) Structural and functional aspects of liver sinusoidal endothelial cell fenestrae: a review. Comp Hepatol 1:1–12

64. Vidal-Vanaclocha F (1997) Role of sinusoidal endothelium in the pathogenesis of liver disease. In: Vidal-Vanaclocha F (ed) Functional heterogeneity of liver tissue. Springer GmbH & Co. KG, Heidelberg, pp 109–118

65. Deleve LD, Wang X, Guo Y (2008) Sinusoidal endothelial cells prevent rat stellate cell activation and promote reversion to quiescence. Hepatology 48:920–930

66. DeLeve LD, Wang X, Guo Y et al (2005) Capillarization is due to the loss of paracrine and autocrine control of the sinusoidal endothelial cell (SEC) phenotype. Hepatology 42:266A

67. March S, Hui EE, Underhill GH et al (2009) Microenvironmental regulation of the sinusoidal endothelial cell phenotype in vitro. Hepatology 50:920–928

68. Smedsrod B, Pertoft H, Gustafson S et al (1990) Scavenger functions of the liver endothelial cell. Biochem J 266:313–327

69. Smedsrod B, Johansson S, Pertoft H (1985) Studies in vivo and in vitro on the uptake and degradation of soluble collagen alpha 1(I) chains in rat liver endothelial and Kupffer cells. Biochem J 228:415–424

70. Melkko J, Hellevik T, Risteli L et al (1994) Clearance of NH2-terminal propeptides of types I and III procollagen is a physiological function of the scavenger receptor in liver endothelial cells. J Exp Med 179:405–412

71. Smedsrod B, Melkko J, Risteli L et al (1990) Circulating C-terminal propeptide of type I procollagen is cleared mainly via the mannose receptor in liver endothelial cells. Biochem J 271:345–350

72. McCourt PA, Smedsrod BH, Melkko J et al (1999) Characterization of a hyaluronan receptor on rat sinusoidal liver endothelial cells and its functional relationship to scavenger receptors. Hepatology 30:1276–1286

73. Mousavi SA, Sporstol M, Fladeby C et al (2007) Receptor-mediated endocytosis of immune complexes in rat liver sinusoidal endothelial cells is mediated by Fc gammaRIIb2. Hepatology 46:871–884

74. Stahl PD, Ezekowitz RA (1998) The mannose receptor is a pattern recognition receptor involved in host defense. Curr Opin Immunol 10:50–55

75. Malovic I, Sorensen KK, Elvevold KH et al (2007) The mannose receptor on murine liver sinusoidal endothelial cells is the main denatured collagen clearance receptor. Hepatology 45:1454–1461

76. Elvevold K, Simon-Santamaria J, Hasvold H et al (2008) Liver sinusoidal endothelial cells depend on mannose receptor-mediated recruitment of lysosomal enzymes for normal degradation capacity. Hepatology 48:2007–2015

77. Lohse AW, Knolle PA, Bilo K et al (1996) Antigen-presenting function and B7 expression of murine sinusoidal endothelial cells and Kupffer cells. Gastroenterology 110:1175–1181

78. Diehl L, Schurich A, Grochtmann R et al (2008) Tolerogenic maturation of liver sinusoidal endothelial cells promotes B7-homolog 1-dependent CD8? T cell tolerance. Hepatology 47:296–305

79. Feder LS, Mc Closkey TW, Laskin DL (1991) Characterization of interleukin-1 (IL-1) and interleukin-6 (IL-6) production by resident and lipopolysaccharide (LPS) activated hepatic macrophages and endothelial cells. In: Wisse E, Knook DL, McCuskey RS (eds) Cells of the hepatic sinusoid. Kupffer Cell Foundation, The Netherlands, pp 37–39

80. Shah V, Haddad FG, Garcia-Cardena G et al (1997) Liver sinusoidal endothelial cells are responsible for nitric oxide modulation of resistance in the hepatic sinusoids. J Clin Invest 100:2923–2930

81. Yokomori H, Oda M, Ogi M et al (2001) Endothelial nitric oxide synthase and caveolin-1 are co-localized in sinusoidal endothelial fenestrae. Liver 21:198–206

82. Yokomori H, Oda M, Ogi M et al (2003) Endothelin-1 suppresses plasma membrane Ca11-ATPase, concomitant with contraction of hepatic sinusoidal endothelial fenestrae. Am J Pathol 162:557–566

83. Couvelard A, Scoazec JY, Feldmann G (1993) Expression of cell-cell and cell matrix adhesion proteins by sinusoidal endothelial cells in the normal and cirrhotic human liver. Am J Pathol 143:738–752

84. Karrar A, Broomé U, Uzunel M et al (2006) Human liver sinusoidal endothelial cells induce apoptosis in activated T cells: a role in tolerance induction. Gut 56:243–252

85. Arteta B, Lasuen N, Lopategi A et al (2010) Colon carcinoma cell interaction with liver sinusoidal endothelium inhibits organ-specific anti-tumor immunity via IL-1-induced mannose receptor. Hepatology 51:2172–2182

86. Schaffner F, Popper H (1963) Capillarization of hepatic sinusoids in man. Gastroenterology 44:239–242

87. Horn T, Christoffersen P, Henriksen JH (1987) Alcoholic liver injury: defenestration in noncirrhotic livers-a scanning electron microscopic study. Hepatology 7:77–82

88. Muro H, Shirasawa H, Kosugi I et al (1993) Defect of Fc receptors and phenotypical changes in sinusoidal endothelial cells in human liver cirrhosis. Am J Pathol 143: 105–120

89. Wisse E, Knook DL (1979) The investigation of sinusoidal cells: a new approach to the study of liver function. In: Popper H, Schaffner F (eds) Progress in liver diseases. Grune and Stratton, New York, NY, pp 153–171

90. Wisse E, Braet F, Luo D et al (1996) Structure and function of sinusoidal lining cells in the liver. Toxicol Pathol 24:100–111

91. Decker K (1990) Biologically active products of stimulated liver macrophages. Eur J Biochem 192:245–261

92. Blouin A (1977) Morphometry of the liver sinusoidal cells. In: Wisse E, Knook DL (eds) Kupffer cells and other liver sinusoidal cells. Elsevier Biomedical, Amsterdam, pp 61–71

93. McCuskey RS, McCuskey PA (1990) The fine structure and function of Kupffer cells. J Electron Microsc Tech 14:237–246

94. Sleyster EC, Knook DL (1982) Relation between localization and function of rat liver Kupffer cells. Lab Invest 47:484–490

95. Bouwens L, Baekeland M, Zanger RD et al (1986) Quantitation, tissue distribution and proliferation kinetics of Kupffer cells in normal rat liver. Hepatology 6:718–722

96. Hoedemakers RM, Morselt HW, Scherphof GL et al (1995) Heterogeneity in secretory responses of rat liver macrophages of different size. Liver 15:313–319

97. Barberá-Guillem E, Ayala R, Vidal-Vanaclocha F (1989) Differential location of hemopoietic cells within liver acini of postnatal and phenylhydrazine treated adult mice. Hepatology 9:29–36

98. Widmann JJ, Fahimi HD (1975) Proliferation of mononuclear phagocytes (Kupffer cells) and endothelial cells in regenerating rat liver: a light and electron microscopic cytochemical study. Am J Pathol 80:349–366

99. Deimann W, Fahimi H (1979) The appearance of transition forms between monocytes and Kupffer cells in the liver of rats treated with glucan. J Exp Med 149:883

100. Bouwens L, Baekeland M, Wisse E (1984) Importance of local proliferation in the expanding Kupffer cell population of rat liver alter zymosan stimulation and partial hepatectomy. Hepatology 4:213–229

101. Rogoff TM, Lipsky PE (1980) Antigen presentation by isolated guinea pig Kupffer cells. J Immunol 124:1740–1744

102. Wiegard C, Frenzel C, Herkel J et al (2005) Murine liver antigen presenting cells control suppressor activity of CD4+CD25+ regulatory T cells. Hepatology 42:193–199

103. Ju C, Pohl LR (2005) Tolerogenic role of Kupffer cells in immune-mediated adverse drug reactions. Toxicology 209:109–112

104. Seki S, Habu Y, Kawamura T et al (2000) The liver as a crucial organ in the first line of host defense: the roles of Kupffer cells, natural killer (NK) cells and NK1.1 Ag+ T cells in T helper 1 immune responses. Immunol Rev 174:35–46

105. Bayon LG, Izquierdo MA, Sirovich I et al (1996) Role of Kupffer cells in arresting circulating tumor cells and controlling metastatic growth in the liver. Hepatology 23:1224–1231

106. Crofton RW, Diesselhoff-den Dulk MM, van Furth R (1978) The origin, kinetics, and characteristics of the Kupffer cells in the normal steady state. J Exp Med 148:1–17

107. Diesselhoff-den Dulk MM, Crofton RW, van Furth R (1979) Origin and kinetics of Kupffer cells during an acute inflammatory response. Immunology 37:7–14

108. van Furth R (1980) Monocyte origin of Kupffer cells. Blood Cells 6:87–92

109. Bouwens L, Knook DL, Wisse E (1986) Local proliferation and extrahepatic recruitment of liver macrophages (Kupffer cells) in partial-body irradiated rats. J Leukoc Biol 39:687–697

110. Yamamoto T, Naito M, Moriyama H et al (1996) Repopulation of murine Kupffer cells after intravenous administration of liposome-encapsulated dichloromethylene diphosphonate. Am J Pathol 149:1271–1286

111. Klei, I, Cornejo JC, Polakos NK et al (2007) Kupffer cell heterogeneity: functional properties of bone marrow-derived and sessile hepatic macrophages. Blood 110:4077–4085

112. Wisse E, Noordende JMVt, Meulen JVD et al (1976) The pit cell: description of a new type of cell occurring in rat liver and peripheral blood. Cell Tissue Res 173:423–435

113. Kaneda K, Dan C, Wake K (1983) Pit cells as natural killer cells. Biomed Res 4:567–576

114. Winnock M, Barcina MG, Lukomska B et al (1993) Liver-associated lymphocytes: role in tumor defense. Semin Liver Dis 13:81–92

115. Bouwens L, Remels L, Baekeland M et al (1987) Large granular lymphocytes or "pit cells" from rat liver: isolation, ultrastructural characterization and natural killer activity. Eur J Immunol 17:37–42

116. Nakatani K, Kaneda K, Seki S et al (2004) Pit cells as liver associated natural killer cells: morphology and function. Med Electron Microsc 37:29–36

117. Mehal WZ, Juedes AE, Crispe IN (1999) Selective retention of activated CD8+ T cells by the normal liver. J Immunol 163:3202–3210

118. John B, Crispe IN (2005) TLR-4 regulates CD8+ T cell trapping in the liver. J Immunol 175:1643–1650

119. Crispe IN, Giannandrea M, Klein I et al (2006) Cellular and molecular mechanisms of liver tolerance. Immunol Rev 213:101–118

120. O'Connell J, Bennett MW, Nally K et al (2000) Altered mechanisms of apoptosis in colon cancer: Fas resistance and counterattack in the tumor-immune conflict. Ann NY Acad Sci 910:178–192; discussion 193–195

121. Kudo S, Matsuno K, Ezaki T et al (1997) A novel migration pathway for rat dendritic cells from the blood: hepatic sinusoids-lymph translocation. J Exp Med 185:777–784

122. Cyster JG (1999) Chemokines and the homing of dendritic cells to the T cell areas of lymphoid organs. J Exp Med 189:447–450

123. Yoneyama H, Matsuno K, Zhang Y et al (2001) Regulation by chemokines of circulating dendritic cell precursors, and the formation of portal tract-associated lymphoid tissue, in a granulomatous liver disease. J Exp Med 193:35–49

124. Grant AJ, Goddard S, Ahmed-Choudhury J et al (2002) Hepatic expression of secondary lymphoid chemokine (CCL21) promotes the development of portal-associated lymphoid tissue in chronic inflammatory liver disease. Am J Pathol 160:1445–1455

125. Bertolino P, McCaughan GW, Bowen DG (2002) Role of primary intrahepatic T-cell activation in the 'liver tolerance effect'. Immunol Cell Biol 80:84–92

126. Triger DR, Cynamon MH, Wright R (1973) Studies on hepatic uptake of antigen. I. Comparison of inferior vena cava and portal vein route of immunization. Immunology 25:941–950

127. Yang R, Liu Q, Grosfeld JL et al (1994) Intestinal venous drainage through the liver is a prerequisite for oral tolerance induction. J Pediatr Surg 29:1145–1148

128. Schaffner F, Barka T, Popper H (1963) Hepatic mesenchymal cell reaction in liver disease. Exp Mol Pathol 31:419–441
129. Popper H, Uenfriend S (1970) Hepatic fibrosis. Correlation of biochemical and morphologic investigations. Am J Med 49:707–721
130. Kinnman N, Housset C (2002) Peribiliary myofibroblasts in biliary type liver fibrosis. Front Biosci 7:d496–d503
131. Beaussier M, Wendum D, Schiffer E et al (2007) Prominent contribution of portal mesenchymal cells to liver fibrosis in ischemic and obstructive cholestatic injuries. Lab Invest 87:292–303
132. Kinnman N, Francoz C, Barbu V et al (2003) The myofibroblastic conversion of peribiliary fibrogenic cells distinct from hepatic stellate cells is stimulated by platelet-derived growth factor during liver fibrogenesis. Lab Invest 83:163–173
133. Ramadori G, Saile B (2004) Portal tract fibrogenesis in the liver. Lab Invest 84:153–159
134. Cassiman D, Libbrecht L, Desmet V et al (2002) Hepatic stellate cell/myofibroblast subpopulations in fibrotic human and rat livers. J Hepatol 36:200–209
135. Ramadori G, Saile B (2004) Portal tract fibrogenesis in the liver. Lab Invest 84:153–159
136. Guyot C, Lepreux S, Combe C et al (2006) Hepatic fibrosis and cirrhosis: the (myo)fibroblastic cell subpopulations involved. Int J Biochem Cell Biol 38:135–151.
137. Desmouliere A, Darby I, Costa AM et al (1997) Extracellular matrix deposition, lysyl oxidase expression, and myofibroblastic differentiation during the initial stages of cholestatic fibrosis in the rat. Lab Invest 76:765–778
138. Lorena D, Darby IA, Reinhardt DP et al (2004) Fibrillin-1 expression in normal and fibrotic rat liver and in cultured hepatic fibroblastic cells: modulation by mechanical stress and role in cell adhesion. Lab Invest 84:203–212
139. Villeneuve J, Pelluard-Nehme F, Combe C et al (2009) Immunohistochemical study of the phenotypic change of the mesenchymal cells during portal tract maturation in normal and fibrous (ductal plate malformation) fetal liver. Comp Hepatol 8:5
140. Libbrecht L, Cassiman D, Desmet V et al (2002) The correlation between portal myofibroblasts and development of intrahepatic bile ducts and arterial branches in human liver. Liver 22:252–258
141. Suzuki K, Tanaka M, Watanabe N et al (2008) p75 Neurotrophin receptor is a marker for precursors of stellate cells and portal fibroblasts in mouse fetal liver. Gastroenterology 135:270–281
142. Asahina K, Tsai SY, Li P et al (2009) Mesenchymal origin of hepatic stellate cells, submesothelial cells, and perivascular mesenchymal cells during mouse liver development. Hepatology 49:998–1011
143. Desmouliere A, Darby I, Costa AM et al (1997) Extracellular matrix deposition, lysyl oxidase expression, and myofibroblastic differentiation during the initial stages of cholestatic fibrosis in the rat. Lab Invest 76:765–778
144. Li Z, Dranoff JA, Chan EP et al (2007) Transforming growth factor-beta and substrate stiffness regulate portal fibroblast activation in culture. Hepatology 46:1246–1256
145. Hellerbrand C, Stefanovic B, Giordano F et al (1999) The role of TGFbeta1 in initiating hepatic stellate cell activation in vivo. J Hepatol 30:77–87
146. Tomasek JJ, Gabbiani G, Hinz B et al (2002) Myofibroblasts and mechano-regulation of connective tissue remodeling. Nat Rev Mol Cell Biol 3:349–363
147. Beaussier M, Wendum D, Schiffer E et al (2007) Prominent contribution of portal mesenchymal cells to liver fibrosis in ischemic and obstructive cholestatic injuries. Lab Invest 87:292–303
148. Richardson MM, Jonsson JR, Powell EE et al (2007) Progressive fibrosis in nonalcoholic steatohepatitis: association with altered regeneration and a ductular reaction. Gastroenterology 133:80–90
149. Fabris L, Cadamuro M, Guido M et al (2007) Analysis of liver repair mechanisms in Alagille syndrome and biliary atresia reveals a role for notch signaling. Am J Pathol 171:641–653

150. Yasoshima M, Kono N, Sugawara H et al (1998) Increased expression of interleukin-6 and tumor necrosis factor-alpha in pathologic biliary epithelial cells: in situ and culture study. Lab Invest 78:89–100

151. Yu J, Lavoie EG, Sheung N et al (2008) IL-6 downregulates transcription of NTPDase2 via specific promoter elements. Am J Physiol Gastrointest Liver Physiol 294:G748–G756

152. Dranoff JA, Kruglov EA, Robson SC et al (2002) The ecto-nucleoside triphosphate diphosphohydrolase NTPDase2/CD39L1 is expressed in a novel functional compartment within the liver. Hepatology 36:1135–1144

153. Dranoff JA, Kruglov EA, Toure J et al (2004) Ectonucleotidase NTPDase2 is selectively down-regulated in biliary cirrhosis. J Invest Med 52:475–482

154. Jhandier MN, Kruglov EA, Lavoie EG et al (2005) Portal fibroblasts regulate the proliferation of bile duct epithelia via expression of NTPDase2. J Biol Chem 280:22986–22992

155. Marra F, DeFranco R, Grappone C et al (1998) Increased expression of monocyte chemotactic protein-1 during active hepatic fibrogenesis: correlation with monocyte infiltration. Am J Pathol 152:423–430

156. Kruglov EA, Nathanson RA, Nguyen T et al (2006) Secretion of MCP-1/CCL2 by bile duct epithelia induces myofibroblastic transdifferentiation of portal fibroblasts. Am J Physiol Gastrointest Liver Physiol 290:G765–771

157. Seki E, de Minicis S, Inokuchi S et al (2009) CCR2 promotes hepatic fibrosis in mice. Hepatology 50:185–197

158. Ito T (1951) Cytological studies on stellate cells of Kupffer and fat storing cells in the capillary wall of human liver. Acta Anat Nippon 26:2–11

159. Wake K (1971) "Sternzellen" in the liver: perisinusoidal cells with special reference to storage of vitamin A. Am J Anat 132:429–462

160. Bronfenmajer S, Schaffner F, Popper H (1966) Fat-storing cells (lipocytes) in human liver. Arch Path 82:447–453

161. Friedman SL (2008) Hepatic stellate cells: protean, multifunctional, and enigmatic cells of the liver. Physiol Rev 88:125–172

162. Friedman SL, Arthur MJ (2002) Reversing hepatic fibrosis. Sci Med 8:194–205

163. Vidal-Vanaclocha F (2008) The prometastatic microenvironment of the liver. Cancer Microenviron 1:113–129

Chapter 3
The Tumor Microenvironment at Different Stages of Hepatic Metastasis

Fernando Vidal-Vanaclocha

Abstract This chapter summarizes current knowledge on the contribution of architectural and functional aspects of the hepatic tissue to cancer cell regulation during the process of hepatic metastasis. To this end, four consecutive phases in the process, each with distinct mechanisms, have been considered: (1) The microvascular phase of liver-infiltrating cancer cells that includes mechanisms of intravascular arrest, death or survival of cancer cells at specific sites of the hepatic microcirculation and their interactions with organ-specific microvascular endothelial and blood cells; (2) The pre-angiogenic, intralobular micrometastatic phase that includes activation of cancer cell growth, regional anti-tumor immune response impairment and stromal cell recruitment into avascular micrometastases; (3) The angiogenic panlobular micrometastatic phase that includes hypoxic stromal myofibroblasts–induced recruitment of endothelial cells, blood vessel formation and hepatic tissue replacement or "pushing-type" cancer cell growth; and (4) The lobar growth phase of hepatic metastases. During this final phase, the clinical impact and prognostic significance of the metastatic process are determined by multiple factors including the intratumoral stroma and angiogenic patterns, the phenotypes of tumor-infiltrating lymphocytes and the specific gene expression profiles of the metastatic cancer cells. In addition, alterations in the local microenvironment during liver inflammation, regeneration and fibrosis provide a favorable milieu for cancer metastasis and their impact is therefore also discussed. Resident hepatic cells and invading cancer cells can reciprocally alter each other's gene expression profiles and functional activities during the metastatic process. The characterization of these molecular changes could lead to identification of novel biomarkers and therapeutic targets that are involved at discrete stages of hepatic metastasis and thereby impact the clinical management of liver metastases.

F. Vidal-Vanaclocha (✉)
Institute of Applied Molecular Medicine (IMMA), CEU-San Pablo University School of Medicine,
Urb. Montepríncipe, Boadilla del Monte, 28668 Madrid, Spain
e-mail: fernando.vidalvanaclocha@ceu.es

P. Brodt (ed.), *Liver Metastasis: Biology and Clinical Management*, Cancer
Metastasis – Biology and Treatment 16, DOI 10.1007/978-94-007-0292-9_3,
© Springer Science+Business Media B.V. 2011

Keywords Tumor microenvironment · Liver sinusoidal cells · Hepatocytes · Tumor stroma · Metastasis-related genes

Abbreviations

SMA   α-smooth muscle actin
CEA   carcinoembryonic antigen
COX   cyclooxygenase
DDR2   discoidin domain receptor-2
HSEC   hepatic sinusoidal endothelial cells
HSC   hepatic stellate cells
ICE   IL-1 converting enzyme
ManR   mannose receptor
NK   natural killer
TLR   toll-like receptor

Contents

3.1 Introduction

The liver is a major metastasis-susceptible site and the majority of patients with hepatic metastases die from the disease in the absence of effective treatment. Currently, a focal liver lesion is more likely to represent a metastatic tumor than a primary malignancy. However, the majority of patients develop multiple liver metastases in both lobes that vary in diameter, suggesting that cancer cell seeding and growth occurs in episodes. Numerous experimental and clinical studies have focused on factors that regulate metastasis recurrence to the liver. However, at present, the genetic and phenotypic properties of specific cancer cells able to implant and grow in the liver have not yet been established for any tumor type. Neither is the contribution of the patient's genetic and physiologic backgrounds to the incidence and progression of hepatic metastases presently understood.

The development of hepatic metastases is associated with an aberrant tissue-reconstitution process that results from the bidirectional interaction between the cancer cells and resident hepatic cells. On the one hand, cancer cells and their molecular products can regulate gene expression in hepatic cells residing in, or infiltrating into the sites of metastases. At these sites, cancer cells exert selective pressures on hepatic cells, thereby shaping their functional phenotypes. Conversely, constituents of the liver microenvironment can also regulate gene expression in the cancer cells, thereby controlling their fate and determining their ability to progress towards metastases formation. Additionally, there are pathophysiological processes such as aberrant hepatic regeneration, inflammation and fibrosis that can change the hepatic microenvironment and affect the development of metastases. Therefore, the tumor microenvironment regulating hepatic metastasis in a given patient consists of structural and functional factors resulting from both hepatic-cancer cell interactions and previous or concurrent hepatic diseases.

In this chapter, a detailed description of the tumor microenvironment at different stages of hepatic metastasis is provided. Specific attention has been paid to the underlying mechanisms, their cellular and molecular mediators and their genetic regulation. Because hepatic and cancer cells mutually alter each other's functional profiles at different phases of the metastatic process, an understanding of these mechanisms may identify biomarkers and therapeutic targets with clinical/therapeutic applications. However, many of the conclusions are based on animal studies and hepatic-cancer cell interactions analyzed in vitro and these will need further clinical validation.

3.2 Phases of the Hepatic Metastasis Process

Once circulating cancer cells reach the liver, their ability to form metastases will depend on the outcome of well-defined colonization steps that only a small fraction of the cells can successfully complete. The complexity of the mechanisms involved and the control exerted by the microenvironment render hepatic metastasis a highly inefficient process [1, 2] that will frequently abort and will have no clinical consequences due to stromal and/or angiogenic deficiencies (Fig. 3.1). A sequence of interrelated processes contributes to the completion of hepatic colonization. These can be divided into four pathophysiological rate-limiting steps [3] that may require different diagnostic and treatment strategies (summarized Table 3.1): (1) *the microvascular phase* of liver-infiltrating cancer cells, consisting of mechanisms of intravascular arrest, followed by death or survival of cancer cells at specific sites of the hepatic microcirculation, their interactions with organ-specific microvascular endothelial and blood cells, their extravascular migration and interaction with perivascular liver cells; (2) *the intralobular pre-angiogenic phase* that includes growth regulation of cancer cells, regional anti-tumor immune response impairment and stromal cell recruitment into avascular micrometastases; (3) *the panlobular angiogenic phase* that consists of endothelial cell recruitment and blood vessel formation induced by hypoxic stromal myofibroblasts and the development of early metastases by hepatic tissue replacement-type or "pushing-type" cancer cell growth; and (4) *the lobar growth phase* of hepatic metastasis. This is the

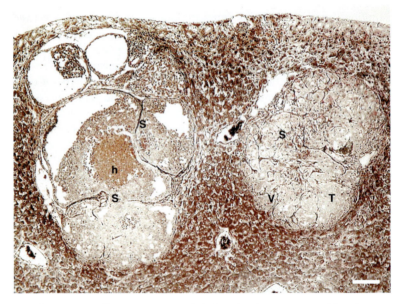

Fig. 3.1 Efficient and inefficient stromagenesis in hepatic micrometastases. The micrometastasis shown on the *left* side has an inefficient stroma (S) with poor angiogenesis. The cancerous tissue becomes necrotic, leading to intrametastatic cavities and hemorrhagic spaces (h). The micrometastasis on the *right* has a solid tumor mass (T) with a well-organized stroma (S) and more efficient angiogenesis (V). No cancer cell death is observed in this metastasis. Bar: 50 μm

Table 3.1   Phases and major mechanisms in the process of hepatic metastasis

1. *Hepatic metastasis microvascular phase*
   o Cancer cell retention and death in the hepatic microvasculature
   o Micro-infarcts and ischemia/reperfusion of hepatic sinusoids
   o Inflammatory factor release by sinusoidal endothelium and Kupffer cells
   o Adhesion molecule expression by microvascular endothelium
   o Cancer cell adhesion to portal vein and sinusoidal endothelium
   o Activation of mannose receptor-mediated endocytosis
   o Anti-tumor cytotoxicity of liver-associated lymphocytes
   o Myofibroblast transdifferentiation of perisinusoidal stellate cells and portal tract fibroblasts at sites of cancer cell arrest
   o Extravascular migration of cancer cells

2. *Hepatic metastasis intralobular pre-angiogenic phase*
   o Onset of cancer cell growth at metastatic niches in the portal space and sinusoidal segments of hepatic lobules
   o Stromal cell recruitment into avascular micrometastases
      ▪ Myofibroblast transdifferentiation of tumor-activated hepatic stellate cells and portal tract fibroblasts
      ▪ Epithelial-to-mesenchymal transition of perimetastatic hepatocytes
   o Immune suppression of anti-tumor hepatic immunity

3. *Hepatic metastasis panlobular angiogenic phase*
   o Angiogenic activation of hypoxic stromal myofibroblasts
   o Angiogenic activation of 3D-growing metastatic cancer cells
   o Hepatic secretion of endogenous anti-angiogenic factors
   o Hepatic metastasis and angiogenic patterns
      ▪ Replacement/Sinusoidal-type metastasis
      ▪ Pushing/Portal-type metastasis

4. *Hepatic metastasis lobar growth phase*
   o Role of tumor-infiltrating stromal cells
   o Pathophysiology of unaffected hepatic areas
   o Hepatic metastasis-related genes
      ▪ Cancer cell genes already encoded at the primary tumor
      ▪ Hepato-mimetic cancer cell genes
      ▪ Tumor-mimetic hepatic cell genes
      ▪ Hepatic microenvironment-dependent genes

"clinical" phase of the process and its outcome (and patient prognosis) are affected by the type of intratumoral stroma, angiogenic patterns, the phenotype of tumor-infiltrating lymphocytes, and the specific gene expression profile of the metastatic cancer cells [3].

Clearly, the tissue architecture and microenvironments encountered by the infiltrating cancer cells at each of these phases and therefore the interactions that ensue are distinct (For more on tumor dormancy, see Chapter 8 in this volume). Namely, at the microvascular phase, cancer cells are affected by organ-specific properties of terminal portal veins, sinusoidal segments and centrilobular veins. At the intralobular phase, cancer cells interact with hepatic parenchymal and non-parenchymal cells prior to the architectural disturbance of the hepatic lobules by tumor growth. At the panlobular angiogenic phase, cancer cells are primarily affected by infiltrating stromal cells and their surrounding hepatic parenchymal cells whose function may have been altered by tumor-derived factors. At the lobar growth phase, cancer cells are affected by specific intrametastatic stromal cells (including tumor-infiltrating lymphocytes, macrophages and myofibroblasts), and abnormal concentrations of hepatic and extrahepatic soluble factors generated by the pathophysiological changes occurring in the liver and outside the liver, as a consequence of cancer growth. These dynamically changing microenvironments are discussed at greater length below.

3.3 The Tumor Microenvironment During the Microvascular Phase of Liver-Infiltrating Cancer Cells

3.3.1 Microvascular Entrapment and Death of Liver-Infiltrating Cancer Cells

The hepatic metastasis process begins with the microvascular retention of circulating cancer cells (Fig. 3.2). Deformation-associated trauma and mechanical stress, experienced by the cancer cells upon entry and residence in the hepatic microvasculature contribute to cancer cell death [4, 5]. Infiltrating cancer cells can also induce obstruction of sinusoids, leading to transient micro-infarcts that damage hepatic cells. In turn, re-oxygenation of ischemic sinusoids can induce the proinflammatory activation of sinusoids [6], leading to additional killing of cancer cells as a result of nitric oxide [7] and reactive oxygen intermediates [8] released from hepatic sinusoidal endothelial cells (HSECs). Kupffer cells also contribute to this tumoricidal microenvironment [9] by phagocytosing the cancer cells [10–12], by producing the pro-apoptotic cytokine TNFα or by releasing immune-stimulating factors such as IFN$_\gamma$ that activate hepatic natural killer (NK) cells [13, 14]. The NK cells can in turn mediate anti-tumor cytotoxicity via secretion of perforin/granzyme-containing granules or through death receptor-mediated mechanisms including the Fas/Fas ligand pathway [15, 16].

3.3.2 The Inflammatory Response of the Tumor-Activated Hepatic Microcirculation

During hepatic colonization by cancer cells, HSECs adopt a tumor-activated phenotype that is manifest as decreased fenestration (pseudo-capillarized phenotype) [17], activation of mannose receptor-mediated endocytosis [18], induction of adhesion molecules [19], and release of proinflammatory factors [20, 21] and reactive oxygen species [22]. Resident Kupffer cells similarly become activated and new ones are recruited from the circulating precursor cell compartment into the tumor-infiltrated hepatic microvasculature. Therefore, cytokine release from tumor-activated hepatic microvascular cells can be identified as an early, tumor-specific, inflammatory response to liver-invading cancer cells that may influence metastasis occurrence. Consequently, factors that attenuate the tumor-induced host

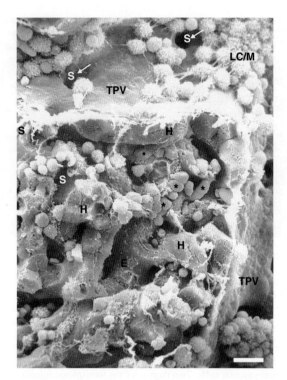

Fig. 3.2 The microvascular phase of hepatic metastasis as shown by scanning electron micro-scopy. Shown is a section of mouse liver tissue on the 5th day after intrasplenic injection of Lewis lung carcinoma cells. Circulating cancer cells first interact with non-fenestrated endothelial cells, adherent leukocytes and macrophages (LC/M) at perilobular terminal portal veins (TPV). Pre-sinusoidal gates (S with *arrows*) provide intralobular access for cancer cells. Intrasinusoidal retention of cancer cells (*) within the periportal area of the hepatic lobule can be seen. Surrounding hepatocytes (H) and endothelial cells (E) lining sinusoids (S) are shown. Bar: 20 μm. Reproduced with permission from [3]

proinflammatory response or block adhesion receptors for cancer cells may have a therapeutic potential in the prevention of liver metastasis [23, 24]. The prometastatic implications of the inflammatory microenvironment elicited by tumor-activated hepatic sinusoidal cells are described in greater detail below.

3.3.2.1 Microvascular Adhesion of Liver-Infiltrating Cancer Cells: Critical Role of IL-18-Induced Endothelial Cell Adhesion Molecules

Liver-infiltrating cancer cells that survive in the inflammatory microenvironment generated by the tumor-activated hepatic microvasculature are able to interact with the sinusoid-lining endothelium and Kupffer cells, leading to firm adhesion of certain cancer cell subpopulations to the sinusoidal wall (Fig. 3.3a). The adhesion mechanism is regulated by proinflammatory cytokines and reactive oxygen metabolites, released by cancer cells and tumor-activated hepatic sinusoidal cells.

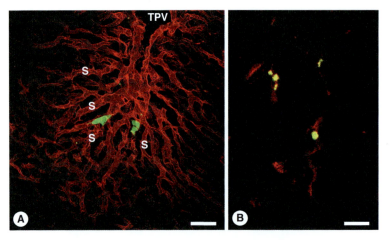

Fig. 3.3 (**a**) Cancer cell entry and residence in the hepatic microvasculature. Carboxyfluorescein (CF)-labeled C26 murine colorectal carcinoma cells were intrasplenically injected into syngeneic mice and their livers were perfused on the 24th and 48th h with fluorescence-labeled wheat germ agglutinin (WGA) for specific staining of hepatic microvascular walls (C26 cells do not bind this lectin). Cryostat sections were then analyzed by confocal laser microscopy. Shown are cancer cells (in *green*) retained in the lumen of a hepatic sinusoid (S, in *red*) near a terminal portal venule (TPV, in *red*). The body of the cancer cell may be attached to the sinusoidal endothelium or in the process of extravasation because endothelial cell labeling with perfused lectin beyond the point of attachment was not blocked. Bar: 25 μm. (**b**) Intrahepatic co-localization of C26 and SMA-expressing microvascular cells. Two days after the intrasplenic injection, the microvascular coordinates of CF-labeled C26 cells (in *green-yellow*) and SMA-expressing cells (in *red*) were determined by immunohistochemistry. SMA-expressing cells co-localized with intrasinusoidally-arrested C26 cells, but were rarely found near tumor-unaffected sinusoidal segments. At this time interval, up to 35% of the arrested cancer cells were not associated with SMA-expressing cells. Bar: 10 μm

Endotoxins released by gastrointestinal bacteria into the portal circulation can also stimulate tumor-endothelial cell adhesion and promote hepatic metastasis prior to cancer cell dissemination from a primary tumor [25] (For a comprehensive discussion on the crosstalk between inflammation and liver metastasis, see Chapters 6 and 7 in this volume).

Experimental studies on the hepatic colonization by B16 melanoma cells support the important prometastatic effects of inflammatory cytokine-dependent cancer-sinusoidal cell interactions [22]. Using intrasplenically injected B16F10 melanoma cells, our group showed that the expression of VCAM-1 significantly increased in HSECs within the first 24 h of metastatic cancer cell infiltration into the liver [20]. *In vivo* VCAM-1 blockade with specific antibodies decreased microvascular retention of luciferase-transfected B16 melanoma cells by 85%, and metastasis development by 75%, indicating that VCAM-1 expression on tumor-activated HSECs had a prometastatic effect [20, 24], while blockade of the VCAM-1-VLA-4 interaction may have anti-metastatic benefits [26].

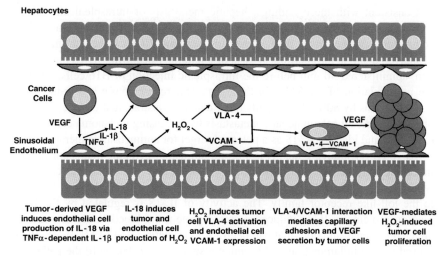

Fig. 3.4 Tumor-induced proinflammatory factors regulate melanoma cell adhesion to the hepatic sinusoidal endothelium prior to experimental metastases formation. Shown is a schematic representation of early events triggered by B16 melanoma cell entry into the hepatic sinusoids. The model is based on data described in [19, 20, 22–26, 84]

Cell adhesion molecule expression on tumor-activated HSECs is regulated by a proinflammatory cytokine cascade (Fig. 3.4), whereby TNF-$_\alpha$ induces IL-1β; and IL-1β either alone or together with TNFα, induce the release of IL-18 [19]. Neither TNF-binding protein nor IL-1 receptor antagonists were able to inhibit the increase in adhesiveness in IL-18-treated HSECs, confirming that neither endogenous TNFα, nor IL-1β mediate IL-18-induced endothelial cell adhesiveness. Conversely, IL-18 neutralization by an IL-18 binding protein [24] did not alter tumor-induced TNFα or IL-1β release from HSECs, suggesting that their production was IL-18-independent. This suggests that TNFα and IL-1β mediate the upregulation of VCAM-1 expression in HSECs via IL-18 and thereby increase cancer cell arrest during transit through the hepatic microvasculature.

The proadhesive response of HSECs to B16 melanoma cell-conditioned medium could also be abrogated by catalase, although this did not affect the release of major proinflammatory cytokines by tumor-activated HSECs [19]. In turn, hydrogen peroxide production by endothelial cells treated with B16-melanoma conditioned medium was found to be regulated by IL-18. The results suggested that liver-infiltrating B16 melanoma cells promote their adhesion to HSECs through a sequential process involving TNFα-dependent IL-1β that in turn induces IL-18 to up-regulate VCAM-1 via hydrogen peroxide. The pivotal role of IL-18-induced hydrogen peroxide is also supported by the finding that incubation of HSECs with nontoxic concentrations of hydrogen peroxide could directly enhance VCAM-1-dependent B16 melanoma cell adhesion *in vitro*, in the absence of proinflammatory cytokines. This highlights the key role that oxidative stress plays in the pathogenesis of IL-18-dependent hepatic metastasis (Fig. 3.4).

Consistent with these findings, hepatic metastasis of intrasplenically-injected B16 melanoma cells was dramatically reduced in IL-1β deficient mice and almost completely abrogated in IL-1 converting enzyme (ICE) knockout mice [20]. Moreover, a single intraperitoneal dose of a naturally occurring IL-18 binding protein, administered 30 min before the intrasplenic injection of B16 cells, abolished the up-regulation of VCAM-1 in the hepatic microvasculature and reduced hepatic metastasis by 80% [24]. Together, the data demonstrate that endogenous IL-18 plays a significant role in hepatic metastasis by increasing melanoma cell adhesion to HSECs and identify IL-18 as a potential target for antimetastatic therapy.

IL-18 (IFNγ inducing factor) is a proinflammatory cytokine that is converted to its biologically active form by the ICE. A wide range of normal and cancer cell types can produce and/or respond to IL-18 through a specific receptor belonging to the toll-like receptor family. The activity of IL-18 is regulated by the IL-18-binding protein, an IFNγ-induced secreted protein the blood levels of which are affected by renal function, that can neutralize circulating IL-18 [27]. IL-18 plays a central role in inflammation and immune response, contributing to the pathogenesis of infectious and inflammatory diseases [28]. Because the immune-stimulating effects of IL-18 have anti-neoplastic consequences, IL-18 has been proposed as a novel adjuvant therapy against cancer (for review, see [29]). However, circulating IL-18 levels were shown to increase in the majority of cancer patients and have been shown to correlate with disease progression and, in some cancer types, with risk of metastatic recurrence and poor clinical outcome (for review, see [29]). Under experimental conditions, cancer cells can also escape immune recognition, increase their adherence to the microvascular wall and even induce production of angiogenic and tumor growth-stimulating factors via IL-18-dependent mechanisms. This is particularly relevant for hepatic metastasis of murine B16 melanoma, where IL-18 has demonstrated prometastatic and proangiogenic effects while IL-18 binding protein could inhibit cancer metastasis (for review, see [29]).

Khatib et al. [21] also found that metastatic murine lung carcinoma H-59 or human colorectal carcinoma CX-1 cells triggered TNFα production by Kupffer cells located in sinusoids around the invading cancer cells, during the initial stages of liver metastasis. This was followed by increased expression of E-selectin, P-selectin, VCAM-1, and ICAM-1 on HSECs. This proinflammatory response was tumor-specific and was not observed with non-metastatic cancer cells. Again, these results identify sinusoidal cell-mediated TNFα production as an early, tumor-selective host inflammatory response to liver-invading cancer cells that may influence the course of metastasis. Interestingly, over-expression of secretory leukocyte protease inhibitor – a factor attenuating inflammatory response by blocking Nuclear Factor-kappaB-mediated TNFα production – in a highly metastatic subline markedly decreased the ability of these cells to elicit a proinflammatory response in the liver and to form hepatic metastases [30].

Using a combination of immunohistochemistry, confocal microscopy, and three-dimensional reconstruction, Auguste et al. [31] detected E-selectin expression mainly on sinusoids by 6 and 10 h, respectively, following murine and human carcinoma cell injection. Cancer cells arrested in E-selectin-expressing microvessels and appeared to flatten and traverse the sinusoidal lining, away from sites of intense E-selectin staining. This process was evident by 8 to 12 h after inoculation, coincided with increased endothelial VCAM-1 expression, and involved tumor cell attachment in areas of intense VCAM-1 and PECAM-1 expression. Non-metastatic human and murine cancer cells induced a weaker response and could not be seen to extravasate, suggesting that only metastatic cancer cells used newly expressed HSEC receptors to arrest and extravasate.

3.3.2.2 Activation of Mannose Receptor-Mediated Endocytosis: Implications for Anti-tumor Immune Suppression

Tumor-induced hepatic inflammation also involves increased mannose receptor (ManR)-mediated endocytosis in HSECs [18] (Fig. 3.5a). The ManR mediates uptake of glycoconjugates carrying mannose in a terminal position and contributes to the adhesion of cancer cells to HSECs [25]. The ManR is also involved in antigen uptake, processing and presentation to T cells by HSECs [32], and it has been suggested that this process diminishes local immune responses in the liver [33]. Based on the inflammatory status of tumor-infiltrated hepatic sinusoids and the inflammatory regulation of hepatic ManR-mediated endocytosis, we recently hypothesized that IL-1-induced ManR-mediated endocytosis may contribute to the pro-metastatic role of tumor-activated HSECs by inhibiting T-cell mediated anti-tumor activity. Using murine C26 colon carcinoma cells, we showed that upon direct

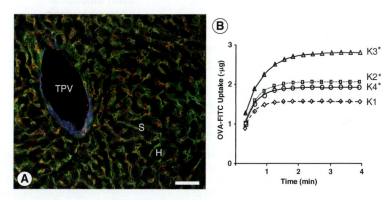

Fig. 3.5 Upregulation of mannose receptor-mediated endocytosis in hepatic sinusoidal endothelium activated by tumor cells. (**a**) Shown are confocal microscopy images of liver sections labeled with antibodies to mouse ManR (*red fluorescence*), ICAM-1(*green fluorescence*) and SMA (*blue fluorescence*). Liver sections were from tumor C26-injected mice and were obtained 96 h post injections. H: hepatocytes; S: sinusoidal lumen; TPV: terminal portal venule. Bar: 50 μm. (**b**) The effect of the IL-1 receptor antagonist (IL-1Ra) on C26-stimulated ManR activity in vivo was measured by intraportal perfusion of FITC-conjugated ovalbumin (OVA-FITC) 36 h after the intrasplenic injection of C26 cells into vehicle- and recombinant human IL-1Ra-treated mice (5 mg/kg). Shown are OVA-FITC clearance values for untreated tumor-free mice (K1), IL-1Ra-treated tumor-free mice (K2) C26-bearing mice (K3) and IL-1Ra-treated C26-bearing mice (K4). (*-$p < 0.05$ as compared to untreated tumor-free mice)

interaction with cancer cells, ManR-mediated endocytosis in HSECs increased and this required a cyclooxygenase (COX)-2-dependent production of IL-1-stimulating factors by the cancer cells [18]. In response to IL-1, ManR-mediated endocytosis was enhanced (Fig. 3.5b), resulting in increased IL-10 and decreased IFNγ production and a reduced anti-tumor cytotoxicity of liver sinusoidal lymphocytes (Fig. 3.6a–e). Therefore, C26 cancer cell-derived factors impaired the liver-specific lymphocyte-stimulating effects of HSECs, leading to inhibition of anti-tumor cytotoxicity and a decrease in the secreted IFNγ/IL-10 ratio. Moreover, ManR deficiency in ManR knockout mice and blockade of ManR on tumor-stimulated HSECs – either directly with specific neutralizing antibodies, or indirectly through IL-1 and COX-2 inhibitors – restored the anti-tumor cytotoxicity of HSEC-interacting lymphocytes,

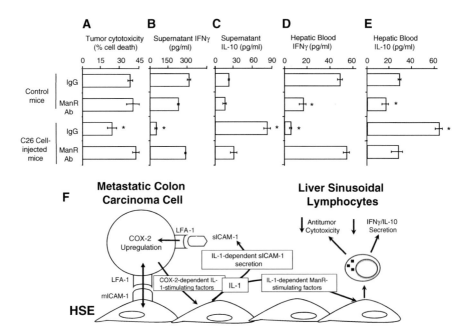

Fig. 3.6 Colon carcinoma cell interaction with the liver sinusoidal endothelium inhibits organ-specific anti-tumor immunity via IL-1-induced mannose receptor. Shown in (**a–c**) are the ex vivo anti-tumor cytotoxic activity and IFNγ and IL-10 secretion by liver sinusoidal lymphocytes (LSLs) isolated from C26 carcinoma-bearing mice. Mice received one single intraperitoneal injection of 400 μg/kg anti-murine ManR antibody 30 min prior to and 24 and 48 h post injection of C26 cells. Changes in anti-tumor cytotoxicity (**a**), IFNγ (**b**) and IL-10 (**c**) production by LSLs derived from control mice versus those derived from C26-bearing mice were statistically significant (*-$p < 0.05$). (**d, e**) IFNγ and IL-10 concentrations were measured in the portal blood of untreated and anti-ManR antibody-treated control and C26 carcinoma cell-injected mice. Changes in IFNγ and IL-10 levels in the portal blood were statistically significant (*-$p < 0.05$) as compared to saline injected mice. Shown in (**f**) is a schematic representation of the interaction between LFA-1-expressing C26 colon carcinoma cells and ICAM-1 expressing HSECs that increases tumor COX-2 activity. Tumor COX-2-dependent paracrine factors stimulate the release of sICAM-1 and IL-1 from HSECs, and this in turn upregulates ManR. The decrease in the anti-tumor cytotoxicity and IFNγ/IL-10 secretion ratio in LSL is induced by a ManR-dependent mechanism

and increased the ratio of IFNγ/IL-10 produced by the liver sinusoidal lymphocytes (Fig. 3.6f).

At present, the relationship between increased ManR-mediated endocytosis and inhibition of liver sinusoidal lymphocyte-mediated anti-tumor activity is not clear. Possible mechanisms include: (i) ManR trapping of tumor-derived antigens and other circulating soluble ligands to which hepatic lymphocytes would normally respond and (ii) activation of ManR-dependent signaling pathways that promote production of immunosuppressive factors by HSECs and/or decrease production of immune-stimulatory molecules. Our findings are in agreement with other reports that identified an immunosuppressive effect of ManR-mediated endocytosis in the hepatic sinusoidal microenvironment [33]. Taken together, these findings identified ManR as a contributor to the prometastatic effects of IL-1 and COX-2 in the liver, and implicated tumor-derived inflammatory factors in the subclinical, and even remote, activation of ManR-mediated localized immune suppression in the liver (Fig. 3.6f). ManR and ManR-stimulating factors may therefore be novel molecular targets whose direct or indirect blockade via IL-1 and/or COX-2 inhibitors may restore hepatic immune defense mechanisms against metastatic colon carcinoma [18].

3.3.2.3 The Prometastatic Effects of Hepatic ICAM-1

ICAM-1 is constitutively expressed on, and secreted by HSECs but it is upregulated in response to tumor-induced inflammation, during the experimental hepatic colonization of colon cancer cells [18], while human and murine colon cancer cells may express the counter-receptor LFA-1 (Fig. 3.7). The role of LFA-1 in liver colonization by colon carcinoma cells is however, unclear. Previously, it was reported that CD44 induces HT-29 cancer cell adhesion and migration via upregulation of LFA-1 [34]. Recently, we detected enhanced expression of LFA-1 in C26 colon carcinoma cells growing as spheroids in a 3D in vitro culture and this led to increased VEGF production in these cells, in response to soluble ICAM-1 [35], thereby potentially increasing angiogenesis. Tumor-activated hepatic stellate cells (HSCs) also express and secrete ICAM-1, and this may further activate LFA-1-expressing colorectal cancer cells at metastatic sites. Interestingly, LFA-1-expressing cancer cells also produce ManR-stimulating factors in response to hepatic ICAM-1, leading to immunosuppression as discussed above [18]. Therefore, increased LFA-1 expression can promote metastasis both through stimulation of angiogenesis and through induction of immunosuppression in response to HSEC and/or HSC-derived ICAM-1. In addition to its proangiogenic effects, VEGF may also be one of the COX-2-dependent ManR-stimulating factors because it could induce IL-1 production in HSECs via a TNFα-dependent mechanism [35].

Other data also implicate the LFA-1/ICAM-1 interaction in the promotion of hepatic metastasis. Soluble ICAM-1 levels increase in patients with hepatic metastases [36] and tumor- and host-derived soluble ICAM-1 were shown to promote immune escape [37] and angiogenesis [38] thereby supporting tumor growth. Moreover, tumor expression of LFA-1 was shown to contribute to hepatic metastasis of

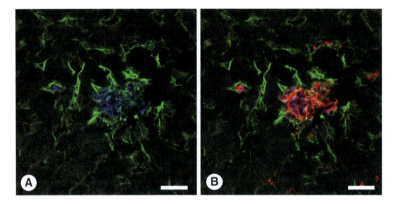

Fig. 3.7 Identification of an intralobular hepatic metastasis niche containing LFA-1[+]C26 colon cancer cells by confocal laser microscopy. Immunostaining was as described in the legend to Fig. 3.5. Shown in (**a**) is a metastatic niche without cancer cell staining. Note the exclusive recruitment of SMA (*blue*) and ICAM-1 (*green*)-expressing hepatic stromal cells to the niche. Shown in (**b**) is the same metastatic niche with cancer cells stained with anti-murine LFA-1 antibodies. Bar: 25 μm

lymphoma, leukemia and breast cancer cells [39, 40] whereas LFA-1 blockade [41] and an ICAM-1 deficiency [42] reduced hepatic metastasis.

3.3.3 Microvascular Survival Mechanisms of Liver-Infiltrating Cancer Cells

Cancer cells that arrest in the hepatic microvessels may have mechanisms to resist and even inactivate the "hostile" microenvironment induced by the inflammatory response. For example, colorectal carcinoma cell-derived carcinoembryonic antigen (CEA) can prevent cancer cell death by inducing IL-10 production and thereby inhibiting inducible NO synthase upregulation in the hepatic cells and NO-dependent cancer cell death [43, 44]. Expression of major histocompatibility complex class I antigen on colon carcinoma cells is a mechanism of immune escape that can also negatively regulate hepatic NK cell-mediated apoptosis and cytolysis by blocking the perforin/granzyme pathway [45]. A high intracellular level of glutathione can also protect cancer cells from oxidative stress induced by hepatic sinusoidal cell-derived reactive oxygen metabolites [46]. This mechanism appears highly dependent on the glutathione peroxidase/reductase system required to eliminate hydrogen peroxide [47].

3.3.4 Myofibroblast Transdifferentiation of Perisinusoidal Stellate Cells at Sites of Microvascular Cancer Cell Arrest

The complex endothelial cell reaction to liver-infiltrating cancer cells also affects the HSC, as evident from their association with small avascular micrometastases prior to angiogenic cell recruitment [48, 49]. HSCs are pericytes of hepatic sinusoids whose functional phenotype is controlled, under normal physiological conditions, by neighboring parenchymal and non-parenchymal cells, including HSECs and Kupffer cells [50, 51]. Because inflammatory factors contribute to HSC transdifferentiation into myofibroblasts [52], we recently hypothesized that tumor-activated HSECs may produce soluble factors that contribute to HSC differentiation and myofibroblast recruitment into hepatic micrometastases. Confocal microscopy was used to study the location of α-smooth muscle actin (SMA)-expressing cells 48 h after intrasplenic injection of C26 colon cancer cells. Interestingly, α-SMA-expressing cells co-localized with 65% of intra-sinusoidally-arrested C26 cells, while rarely found around cancer cell-devoid sinusoids (Fig. 3.3b). Next, primary cultures of HSECs were treated with C26-conditioned medium to mimic HSEC activation during hepatic trafficking of cancer cells, and HSC then treated with activated HSE-conditioned medium and analyzed for α-SMA expression (i.e. transdifferentiation), chemotactic migration and VEGF secretion. We found that conditioned medium from tumor-activated HSECs increased the number of α-SMA-expressing HSCs 2-fold relative to controls. It has been shown previously that the regulatory effect that differentiated HSECs exert on HSCs requires NO and that capillarized HSECs that produce less NO, due to loss of VEGF responsiveness, loose the ability to maintain HSC quiescence or promote reversion [50]. During the hepatic infiltration of colon cancer cells, CEA was shown to stimulate the release of the anti-inflammatory cytokine IL-10 that strongly inhibited NO and reactive species production by the ischemic/reoxygenated liver, reducing the toxicity of hepatic ischemia-reperfusion injury and indirectly stimulating cancer cell survival and liver colonization [43, 44]. Interestingly, we have recently demonstrated that IL-10 concentration in the hepatic circulation increases by 2-fold during the earliest stage of the hepatic colonization by C26 cancer cells [18], suggesting that the increase in the proportion of α-SMA-expressing HSCs in C26-injected mice may be attributable to the decline in NO production due to IL-10 release in the microvascular milieu of the liver. Therefore, tumor-induced production of IL-10 may be a key prometastatic factor in the microvascular phase of hepatic metastasis. By abrogating NO production by tumor-activated sinusoids, IL-10 may first promote the ability of circulating cancer cells to survive the ischemia-reperfusion injury of implantation [44], then contribute to ManR-dependent anti-tumor immunosuppression [18] and finally generate a permissive microenvironment for HSC activation and recruitment into avascular micrometastases. It appears therefore, that the response of HSC-derived myofibroblasts to paracrine factors released by tumor-activated HSECs may constitute the earliest event in stromal cell recruitment that occurs as the metastatic cancer cells begin to divide in the microvascular microenvironment and prior to initiation of angiogenesis.

3.4 The Microenvironment of the Intralobular Micrometastasis

This phase begins as cancer cells that survived the microvascular phase and successfully evaded hepatic immune defenses begin to proliferate. These cancer cells are normally located at metastatic niches consisting of a constellation of structural and functional factors that are communicated to the cancer cells by tumor-activated hepatic sinusoidal cells. Other major players during this phase are tumor-activated HSCs that have differentiated into myofibroblasts, portal tract fibroblasts and hepatocytes around cancer cell foci that undergo epithelial-to-mesenchymal transition. Intrametastatic recruitment of these hepatic cell types is promoted by tumor-derived factors, suggesting that those cancer cells unable to induce a stromal reaction at metastatic niches may not be able to progress into intralobular micrometastases. The evidence shows that hepatic stromal cells can infiltrate the site of metastatic cell arrest forming a symbiotic microenvironment that serves to stimulate the production, by cancer cells, of motility and growth factors that mediate the recruitment of pre-angiogenic stromal cells. Proliferation of cancer cells at metastatic niches occurs mainly in periportal areas of the liver lobule [53] and results in the formation of subclinical, avascular micrometastases. This phase concludes when growing micrometastases have a larger diameter than the hepatic lobule and, therefore, can invade neighboring lobules.

3.4.1 Cancer Cell Growth at Liver Metastatic Niches

The induction of cancer cell proliferation at liver metastatic niches is a key step leading to subclinical avascular micrometastases. Whether these metastatic niches precede cancer cell entry into the liver – the pre-metastatic niche concept, as proposed by Kaplan et al. [54] – or are, in fact, induced by arrested cancer cell – metastatic niche – is unclear. However, the microvascular spatial coordinates of surviving cancer cells within the hepatic tissue determine three major metastatic niche types, each with distinct molecular and cellular components and, therefore distinct microenvironments for the metastatic cells. The characteristics of these microenvironments are described below, summarized in Table 3.2 and shown in Fig. 3.8a, b.

3.4.1.1 The Intra-sinusoidal Metastatic Niche

The site of cancer cell location in these niches is intravascular and therefore, cancer cells are surrounded by HSECs (Figs. 3.2 and 3.8a). Other cells in the composition of this microenvironment are Kupffer cells, hepatic lymphocytes, platelets, and infiltrating granulocytes. The molecular composition of this microenvironment includes low-oxygenated portal blood with high concentrations of metabolic substrates, proinflammatory cytokines and reactive oxygen species. Cancer cells in this niche may be incompetent for endothelial cell adhesion and extravascular migration but possess cellular mechanisms for intravascular survival. Metastatic progression depends on intra-capillary proliferation of the cancer cells and leads to mechanical destruction of the sinusoid, followed by replacement-type metastatic growth.

Table 3.2 Anatomic and functional features of the hepatic metastasis niches

	Metastatic niches in the liver		
	Intrasinusoidal niche	Perisinusoidal niche	Periportal tract niche
Site of cancer cell location	Intravascular, surrounded by hepatic sinusoidal endothelium	Perivascular, space of Disse, surrounded by hepatocytes and sinusoidal wall	Portal space, surrounded by connective tissue fibroblasts
Composition of the cellular microenvironment	Kupffer cells, hepatic lymphocytes, platelets, leukocytes, and hepatic sinusoidal endothelium	Myofibroblasts derived from trans-differentiated hepatic stellate cells and hepatocytes undergoing epithelial-mesenchymal transition	Portal tract myofibroblasts, cholangiocytes and hepatocyte progenitor cells
Molecular microenvironment	Low oxygenated portal blood with high concentration of metabolic substrates, proinflammatory cytokines and reactive oxygen species	Low oxygenated interstitial plasma filtered by HSE fenestrae, subendothelial extracellular matrix and high concentration of growth factors from hepatocytes and hepatic stellate cells	Highly oxygenated interstitial plasma from portal tract capillaries and connective tissue extracellular matrix
Cancer cell growth pattern	Intra-capillary proliferation of cancer cells leading to the mechanical destruction of the sinusoid and replacement-type metastatic growth	Peri-capillary proliferation of cancer cells leading to invasion of hepatocyte plates and pushing-type metastatic growth	Periportal proliferation of cancer cells leading to portal vein invasion and pushing-type metastatic growth

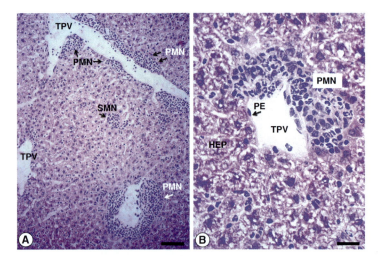

Fig. 3.8 Periportal and sinusoidal implantation of liver-colonizing cancers. Shown in (**a**) is a low magnification image of periportal (PMN) and sinusoidal (SMN) metastatic niches developing by 4T1 murine breast cancer cells. Bar: 50 μm. Shown in (**b**) is a high power image of a periportal metastatic niche (PMN) containing cancer cells beneath the portal endothelium (PE) of terminal portal venules (TPV). While cancer cells are the main cell subpopulation within these niches, recruited leukocytes can also be observed. The niches are surrounded by hepatocytes (HEP). Bar: 15 μm

3.4.1.2 The Perisinusoidal Metastatic Niche

In this type of niche, the cancer cells are located in the perivascular space of Disse, where they are surrounded by hepatocytes and sinusoidal walls. Other cells in the microenvironment are myofibroblasts recruited through HSC transdifferentiation and hepatocytes undergoing epithelial-mesenchymal transition. Molecular features of this microenvironment are low oxygenated, interstitial plasma filtered by HSE fenestrae, a subendothelial extracellular matrix and a high concentration of growth factors from tumor-activated hepatocytes and HSCs. Cancer cells in this niche are competent for endothelial cell adhesion and extravascular migration. Metastasis progression depends on pericapillary proliferation of cancer cells leading to invasion of parenchymal cell plates and thereafter to "pushing-type" metastatic growth.

3.4.1.3 The Periportal Metastatic Niche

The location of the cancer cells in this niche is the portal space, where they are surrounded by subendothelial connective tissue (Fig. 3.8a, b). Other relevant host cells in the microenvironment are cholangiocytes of the bile ducts, hepatocyte progenitor cells and portal tract-specific fibroblasts and hepatic lymphocytes. The molecular composition of this microenvironment includes highly-oxygenated interstitial plasma from portal tract capillaries and connective tissue matrix. Cancer cells in this niche are competent for endothelial cell adhesion and extravascular migration at terminal portal venules. Metastasis progression depends on the periportal proliferation of the cancer cells, leading to portal vein invasion and "pushing-type" metastatic growth.

Importantly, many liver-infiltrating cancer cells can remain dormant at any of these metastatic niches and, therefore, activation of solitary dormant cancer cell proliferation is a key event for hepatic metastasis progression. Both intra- and perisinusoidal metastatic niches, but not periportal metastatic niches, are markedly affected by the phenotypic diversity of hepatic cells [55] and the gradient of oxygen, metabolic substrates, hormones, and extracellular matrix proteins across the liver lobule [56].

Several mechanisms may operate at metastatic niches. First, proliferation of intra-vascularly located cancer cells can be activated by paracrine growth factors released by neighboring tumor-activated endothelial cells – a mechanism significantly enhanced by proinflammatory cytokines [20, 21, 23]. Secondly, proliferation of extravascularly located cancer cells can be activated by paracrine growth factors released by neighboring tumor-activated hepatocytes and HSCs. This is facilitated by adhesive mechanisms [57] and junctional specializations, such as desmosomes, formed between cancer cells and hepatocytes, soon after invasion of the parenchymal cell plate [58, 59]. Significantly, however, early micrometastatic foci may disappear after a few days, with only a small subset continuing to grow [60], suggesting that mechanisms responsible for cancer cell elimination and metastatic inefficiency may play a role at this phase of the process.

3.4.2 Stromal Cell Recruitment into Avascular Micrometastases

A rich, tumor-stimulating stroma, generated from tumor-activated hepatic cells develops during the intralobular phase, prior to recruitment of angiogenic endothelial cells [61]. This host cell recruitment is driven by the ability of cancer cells to produce stromal cell migration- and proliferation-stimulating factors. The main sources of tumor-associated stromal cells at this stage are HSCs, portal tract fibroblasts and hepatocytes. Circulating bone marrow-derived mesenchymal cells may also contribute, but their role has not yet been confirmed.

3.4.2.1 Hepatic Stellate Cell-Derived Myofibroblasts

HSCs transdifferentiate into myofibroblasts in response to paracrine factors released from cancer cells, tumor-activated HSECs and Kupffer cells [48]. This specific source of hepatic myofibroblasts contributes to those micrometastases that develop at the sinusoidal area of hepatic lobules (intrasinusoidal/perisinusoidal metastatic niches). As discussed above, α-SMA-expressing HSCs can first be detected in association with HSECs that interact with metastatic cancer cells prior to extravascular migration (see Fig. 3.9). In agreement with findings based on immunohistochemistry (see Fig. 3.3b), we found that conditioned media harvested from tumor-activated HSECs could induce α-SMA expression in quiescent HSCs, stimulate HSC migration in an IL-18-dependent manner and induce HSCs to secrete VEGF. These findings are consistent with the reported prometastatic effects of IL-18 in the

I) Myofibroblast Transdifferentiation in the Microvascular Phase of Hepatic Metastasis

II) Myofibroblast Recruitment in the Avascular Phase of Hepatic Micrometastasis

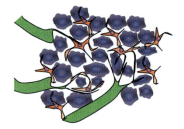

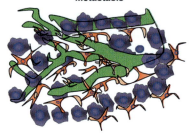

III) Proangiogenic Effects of Tumor-activated Myofibroblasts from Hypoxic Micrometastasis

IV) Myofibroblast-Induced Cancer Cell Growth in the Post-angiogenic phase of Hepatic Metastasis

Fig. 3.9 Hepatic stellate cell activation and activities during the progression of hepatic metastasis. The hepatic colonization process of circulating cancer cells has been schematically represented in four consecutive stages with respect to the activation, intratumoral recruitment and pro-tumorigenic effects of perisinusoidal hepatic stellate cell-derived myofibroblasts

liver [20, 24, 29] and the documented ability of HSCs to stimulate endothelial cell migration [49]. They are also in agreement with other reports on the proangiogenic role of intra-metastatic HSC-derived myofibroblasts [59]. Therefore, the response of HSCs to transdifferentiation-stimulating factors from HSECs located at specific sites of cancer cell arrest may represent the earliest stage of tumor stroma formation during the sinusoidal phase of hepatic metastases. Later on, additional recruitment of HSCs may occur in most precocious micrometastases by direct effect of tumor-derived factors or even by factors such as VEGF, PDGF-AB, HGF, PGE2, NGF and TGF-β, secreted by the recruited HSCs themselves [61].

3.4.2.2 Portal Tract Fibroblast-Derived Myofibroblasts

Portal tract fibroblasts can also contribute to the intra-metastatic stroma when invading cancer cells are located in portal tracts and are unable to activate the HSC-dependent stromagenesis. Portal tract-derived fibroblasts produce IL-8, a chemokine implicated in invasion and angiogenesis, in response to TNF-α-induced NFκB signaling [62].

3.4.2.3 Hepatocyte-Derived Myofibroblasts

Perimetastatic hepatocytes can undergo epithelial-to-mesenchymal transition in response to tumor and HSC-derived factors (Fig. 3.10a, b). The epithelial-to-mesenchymal transition occurs at peripheral areas of hepatic micrometastases, while they are recruited into metastatic tissue [63]. Upregulation of vimentin, SNAIL and nerve growth factor expression, and down-regulation of cadherin-H1 expression are early markers of the hepatocyte transdifferentiation into myofibroblasts during growth of hepatic metastases [64].

3.4.3 Targeting Myofibroblasts in Hepatic Micrometastases

Because of their central role in the progression of liver metastasis, the hepatic myofibroblasts represent an attractive therapeutic target. Moreover, their multifunctional involvement in the course of metastasis provide an opportunity to disrupt several key steps in the process namely (A) the transdifferentiation of tumor-activated HSC into myofibroblasts; (B) the intra-tumoral recruitment (chemotactic migration) and proliferation of HSC-derived myofibroblasts; (C) the pro-angiogenic

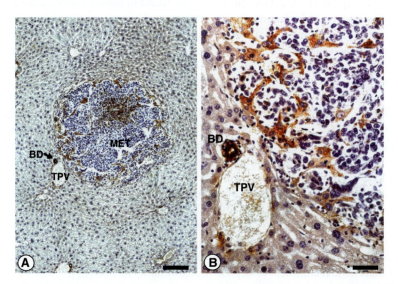

Fig. 3.10 The intratumoral recruitment of hepatocytes in a C26 colon carcinoma intralobular micrometastasis (MET). Tumor-activated perimetastatic and intrametastatic hepatocytes (in *brown*) were immunohistochemically revealed by staining with an anti-mouse nerve growth factor (NGF) antibody. Low (**a**) and high (**b**) magnification images are shown. Under normal physiological conditions, only cholangiocytes within the perilobular bile ducts (BD) and periportal hepatocytes express NGF. However, tumor microenvironmental factors induce NGF expression in the hepatocytes (brown polygonal cytoplasm with large-size round nuclei) and hepatic stellate cells (brown cytoplasm with small nuclei and condensed chromatin). TPV-terminal portal venule. Bar: 100 μm (**a**) and 10 μm (**b**). Reproduced with permission from [3]

effects of tumor-associated myofibroblasts on endothelial cells; and (D) the release and/or stimulating effects of myofibroblast-derived paracrine factors on cancer cell invasion and proliferation.

Based on the increased awareness of the important role played by hepatic tumor-associated myofibroblasts in the metastatic process, we and other groups have studied the localization and phenotype of hepatic myofibroblasts in the hepatic tumor tissue of animals receiving anti-neoplastic agents. Results demonstrate a statistically significant decrease in the number of tumor-associated hepatic myofibroblasts in treated animals as compared to controls, suggesting that some drugs may exert their anti-tumoral effects in part, through inhibitory actions on tumor-activated HSCs. For example, decreased pericytic coverage of angiogenic vessels from colon cancer liver metastases has been correlated with the anti-tumoral effects of the anti-angiogenic tyrosine-kinase inhibitor Su6668 [65]. The integrin αV/β3 and αV/β5 inhibitor S247 also diminished intra-tumoral angiogenesis with a reduction in pericyte coverage [66] and TNP470 – a very popular semi-synthetic analogue of fumagillin with demonstrated ability to inhibit in vitro HSC transdifferentiation [67] – significantly decreased liver tumor angiogenesis [68] and intra-metastatic recruitment of hepatic myofibroblasts in vivo (Vidal-Vanaclocha, unpublished data). Other examples include endostatin, a potent antiangiogenic compound that targets sinusoidal-type liver metastases [60], that was found to inhibit tumor-induced HSC migration in vitro and intrametastatic recruitment of hepatic myofibroblasts in vivo; Resveratrol – a natural antioxidant product derived from grapes, with cyclooxygenase (COX) and human HSC inhibitory activities [69] that reduced the prometastatic and pro-angiogenic activities of tumor-associated myofibroblasts, both in vitro and in vivo (Vidal-Vanaclocha, unpublished data); and interestingly, the COX-2 inhibitors Celecoxib and Rofecoxib that had the same effects as Resveratrol [70, 71]. In addition, sodium salicylate – a hypoxia inducible factor-1α inhibitor that reduces experimental liver tumors as reported by Yang et al. [72] – reduced VEGF expression and intratumoral recruitment of hepatic myofibroblasts in vivo, Adaphostin – a tyrosine kinase inhibitor with proapoptotic effects on cancer cells [73] – inhibited VEGF production from tumor-activated HSCs in vitro (Vidal-Vanaclocha, unpublished data), and another pro-apoptotic agent – the heat shock protein-90 inhibitor 17-Dimethylaminoethylamino-17-desmethoxygeldanamycin [74] – also significantly decreased intra-metastatic recruitment of hepatic myofibroblasts in vivo (Vidal-Vanaclocha, unpublished data). Finally, recombinant human IL-18 binding protein inhibited the migration of tumor-activated human HSCs in vitro and intra-metastatic recruitment of hepatic myofibroblasts in vivo [29].

The targeting of stromal-tumor cell interactions that stimulate cancer cell growth in the liver with new types of anti-cancer therapies offers some distinct advantages. Cancer-stromal cell interactions may occur in a similar fashion in a wide range of liver-metastasizing cancer cell types and therefore these therapies may be broadly relevant. Moreover, the stromal cells appear to have a normal, relatively stable genetic make-up in contrast to diverse and unstable genomes of the metastatic cancer cells and therefore targeting the stromal cells may result in more effective responses. However, therapeutic targeting of tumor-activated hepatic myofibroblasts may only serve to arrest cancer development and may not be effective at causing cancer cell death. Therefore, targeting these stromal cells or their heterotypic interactions will probably be most effective in combination with other therapies that are cytotoxic to the cancer cells. However, before such therapies can be developed, a better understanding of the precise role of these interactions in liver metastasis is essential. Interest in this area can be expected to increase in the coming years.

3.4.4 Contribution of Hepatic-Derived Nerve Growth Factor to the Microenvironment of Intralobular Hepatic Micrometastases

It has been reported that nerve growth factor (NGF) increases during hepatic regeneration and carcinogenesis [75, 76], but its role during hepatic metastasis is unknown. We investigated NGF and neurotrophin receptor expression by cancer and stromal cells using a tissue-array of metastases from 24 patients who had undergone hepatic excision of colorectal adenocarcinoma metastases. We have observed that NGF immunostaining of cancer cells only occurred in 2 out of 24 patients with hepatic metastases, while approximately 80% of patients had metastases with NGF-expressing stromal cells. Conversely, high affinity TrkA neurotrophin receptor immunoreactivity was mainly concentrated in cancer cells, with low expression occurring in the tumor stroma. However, NGF immunostaining of tumor stroma and cancer cell immunostaining with anti-ki67 antibodies did not correlate, suggesting that NGF was not associated with metastatic cell proliferation. Interestingly, NGF immunoreactivity was unequivocally localized to desmin-expressing HSCs and perimetastatic hepatocytes, located at the invasion front of metastases. NGF-expressing hepatocytes had phenotypic features suggestive of epithelial-to-mesenchymal transition, including cadherin-1 downregulation and vimentin and SNAIL upregulation. A similar immunostaining pattern was observed during the experimental hepatic colonization by C26 and 51b murine colorectal carcinoma cells (Fig. 3.10). Consistent with the in situ findings, NGF levels increased by two-fold in hepatic blood derived from metastasis-bearing mice. NGF also significantly increased in the supernatants of HSCs treated with tumor cell-conditioned medium, and of hepatocytes treated with tumor-activated HSCs, but not tumor cell-conditioned medium. Recombinant NGF increased chemotactic migration of neurotrophin receptor-expressing cancer cells in a dose-dependent manner but did not affect their proliferation or adhesion in vitro. In addition, the HSC migration-stimulating activities of VEGF and tumor-activated hepatocytes were also NGF-mediated because they could be neutralized by anti-NGF antibodies. The data suggest that HSC- and hepatocyte-derived myofibroblasts secrete NGF that in turn, contributes to hepatic metastasis by activating tumor and stromal cell migration [63, 64].

3.5 The Tumor Microenvironment During the Angiogenic Phase of Hepatic Metastasis

3.5.1 Angiogenic Patterns of Hepatic Metastases

The tumor microenvironment also influences the process of angiogenesis. Angiogenesis starts at the pre-vascular stromagenic micrometastases phase, when the metastases have an average diameter ≥ 300 μm and grow beyond the limits of the liver lobule. Proangiogenic factors secreted by hypoxic, tumor-activated myofibroblasts and/or cancer cells promote angiogenesis associated with this phase, while endogenous, liver-derived anti-angiogenic factors such as endostatin can inhibit it [60]. Endothelial cell migration can be seen to occur selectively towards avascular micrometastases with a dense myofibroblastic infiltrate. Moreover, myofibroblasts and endothelial cells co-localize within the metastases, and their respective densities consistently correlate in well-vascularized metastases.

Two predominant angiogenic patterns have been recognized in hepatic metastases, each associated with distinct stromal cell types, invasion and growth patterns, and response to treatment [60, 77, 78]:

3.5.1.1 Sinusoidal-Type Angiogenesis

This is associated with reticularly-arranged, infiltrating, but not encapsulating myofibroblasts. It occurs in metastases with replacement growth-pattern, where the liver architecture is preserved because invasive cancer cells co-opt the existing network of sinusoids, and, thus, the interface between tumor and normal tissue is ill-defined. The predominant expression of desmin and glial fibrillary acidic protein – two HSC markers – by myofibroblasts located in sinusoidal-type metastases suggests that HSCs represent the main source of myofibroblasts for this type of metastasis (Fig. 3.11a).

3.5.1.2 Portal-Type Angiogenesis

This is associated with encapsulating, but not infiltrating, fibrous tract-arranged myofibroblasts. It occurs in metastases with desmoplastic and "pushing growth"-patterns, where the architecture of the liver parenchyma is not preserved and the enlarging mass of cancer cells compresses the surrounding parenchyma, causing the formation of tumor lobules delineated by desmoplastic stroma. Myofibroblasts located in portal-type metastases display a vimentin and Thy-1 phenotype, suggesting that resident portal tract fibroblasts constitute the stromal support for these metastases [66] (Fig. 3.11b).

The data presented above on the key proangiogenic role that HSCs play during hepatic metastasis, identifies them as a potential therapeutic target and a useful indicator in the preclinical testing of anti-angiogenic drugs for liver metastasis. Accordingly, we propose a two-step protocol for the screening of anti-angiogenic

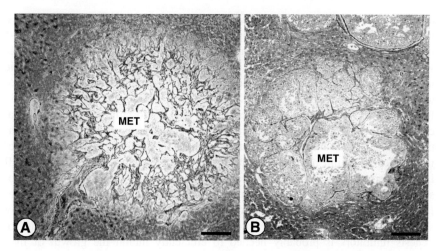

Fig. 3.11 Angiogenic patterns within hepatic metastases. (**a**) Shown is a sinusoidal-type hepatic micrometastasis (MET) in the angiogenic phase, containing a dense network of sinusoidal neovessels, as revealed by a reticulin stain according to the Gordon-Sweets silver impregnation technique (60). Recruited microvessels forming concentric interconnections are evident. The liver architecture is not disturbed at this stage and the cancer cells co-opt the supportive fibrilar network of the sinusoids. Bar: 100 μm. (**b**) Portal-type micrometastasis (MET) at the angiogenic phase. Here, the reticulin network supporting intratumoral angiogenesis is not conserved. A desmoplastic stroma surrounds and traverses the metastasis, facilitating invasion of vascular-type angiogenic vessels. Necrotic areas frequently develop in this type of metastases. Bar: 100 μm. Reproduced with permission from [3]

drugs namely, (A) in situ analyses of their effect on HSC recruitment and co-localization with neo-angiogenic tracts (perivascular coverage) in association with liver tumor development, and (B) *in vitro* analyses of the drug effect on the proangiogenic activity of tumor-activated HSCs, and their ability to activate primary cultured hepatic endothelial cells.

3.5.2 Role of Endogenous, Liver-Derived Antiangiogenic Factors in Metastasis

The angiogenic phase of hepatic metastasis is the result of an altered balance between the positive and negative regulators of neovascularization. Several angiogenic factors contribute to this process, including VEGF, angiopoietins, TGF-α, IL-18, insulin-like growth factor-II, and hepatocyte growth factor. However, the liver is also a rich source of precursors for several angiogenesis inhibitors such as thrombospondin, angiostatin, and endostatin [79]. These molecules are naturally present in the body fluids or tissues and possess anti-angiogenic activity, potentially providing a counterbalance for the pro-angiogenesis factors, and maintaining a physiological balance. Thrombospondin-1 (TSP-1) is a secreted glycoprotein with anti-angiogenic activity found in the extra- and pericellular matrix. TSP-1 regulates the extracellular milieu by a direct interaction with extracellular matrix proteins, influencing levels of extracellular proteases and activating latent TGF-β. TSP-1 inhibits endothelial cell proliferation and migration, thus suppressing angiogenesis. Expression of TSP-1 inversely correlates with tumor vascularity and hepatic metastasis in colon cancer [80]. Endostatin is the C-terminal noncollagenous proteolytic fragment (20-kDa) of type XVIII collagen, a basement membrane protein found in most vascular basement membranes [81]. Endostatin inhibits endothelial cell migration and induces apoptosis, thereby decreasing intra-tumoral vascularization. Endostatin has attracted much attention since its discovery in 1997 because of its potency to inhibit neovascularization and tumor growth [81]. Collagen XVIII is produced mainly by HSC and hepatocytes [79, 82]. The finding that endostatin stably transfected into carcinoma cells blocked tumor formation in the liver [83] suggested that antiangiogenic molecules released from liver cells were not sufficient to reduce tumor angiogenesis, and that treatment with exogenous angiogenesis inhibitors is probably needed to efficiently inhibit the growth of liver tumors.

We analyzed the endogenous levels of endostatin in the peripheral and hepatic blood during progression of experimental hepatic metastasis and investigated the effect of recombinant endostatin on hepatic colonization by intrasplenically injected murine cancer cells. We found a significant increase in endogenous endostatin production in the liver in response to B16 melanoma and 51b colon carcinoma growth [60, 84]. This is in agreement with recent reports showing an increase in endostatin levels in peripheral blood from patients with advanced cancer or disease recurrence [85, 86]. We also found that endogenous endostatin was generated by liver cells, but not by B16 melanoma and 51b colon carcinoma cells. Thus, it is tempting to speculate that the first peak of endostatin in the hepatic blood that coincides with the onset of micrometastatic disease may be the consequence of HSC activation and recruitment by tumor-derived factors within avascular micrometastases. Subsequent increases in endostatin levels in the hepatic blood seen when macroscopic metastases are evident may be due to sustained tumor-induced hepatic myofibroblast recruitment as well as to collagen XVIII processing by tumor- and stromal cell-derived proteases [60]. Because angiogenic activity during the micrometastatic stage does not occur prior to myofibroblast recruitment, and neovascularization is not observed in myofibroblast free-hepatic metastases [48], elevation of endostatin levels in the serum may be an indication of a preangiogenic status in those patients with occult micrometastases in the liver. However, high levels of circulating endostatin are not unique to patients with cancer, and their clinical significance should be elucidated.

We also found that despite local production of endostatin in the liver, systemic administration of exogenous endostatin was still necessary to efficiently decrease the formation of micrometastases and the growth of macrometastases. It is possible that the endostatin produced endogenously in the liver of 51b carcinoma-bearing mice is in an inactive, preprocessed or cleaved form with impaired function [87] or its concentration may be too low to inhibit metastasis, or both. Indeed, exogenous endostatin had inhibitory effects at different stages of hepatic colonization by cancer cells. On the one hand, when injected as a single dose before cancer cell injection, it decreased the number of metastases by 30%. Because systemically administered endostatin has a half-life of about 5 h in mice, its antimetastatic effect in this setting likely occurred during the first 24 h post tumor cell injection. This early stage of metastasis is regulated mostly by a proinflammatory microenvironment induced by tumor-derived factors. However, endogenous endostatin levels are not as yet increased at this stage, and the antimetastatic effect of exogenous endostatin may therefore depend on its ability to inhibit tumor cell adhesion to endothelium and/or its extravascular migration [84]. Not surprisingly, endostatin can inhibit tumor cell invasion by blocking the activation and catalytic activity of matrix metalloproteinase 2 [88] and has been shown to modulate cell migration and survival in an integrin-dependent manner [88]. However, this chemopreventive effect of endostatin needs to be confirmed in a clinical setting and may selectively affect those cancer cells metastasizing via inflammation-dependent mechanisms.

When endostatin was administered 10–20 days post cancer cell injection, a significant decrease in the number of metastases was also observed, suggesting an additional inhibitory effect on a significant fraction of micrometastases that had developed before drug administration [60]. The decrease of CD31-expressing intra-metastatic microvessels, together with the increase in small-size metastases containing a large necrotic area suggests that endostatin may inhibit tumor progression through an efficient blockade of the transition from an avascular to a vascular stage of micrometastases. This may lead to tumor regression, explaining the decrease in the overall number of metastases, or to growth inhibition, as suggested by the increase in the ratio of micro to macrometastases and by the decrease in overall liver volume occupied by metastases [60].

The fact that some metastases were able to progress irrespective of the endostatin treatment prompted us to analyze their histological characteristics. We found that large metastases that developed in endostatin-treated mice had a portal-type angiogenic pattern, whereas the sinusoidal-type metastases that represent approximately 60% of all the metastases, were reduced in number and size [60]. Portal tract-derived endothelial cells are phenotypically different than sinusoidal (scavenger-type) endothelial cells. The fact that endostatin inhibited sinusoidal-type, but not portal-type metastases, indicates that at least two different angiogenic mechanisms with different sensitivities to endostatin may be activated by the same cancer cells in the liver.

3.6 The Tumor Microenvironment at the Lobar Stage of the Hepatic Metastasis Process

At the lobar stage, hepatic metastases are clinically detectable. Depending on their location, they may alter the whole hepatic organ in terms of tissue structure, blood supply and metabolic substrate availability, jeopardizing parenchymal cell function. However, cancer cells can still be microenvironmentally modulated at this stage by both tumor-infiltrating lymphocytes [89] including immunosuppressive CD4/CD25 regulatory T cells [90] and by stromal myofibroblasts [91] whose specific phenotypes have prognostic implications. In addition, high concentrations of hepatic soluble factors, such as proinflammatory and angiogenic cytokines [92], type I-insulin-like growth factor [93], and immunosuppressive factors (TGF-β, IL-10, soluble ICAM-1, etc.) also regulate cancer cells growth at this stage.

3.6.1 Regulation of "Hepatic Metastasis" Gene Expression by the Microenvironment

Distinct alterations in gene expression underlie metastasis to specific organ sites. However, the genetic and phenotypic properties of specific cancer cells able to implant and grow in the liver have not yet been established for any tumor type. Neither is the contribution of the diverse genetic background of different patients to hepatic metastasis well understood. At the transcriptional level, the clinical phase of hepatic metastasis is associated with marked changes to gene expression including up- and down-regulation of multiple genes. Some of the gene alterations may originate in the primary tumor and may promote hepatic metastasis [94]. However, other changes in gene expression may occur in the liver and may be regulated by tumor-activated hepatic cells. Recently, we analyzed the gene expression profiles of hepatic colorectal carcinoma metastases and tumor-unaffected liver tissue from the same patients. In addition, HT-29 human colon carcinoma and primary cultured human hepatocytes and liver myofibroblasts were used to determine if both tumor and liver cells are mutually influencing the expression of metastasis-associated genes. Three microenvironment-related gene expression categories were identified (Table 3.3):

3.6.1.1 Hepatic Metastasis Genes Not Expressed in Tumor-Unaffected Liver

Some of these genes were also expressed in the primary tumors particularly in a group of patients that developed metastases within 5 years of diagnosis. They were also expressed in HT-29 cells treated with cultured liver cell-conditioned media and in liver cells treated with HT-29 cell-conditioned media.

3.6.1.2 Genes Co-expressed in Hepatic Metastases and Tumor-Unaffected Liver Tissue

This gene group was not expressed in the primary tumors. This category also included both liver-specific genes expressed by HT-29 cells treated with liver cell-conditioned media and colon cancer-specific genes expressed by liver cells receiving HT-29-conditioned media.

Table 3.3 Microenvironment-related gene expression categories in hepatic colorectal cancer metastasis: examples of overexpressed genes

	Hepatic metastases genes not expressed in tumor-unaffected liver	Genes expressed in hepatic metastases and in tumor-unaffected liver tissue	Genes of tumor-unaffected liver tissue not expressed in hepatic metastases
Genes from primary tumors of colorectal carcinoma patients that developed hepatic metastases in less than five years from first diagnosis	• Cadherin CDH1 • S100P	• Macrophage migration inhibitory factor • Peroxiredoxin-IV • Cellular apoptosis susceptibility	• Metalotionein-1e • Ribosomal Protein L23a
Hepatic colorectal cancer metastases genes not expressed at the primary tumors	• Osteopontin	• Haptoglobin • TNF superfamily-member 14	• Alcohol dehydrogenase 1B • APOE • Cytochrome P450 CYP2E1 • Kininogen-1
Genes expressed in hepatic metastases that were not expressed by normal liver tissue	• TGFβ-induced protein ig-h3 (keratoepithelin) • Thioredoxin-1 • S100A6	Ephrin-α1	• Vitronectin • Metallopanestimulin-1

cDNA microarrays and reverse transcription-polymerase chain reaction were used to determine the gene expression profiles of hepatic colorectal carcinoma metastases and their corresponding tumor-unaffected liver tissue from the same patients. Genes overexpressed by a factor of ≥ 3 fold were classified into three distinct groups: Genes not expressed in tumor-unaffected liver tissue (left column), co-expressed by hepatic metastases and tumor-unaffected liver tissue (central column) and expressed by tumor-unaffected liver tissue but not in hepatic metastases (right column). Interestingly, for every subgroup, some genes occurred at the primary tumors of colorectal carcinoma patients that developed hepatic metastases in less than five years from first diagnosis (upper row); some exclusively occurred in hepatic colorectal cancer metastases but not in the primary tumors (middle row) and finally, some occurred in hepatic metastases but not in the normal liver tissue

3.6.1.3 Genes of Tumor-Unaffected Liver Tissue Not Expressed in Hepatic Metastases

This gene group was expressed in liver cells, but not in colon cancer cells, and represented the genetic background of the liver microenvironment before it was altered by tumor growth.

These results suggest that although some hepatic metastasis genes may already be expressed in the primary colorectal tumors and may be predictive of metastasis risk in the cancer patients, additional changes to gene expression take place in the liver under the control of tumor-activated hepatic cells. While this microenvironmental regulation of hepatic metastasis genes may occur at the earliest stages of metastasis, it is likely that some of the altered genes are still under microenvironmental control even at an advanced phase of the metastatic process and may therefore have implications for therapy.

In addition, using HT-29 colon carcinoma cells treated with conditioned media derived from primary cultured human hepatocytes or HSC-derived myofibroblasts, we were able to distinguish between gene expression changes induced in hepatic metastases by these two liver cell types (Fig. 3.12). Not surprisingly, we found that close to 50% of the genes regulated by soluble factors produced by hepatic cells belonged to a subgroup of cell cycle-regulating genes, further supporting the role of these hepatic cells in the control of metastatic cell proliferation.

The finding that the gene expression profiles of hepatic metastases had some similarities to profiles seen in tumor-unaffected hepatic tissue, suggest that metastatic

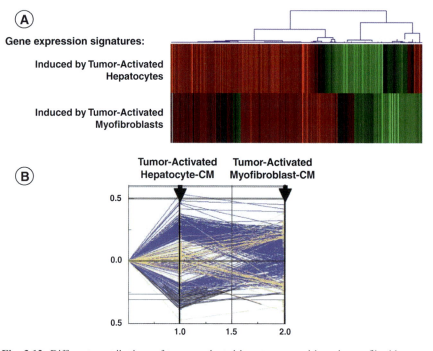

Fig. 3.12 Different contributions of tumor-activated hepatocytes and hepatic myofibroblasts to changes in gene expression in HT-29 human colon carcinoma cells. (**a**) Signature genes characterizing the transcriptional responses of HT-29 cancer cells to conditioned media (CM) from tumor-activated primary cultured human hepatocytes and hepatic stellate cell-derived myofibroblasts. The level of expression of each gene in each treated HT-29 cell sample, relative to the level of expression of that gene in untreated control samples, is presented in the form of a heat map, using a *red-black-green* color scale (*green*: below control sample; *black*: equal to control sample; *red*: above control sample). (**b**) Shown are gene expression changes in HT-29 cancer cells cultured in tumor-activated hepatocyte-CM as compared to basal medium and in HT-29 cells cultured in tumor-activated hepatic myofibroblast-CM as compared to basal medium. *Blue lines*: genes exclusively up/down regulated by tumor-activated hepatocytes. *Yellow lines*: genes exclusively up/down regulated by tumor-activated hepatic myofibroblasts

colon cancer cells have hepatomimetic properties. Conversely, we also found in our model that hepatic tissue expressed colon cancer-specific genes under the regulation of tumor-derived factors. This suggests that mutual gene expression mimicking occurs when metastatic cells are exposed to the hepatic microenvironment and *vice versa*. The identification of distinct microenvironment-related hepatic metastasis genes in clinical specimens from primary tumors implicates them in the hepatotropism of colorectal carcinoma and metastases formation.

3.7 Altered Hepatic Microenvironments and Metastasis

It is generally accepted that alterations in the local microenvironment during inflammation, wound healing or organ growth provide a favorable climate for cancer cell growth and metastasis [95–98]. This is best illustrated in models of liver regeneration following partial hepatectomy and in liver fibrosis and cirrhosis models. These models of prometastatic microenvironments offer opportunities for identification of new molecular targets for anti-metastatic therapy. Their major features are therefore summarized below.

3.7.1 The Regenerating Liver and Metastasis Development

Surgical resection of hepatic tumors remains the first choice for curative treatment of hepatic metastases, giving the patient the only chance for long-term survival [99, 100]. However, in up to 45% of tumors, extended liver resection is necessary to achieve clear resection margins and unresectability is often due to the fact that the remnant liver is of insufficient volume to support postoperative liver function. In these cases, a surgical procedure combining preoperative portal vein embolization that reduces blood flow to the resected hepatic segments and increases blood supply to the remaining liver can be used. This reduces the risk of postoperative liver failure after major liver resection and thereby increases the number of patients that can undergo resection [101–104] (The reader is referred to Chapters 12 and 13 for further discussion on resection criteria and treatment options). However, partial hepatectomy for patients with liver metastases is associated with a tumor recurrence rate approaching 80%. There are cases in which accelerated hepatic tumor growth occurs even after portal vein embolization [105], suggesting that factors involved in liver regeneration may stimulate the reactivation of dormant hepatic micrometastases and even the hepatic implantation of circulating cancer cells. Therefore, despite the known survival benefits for patients undergoing partial hepatectomy for colorectal liver metastases, questions have arisen regarding the potential effects of the regeneration process on the growth of any residual tumor deposits.

In an experimental rat model, excision of 70% of total liver mass was shown to induce rapid hyperplastic growth of remnant liver tissue that restored initial organ mass within two weeks post-surgery [106]. The same surgical procedure significantly increased the number of liver metastases following intravenous injection of syngeneic cancer cells, enhanced growth of liver implanted tumor, promoted outgrowth of dormant micrometastases, and accelerated tumor growth at distant sites [107–111]. However, when cancer cells were introduced after liver regeneration was complete, the tumor load was comparable to that of non-surgical controls. Thus, stimulation of tumor growth consequent to partial hepatectomy appears to depend on factors associated with active liver regeneration. Not surprisingly, cellular and molecular changes resulting from partial hepatectomy and the subsequent liver regeneration process can influence the kinetics of cancer cell growth and contribute to recurrence. Several groups have explored the mechanisms underlying the rapid tumor growth after portal vein embolization. Kokudo et al. [112] assessed the proliferative activity of intrahepatic metastases in the embolized liver after portal vein embolization in 18 patients with colorectal carcinoma metastases and found a significantly increased tumor Ki-67 labeling index in the metastases of the portal vein embolization group as compared to those not treated by portal vein embolization. It was postulated that the tumor growth after portal vein embolization may be controlled by three factors namely, the malignant potential of the tumors, changes in the blood supply after portal vein embolization and changes in the levels of cytokines or growth factors induced by portal vein embolization [112]. For example, cytokines such as HGF, IL-6 and IGF-I and prostaglandins have been implicated in promoting hepatic regeneration, while other factors such as TGFβ, glucagon, and glucocorticoids are known to be inhibitory.

HGF is one of the most powerful hepatotropic factors identified to date. However, the ability of HGF to promote cancer cell "scattering" and invasion raises some concern about its therapeutic safety. Animal models of portal vein branch ligation showed that HGF mRNA levels markedly increased in the non-ligated growing lobe, but was increased only slightly in the ligated shrinking lobe. Increased tissue levels of HGF may also increase plasma levels, thereby stimulating the growth of hepatic tumors. Takahara et al. [113] compared the therapeutic efficacy of HGF with that of an engineered cytokine (Metron Factor-1) derived from HGF and the HGF-like factor, macrophage stimulating protein. Metron factor-1 was as effective as HGF at preventing liver injury and at promoting hepatocyte regeneration. However, it was therapeutically safer than HGF because it lacked proangiogenic and prometastatic activity during intrahepatic dissemination of orthotopically-injected hepatocarcinoma cells. Therefore, a better understanding of underlying microenvironmental changes in the liver resulting from hepatectomy and the subsequent liver regeneration process is essential. This may enable alternative strategies to minimize tumor recurrence and improve patient survival after hepatectomy.

3.7.2 The Fibrotic Microenvironment of the Liver and Metastasis

Liver damage leads to an inflammatory response and to the activation and proliferation of mesenchymal cell populations within the liver that remodel the extracellular matrix as part of an orchestrated wound-healing response [52]. Chronic damage results in a progressive accumulation of scarring proteins (fibrosis) that alters tissue structure and function with increasing severity, leading to cirrhosis and liver failure. Frequently, circulating cancer cells colonize this altered microenvironment of the cirrhotic liver. However, at the moment it is unclear whether changes in the architecture and function of cirrhotic livers are preventing or promoting metastasis.

3.7.2.1 Cirrhosis and Hepatic Metastasis

Malignant cancers rarely metastasize to livers with cirrhosis and autopsies have confirmed that the rate of metastasis to cirrhotic liver is lower than that to normal liver, suggesting that cirrhosis may inhibit metastasis formation [114–118]. A possible explanation is that venous shunting in cirrhosis prevents cancer cells from reaching the liver, and that changes in the architecture of cirrhotic sinusoids may reduce metastasis [117]. Moreover, the activation of Kupffer cells in cirrhosis may also inhibit the formation of hepatic metastases due to their tumoricidal effects [119]. However, the mechanisms responsible for reduced tumor growth remain unclear and as suggested by Vanbockrijck and Kloppel [120], the lower incidence of metastases may actually be due to a shorter life expectancy of patients with cirrhosis. Moreover, recent observations argue against antimetastatic effects of cirrhosis. For example, using intravital videomicroscopy Qi et al. [121] showed that the hepatic sinusoids were narrower in cirrhotic livers and more cancer cells were retained in terminal portal veins. This was also consistent with the increased expression of vascular adhesion molecules by sinusoids of cirrhotic livers. Interestingly, using confocal microscopy and the fluorescent nitric oxide probe 4,5-diaminofluorescein diacetate, the same authors detected a significantly lower level of NO release in livers with cirrhosis both under basal conditions and after cancer cell arrest, and a lower percentage of apoptotic cancer cells could be observed in the sinusoids of cirrhotic than normal livers. Consistent with these findings, more mitotic and Ki-67$^+$ cancer cells were detected in the cirrhotic livers. Taken together, the results suggest that microenvironmental changes in the architecture, adhesion molecule expression and NO production levels may cause more cancer cells to arrest, survive and proliferate in the microvasculature of livers with cirrhosis.

3.7.2.2 Discoidin Domain Receptor-2 Deficiency and Hepatic Metastasis Predisposition

Activation of HSC is a central event in the fibrogenic response to hepatic injury and cirrhosis. Major features of HSC activation include cell proliferation and recruitment into areas of injury, remodeling of surrounding extracellular matrix and release of proliferative and chemotactic factors [52]. Activated HSC display myofibroblastic features, such as α-SMA expression and induction of tyrosine kinase receptors such as PDGF receptor-β and discoidin domain receptor-2 (DDR2). However, the transdifferentiation of HSCs into myofibroblasts is also a key event for the development of stroma and angiogenesis during the development of hepatic metastases [48, 49]. Liver myofibroblasts promote cancer cell growth and migration in primary and metastatic hepatic tumors and contribute to the tumor stroma supporting intra-metastatic neoangiogenesis and growth by deposition of tumor-associated extracellular matrix and secretion of migratory and proliferative factors [3].

DDR2 is a tyrosine kinase receptor for fibrillar collagen whose expression increases during the HSC activation associated with hepatic fibrosis [122]. Type I collagen-dependent upregulation of DDR2 expression establishes a positive feedback loop in activated HSCs, leading to further proliferation and enhanced release of matrix metalloproteinases. However, mice lacking the DDR2 gene ($DDR2^{-/-}$) had an enhanced susceptibility to carbon-tetrachloride-induced hepatic fibrosis, suggesting that DDR2-dependent genes may also be anti-fibrogenic [123]. Based on these findings, we hypothesized that tumor stroma formation by transdifferentiated HSCs may be enhanced by DDR2 deficiency, predisposing hepatic tissue to cancer metastasis. Interestingly, experimental hepatic metastasis of murine MC38 colon carcinoma cells significantly increased in $DDR2^{-/-}$ as compared to wild type mice. Immunohistochemical analysis showed that hepatic metastases in $DDR2^{-/-}$ mice had a higher density of HSC-derived myofibroblasts, neoangiogenic vessels and proliferating cancer cells than those in $DDR2^{+/+}$ littermates. Consistent with the in vivo findings, secretion of endothelial cell adhesion- and migration-stimulating factors, and of tumor cell proliferation enhancing factors significantly increased in supernatants derived from primary cultures of $DDR2^{-/-}$ HSCs, as compared to wild-type HSCs. These secreted factors further increased in the supernatants of $DDR2^{-/-}$ HSC cultures pretreated with cancer cell-conditioned media. Moreover, gene profiling of $DDR2^{-/-}$ HSC showed increased expression of a cluster of genes, associated with inflammation and extracellular matrix remodeling that have been clinically correlated with hepatic metastasis occurrence, including IL-10, TGFβ, syndecan-1, integrin α2, thrombopoietin and BMP7 [123]. These results demonstrate that DDR-2 deficiency predisposes hepatic tissue to colon carcinoma metastasis in this murine model and suggest that this is due to the loss of DDR2-dependent factors that normally prevent cancer cell adhesion and proliferation and endothelial cell migration.

3.8 Conclusions

The availability of methods for isolating and culturing hepatic parenchymal and non-parenchyma cells has greatly facilitated the research on molecular mechanisms of cancer-host cell interactions in the liver by providing in vitro models that can mimic these interactions. New features of the microenvironment of hepatic metastases could be revealed and molecular targets of interest for anti-tumor therapeutics identified using these experimental models. However, further preclinical research is necessary to determine whether the same microenvironmental factors operate for every metastasis, irrespective of the tumor type, and whether hepatic metastases can be prevented or treated by blocking prometastatic factors or upregulating endogenous anti-metastatic factors in the hepatic microenvironment.

Some circulating cancer cells are resistant to the specialized anti-tumoral mechanisms of the liver microvasculature, while concurrently taking advantage of the growth-promoting effects of the hepatic microenvironment for developing metastases. The influence of the hepatic microenvironment on the metastatic process can change as the metastatic process advances and based on the location of the cancer cells, and can be classified into three major stages, each providing different opportunities for therapy (Table 3.4).

3.8.1 Hepatic Metastasis Stage I

At this stage the behavior of liver-infiltrating cancer cells is affected mainly by the microvascular anatomy and the functional zonation occurring within the hepatic lobules or acini. This stage begins with the initial arrest of circulating cancer cells in the hepatic microvasculature and lasts until the formation of an avascular micrometastasis that has not yet progressed beyond the limits of the hepatic lobule because its diameter is smaller than 300 μm. At this stage, cancer cells interact with hepatic cells located in their normal physiological site. This stage includes both microvascular and intralobular micrometastases that are completely subclinical, avascular, sometimes even stroma-free, and do not yet have a significant impact on the functionality of the whole organ. Therapeutic targets at this stage may include molecular mediators that induce tumor-dependent hepatic inflammation, immune response suppression, intrametastatic myofibroblast recruitment and up regulation of the endogenous antioxidant machinery in cancer cells.

3.8.2 Hepatic Metastasis Stage II

This stage begins when liver-infiltrating cancer cells have formed a micrometastasis whose further development is no longer affected by hepatic microvasculature and zonation. However, the process is still strongly microenvironment-dependent and requires the cooperation of hepatic cells to develop the intrametastatic stroma and induce angiogenesis. This is the panlobular stage of hepatic metastasis because it involves several hepatic lobules. Here, cancer cells interact mainly with migratory hepatic parenchymal and non-parenchymal cells that have lost their original positional coordinates in the hepatic tissue microarchitecture and are recruited into the metastatic lesion to form the tumor stroma. This stage corresponds to the angiogenic phase of the metastatic process and entails a transition from avascular to vascularized metastases. Metastases at this stage can be detectable by non-invasive methods [124] but they are still considered subclinical because their size ranges between 0.3 and 5 mm. These metastases have the potential of becoming clinically relevant and, if multifocal, they may affect liver functions and hemodynamic parameters. Therapeutic targets at this stage are cancer cell invasion and proliferation-stimulating factors and mediators of tumor-induced angiogenesis and stromagenesis.

Table 3.4 Clinical, microenvironmental and therapeutic features at different stages of the process of hepatic metastasis

	Stage I hepatic metastasis	Stage II hepatic metastasis	Stage III hepatic metastasis
Metastasis size Clinical impact	< 300 μm: Not detectable – Subclinical effects/Reversible Metastasis – Disturbance of hepatic microcirculation – Increase of proinflammatory cytokines, soluble ICAM-1 and endostatin in hepatic blood	0.3–5 mm: Sometimes detectable – Subclinical effects/Reversible metastasis – Disturbance of hepatic lobules – Regional effects on the perimetastatic hepatic microenvironment – Risk of intrahepatic micrometastasis spread	>5 mm: Detectable – Clinical effects/Irreversible metastasis – Disturbance of main liver functions – Hepatic and systemic functional effects – Risk of extrahepatic dissemination
Metastasis status	– Microvascular and intralobular preangiogenic phases – From hepatic microvascular infiltration of circulating cancer cells to the avascular micrometastasis growth	– Panlobular angiogenic phase – From stromagenic avascular micrometastasis to angiogenic small-size metastasis	– Lobar growth phase – Invasive metastasis
Microenvironmental interactions	– Cancer cells interact with hepatic cells located in their original tissue organization	– Cancer cells interact with tumor-infiltrating migratory hepatic cells and promote intrametastatic stroma and angiogenesis development	– Cancer cells are influenced by factors from both tumor-unaffected hepatic areas, and tumor-infiltrating hepatic cells

Table 3.4 (continued)

	Stage I hepatic metastasis	Stage II hepatic metastasis	Stage III hepatic metastasis
Intrahepatic impact	– Transient microcirculatory disturbance – Microvascular inflammation – Oxidative stress-mediated tissue damage – Hepatic recruitment of circulating leukocytes and mesenchymal cells	– Intrametastatic recruitment of hepatic myofibroblasts – Anti-tumor immune response impairment – Tumor angiogenesis	– Hepatic tissue structure disturbance – Altered hepatic blood supply – Altered hepatic parenchymal cell function
Therapeutic targets	– Proinflammatory cytokines – Oxidative stress-inducing factors – Mannose receptor-stimulating factors – Gene products from tumor-unaffected hepatic tissue	– Angiogenic factors – Immune suppressant factors – Myofibroblast-stimulating factors – Metastasis suppressor genes – Gene products from tumor-unaffected hepatic tissue	– Angiogenic factors – Immune suppressant factors – Myofibroblast-stimulating factors – Tumor-growth factors – Gene products from hepatic metastasis-specific tissue

Three major hepatic metastasis stages, each providing different opportunities for therapy, were considered: Stage I: from initial arrest of circulating cancer cells in the hepatic microvasculature up to formation of avascular micrometastases that do not progress beyond hepatic lobule limits; Stage II: the panlobular angiogenic metastases and Stage III: clinically detectable lobar metastases. Clinical, biological and therapeutic features at each of these stages were used to demonstrate that specific microenvironmental changes require tailored therapeutic approaches for each stage.

3.8.3 Hepatic Metastasis Stage III

This stage begins when liver-infiltrating cancer cells have formed a clinically detectable lobar metastasis larger than 5 mm in diameter, whose development is no longer affected by hepatic tissue organization. This is the most advanced stage of the metastatic process. It involves the whole liver, which it affects through the secretion of tumor-derived factors. During this stage, the tumor progressively alters hepatic tissue structure, blood supply and metabolic substrate availability, jeopardizing parenchymal cell function. However hepatic metastases are still microenvironmentally modulated at this stage. On one hand, metastases contain tumor-infiltrating lymphocytes [89] – including immunosuppressive CD4/CD25 regulatory T cells [89] – as well as stromal cells derived mainly from hepatic tissue [3], whose specific phenotypes have prognostic implications. On the other hand, both normal and cancer cells within the metastatic lesions are also transcriptionally regulated by liver-derived soluble factors including proinflammatory and angiogenic cytokines [92], IGF-I [93], and immunosuppressive factors (TGFβ, IL-10, soluble ICAM-1, etc.), whose levels in the hepatic circulation are elevated. At this stage, therefore, hepatic metastases are also affected by two interrelated microenvironments whose control may require different therapeutic approaches namely, parenchymal and nonparenchymal cells residing in tumor-unaffected hepatic areas, and tumor-activated hepatic cells recruited into the metastatic site.

In summary, the liver can exert opposing effects on the metastatic cells. While on one hand these cells can be eliminated by hepatic antitumor defense mechanisms, their growth can also be enhanced by the prometastatic effects of the liver, possibly accounting for the high incidence and aggressiveness of hepatic metastases. Our growing understanding of the molecular basis for the regulation of metastases by the hepatic microenvironment opens new avenues for prevention of metastases at a subclinical stage and for their treatment at more advanced stages. In addition, while the identification of metastasis-related gene profiles may assist in determining the liver metastatic potential of primary tumors, it should be recognized that some gene expression patterns in metastatic cells are liver cell-dependent. New biomarkers are therefore needed in order to predict the liver capacity to provide a prometastatic microenvironment and to individualize the assessment of hepatic metastasis risk in cancer patients. One should bear in mind however, that many of the conclusions outlined herein are based on animal and in vitro studies. While these models are essential to access and analyze very early events in the process of liver metastasis (generally not accessible in the clinical setting), animal models are generally based on experimental assays that do not always accurately mimic the clinical scenario (e.g. in time scale of the metastatic process, mode of inoculation and tumor cell entry into the liver and use of established cell lines). Their translational relevance remains therefore to be validated in the clinical setting.

Acknowledgements The author acknowledges with gratitude Dr. Pnina Brodt's significant editorial contribution to this chapter.

References

1. Weiss L (1994) Inefficiency of metastasis from colorectal carcinomas. Relationship to local therapy for hepatic metastasis. Cancer Treat Res 69:1–11
2. Chambers AF, Naumov GN, Vantyghem SA, Tuck AB (2000) Molecular biology of breast cancer metastasis. Clinical implications of experimental studies on metastatic inefficiency. Breast Cancer Res 2:400–407
3. Vidal-Vanaclocha F (2008) The prometastatic microenvironment of the liver. Cancer Microenviron 1:113–129
4. Weiss L (1992) Biomechanical interactions of cancer cells with the microvasculature during hematogenous metastasis. Cancer Met Rev 11:227–235
5. Barberá-Guillem E, Smith I, Weiss L (1993) Cancer-cell traffic in the liver. II. Arrest, transit and death of B16F10 and M5076 cells in the sinusoids. Int J Cancer 53:298–301
6. Jessup J, Battle P, Waller H et al (1999) Reactive nitrogen and oxygen radicals formed during hepatic ischemia-reperfusion kill weakly metastatic colorectal cancer cells. Cancer Res 59:1825–1829
7. Wang H, McIntosh A, Hasinoff B et al (2000) B16 melanoma cell arrest in the mouse liver induces nitric oxide release and sinusoidal cytotoxicity: a natural hepatic defense against metastasis. Cancer Res 60:5862–5869
8. Anasagasti MJ, Alvarez A, Avivi C et al (1996) Interleukin-1-mediated H2O2 production by hepatic sinusoidal endothelium in response to B16 melanoma cell adhesion. J Cell Physiol 167:314–323
9. Roos E, Dingemans KP, Van de Pavert IV et al (1978) Mammary-carcinoma cells in mouse liver: infiltration of liver tissue and interaction with Kupffer cells. Br J Cancer 38:88–99
10. Kan Z, Ivancev K, Lunderquist A et al (1995) In vivo microscopy of hepatic metastases: dynamic observation of tumor cell invasion and interaction with Kupffer cells. Hepatology 21:487–494
11. Bayón LG, Izquierdo MA, Sirovich I et al (1996) Role of Kupffer cells in arresting circulating tumor cells and controlling metastatic growth in the liver. Hepatology 23:1224–1231
12. Timmers M, Vekemans K, Vermijlen D et al (2004) Interactions between rat colon carcinoma cells and Kupffer cells during the onset of hepatic metastasis. Int J Cancer 112:793–802
13. Bouwens L, Jacobs R, Remels L (1988) Natural cytotoxicity of rat hepatic natural killer cells and macrophages against a syngeneic colon adenocarcinoma. Cancer Immunol Immunother 27:137–141
14. Gardner CR, Wasserman AJ, Laskin DL (1991) Liver macrophage mediated cytotoxicity toward mastocytoma cells involves phagocytosis of tumor targets. Hepatology 14:318–324
15. Vermijlen D, Luo D, Robaye B et al (1999) Pit cells (Hepatic natural killer cells) of the rat induce apoptosis in colon carcinoma cells by the perforin/granzyme pathway. Hepatology 29:51–56
16. Vekemans K, Timmers M, Vermijlen D et al (2003) CC531 colon carcinoma cells induce apoptosis in rat hepatic endothelial cells by the Fas/FasL-mediated pathway. Liver Int 23:283–293
17. Vidal-Vanaclocha F, Alonso A, Barberá-Guillem E (1990) Functional variations of liver tissue during the hepatic colonization by metastatic tumor cells. Virchows Arch A Pathol Anat 416:189–195
18. Arteta B, Lasuen N, Lopategi A et al (2010) Colon carcinoma cell interaction with liver sinusoidal endothelium inhibits organ-specific anti-tumor immunity via IL-1-induced mannose receptor. Hepatology 51:2172–2182
19. Mendoza L, Carrascal T, de Luca M et al (2001) Hydrogen peroxide mediates vascular cell adhesion molecule-1 expression from IL-18-activated hepatic sinusoidal endothelium: implications for circulating cancer cell arrest in murine liver. Hepatology 34:298–310

20. Vidal-Vanaclocha F, Fantuzzi G, Mendoza L et al (2000) IL-18 regulates IL-1 beta-dependent hepatic melanoma metastasis via vascular adhesion molecule-1. Proc Natl Acad Sci USA 97:734–739

21. Khatib AM, Auguste P, Fallavollita L et al (2005) Characterization of the host proinflammatory response to tumor cells during the initial stages of liver metastasis. Am J Pathol 167:749–759

22. Anasagasti MJ, Alvarez A, Martin JJ et al (1997) Sinusoidal endothelium release of hydrogen peroxide enhances very late antigen-4-mediated melanoma cell adherence and tumor cytotoxicity during interleukin-1 promotion of hepatic melanoma metastasis in mice. Hepatology 25:840–846

23. Vidal-Vanaclocha F, Amézaga C, Asumendi A et al (1994) Interleukin-1 receptor blockade reduces the number and size of murine B16 melanoma hepatic metastases. Cancer Res 54:2667–2672

24. Carrascal T, Mendoza L, Vacarcel M et al (2003) Interleukin-18 binding protein reduces B16 melanoma hepatic metastasis by neutralizing the adhesiveness and growth factors of sinusoidal endothelial cell. Cancer Res 63:491–497

25. Vidal-Vanaclocha F, Alvarez A, Asumendi A et al (1996) Interleukin 1 (IL-1)-dependent melanoma hepatic metastasis in vivo; increased endothelial adherence by IL-1-induced mannose receptors and growth factor production in vitro. J Natl Cancer Inst 88:198–205

26. Zubia A, Mendoza L, Vivanco S et al (2005) Application of stereocontrolled stepwise [3+2]. Cycloadditions to the preparation of inhibitors of alpha(4)beta(1)-integrin-mediated hepatic melanoma metastasis. Angew Chem Int Ed Engl 44:2903–2907

27. Moller B, Paulukat J, Nold M et al (2003) Interferon-gamma induces expression of interleukin-18 binding protein in fibroblast-like synoviocytes. Rheumatology (Oxford) 42:442–445

28. Dinarello, CA, Novick D, Puren AJ et al (1998) Overview of interleukin-18: more than an interferon-gamma inducing factor. J Leukocyte Biol 63:658–666

29. Vidal-Vanaclocha F, Mendoza L, Telleria N et al (2006) Clinical and experimental approaches to the pathophysiology of interleukin-18 in cancer progression. Cancer Metastasis Rev 25:417–434

30. Wang N, Thuraisingam T, Fallavollita L et al (2006) The secretory leukocyte protease inhibitor is a type 1 insulin-like growth factor receptor-regulated protein that protects against liver metastasis by attenuating the host proinflammatory response. Cancer Res 66:3062–3070

31. Auguste P, Fallavollita L, Wang N et al (2007) The host inflammatory response promotes liver metastasis by increasing tumor cell arrest and extravasation. Am J Pathol 170:1781–1792

32. Stahl PD, Ezekowitz RA (1998) The mannose receptor is a pattern recognition receptor involved in host defense. Curr Opin Immunol 10:50–55

33. Knolle PA, Gerken G (2000) Local control of the immune response in the liver. Immunol Rev 174:21–34

34. Fujisaki T, Tanaka Y, Fujii K et al (1999) CD44 stimulation induces integrin mediated adhesion of colon cancer cell lines to endothelial cells by up-regulation of integrins and c-Met and activation of integrins. Cancer Res 59:4427–4434

35. Valcárcel M, Arteta B, Jaureguibeitia A et al (2008) Three-dimensional growth as multicellular spheroid activates the proangiogenic phenotype of colorectal carcinoma cells via LFA-1-dependent VEGF: implications on hepatic micrometastasis. J Transl Med 9:57–69

36. Kamekazi S, Kurozawa Y, Iwai N et al (2005) Serum levels of soluble ICAM-1 and VCAM-1 predict pre-clinical cancer. Eur J Cancer 41:2355–2359

37. Kooy AJ, Tank B, Vuzevski VD et al (1998) Expression of interferon-gamma receptors and interferon-gamma-induced up-regulation of intercellular adhesion molecule-1 in basal cell carcinoma; decreased expression of IFN-gamma R and shedding of ICAM-1 as a means to escape immune surveillance. J Pathol 184:169–176

38. Gho YS, Kleinman HK, Sosne G (1999) Angiogenic activity of human soluble intercellular adhesion-1. Cancer Res 59:5128–5132

39. Roossien FF, de Rijk D, Bikker A et al (1989) Involvement of LFA-1 in lymphoma invasion and metastasis demonstrated with LFA-1 deficient mutants. J Cell Biol 108: 1979–1985

40. Wang HS, Hung Y, Su CH et al (2005) CD44 cross-linking induces-integrin mediated adhesion and transendothelial migration in breast cancer cell line by up-regulation of LFA-1 (alphaL beta2) and VLA-4 (alpha4 beta 1). Exp Cell Res 304:116–126

41. Cohen S, Haimovich J, Hollander N (2003) Anti-idiotype x anti-LFA-1 bispecific antibodies inhibit metastasis of B cell lymphoma. J Immunol 170:2695–2701

42. Aoudjit F, Potoworowski EF, Springer TA et al (1998) Protection from lymphoma cell metastasis in ICAM-1 mutant mice: a posthoming event. J Immunol 161:2333–2338

43. Jessup JM, Laguinge L, Lin S et al (2004) Carcinoembryonic antigen induction of IL-10 and IL-6 inhibits hepatic ischemic/reperfusion injury to colorectal carcinoma cells. Int J Cancer 111:332–337

44. Jessup JM, Samara R, Battle P et al (2004) Carcinoembryonic antigen promotes tumor cell survival in liver through an IL-10-dependent pathway. Clin Exp Metastasis 21:709–717

45. Luo D, Vermijlen D, Kuppen PJ et al (2002) MHC class I expression protects rat colon carcinoma cells from hepatic natural killer cell-mediated apoptosis and cytolysis, by blocking the perforin/granzyme pathway. J Comp Hepatol 1:2

46. Anasagasti MJ, Martin JJ, Mendoza L et al (1998) Glutathione protects metastatic melanoma cells against oxidative stress in the murine hepatic microvasculature. Hepatology 27: 1249–1256

47. Estrela JM, Ortega A, Obrador E (2006) Glutathione in cancer biology and therapy. Crit Rev Clin Lab Sci 43:143–181

48. Olaso E, Santisteban A, Bidaurrazaga J et al (1997) Tumor-dependent activation of rodent hepatic stellate cells during experimental melanoma metastasis. Hepatology 26: 634–642

49. Olaso E, Salado C, Egilegor E et al (2003) Proangiogenic role of tumor-activated hepatic stellate cells in experimental melanoma metastasis. Hepatology 37:674–685

50. Deleve LD, Wang X, Guo Y (2008) Sinusoidal endothelial cells prevent rat stellate cell activation and promote reversion to quiescence. Hepatology 48:920–930

51. Gressner AM, Bachem MG (1995) Molecular mechanisms of liver fibrogenesis – a homage to the role of activated fat-storing cells. Digestion 56:335–346

52. Friedman SL (2008) Mechanisms of hepatic fibrogenesis. Gastroenterology 134:1655–1669

53. Barberá-Guillem E, Alonso-Varona A, Vidal-Vanaclocha F (1989) Selective implantation and growth in rats and mice of experimental liver metastasis in acinar zone one. Cancer Res 49:4003–4010

54. Kaplan RN, Rafii S, Lyden D (2006) Preparing the "soil": the premetastatic niche. Cancer Res 66:11089–11093

55. Jungermann K (1995) Zonation of metabolism and gene expression in liver. Histochem Cell Biol 103:81–91

56. Jungermann K, Kietzmann T (2000) Oxygen: modulator of metabolic zonation and disease of the liver. Hepatology 31:255–260

57. Kemperman H, Wijnands Y, Meijne AM et al (1994) TA3/St, but not TA3/Ha, mammary carcinoma cell adhesion to hepatocytes is mediated by alpha 5 beta 1 interacting with surface-associated fibronectin. Cell Adhes Commun 2:45–58

58. Shimizu S, Yamada N, Sawada T et al (2000) Ultrastructure of early phase hepatic metastasis of human colon carcinoma cells with special reference to desmosomal junctions with hepatocytes. Pathol Int 50:953–959

59. Shimizu S, Yamada N, Sawada T et al (2000) In vivo and in vitro interactions between human colon carcinoma cells and hepatic stellate cells. Jpn J Cancer Res 91:1285–1295

60. Solaun MS, Mendoza L, de Luca M et al (2002) Endostatin inhibits murine colon carcinoma sinusoidal-type metastases by preferential targeting of hepatic sinusoidal endothelium. Hepatology 35:1104–1116
61. Olaso E, Arteta B, Salado C (2006) Proangiogenic implications of hepatic stellate cell trans-differentiation into myofibroblasts induced by tumor microenvironment. In: Chaponnier C (ed) Tissue repair, contraction and the myofibroblast. Landes Publication, Austin
62. Mueller L, Goumas FA, Affeldt M et al (2007) Stromal fibroblasts in colorectal liver metastases originate from resident fibroblasts and generate an inflammatory microenvironment. Am J Pathol 171:1608–1618
63. Basaldua F, Vidal-Vanaclocha F (2008) Nerve growth factor expression by hepatic parenchymal and non-parenchymal cells during metastatic colorectal development in human and murine liver. Proceedings of the 14th International Symposium on Cells of the Hepatic Sinusoid (ISCHS), Tromso (Norway)
64. Basaldua F, Lopategi A, Arteta B et al (2008) Tumor-induced liver nerve growth factor (NGF): a new target for stromal cell inhibition during metastatic colorectal carcinoma growth. Eur J Cancer 12:55
65. Shaheen RM, Tseng W, Davis DW et al (2001) Tyrosine kinase inhibition of multiple angiogenic growth factors receptors improves survival in mice bearing colon cancer liver metastases by inhibition of endothelial cell survival mechanism. Cancer Res 61:1464–1468
66. Reinmuth N, Liu W, Ahmad SA et al (2003) AlphaVbeta3 integrin antagonist S247 decreases colon cancer metastasis and angiogenesis and improves survival in mice. Cancer Res 63:2079–2087
67. Wang YQ, Ikeda K, Ikebe T et al (2000) Inhibition of hepatic stellate cell proliferation and activation by the semisynthetic analogue of fumagillin TNP-470 in rats. Hepatology 32:980–989
68. Kinoshita S, Hirai R, Yamano T et al (2004) Inhibitor TNP-470 can suppress hepatocellular carcinoma growth without retarding liver regeneration after partial hepatectomy. Surg Today 34:40–46
69. Godichaud S, Krisa S, Couronne et al (2000) Deactivation of cultured human liver myofibroblasts by trans-resveratrol, a grapevine-derived polyphenol. Hepatology 31:922–931
70. Fenwick SW, Toogood GJ, Lodge JP et al (2003) The effect of the selective cyclooxygenase-2 inhibitor rofecoxib on human colorectal cancer liver metastases. Gastroenterology 125:716–729
71. Wei D, Wang L, He Y et al (2004) Celecoxib inhibits VEGF expression in and reduces angiogenesis and metastasis of human pancreatic cancer via suppression of Sp1 transcription factor activity. Cancer Res 64:2030–2038
72. Yang ZF, Poon RT, To J et al (2004) The potential role of HIF1-alpha in tumor progression after hypoxia and chemotherapy in hepatocellular carcinoma. Cancer Res 64:5496–5503
73. Yu C, Rahmani M, Almenara J et al (2004) Induction of apoptosis in human leukemia cells by the tyrosine kinase inhibitor adaphostin proceeds through a RAF-1/MEK/ERK- and AKT-dependent process. Oncogene 23:1364–1376
74. Snader KM, Vishnuvajjala BR, Sausville EA et al (2002) 17-Dimethylaminoethylamino-17-desmethoxygeldanamycin (17-DMAG), a potent Hsp90 inhibitor with improved pharmaceutical and antitumor properties. In: 1st International symposium on signal transduction modulators in cancer therapy, Amsterdam
75. Kishibe K, Yamada Y, Ogawa K (2002) Production of nerve growth factor by mouse hepatocellular carcinoma cells and expression of TrkA in tumor-associated arteries in mice. Gastroenterology 122:1978–1986
76. Rasi G, Serafino A, Bellis L et al (2007) Nerve growth factor involvement in liver cirrhosis and hepatocellular carcinoma. World J Gastroenterol 13:4986–4995
77. Paku S, Lapis K (1993) Morphological aspects of angiogenesis in experimental liver metastases. Am J Pathol 143:926–936

78. Vermeulen PB, Colpaert C, Salgado R et al (2001) Liver metastases from colorectal adenocarcinomas grow in three patterns with different angiogenesis and desmoplasia. J Pathol 195:336–342
79. Clement B, Musso O, Lietard J et al (1999) Homeostatic control of angiogenesis: a newly identified function of the liver? Hepatology 29:621–623
80. Maeda K, Nishiguchi Y, Kang SM et al (2001) Expression of thrombospondin-1 inversely correlated with tumor vascularity and hematogenous metastasis in colon cancer. Oncol Rep 8:763–766
81. O'Reilly MS, Boehm T, Shing Y et al (1997) Endostatin: an endogenous inhibitor of angiogenesis and tumor growth. Cell 88:277–285
82. Musso O, Theret N, Heljasvaara R et al (2001) Tumor hepatocytes and basement membrane-producing cells specifically express two different forms of the endostatin precursor, collagen XVIII, in human liver cancers. Hepatology 4:868–876
83. Yoon SS, Eto H, Lin C-M et al (1999) Mouse endostatin inhibits the formation of lung and liver metastases. Cancer Res 59:6251–6256
84. Mendoza L, Valcárcel M, Carrascal T et al (2004) Inhibition of cytokine-induced microvascular arrest of tumor cells by recombinant endostatin prevents experimental hepatic melanoma metastasis. Cancer Res 64:304–310
85. Feldman AL, Tamarkin L, Paciotti GF et al (2000) Serum endostatin levels are elevated and correlate with serum vascular endothelial growth factor levels in patients with stage IV clear cell renal cancer. Clin Cancer Res 6:4628–4634
86. Kuroi K, Tanaka C, Toi M (2001) Circulating levels of endostatin in cancer patients. Oncol Rep 8:405–409
87. Iughetti P, Suzuki O, Godoi PH et al (2001) A polymorphism in endostatin, an angiogenesis inhibitor, predisposes for the development of prostatic adenocarcinoma. Cancer Res 61:7375–7378
88. Kim YM, Jang JW, Lee OH et al (2000) Endostatin inhibits endothelial and tumor cellular invasion by blocking the activation and catalytic activity of matrix metalloproteinase. Cancer Res 60:5410–5413
89. Winnock M, Garcia-Barcina M, Huet S et al (1993) Functional characterization of liver-associated lymphocytes in patients with liver metastasis. Gastroenterology 105:1152–1158
90. Kobayashi N, Hiraoka N, Yamagami W et al (2007) FOXP3+ regulatory T cells affect the development and progression of hepatocarcinogenesis. Clin Cancer Res 13:902–911
91. Ooi LP, Crawford DH, Gotley DC et al (1997) Evidence that "myofibroblast-like" cells are the cellular source of capsular collagen in hepatocellular carcinoma. J Hepatol 26:798–807
92. Stoeltzing O, Liu W, Reinmuth N et al (2003) Angiogenesis and antiangiogenic therapy of colon cancer liver metastasis. Ann Surg Oncol 10:722–733
93. Bauer TW, Fan F, Liu W et al (2007) Targeting of insulin-like growth factor-I receptor with a monoclonal antibody inhibits growth of hepatic metastases from human colon carcinoma in mice. Ann Surg Oncol 14:2838–2846
94. Yamasaki M, Takemasa I, Komori T et al (2007) The gene expression profile represents the molecular nature of liver metastasis in colorectal cancer. Int J Oncol 30:129–138
95. Murthy SM, Goldschmidt RA, Rao LN et al (1989) The influence of surgical trauma on experimental metastasis. Cancer 64:2035–2044
96. Murthy MS, Scanlon EF, Jelachich ML et al (1995) Growth and metastasis of human breast cancers in athymic nude mice. Clin Exp Metastasis 13:3–15
97. Bogden AE, Moreau J-P, Eden PA (1997) Proliferative response of human animal tumors to surgical wounding of normal tissues: onset, duration and inhibition. Br J Cancer 75:1021–1027
98. Hofer SO, Shrayer D, Reichner JS et al (1998) Wound-induced tumor progression: a probable role in recurrence after tumor resection. Arch Surg 133:383–389

99. Nordlinger B, Guiguet M, Vaillant JC et al (1996) Surgical resection of colorectal carcinoma metastases to the liver: a prognostic scoring system to improve case selection, based on 1568 patients. Cancer 77:1254–1262

100. Jaeck D, Bachellier P, Guiguet M et al (1997) Long-term survival following resection of colorectal hepatic metastases. Br J Surg 84:977–980

101. Makuuchi M, Le Thai B, Takayasu K et al (1990) Preoperative portal embolization to increase safety of major hepatectomy for hilar bile duct carcinoma: a preliminary report. Surgery 107:521–527

102. Elias D, Roche A, Vavasseur D et al (1992) Induction of hypertrophy of a small left hepatic lobe by preoperative right portal embolization, preceding extended right hepatectomy. Ann Chir 46:404–410

103. Azoulay D, Castaing D, Smail A et al (2000) Resection of non resectable liver metastases from colorectal cancer after percutaneous PVE. Ann Surg 231:480–486

104. Liu H, Zhu S (2009) Present status and future perspectives of preoperative portal vein embolization. Am J Surgery 197:686–690

105. Elias D, de Baere T, Roche A et al (1999) During liver regeneration following right portal embolization the growth rate of liver metastases is more rapid than that of the liver parenchyma. Br J Surg 86:784–788

106. Higgins GM, Anderson RM (1931) Experimental pathology of the liver. I. Restoration of the liver of the white rat following partial surgical removal. Arch Pathol 12:186–202

107. Ichihashi H, Mabuchi H, Suenaga M et al (1984) Liver regeneration and tumor growth in the rat after partial hepatectomy. Jpn J Surg 14:510–514

108. Morimoto H, Nio Y, Imai S et al (1992) Hepatectomy accelerates the growth of transplanted liver tumor in mice. Cancer Detec Prev 16:137–147

109. Panis Y, Ribeiro J, Chretien Y et al (1992) Dormant liver metastases: an experimental study. Br J Surg 79:221–223

110. Gutman M, Singh RK, Price JE et al (1994) Accelerated growth of human colon cancer cells in nude mice undergoing liver regeneration. Inv Metastasis 14:362–371

111. Asaga T, Suzuki K, Umeda M et al (1991) The enhancement of tumor growth after partial hepatectomy and the effect of sera obtained from hepatectomized rats on tumor cell growth. Jpn J Surg 21:669–675

112. Kokudo N, Tada K, Seki M et al (2001) Proliferative activity of intrahepatic colorectal metastases after preoperative hemihepatic portal vein embolization. Hepatology 34:267–272

113. Takahara T, Xue F, Mazzone M et al (2008) Metron factor-1 prevents liver injury without promoting tumor growth and metastasis. Hepatology 47:2010–2025

114. Gervaz P, Pak-art R, Nivatvongs S et al (2003) Colorectal adenocarcinoma in cirrhotic patients. J Am Coll Surg 196:874–879

115. Melato M, Laurino L, Mucli E et al (1989) Relationship between cirrhosis, liver cancer, and hepatic metastases. An autopsy study. Cancer 64:455–459

116. Pereira-Lima JE, Lichtenfels E, Barbosa FS et al (2003) Prevalence study of metastases in cirrhotic livers. Hepatogastroenterology 50:1490–1495

117. Seymour K, Charnley RM (1999) Evidence that metastasis is less common in cirrhotic than normal liver: a systematic review of post-mortem case-control studies. Br J Surg 86:1237–1242

118. Song E, Chen J, Ouyang N et al (2001) Kupffer cells of cirrhotic rat livers sensitize colon cancer cells to Fas-mediated apoptosis. Br J Cancer 84:1265–1271

119. Uetsuji S, Yamamura M, Yamamichi K et al (1992) Absence of colorectal cancer metastasis to the cirrhotic liver. Am J Surg 164:176–177

120. Vanbockrijck M, Kloppel G (1992) Incidence and morphology of liver metastasis from extrahepatic malignancies to cirrhotic livers. Zentralbl Pathol 138:91–96

121. Qi K, Qiu H, Sun D et al (2004) Impact of cirrhosis on the development of experimental hepatic metastases by B16F1 melanoma cells in C57BL/6 mice. Hepatology 40:1144–1150

122. Olaso E, Ikeda K, Eng FJ et al (2001) DDR2 receptor promotes MMP-2-mediated proliferation and invasion by hepatic stellate cells. J Clin Invest 108:1369–1378
123. Badiola I, Vidal-Vanaclocha F, Olaso E (2010) Discoidin domain receptor 2 deficiency predisposes hepatic tissue to colon carcinoma metastasis. 15th ISCHS, Pasadena (CA)
124. Nomura K, Kadoya M, Ueda K et al (2007) Detection of hepatic metastases from colorectal carcinoma: comparison of histopathologic features of anatomically resected liver with results of preoperative imaging. J Clin Gastroenterol 41:789–795

Chapter 4
The Colorectal Cancer Initiating Cell: Markers and Their Role in Liver Metastasis

Margot Zöller and Thorsten Jung

Abstract Colorectal cancer is one of the leading cancers in the Western world with a steadily increasing incidence. The most common site of metastasis is the liver, where the appearance of metastases strongly correlates with survival time and survival rates. After a brief overview on colorectal cancer and the metastatic process, this chapter will focus on the possible impact of the cancer initiating cell and the markers EpCAM and CD44 on metastasis formation. This will include a discussion on the importance of the tumor matrix and of exosomes in angiogenesis and in preparing the metastatic niche.

Keywords Colorectal cancer · Metastasis · Cancer-initiating cells · CD44 · EpCAM · Exosomes

Abbreviations

ALDH	aldehydedehydrogenase
ASC	adult stem cell
bFGF	basic fibroblast growth factor
C	complement component
CD44s/CD44v	CD44 standard/variant isoform
CEA	carcinoembryonic antigen
CIC	cancer initiating cell
CM	conditioned medium
CoCIC	colorectal cancer initiating cells
COX	cyclooxygenase
CRC	colorectal carcinoma
CXCR	CXC chemokine receptor
DJ-1	Parkinson disease protein-7
EC	endothelial cells
ECM	extracellular matrix

M. Zöller (✉)
Department of Tumor Cell Biology, University Hospital of Surgery, Im Neuenheimer Feld 365, D-69120 Heidelberg, Germany; German Cancer Research Centre, Heidelberg, Germany
e-mail: margot.zoeller@uni-heidelberg.de

P. Brodt (ed.), *Liver Metastasis: Biology and Clinical Management*, Cancer Metastasis – Biology and Treatment 16, DOI 10.1007/978-94-007-0292-9_4, © Springer Science+Business Media B.V. 2011

EGF/EGFR	epidermal growth factor/-receptor
EMT	epithelial-mesenchymal transition
EpCAM	epithelial cell adhesion molecule
ERM	ezrin, radixin, moesin
ESC	embryonic stem cell
FAK	focal adhesion kinase
FHL2	four and half LIM only
FGFR	fibroblast growth factor receptor
GEM	glycolipid-enriched membrane domain
GPCR	G-protein coupled receptor
HA	hyaluronan
HAS	HA synthase
HDGF	hepatoma-derived growth factor
HGF	hepatocyte growth factor
Hsp	heat shock protein
ICAM	intercellular adhesion molecule
IFN	interferon
IL	interleukin
JAK	Janus family kinases
MHC	major histocompatibility locus
MMP	matrix metalloproteinase
MT1-MMP	membrane type1 MMP
MVB	multivesicular body
PDGF/PDGFR	platelet-derived growth factor /-receptor
PDZ domain	named according to three proteins containing the domain (*PSD*-95, *D*isks-large, *ZO*1)
PGE2	prostaglandin E2
PI3K	phosphoinositol-3-kinase
PPAR	peroxisomal proliferator-activator receptor
PS2-NTF	presenilin-2 N-terminal fragment
Pten	phosphatase and tensin homolog
PTK	phosphotyrosine kinase
SC	stem cell
SDF-1	stromal-derived factor-1
SMA	smooth muscle actin
STAT	signal transducers and activators of transcription
TACE	TNFα converting enzyme
TGF/TGF-R	transforming growth factor/-receptor
TEM	tetraspanin-enriched membrane domain
TIMP	tissue inhibitor of MMP
TNF	tumor necrosis factor
uPA/uPAR	plasminogen activator/-receptor
VCAM	vascular cell adhesion molecule
VEGF/VEGFR	vascular endothelial growth factor/-receptor
Wnt	wingless

Contents

4.1 Colorectal Cancer and Metastasis

Colorectal cancer is one of the most frequent cancers in the Western World and the incidence is increasing in other countries [1–3]. The incidence is higher in men than women and it is mostly a disease of older age with a peak incidence between the 6th and 7th decades of life [4]. Though the death rate is modestly decreasing, mostly due to improved surgical intervention including for liver metastases, it is still a leading cause of mortality [5]. The survival and prognosis of patients depends on the stage of the tumor at the time of detection. Unfortunately, over 57% have regional or distant spread of their tumor at the time of diagnosis [6]. Colorectal cancer can disseminate by continuity, via the lymphatics or hematogeneously. In 12–41% of patients with colorectal cancer, tumor cells are found in the peritoneal cavity. Lymphatic spread starts from the small lymphatic vessels in the mucosa from where it proceeds to the lymphatics in the submucosa, finally reaching the mesenteric lymph nodes. Hematogeneous spread can occur subsequently to lymphatic spread, as a result of tumor cells invading preexisting vessels or utilizing the tumor vasculature [7–9]. Thus, abundant angiogenesis, crucial to supply the growing tumor with nutrients and oxygen also facilitates metastatic spread. Tumor vessels are frequently leaky, which allows the extravasation of plasma proteins that form a scaffold for newly migrating endothelial cells (EC) and facilitate initiation of thrombus formation and spontaneously occurring focal hemorrhages that can promote the arrest of isolated tumor cells and thereby metastasis formation [10].

According to the blood supply, colon cancer and upper rectum cancer metastasize via the venae mesenterica inferior or superior and the vena portae to the liver. Carcinomas of the lower rectum metastasize via the venae rectales media and inferior to the lung and can, via venal plexi and the venae vertebralis metastasize to the vertebrae. About 25% of colorectal carcinoma (CRC) patients have detectable liver metastases at the time of presentation and another 25% develop liver metastases, mostly within the first 2 years post surgery. The survival rate is closely related to the tumor burden. Patients with unilobular liver metastases have a median survival time of less than 24 months and for those with bilobular metastases, the mean survival time decreases to <18 months. With partial hepatectomy the 5 years survival rate increases to 35–40% [11, 12]. Therefore, detection of disseminated tumor cells in the liver could be helpful for prognosis. In colorectal cancer, disseminated tumor cells have been detected in 5–69% of samples in different studies. With the exception of 1 study, the presence of disseminated colorectal cancer cells correlated with prognosis [13]. Thus, it is essential to further improve the sensitivity and specificity of assays for the detection of disseminated tumor cells. Several methods can be used for the detection of disseminated tumor cells in the liver ex vivo. Immunohistology is based mainly on the detection of CEA (carcinoembryonic antigen), EpCAM (epithelial cell adhesion molecule) or cytokeratin 20 in liver specimens. The limitation of this approach is its reliance on a small number of liver sections. mRNA based studies frequently use the same markers and, in addition, guanylcyclase, which is expressed at the apical brush border of colonic cells [14–17]. To increase the sensitivity and to avoid false positive results, it has been proposed that multiple markers should be used simultaneously [14, 18–21]. Screening studies for disseminated colorectal cancer cells in the liver based on aberrant DNA have also been used and they mostly evaluate point mutations of K-ras and p53 and fragment length polymorphism. Though highly sensitive, the disadvantage of these analyses is that these mutations can be found in only 50% of the primary tumors. More recently the recovery of exosomes and of microRNA in body fluids was suggested as the most valuable, non-invasive diagnostic tool for different malignancies, including colorectal cancer [23–26].

4.2 Liver Metastases in Colorectal Cancer

The metastatic cascade is initiated by the epithelial-mesenchymal transition of cancer stem cells/cancer initiating cells [27–29]. The different steps of the metastatic cascade namely, detachment from the primary tumor, intravasation, extravasation, arrest and growth in distant organs, are well documented [7, 30–33]. Among the molecular mediators involved in tumor progression are cell-cell and cell-matrix adhesion molecules, matrix degrading enzymes and their inhibitors, chemotactic factors released from the degraded matrix or by host stromal and parenchymal cells and corresponding chemokine receptors expressed on the metastasizing tumor cells, as well as mediators of apoptosis resistance and inducers of angiogenesis [34–37].

The final step of the metastatic cascade, i.e. colonizing a "premetastatic organ" is a highly selective process, first described by Paget in his "seed and soil" hypothesis, postulating that a tumor cell may only settle in preferred compatible organs. Recently, evidence has been documented that the small population of cancer initiating cells (CIC) [38, 39] is also responsible for organizing a niche in the metastatic organ, possibly in advance of tumor cell arrival [39–41].

As outlined above, the liver, for anatomical and hemodynamic reasons, is the preferred metastatic site for colorectal cancer cells. In addition, the environment of the liver supports colorectal cancer cell arrest and growth.

The liver is a common site of arrest for tumor cell emboli carried by the blood. The liver filters the venous drainage from the majority of intra-abdominal organs including the colon and the upper part of the rectum. In addition, 30% of the cardiac output passes through the liver [42]. The hepatic microcirculation is slow and tortuous due to the anastomotic arrangement of networking sinusoidal capillaries within hepatic lobes and the control of blood flow by Kupffer and stellate cells [43]. Three features are particularly important considering the microcirculation in the liver. First, endothelial cells of hepatic sinusoids are fenestrated (150–175 nm) [44–46] and lack a diaphragm and a basal lamina shielding the vessel endothelium. These features greatly facilitate extravasation of tumor cells. Secondly, Kupffer cells, which are anchored in the periportal zone of the liver lobules and line hepatic sinusoids, express various surface oligosaccharides and cell adhesion proteins that support tumor cell adhesion. Kupffer cells also display recognition patterns for a variety of pathogen-associated molecular determinants [47–49]. In this context, it should also be mentioned that the liver contains relatively large resident populations of activated dendritic cells, mast cells, NK cells and T lymphocytes [50, 51]. This abundance of immune defense cells likely accounts for the fact that many solitary tumor cells, reaching the liver are eliminated and never form a metastasis. Thirdly, portal fibroblasts and liver sinusoidal stellate cells contribute to intratumoral stroma and blood vessel generation in response to tumor-derived factors, providing a favorable milieu for tumor cell survival and growth. Stellate cells are found within the space of Disse. They secrete matrix proteins and upon activation change to myofibroblasts [52–55]. In response to the appropriate stimuli, such as tumor cells or tumor cell conditioned medium, gene expression in the stellate cells is strikingly changed. Thus, close to 2000 genes were found to be differentially expressed in hepatic stellate cells in response to tumor cell conditioned medium [56]. Activated hepatic stellate cells display proangiogenic features. They secrete vascular endothelial growth factor (VEGF), and have an upregulated expression of cyclooxygenase (COX)-2 and prostaglandin (PG)-E2 that stimulate the hepatic sinusoidal endothelium [57]. Hepatic stellate cells also secrete stroma-derived factor (SDF)-1-a ligand of the chemokine receptor CXCR4 whose expression is increased in colorectal liver metastases as compared to the primary tumor [58] (For a more extensive discussion on the role of the hepatic stellate cells and of chemokine/chemokine receptor signaling in liver metastasis see Chapters 3 and 5, respectively in this volume).

The process of hepatic metastasis begins with the retention of circulating tumor cells in the microvasculature. Clumps of tumor cells may arrest in the proximal segments of sinusoids located in the periportal area of hepatic lobules [59–61]. Infiltrating cancer cells can also induce obstruction of affected sinusoidal segments, leading to a blockade of the blood flow and transient micro-infarcts [62]. Migrating cancer cells that arrest in the liver microvasculature adhere to the sinusoidal endothelium and Kupffer cells, where adhesion is promoted by inflammatory factors and reactive oxygen metabolites [63, 64]. E-selectin and vascular cell adhesion molecule (VCAM)-1 [65–68] are upregulated and a cytokine cascade with interleukin (IL)-1β, tumor necrosis factor (TNF)α and IL-18 is initiated, IL-1β and TNFα, in particular, promoting micrometastases formation [69–72]. The formation of these still avascular micrometastases is supported by the recruitment of stromal cells. Liver zonation is characterized by phenotypic diversity of hepatocytes and sinusoidal cells along the length of the sinusoid from the portal to the central vein [57, 73] and influenced by fenestration and differential expression of adhesion molecules [46, 74]. Recruitment of stromal cells is driven by tumor-released factors favoring migration and proliferation of stromal cells, perisinusoidal hepatic stellate cells, portal fibroblasts and hepatocytes. The stromal cells are then activated in a paracrine fashion by tumor-derived growth factors and this results in the establishment of a proangiogenic stroma in the periportal areas [57, 75]. Hepatic stellate cells that migrate in response to tumor factors differentiate into myofibroblasts [55, 76, 77]. Stellate cell-derived myofibroblasts secrete VEGF, platelet-derived growth factor (PDGF) and transforming growth factor (TGF)β. Thus, the angiogenic phase of a liver metastasis greatly depends on the myofibroblasts that assume the function of pericytes in other organs [78]. In addition, it is well documented that these cells display tumor promoting activity [79–81]. Finally, it should be mentioned that fibrotic capsule formation can be observed in colorectal cancer liver metastases and is thought to be an indicator of good prognosis. However, the capsule consists of myofibroblasts (stellate cells) and α-SMA$^+$ (smooth muscle actin) cells that secrete collagen I and the metalloproteinases (MMP)-1 and -2 and tissue inhibitor of metalloproteinases (TIMP)-1. The fibrotic capsule could therefore also support infiltration and destruction of the surrounding tissue through the release of extracellular matrix (ECM) degrading proteinases, and the prognostic significance of the fibrotic stromal response remains therefore to be clarified [82] (For a more extensive discussion of the role of the stroma in liver metastasis, see Chapter 3 in this volume).

In summary, in addition to anatomical considerations, hemodynamic factors also facilitate the arrest and invasion of dispersed tumor cells in the liver. These include a sluggish blood flow, fenestration of the vessel endothelium and the differentiation of stellate cells into myofibroblasts that can secrete chemoattractants and angiogenesis-promoting factors all acting in concert to promote metastasis.

4.3 Molecular Features of Metastasis Formation: Cancer Initiating Cell Markers

4.3.1 Definition of Cancer Initiating Cells (CIC)

There is compelling evidence that tumors contain a small population of CIC [38, 39, 83]. These cells are functionally defined by their high potency to regenerate cancer in xenograft models, and their capacity to initiate metastatic growth [84], recapitulate the heterogeneity of the parental tumor at a secondary site [85] and form metastases after prolonged periods of tumor dormancy [86]. CIC have the ability for self renewal and differentiation, are drug resistant and likely require a niche for growth [87–89]. In addition to their functional definition, CIC are also defined by so called "CIC markers" [85, 90, 91]. CIC can be enriched from primary tumors by soft agar cloning, spheroid growth [92], selection for cells expressing CIC markers

[85] and enzymatic markers such as aldehyde dehydrogenase (ALDH) [93] or by Hoechst 33342 dye efflux. Cells that rapidly extrude dyes such as Hoechst 33342, the so called "side population", have been found to share with CIC the tumor initiating capacity, expression of stem-like genes and chemotherapeutic drug resistance [94].

CIC share many features with embryonic (ESC) and adult (ASC) stem cells, including signaling pathways that regulate "stemness" versus those that induce differentiation [95, 96], including gene expression profiles that point to a major role for (among others) cell adhesion, matrix interactions and wingless/int-1 (Wnt-1), Janus family kinases/signal transducers and activators of transcription (JAK/STAT) and focal adhesion kinase (FAK) signaling [97]. Thus, CD44 is a hematopoietic stem cell maker and a leukemia initiating cell marker. Accordingly, a blockade of CD44 induces hematopoietic stem cell mobilization [98] and interferes with the embedding of leukemia initiating cells into their niche [99]. CXCR4, expressed on embryonic and adult stem cells of different organs [100–102], as well as on several tumor cell types [103] and its ligand SDF-1 are crucial for hematopoietic stem cell and tumor cell migration. SDF-1 is secreted by stroma and endothelial cells and attracts hematopoietic progenitor cells [104], circulating, tissue-committed stem cells [100] and metastasizing tumor cells [105–107]. HGF/c-Met interactions drive mobilization and emigration of stem cells in the embryo and the adult and high level c-Met expression on many carcinoma cells is important for tumor cell migration and metastases formation. The HGF–c-Met axis is also involved in angiogenesis through HGF expression in mesenchymal stem cells that participate in the process [108–110]. β-catenin is also a key player in stem cell homing/mobilization and in metastasis [111]. Upon activation, β-catenin translocates to the nucleus and interacts with the Tcf/Lef (high motility group box containing transcription factors) complex that in turn, transcriptionally activates cell cycle related genes such as cyclin *D1* and *c-Myc* [112].

While these findings highlight the high degree of similarity between ESC, ASC and CIC [95, 113], relatively little is known about the function of the CIC markers, and even less about the CIC niche. Herein, we will discuss in some detail what is known about the functional contribution of colorectal CIC (CoCIC) markers and how the activities they mediate may facilitate the establishment of the pre-metastatic niche.

4.3.2 Colorectal CIC markers

As alluded to earlier, CIC are characterized not only on the basis of the functional criteria described above but also by defined cell surface markers. Many of these markers are shared with ASC [95, 96], suggesting that they are functionally involved in CIC activity. Colorectal CIC (CoCIC) are EpCAM-, CD44-, CD166-and, possibly CD133-positive [114–117]. These markers are also expressed by other tumors. For example, CD133 is expressed by glioblastoma, prostate cancer, breast and bladder carcinomas. CD166 has been described as a CIC marker of malignant melanoma and is also, together with CD29, CD44 and CD105, a marker of mesenchymal stem cells [118–120]. CD166 is a type I transmembrane protein belonging to the Ig superfamily that mediates homophilic and heterophilic cell-cell adhesion [118]. Because (surprisingly) little is presently known about its potential functions as a CIC marker, this chapter will focus on the better characterized CoCIC markers namely, CD44 and EpCAM that are also expressed in other malignancies. CD44 is a CIC marker in leukemia, prostate, breast and pancreatic cancer. Breast and pancreatic cancer share with CoCIC also the expression of EpCAM, which, in addition, is detected in CIC of ovarian and hepatocellular cancer [115, 116, 121, 122, rev. in 91, 123–126]. Because CIC account for the capacity of a tumor to form metastases, the question arises as to whether and how CIC markers are involved.

4.3.2.1 The CoCIC Marker EpCAM and Claudin-7

EpCAM is expressed on most human epithelial cells [127] and in parallel to its distribution in non-transformed tissue, nearly all carcinoma, as well as myeloma cells express EpCAM [127–133]. EpCAM expression is actually increased in carcinoma cells as compared to non-transformed tissue and is strongly upregulated, among others, in CIC of colorectal cancer.

EpCAM is a type I transmembrane molecule with an epidermal growth factor (EGF)-like domain, followed by a thyroglobulin repeat domain [134], a cystein poor region, a transmembrane domain and a short cytoplasmic tail [135]. Both the EGF-like repeat and the thyroglobulin domain form a globular structure and are required for EpCAM-mediated homophilic cell-cell adhesion. The EGF-like domain is required for the reciprocal cell-cell interaction and the thyroglobulin-like domain for the lateral interaction of EpCAM molecules. Both domains are involved in anchoring the actin microfilaments to the cell membrane via α-actinin, a process regulated by the cytoplasmic tail of EpCAM [136]. Thyroglobulin domains are known to inhibit cathepsins. Whether EpCAM serves as a protease inhibitor, to protect tumor cell products from degradation is unknown.

Based on its function, EpCAM could be expected to prevent metastases formation [137]. However, it was shown to be involved in the abrogation of E-cadherin-mediated cell-cell adhesion by disrupting the link between β-catenin and F-actin [129, 138], and in this capacity could promote tumor progression [139]. Moreover, EpCAM was implicated in signal transduction mediating cell motility [140, 141] – a requirement for metastases formation. EpCAM-induced up-regulation of *c-myc* supports cell proliferation via up-regulated synthesis of cyclin A and E [142, 143] and it was also shown to upregulate epidermal fatty acid binding protein (E-FABP) expression. Upregulated E-FABP has been described in several cancers to correlate with poor survival. FABPs are involved in transporting fatty acids into the cell and cooperate with the PPAR (peroxisome proliferator-activated receptor) nuclear receptors that regulate the transcription of many genes. The molecular mechanisms whereby FABPs contribute to tumor progression are unknown [144]. The phenotype of EpCAM transgenic mice, where EpCAM is over-expressed in mammary glands and this is linked to increased Bcl-2 and Ki67 expression, also supports a role for this molecule in mutagenic signaling [145]. Cross-linking of EpCAM triggers cleavage of its intracellular peptide and this requires the cooperative activity of TACE (TNFα converting enzyme, ADAM17) and PS2-NTF (presenilin 2 N-terminal fragment). The cleaved peptide, termed EpIC, then forms a complex with β-catenin, FHL2 (*f*our-and-*h*alf-*L*IM-only) and Lef-1 that translocates to the nucleus and initiates transcription of *c-myc* by binding to LEF consensus sites [146]. This contribution to the activation of Wnt signaling may be one major aspect of the functional relevance of the marker EpCAM to the CIC phenotype.

An additional feature of EpCAM is likely important to its functional activity as a CIC marker. In metastasizing colon and pancreatic cancer tissues and lines, EpCAM is associated with claudin-7. The family of claudins comprises 24 members of 20–33 kDa. Claudins are 4-transmembrane domain proteins. The C-terminal domain has several potential phosphorylation sites and a PDZ (named according to *P*SD-95, *D*isks-large, *Z*O-1, which contain this motif) binding motif [147]. Originally, claudins have been described as components of tight junctions, membrane domains with close contact to neighboring cells [148] that provide a barrier to intercellular diffusion of solutions and separate the apical from the basolateral membrane regions [149]. The importance of claudins for the maintenance of the epithelial barrier has been well documented [150]. Claudin-1$^{-/-}$ mice die postnatally due to dehydration [151]. The loss of cell polarity in epithelial tumors is frequently accompanied by alterations in claudin expression [152, 153]. In breast cancer, the loss of claudin-7 correlates with dedifferentiation [154]. However, in some cell types, claudins are also detected as diffusely distributed in the basolateral membranes, a phenomenon first described for claudin-7 [155, 156]. This suggests that claudins are not involved only in the maintenance of barriers. In fact, similar to EpCAM, claudin-7 increases TCF/LEF activity and tumorigenicity of colorectal cancer cells [157]. These additional functions of claudins are not well defined [155, 156], but could well contribute to tumor progression.

Claudins have conserved dicystein palmitoylation motifs [158]. Palmitoylated claudins are partitioned into glycolipid-enriched membrane microdomains, where they interact with cytosolic scaffold proteins, forming a platform for the recruitment of signal transducing molecules and a linkage to the cytoskeleton [159]. Furthermore, tight junctions are constantly remodeled by endocytosis [160]. Internalized tight junction proteins/claudins enter the early endosomes but are not recovered from late and recycling endosomes or the Golgi. Thus, there seems to be a distinct storage compartment for these proteins that co-localizes with syntaxin 4 [161]. Claudin endocytosis is enhanced by claudin phosphorylation [162] and claudin phosphorylation negatively regulates their integration into tight junctions [163]. Although it has originally been speculated that epithelial-mesenchymal transition (EMT) is accompanied and facilitated by down-regulation of claudins [164, 165], the above-cited findings indicate that claudins could actively support EMT transition. Namely, in addition to the documented regulation of EMT by claudin-1 through Wnt/β-catenin signaling [166], claudin internalization and, as outlined below, the recovery in exosomes, may also contribute to the metastatic process.

In line with the suggested regulatory activities of claudin-7 are the observations that in colorectal cancer, claudin-7 expression is up-regulated and that phosphorylated claudin-7 associates with EpCAM. The association of EpCAM with claudin-7 is accompanied by relocation of EpCAM into tetraspanin-enriched membrane microdomains (TEM), where the EpCAM-claudin-7 complex associates with the tetraspanins Tspan8 and CD44v6. When correlating co-expression and complex formation of these molecules with clinical variables and chemotherapeutic drug resistance, co-expression and complex formation in TEM inversely correlates with disease-free survival. Claudin-7 is the essential partner for complex formation, because EpCAM does not co-localize or co-immunoprecipitate with CD44v6 and Tspan8 in tumors with low claudin-7 expression. Thus, it is not the expression of the individual molecules, but rather the EpCAM-claudin-7-Tspan8-CD44v6 complex that is decisive for metastatic progression [167].

Because complex formation is similar in primary tumors and metastases and does not vary within different regions of the primary tumor, it is tempting to speculate that the presence of this complex may provide a survival advantage to the isolated tumor cell that has left the primary tumor rather than directly support tumor progression. Indeed, expression of EpCAM and claudin-7 promotes proliferation, which is, in turn accompanied by an increase in ERK1/2 phosphorylation. Cells expressing all four molecules are highly apoptosis-resistant while apoptosis resistance is strongly reduced in cell lines devoid of anyone of the four molecules [168, 169], or upon TEM destruction by partial cholesterol depletion [167]. Apoptosis resistance is accompanied by Akt and BAD phosphorylation and up-regulation of bcl-2 and bcl-Xl expression. Thus, EpCAM-claudin-7 complex formation and recruitment into TEM supports activation of the mitochondrial pathway of apoptosis resistance [170]. Furthermore, homophilic cell-cell adhesion of EpCAM molecules that requires lateral tetramer formation, is inhibited by the association of EpCAM with claudin-7, and the inhibition of cell-cell adhesion results in turn, in increased cell motility [170]. Inhibition of EpCAM-mediated cell-cell adhesion and support of cell motility are also favorable to CIC dispersion from the primary tumor tissue and thereby to metastasis.

In summary, the CIC marker EpCAM, originally described as a cell-cell adhesion molecule, has been identified as a major player in the Wnt signaling pathway. Through its association with claudin-7, it is recruited into TEM, where it associates with tetraspanins and CD44 (Fig. 4.1). TEM are known as signaling platforms prone for internalization. As outlined below, the latter may become important for the recruitment of EpCAM into exosomes and the exosomal crosstalk with the stroma in metastatic organs.

4.3.2.2 The Contribution of CD44 to the Metastatic Process

The lymphocyte homing receptor CD44 attracted considerable interest when it was first shown that the CD44 splice variants (CD44v) suffice to confer a metastatic phenotype onto locally growing tumor cells [171]. The importance of CD44v in tumor progression has since been convincingly demonstrated in many types of cancer [172,

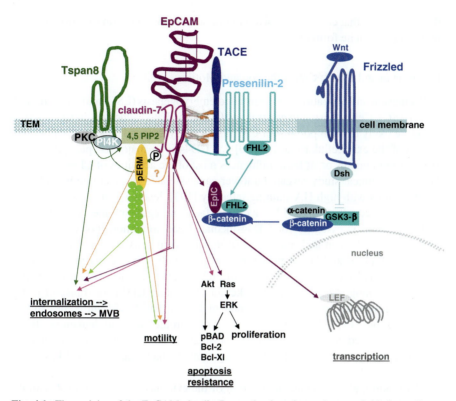

Fig. 4.1 The activity of the EpCAM-claudin-7 complex in colorectal cancer initiating cells – a proposed model. In colorectal cancer, the cleaved cytoplasmic tail of EpCAM (EpIC) forms a complex with β-catenin, FHL2 (*four-and-half-LIM-only*) and Lef-1, which relocates to the nucleus and initiates transcription of *c-myc* by binding to LEF consensus sites. Claudin-7, which is associated with EpCAM, also increases TCF/LEF activity. Furthermore, phosphorylated claudin-7 recruits EpCAM into tetraspanin-enriched membrane microdomains that are prone for internalization

173]. More recently, CD44 has been described as a CIC marker on leukemia and carcinoma cells, including colorectal cancer [114, 121, 174–178]. The functional contribution of CD44 as a CIC marker has not yet been defined.

CD44 comprises a family of glycoproteins encoded by a single gene [179]. The CD44 glycoproteins vary in size due to N- and O-glycosylation and insertion of alternatively spliced variable exon products in the extracellular domains of the molecule [180]. Unlike the rather ubiquitously expressed standard isoform (CD44s), CD44v expression is restricted to some epithelial cells and it is transiently expressed during embryonic development and during lymphocyte maturation and activation. In addition, mounting evidence suggests aberrant expression of CD44v in many tumors including colorectal carcinoma, where it confers metastatic potential resulting in poor prognosis [181–186]. CD44v upregulation appears to be an early event and requires adenomatous polyposis coli gene inactivation [187–189]. While CD44 can mediate multiple activities [33, 171–173], the discussion below will focus on those functions that could be involved in tumor cell crosstalk with the stroma and in premetastatic niche formation.

Hyaluronan and CD44: Cell Adhesion and Motility

Cell adhesion and migration are essential to embryogenesis (ESC) and tissue remodeling (ASC). Cell adhesion in general and CD44-mediated adhesion, in particular, is therefore likely to be important for CIC function. Hyaluronan (HA) is a major component of the extracellular matrix [190] and CD44 is its major receptor [191, 192]. HA binding initiates or, at least, influences most of the activities of CD44. In fact, a large-scale clinical study revealed a lower cancer-related survival rate in Duke's C and D tumors with high HA staining intensity [193], leading to the hypothesis that CD44-mediated adhesion to HA is a critical factor in regulating metastasis [194].

HA binding is essential for CD44-mediated cell migration. For example, the most primitive human and mouse hematopoietic stem cells (HSC) synthesize and express HA [195] and HA expression correlates with selective migration of HSC to the endosteal niche [195, 196]. Accordingly, CD44 also accounts for leukemic stem cell homing. Acute myeloid leukemia SC require CD44 for transport to the stem cell-supportive microenvironmental niche and anti-CD44 antibodies induce differentiation [197]. In a mouse model of chronic myeloid leukemia, BCR-ABL1-transduced progenitors from CD44-mutant donors are defective in bone marrow homing, resulting in decreased engraftment and impaired CML-like disease induction [198].

HA binding also promotes interaction of the cytoplasmic tail of CD44 with the cytoskeleton via ankyrin [199] and members of the ERM (Ezrin/Radixin/Moesin) family [200, 201]. The interaction of CD44 with ERM proteins is regulated by ERM protein phosphorylation, such that only phosphorylated ERM proteins are in a configuration that allows CD44 as well as actin binding, thereby linking CD44 to the cytoskeleton [202]. By its interaction with the actin cytoskeleton, CD44 is guided to the leading edge of the migrating cells and becomes involved in cell motility [203, 204].

HA binding of CD44 may also become important for extravasation of CIC. HA is bound to endothelial cells through CD44, and proinflammatory cytokines that stimulate CD44 expression strengthen HA binding to EC [205, 206]. Both leukocyte extravasation and tumor cell dissemination are facilitated by binding to EC-associated HA [207]. Furthermore, MMP-2 and MMP-9 production is stimulated by the interaction between HA and CD44 [208, 209]. The HA – CD44 interaction promotes MMP-9 binding to the ectodomain of CD44, a process facilitating invasion, TGF-β processing and angiogenesis [209]. MMP-7 binds via the heparan sulfate side chain of CD44 and cleaves heparin binding growth factors, which is a prerequisite for their activation as shown for HER4 in mammary epithelial cells. [210, 211].

Finally, CD44 also contributes to the storage function of the extracellular/peritumoral matrix. The proteoglycan CD44 binds several cytokines and chemokines [212, 213] such as interferon (IFN)γ [214], osteopontin [215],

hepatocyte growth factor/scatter factor (HGF) [216], basic fibroblast growth factor (bFGF) [217], VEGF [218], heparin binding factor [219], MIP-1β [220] and
RANTES [221] and this in turn, can have significant functional consequences for
the HA-providing cell. Binding of bFGF in the developing limb stimulates proliferation of the underlying mesenchymal cells [222]. Similar mechanisms are involved
in the uretric buds and mammary gland development [210]. CD44 binding to osteopontin leads to signals that stimulate activation of PI3-kinase and Akt, promoting
cell survival [223], while HGF binding provides the initiating signal for c-Met
autophosphorylation and activation [224, 225].

These data collectively show that CD44 through its interaction with HA plays
an important role in organogenesis, hematopoiesis and tumor progression. Beyond
its role in adhesion/migration, the impact of this interaction is due to the function
of HA-containing matrix as a reservoir of growth factors, like HGF and hepatoma-
derived growth factor (HDGF) and matrix degrading enzymes, like uPA, several
metalloproteinases, serine peptidases, the dipeptidase CD13 and others that can
trigger CD44-initiated signal transduction [33, 131, 226] (Fig. 4.2).

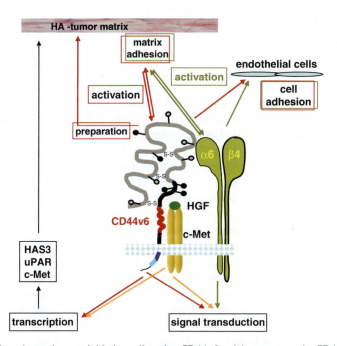

Fig. 4.2 The colorectal cancer initiating cell marker CD44v6 and the tumor matrix. CD44 supports
the assembly of a tumor matrix that promotes adhesion and migration of tumor cells via CD44v6
or α6β4 integrin binding. Because of its interaction with HA, this matrix also has an enhanced
storage capacity for adhesion molecules, chemokines, growth factors and metalloproteinases and
this promotes signal transduction. In an autocrine feedback loop, the matrix initiates CD44v6, c-
Met and α6β4 activation. Upon activation, CD444v6 and c-Met can mediate c-Met, HAS3 and
uPAR transcription and this further supports the assembly of a matrix

CD44-Initiated Signal Transduction

Though CD44 has no catalytic activity, it can initiate signal transduction via associated transmembrane kinases, such as the family of ErbB receptor tyrosine kinases [110, 222, 227] or via interaction of the cytoplasmic tail with non-receptor tyrosine kinases and cytoskeleton linker proteins [199–201]. By interacting with other transmembrane proteins devoid of catalytic activity [33, 172], CD44 can also gain access to signal transduction pathways mediated by protein partners [228].

CD44 can directly associate with receptor tyrosine kinases such as TFGβ receptor(R)I and fibroblast growth factor receptor (FGFR) [229] or through their ligands as is the case with c-Met binding via CD44v3-bound HGF, an important mechanism in colorectal cancer tumorigenesis [230]. CD44v6-initiated c-Met activation via HGF binding requires an interaction of CD44 with ERM proteins [231]. As revealed by haploinsufficiency of c-Met in CD44$^{-/-}$ mice, these interactions are vital, as these mice die at birth due to defects in synaptogenesis and axon myelination [232]. Recruitment of similar complexes has also been described for human cancer, where CD44 upon HA binding recruits a complex of ErbB2, ezrin, PI3K (phosphoinositol-3-kinase), Hsp90 and cdc37 that promotes ErbB2 activation [233]. Thus, CD44 efficiently initiates a cross-talk between receptor and non-receptor tyrosine kinases/linker proteins [234].

Among the non-receptor kinases that function as CD44 partners, the src family of protein tyrosine kinases (PTK) are of particular importance [235]. PTKs play a central role as membrane-attached molecular switches linking a variety of extracellular signals to crucial intracellular signaling pathways [236]. This is facilitated by their location in glycolipid-enriched membrane microdomains (GEM or TEM), providing a scaffold for cytoskeletal linker proteins, adaptors and signal transducing molecules [237]. The variability in CD44-initiated signal transduction depends, at least in part, on the CD44 location in GEM, which varies depending on the state of activation and the association with ERM proteins [238–241]. It is important to note in this context that the CD44v6/matrix interaction is reciprocal. While CD44v6 contributes to matrix assembly, the matrix can, in turn contribute to signal transduction in the metastasizing cell, thereby enhancing motility and apoptosis-resistance. This reciprocal effect can, but may not always proceed directly via CD44v6. We recently demonstrated that it can also be initiated via CD44v-associated molecules. Thus, migration and apoptosis resistance can be promoted by CD44v6-HA binding, but also by c-Met via CD44v6-bound HGF or via the interaction of laminin with α6β4, which in GEM/TEM is CD44v6-associated. Migration proceeds through ERM proteins that link CD44v to the cytoskeleton and through the integrin- and c-Met-mediated association of CD44v with the focal adhesion kinase (FAK). Apoptosis resistance is jointly initiated via activation of the PI3-K and the MAPK pathways downstream of signals that are initiated by the CD44v-α6β4-c-Met complex and converge downstream of CD44v (Zöller et al, unpublished finding).

The link between CD44v6 expression, metastatic progression and a poor prognosis in colorectal cancer [242–244] may indeed be due to the involvement of CD44v6

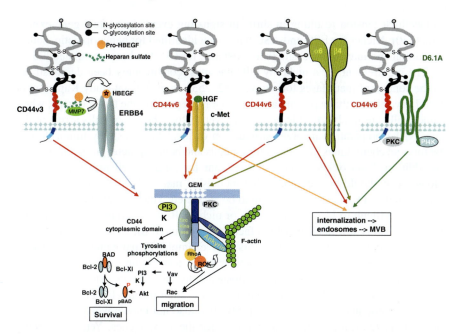

Fig. 4.3 The colorectal cancer initiating cell marker CD44v6 coordinates signal transduction of associated molecules. In colorectal cancer initiating cells CD44v6 associates with receptor tyrosine kinases as well as α6β4. Upon activation, CD44v6 also associates with Src, ankyrin and ERM proteins that are activated (phosphorylated) and bind to actin. Activation of FAK, the PI3K/Akt pathway and the MAPK pathway can be initiated equally well by a CD44v6-dependent matrix, HA, HGF or laminin5. Irrespective of the initiating stimulus, signals converge downstream of CD44. The activated complex is recruited into TEM/GEM, where similarly to the EpCAM-claudin-7 complex, it is internalized together with tetraspanins

in the delivery and assembly of a matrix that in a feedback loop, further promotes tumor cell motility and strengthens apoptosis resistance via CD44v6 and associated molecules (Fig. 4.3). The CD44v6-dependent tumor matrix may also contribute to the communication between the tumor cells and the metastatic niche (see below).

CD44v6-Dependent Matrix Assembly

As early as in 1978, it has been proposed that maintenance of stem cells (SC) requires a niche [245]. The SC niche provides the external control for survival, self-renewal and differentiation of SC through local and systemic signals [246]. The SC niche is a dynamic microenvironment that responds to local and systemic cues, ultimately influencing SC fate [247]. It is composed of extracellular matrix proteins that provide structural, organizational and mechanical cues, stromal cells, soluble factors, blood vessels and several neural inputs [248]. Supporting cells residing in the local microenvironment of SC affect their fate by direct contact, secreted factors and ECM proteins [249]. Perturbation in the matrix can alter cell shape and intracellular tension resulting in shifts in signaling events that affect gene expression [250]. Niches for ESC and ASC have been identified for hematopoietic, neural, epidermal and intestinal SC and their existence for CIC has been postulated [251].

The requirement for a niche by CIC has most convincingly been demonstrated in the context of metastases formation [252, 253]. In an elegant study Kaplan et al. [254] have shown that a pre-metastatic niche is prepared in the target organs, where tumor cells are likely to settle and grow, even before the tumor cells arrive at this site. Niche preparation involves stimulation of local fibroblasts by tumor-derived factors and chemokines that attract tumor cells and hematopoietic progenitors [254]. In addition, lysyl oxidase may be important for marrow cell recruitment [255]. However, it should be mentioned that models of mammalian SC niches are often provisional and key questions remain to be answered. Thus, unlike flies and worms, it is very difficult to identify stem cells or niche cells with certainty in mammalian tissue. It also is still unclear, which factors are required for stem cell maintenance and which cells produce these factors. For example, hematopoietic SC survival relies on an endosteal and/or perivascular niche and requires SDF-1 that is also expressed by both perivascular and endosteal cells. In addition, osteoblasts as well as perivascular mesenchymal progenitors express angiopoietin-1 – a factor that regulates hematopoietic SC quiescence [256]. It is also not known whether ESC/ASC and CIC have different niches or compete for the same niches. Yet, the selective depletion of leukemic SC by anti-CD44 provided evidence that it is, at least, possible to selectively drive CIC out of their niche [105].

Our findings that (i) a CD44v6 knockdown in metastatic tumor cells prevents metastases formation, (ii) CD44v6 is essential for assembling a matrix that allows tumor cell adhesion and (iii) the matrix provides signals that promote tumor cell motility and enhance apoptosis resistance, raised the possibility that the CD44v6-dependent matrix may also contribute to the tumor-induced stromal reaction including the "conditioning" of the premetastatic organ.

Our results confirmed, in fact, that this was the case. When rats received conditioned medium (CM) of a metastasizing pancreatic adenocarcinoma line (ASML^{wt}) in advance of an intrafootpad inoculation of poorly metastatic CD44v4-v7 or CD44v6/v7 knockdown of these cells (ASML-CD44v^{kd}), recruitment of ASML-CD44v^{kd} cells to the draining lymph nodes and lung colonization were strikingly accelerated. A search for "niche-like" structures and characteristic gene expression profiles in lymph nodes and lung revealed a marked upregulation of SDF1, CD31 and CD54 expression, pronounced CD49c, VEGFR1, VEGFR2, MMP9, MMP13 and uPAR expression and clusters of CD49d$^+$ and CD11b$^+$ cells in advance of tumor cell arrival [257]. These findings provide strong evidence that ASML^{wt} CM initiated a process of (pre)metastatic niche preparation.

To further define which subfraction of the CM promoted lymph node and the lung colonization by ASML-CD44v^{kd} cells we separated the matrix from exosomes that are known to support metastases formation [258, 259] and induce angiogenesis at distant sites [260–263]. Separating exosomes from the matrix revealed an essential contribution by the exosomes in preparing the (pre)metastatic niche, but also showed that the exosomes required the contribution of the soluble matrix to exert this effect. As the assembly of this exosome-supporting matrix depended on CD44v6 expression, the underlying mechanism(s) was of interest.

We found that a CD44v-knockdown was accompanied by a greatly reduced expression of HA synthase 3 (HAS3) an enzyme known to promote the malignant phenotype in many types of tumors [264]. Reduced expression of HAS3 in ASML-CD44v^{kd} cells resulted in turn, in a reduced recovery of HA. On the other hand, however, expression of hyaluronidase-1 in these cells increased, possibly accounting for the recovery of shorter HA molecules in the ASML-CD44v^{kd} matrix. Since key functions of HA vary considerably with length [226], the altered balance between HAS3 and hyaluronidase levels could well have contributed to the observed inefficiency of ASML-CD44v^{kd} matrix in supporting niche preparation.

Moreover, the knockdown of CD44v also had significant consequences on c-Met and uPAR expression. Thus, in the absence of CD44v6, c-Met stimulation was hampered resulting in reduced transcription of c-Met regulated genes, including c-Met itself [265]. Plasminogen activator receptor (uPAR) transcription is known to be regulated by c-Met [265, 266] and therefore downregulation of c-Met can affect uPAR levels. In addition HA binding to CD44 was also shown to regulate uPAR transcription [267] and the absence of CD44v6 can therefore directly contribute to uPAR down-regulation. In fact, we observed that uPAR was strongly down-regulated in ASML^{kd} cells. UPAR is involved in uPA binding/plasminogen activation and associates with several integrins, epidermal growth factor receptor (EGFR), PDGFR, caveolin and vitronectin, thereby initiating signal transduction via FAK, Src, Akt, ERK and ras [268]. Thus, uPAR could contribute to (pre)metastatic niche preparation by harboring uPA [257] and/or by binding to integrins or EGFR and initiating signal transduction. In ASML^{wt} cells, CD44v6, c-Met and uPAR co-immunoprecipitate upon treatment with a chemical cross-linker, and CD44 cross-linking by HA induces c-Met activation (unpublished findings). The reduction in HAS3 levels could therefore contribute to reduced c-Met and uPAR induction through reduced HA-c-Met interaction (Fig. 4.2).

Other molecules, whose recovery in the ASML-CD44v^{kd} matrix was greatly reduced were complement component (C)3 [255], several proteases that could well influence matrix assembly such as dipeptidases and MMPs (unpublished findings) and the hepatoma-derived growth factor (HDGF) that can stimulates the growth of fibroblasts, endothelial cells and vascular smooth muscle cells, promote angiogenesis, increase invasion, protect cells from apoptosis and recruit mesenchymal stem cells [269–271]. Strong differences were also observed in the expression of vimentin, enolase-1, clusterin, ECM protein-1, and DJ-1 (Parkinson disease protein-7). These molecules could all contribute to tumor cell communication with the stroma and to metastasis. Thus, clusterin is a prosurvival chaperon-like molecule and in its soluble form can influence chemokine secretion and initiate stromal changes that affect intercellular communication [272]. ECM protein-1 is a secreted glycoprotein that interacts with perlecan, fibulin-1C/D and MMP-9 and can interfere with angiogenesis [273]. DJ-1 is a negative regulator of the tumor suppressor gene PTEN (phosphatase and tensin homolog) and thereby controls PI3K signaling and cell survival [274]. Finally, the loss of the anaphylatoxin C3a [275] and the

CD11b ligand C3b [276] could affect the recruitment of host cells [255]. Though the global relevance of molecular changes induced by altered CD44v6 expression remains to be explored, our findings convincingly demonstrate that via CD44v6 the matrix can provide tumor cells with signals that are advantageous for survival and growth, while also potentially affecting the host stroma and premetastatic niche preparation.

In summary, CD44 has been defined as a CIC marker in colorectal cancer. While it has not been determined whether CIC express CD44s (standard) or CD44v isoforms, there is strong evidence that in colorectal cancer CD44v6 rather than CD44s plays a more dominant role. This is due to multifaceted function of this molecule. It promotes cell and matrix adhesion and is engaged in assembly of a matrix with optimized storage capacities. Although devoid of a catalytic domains, CD44v6 can mediate signal transduction through its association with receptor and cytosolic tyrosine kinases and cytoskeletal linker proteins. Importantly, CD44v6, via signals from the matrix, can induce a milieu that is conducive to remodeling of the surrounding tissue stroma thereby potentially providing niche functions to CIC/solitary tumor cells.

4.4 Exosomes and Metastasis

When metastasizing to distant sites, tumor cells typically require a "prepared environment" in order to successfully implant and grow [41]. As mentioned above, we have shown that that preparation of the host stroma for the successful embedding and growth of solitary tumor cells requires exosomes as well as the tumor matrix [257]. Exosomes recently received attention as possibly the most powerful intercellular communicator and gene delivery vehicle [258, 259, 260]. They are important during embryogenesis [277] and in immunity [261, 278, 279]. They also contribute to tumor angiogenesis [262, 263] and metastatic niche formation [22, 258, 259, 280, 281].

4.4.1 The Exosomes – Origin, Properties and Function

Exosomes are small 30–100 nm vesicles [282] that are derived from multivesicular bodies (MVB) that fuse with the plasma membrane and release their intraluminal vesicles [283]. Many cells release exosomes, but release is most abundant in tumor cells [282]. Exosomes harbor a common set of membrane and cytosolic molecules that include tetraspanins, integrins, intercellular adhesion molecules (ICAM), major histocompatibility (MHC) molecules, molecules associated with vesicle transport, Hsp, cytoskeletal proteins, signal transduction molecules, enzymes and other cell type-specific components [284]. A proteome analysis of immunoaffinity-purified exosomes derived from a colon cancer line revealed, molecules such as cadherin-17, CEA, mucin 13, keratin 18 and enrichment of EpCAM as well as claudins 1, 3 and 7 [26]. Notably, exosomal proteins maintain their functional activities [285] that in turn depend on the exosome origin. Thus, exosomes derived from antigen presenting cells initiate an immune response by their capacity to present peptides in the context of MHC class I and II molecules [286]. In contrast, tumor-derived exosomes suppress immune reactions [287]. Exosomes also contain mRNA and miRNA, which can be transferred to the target cell, where the mRNA can be translated and the miRNA mediate RNA silencing [288–292]. Thus, exosomes can stimulate target cells by binding and by the transfer of membrane receptors, bioactive lipids, mRNA and miRNA [22].

Two features of exosomes suggest that the constitutive recovery of tetraspanins may be of functional importance. First, although the molecular composition of exosomes reflects their origin [293], the relative abundance of proteins differs between exosomes and donor cells. This implies active sorting into MVB [294], which for proteins can be achieved, among others, by localization in cholesterol-rich membrane microdomains, or higher order oligomerization [295, 296]. Secondly, in view of the strong impact that exosomes can have on their target cells, it becomes important that exosomes only interact with selected target cells [278, 283]. The mode of exosome – target cell interactions has not been unequivocally defined. Receptor-ligand interactions [258], attachment, fusion [297, 298] and internalization [299] have been proposed. These processes are not necessarily mutually exclusive [285]. In fact, the selectivity of exosome-target cell interactions indicates that the initial step involves a receptor ligand interaction. For the reasons outlined below, both the selective recruitment of proteins into exosomes and the selective delivery of exosomes could be facilitated by tetraspanins.

Tetraspanins are a family of 34 proteins that span the membrane four times [169, 300–302]. They are organized in TEM. Within TEM, tetraspanins form a network that consists of other tetraspanins and additional transmembrane and intracellular membrane-proximal signaling proteins [303, 304]. The most prominent non-tetraspanin transmembrane partners are the integrins [305]. Tetraspanins also associate with growth factor receptors [306, 307], G protein coupled receptors (GPCR) and their intracellular associated heterotrimeric G-proteins [308], several peptidases [302], Ig superfamily members and, importantly, in colorectal cancer the CIC markers CD44 and EpCAM [115, 309–311]. Notably, though TEM are raft-independent membrane microdomains [169, 312], they are, similarly to rafts prone for internalization [313] a process that for some tetraspanins can become facilitated by a tyrosine-based sorting motif [304, 314]. In fact, the two tetraspanins associated with the metastatic process, CD151 and Tspan8 (formerly CO-029, D6.1A) are abundantly recovered in exosomes together with their network of associating molecules. In colorectal cancer this includes the integrins $\alpha3\beta1$ and, most prominently, $\alpha6\beta4$ as well as the CIC markers CD166, CD44v6 and claudin-7-associated EpCAM (unpublished finding).

Tetraspanins, mostly via their laterally associated partner molecules, are contributing to cell motility, adhesion, invasion, and fusion [315–320]. As outlined below, exosomal tetraspanins maintain these activities. Although the mechanism whereby tetraspanins contribute to the fusion between exosomes and their target cell has not been elucidated, there is convincing evidence that tetraspanins contribute to target cell-selective exosome docking [263, 313, 314], which for endothelial cells proceeds via a Tspan8-CD49d complex [263].

Taken together, tumor cells abundantly release exosomes composed of lipids, proteins, mRNA and miRNA, where differences in the relative levels of these components between exosomes and donor cells implies an active sorting process. Exosomes are recovered in body fluids, including the blood, which allows exosomes to reach premetastatic organs. According to their membrane protein pattern, they only interact with selected target cells. Through the delivery of proteins, mRNA and miRNA, exosomes can profoundly alter/reprogram their target cells.

4.4.2 The Exosomes – Role in Angiogenesis and the Premetastatic Niche Formation

Primary tumors as well as metastases depend on angiogenesis. The crosstalk between a tumor and pre-existing vessels has been intensely explored [321] and is thought to be initiated by the angiogenic switch, defined by a dominance of proangiogenic over anti-angiogenic factors [322, 323]. However, systemic alterations associated with tumor growth, such as thrombi formation are poorly understood [324], but suggested to depend on soluble mediators provided by the tumor [325]. As tumor-derived exosomes are present in all body fluids [298], they can easily become involved in systemic angiogenesis, which can culminate in severe thrombosis [326]. In fact, exosomes have been described to play a crucial role in the haemostatic balance [327], in tumor angiogenesis as well as tumor-associated thrombosis [258, 328, 329]. The latter was first described for platelet-derived exosomes, which transferred the αIIb integrin chain to lung cancer cells, stimulated the MAPK pathway and membrane type (MT)1-MMP expression, increased cyclinD2 expression, stimulated angiogenic factor expression and adhesion to fibrinogen and concomitantly activated human umbilical vein endothelial cells [258]. Melanoma-derived exosomes were shown to interact with endothelial cells and to promote an angiogenic response [280]. Glioblastoma-derived microvesicles that incorporated mRNA, miRNA and pro-angiogenic proteins were also shown to be taken up by normal host cells and could stimulate tube formation by ECs as well as mediate self promoting effects [292]. We have shown that exosomes could efficaciously initiate EC-progenitor maturation and resting EC activation. The proangiogenic activity of the exosomes strongly depended on the presence of the tetraspanin Tspan8 and its association with the $\alpha 4\beta 1$ integrin. Exosomes expressing a Tspan8-$\alpha 4\beta 1$ complex bound preferentially to ECs and EC-progenitors but poorly to cells such as fibroblasts, consistent with the ability of an antibody to the $\alpha 4\beta 1$ counter-receptor VCAM-1 to block exosome binding and uptake. Binding and uptake of exosomes was also inhibited by a Tspan8-specific antibody, but not by antibodies against other tetraspanins that were also enriched in exosomes. Transient recovery of selectively in AS-Tspan8-exosomes enriched mRNA in EC revealed that EC internalized Tspan8-CD49d complex-containing exosomes. Exosome uptake induced VEGF-independent regulation of several angiogenesis-related genes, including von Willebrand factor,

Tspan8, the chemokines CXCL5 and MIF, the chemokine receptor CCR1 and, together with VEGF, VEGFR2. This was accompanied by enhanced proliferation, migration and sprouting of EC and maturation of EC-progenitors [263].

These findings imply that depending on their tetraspanin web and on the target cells ligands, exosomes bind to and are taken up by selective target cells with the consequence of significant alterations in the target cell program. For colorectal cancer-derived exosomes this would imply not only the acquisition of an ability to activate and induce proliferation of endothelial cells, but also the ability to stimulate stellate cells and their transformation into myofibroblasts. Similar effects have also been observed in stromal cells upon uptake of tumor-derived exosomes.

In fact, exosomes have also been described to directly support metastasis formation. A direct transfer of metastatic capacity by exosomes was demonstrated for B16 melanoma cells, where uptake of exosomes of a metastasizing subclone resulted in lung metastases formation by the low metastatic B16F1 line [259]. We described that exosomes derived from a highly metastatic tumor line contributed to metastatic niche formation. Exosomes promoted expression of several adhesion molecules in lymph node cells, lymph node stromal cells, lung fibroblasts and endothelial cells. In addition, several growth factors, including HGF, IGF and PDGF, as well as growth factor- and chemokine receptors became upregulated and proliferation was strongly promoted. Whether this is due to the transfer of exosomal proteins, mRNA translation or exosomal miRNA silencing remains to be explored [257].

Colorectal cancer-derived microvesicles have also been shown to contain several hundred proteins [330, 331]. Moreover, significantly increased levels of exosomal mRNA were detected in the sera of colorectal cancer patients [332, 333]. The exosomal mRNA was enriched in cell-cycle-related mRNAs that promoted proliferation of endothelial cells, suggesting that these exosomes are involved in tumor growth and metastasis by facilitating angiogenesis-related processes [22].

Finally, several studies have been conducted to define the miRNA profile in colorectal cancer [23, 24, 334–340], where both overexpression and silencing of specific miRNAs have been observed [341]. Many profiling studies indicated a general downregulation of miRNA in several cancers, suggesting a negative regulation of tumorigenicity by miRNA [342–345]. This also accounts for reduced recovery of miRNA, such as miR-34a in colorectal cancer, indicating that it acts as a tumor suppressor [346–350]. However, miRNAs can also have tumor-promoting activities. In colon cancer 37 miRNAs were found to be differentially expressed as compared to the normal colonic mucosa, where high miR-21 expression was associated with poor survival due to downregulation of Bcl2, PTEN (phosphatase and tensin homolog) and tropomyosin 1 [345, 351]. These findings are in line with the interpretation that tumor-promoting miRNA in colorectal cancer (miR-20, miR-21 and others, [352, 353]) function by inhibiting tumor suppressor genes [354]. The detection of miRNA in serum has already been proposed as a diagnostic tool. Thus, 69 miRNAs were found in sera of all tested colon cancer patients, but not in sera of healthy donors [355]. It should be noted that these studies focused exclusively on the possible impact of the miRNA on the tumor cells and discussed potential therapeutic manipulations of cancer-related miRNA. Yet, it is our contention that evaluating the impact of exosomal miRNA on target cells in the premetastatic niche may be equally important and may lead to strategies for the prevention of CIC survival or of implantation and growth of isolated CoCIC in the liver. An essential prerequisite for therapeutic considerations for both will be the identification of target structures in the tumor cells and the respective target organ stroma.

Several studies have demonstrated significantly increased exosome levels in serum and other body fluids of cancer patients, including colorectal cancer patients [349, 356, 357]. It has been suggested that exosomal mRNA and miRNA profiling could well be used as a diagnostic strategy [22, 358]. However, limited data are available regarding the potential crosstalk between exosomal mRNA/miRNA and target cells in the metastatic organ. Nonetheless there is in vivo and in vitro evidence for reprogramming of the host stroma by exosomal proteins, mRNA and, likely miRNA to support the metastatic process (Fig. 4.4). Though further studies are urgently needed, there is good reason to propose that unraveling the pathophysiological role of exosomes in colorectal cancer will open new avenues for interfering with angiogenesis and metastases formation.

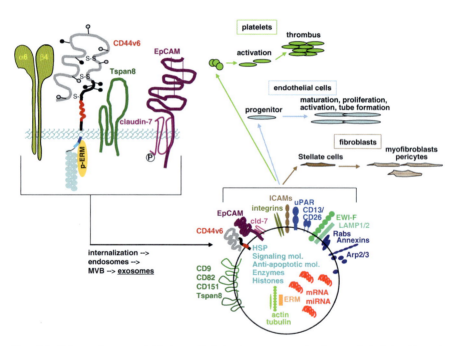

Fig. 4.4 Colorectal cancer initiating cell-derived exosomes stimulate endothelial cells and metastatic organ stromal cells. Colorectal cancer initiating cell-derived exosomes are enriched in tetraspanins and carry the cancer stem cell markers EpCAM, claudin-7, CD44v6, as well as several integrins, uPAR and other proteases. The exosomes also include ERM proteins and cytoskeletal proteins. The exosomes bind to platelets, metastatic organ fibroblasts and endothelial cells. Exosomes are taken up by these cells and this leads to maturation, proliferation and activation of the target cells

4.5 Concluding Remarks

The liver as the blood-draining organ for the colon and the upper rectum offers itself as the first station encountered by tumor cells dispersed from these sites. Although the liver is well equipped for defense, its architecture and particularly the torturous blood flow are also well suited for anchorage of isolated tumor cell. Correspondingly, colorectal cancer initiating cells are optimally equipped to modulate the microenvironment they encounter in the liver and create a niche that supports their survival and growth.

A. Most importantly, they can assemble in a CD44v6-dependent manner, a matrix that promotes cell adhesion and aggregation, and this can facilitate vessel occlusion and tumor cell retention.
B. The CD44v6-dependent matrix promotes tumor cell motility and survival, and the association of CD44v6 with receptor tyrosine kinases, particularly c-Met, and with $\alpha6\beta4$ further amplifies signal transduction and transcription of genes that enhance invasiveness. It is at this point, that the recruitment of CD44v6 as well as of EpCAM via claudin-7 into TEM likely becomes important to promote CIC maintenance and apoptosis resistance.
C. The matrix harbors cytokines, chemokines and growth factors that activate the host stroma and this can also be mediated in a CD44v6-dependent manner.
D. Irrespective of CD44v6 expression, tumor-derived exosomes can promote endothelial cell progenitor maturation and differentiation as well as activation of mature endothelial and other stromal cells in the (premetastatic) organ. There is evidence that reprogramming of stromal cells is a process jointly regulated by exosomal proteins, mRNA and miRNA.

As in most malignancies, the prognosis of patients with colorectal cancer correlates with tumor cell dissemination at the time of diagnosis. Given that CIC are the driving force for metastatic growth, and that metastases formation requires a crosstalk with the target organ stroma, it appears worthwhile to take great effort in defining the components and the molecular mechanisms of this intercellular communication in order to develop therapeutic interventions. The CoCIC markers EpCAM and, particularly, CD44v6, as well as exosomes appear to be critical elements in this process and may provide effective therapeutic targets.

Acknowledgement This work was supported by the Deutsche Forschungsgemeinschaft (SPP1190), the Deutsche Krebshilfe and the Tumorzentrum-Heidelberg/Mannheim (MZ).

References

1. Stein U, Schlag PM (2007) Clinical, biological, and molecular aspects of metastasis in colorectal cancer. Recent Results Cancer Res 176:61–80
2. Shike M, Winawer SJ, Greenwald PH, Bloch A, Hill MJ, Swaroop SV (1990) Primary prevention of colorectal cancer. The WHO Collaborating Centre for the Prevention of Colorectal Cancer. Bull World Health Organ 68:377–385

3. Papagrigoriadis S (2007) Follow-up of patients with colorectal cancer: the evidence is in favour but we are still in need of a protocol. Int J Surg 5:120–128

4. Pasetto LM, Monfardini S (2007) Colorectal cancer screening in elderly patients: when should be more useful? Cancer Treat Rev 33:528–532

5. Huerta S (2008) Recent advances in the molecular diagnosis and prognosis of colorectal cancer. Expert Rev Mol Diagn 8:277–288

6. Figueredo A, Coombes ME, Mukherjee S (2008) Adjuvant therapy for completely resected stage II colon cancer. Cochrane Database Syst Rev:CD005390

7. Ceelen WP, Bracke ME (2009) Peritoneal minimal residual disease in colorectal cancer: mechanisms, prevention, and treatment. Lancet Oncol 10:72–79

8. Royston D, Jackson DG (2009) Mechanisms of lymphatic metastasis in human colorectal adenocarcinoma. J Pathol 217:608–619

9. Sugarbaker PH (1993) Metastatic inefficiency: the scientific basis for resection of liver metastases from colorectal cancer. J Surg Oncol Suppl 3:158–160

10. Iwasaki J, Nihira S (2009) Anti-angiogenic therapy against gastrointestinal tract cancers. Jpn J Clin Oncol 39:543–551

11. Mangnall D, Bird NC, Majeed AW (2003) The molecular physiology of liver regeneration following partial hepatectomy. Liver Int 23:124–138

12. Bird NC, Mangnall D, Majeed AW (2006) Biology of colorectal liver metastases: a review. J Surg Oncol 94:68–80

13. Conzelmann M, Linnemann U, Berger MR (2005) Detection of disseminated tumour cells in the liver of colorectal cancer patients. Eur J Surg Oncol 31:38–44

14. Conzelmann M, Linnemann U, Berger MR (2005) Molecular detection of clinical colorectal cancer metastasis: how should multiple markers be put to use? Int J Colorectal Dis 20: 137–146

15. Yokoyama N, Shirai Y, Ajioka Y, Nagakura S, Suda T, Hatakeyama K (2002) Immunohistochemically detected hepatic micrometastases predict a high risk of intrahepatic recurrence after resection of colorectal carcinoma liver metastases. Cancer 94:1642–1647

16. Linnemann U, Schimanski CC, Gebhardt C, Berger MR (2004) Prognostic value of disseminated colorectal tumor cells in the liver: results of follow-up examinations. Int J Colorectal Dis 19:380–386

17. Topal B, Aerts JL, Roskams T, Fieuws S et al (2005) Cancer cell dissemination during curative surgery for colorectal liver metastases. Eur J Surg Oncol 31:506–511

18. Nordgård O, Aloysius TA, Todnem K, Heikkilä R, Ogreid D (2003) Detection of lymph node micrometastases in colorectal cancer. Scand J Gastroenterol 38:125–132

19. Rosenberg R, Hoos A, Mueller J et al (2002) Prognostic significance of cytokeratin-20 reverse transcriptase polymerase chain reaction in lymph nodes of node-negative colorectal cancer patients. J Clin Oncol 20:1049–1055

20. Bustin SA, Siddiqi S, Ahmed S, Hands R, Dorudi S (2004) Quantification of cytokeratin 20, carcinoembryonic antigen and guanylyl cyclase C mRNA levels in lymph nodes may not predict treatment failure in colorectal cancer patients. Int J Cancer 108:412–417

21. Vlems FA, Diepstra JH, Punt CJ et al (2003) Detection of disseminated tumour cells in blood and bone marrow samples of patients undergoing hepatic resection for metastasis of colorectal cancer. Br J Surg 90:989–995

22. Hong BS, Cho JH, Kim H et al (2009) Colorectal cancer cell-derived microvesicles are enriched in cell cycle-related mRNAs that promote proliferation of endothelial cells. BMC Genomics 10:556

23. Aslam MI, Taylor K, Pringle JH, Jameson JS (2009) MicroRNAs are novel biomarkers of colorectal cancer. Br J Surg 96:702–710

24. Slaby O, Svoboda M, Michalek J, Vyzula R (2009) MicroRNAs in colorectal cancer: translation of molecular biology into clinical application. Mol Cancer 8:102

25. Li M, Marin-Muller C, Bharadwaj U, Chow KH, Yao Q, Chen C (2009) MicroRNAs: control and loss of control in human physiology and disease. World J Surg 33:667–684

26. Mathivanan S, Lim JW, Tauro BJ, Ji H, Moritz RL, Simpson RJ (2010) Proteomics analysis of A33 immunoaffinity-purified exosomes released from the human colon tumor cell line LIM1215 reveals a tissue-specific protein signature. Mol Cell Proteomics 9:197–208

27. Brabletz T, Jung A, Spaderna S, Hlubek F, Kirchner T (2005) Opinion: migrating cancer stem cells – an integrated concept of malignant tumour progression. Nat Rev Cancer 5: 744–749

28. Hlubek F, Spaderna S, Schmalhofer O, Jung A, Kirchner T, Brabletz T (2007) Wnt/FZD signaling and colorectal cancer morphogenesis. Front Biosci 12:458–470

29. Yang J, Weinberg RA (2008) Epithelial-mesenchymal transition: at the crossroads of development and tumor metastasis. Dev Cell 14:818–829

30. Ahmad A, Hart IR (1997) Mechanisms of metastasis. Crit Rev Oncol Hematol 26: 163–173

31. Birchmeier C, Birchmeier W, Gherardi E, Vande Woude GF (2003) Met, metastasis, motility and more. Nat Rev Mol Cell Biol 4:915–925

32. Gassmann P, Enns A, Haier J (2004) Role of tumor cell adhesion and migration in organ-specific metastasis formation. Onkologie 27:577–582

33. Marhaba R, Zöller M (2004) CD44 in cancer progression: adhesion, migration and growth regulation. J Mol Histol 35:211–231

34. Albini A, Mirisola V, Pfeffer U (2008) Metastasis signatures: genes regulating tumor-microenvironment interactions predict metastatic behavior. Cancer Metastasis Rev 27:75–83

35. Friedl P, Wolf K (2003) Tumour-cell invasion and migration: diversity and escape mechanisms. Nat Rev Cancer 3:362–374

36. Kerbel R, Folkman J (2002) Clinical translation of angiogenesis inhibitors. Nat Rev Cancer 2:727–739

37. Mott JD, Werb Z (2004) Regulation of matrix biology by matrix metalloproteinases. Curr Opin Cell Biol 16:558–564

38. Regenbrecht CR, Lehrach H, Adjaye J (2008) Stemming cancer: functional genomics of cancer stem cells in solid tumors. Stem Cell Rev 4:319–328

39. Werbowetski-Ogilvie TE, Bhatia M (2008) Pluripotent human stem cell lines: what we can learn about cancer initiation. Trends Mol Med 14:323–332

40. Alix-Panabières C, Riethdorf S, Pantel K (2008) Circulating tumor cells and bone marrow micrometastasis. Clin Cancer Res 14:5013–5021

41. Bidard FC, Pierga JY, Vincent-Salomon A, Poupon MF (2008) A "class action" against the microenvironment: do cancer cells cooperate in metastasis? Cancer Metastasis Rev 27:5–10

42. Lautt WW, Greenway CV (1987) Conceptual review of the hepatic vascular bed. Hepatology 7:952–963

43. Oda M, Yokomori H, Han JY (2006) Regulatory mechanisms of hepatic microcirculatory hemodynamics: hepatic arterial system. Clin Hemorheol Microcirc 34:11–26

44. Simionescu N, Lupu F, Simionescu M (1983) Rings of membrane sterols surround the openings of vesicles and fenestrae, in capillary endothelium. J Cell Biol 97:1592–1600

45. Vekemans K, Braet F (2005) Structural and functional aspects of the liver and liver sinusoidal cells in relation to colon carcinoma metastasis. World J Gastroenterol 11:5095–5102

46. Smedsrød B, Le Couteur D, Ikejima K et al (2009) Hepatic sinusoidal cells in health and disease: update from the 14th International Symposium. Liver Int 29:490–501

47. Bouwens L, Baekeland M, De Zanger R, Wisse E (1986) Quantitation, tissue distribution and proliferation kinetics of Kupffer cells in normal rat liver. Hepatology 6:718–722

48. Ishibashi H, Nakamura M, Komori A, Migita K, Shimoda S (2009) Liver architecture, cell function, and disease. Semin Immunopathol 31:399–409

49. Baffy G (2009) Kupffer cells in non-alcoholic fatty liver disease: the emerging view. J Hepatol 51:212–223

50. Gao B, Jeong WI, Tian Z (2008) Liver: an organ with predominant innate immunity. Hepatology 47:729–736

51. Crispe IN (2009) The liver as a lymphoid organ. Annu Rev Immunol 27:147–163

52. Mann J, Mann DA (2009) Transcriptional regulation of hepatic stellate cells. Adv Drug Deliv Rev 61:497–512
53. Atzori L, Poli G, Perra A (2009) Hepatic stellate cell: a star cell in the liver. Int J Biochem Cell Biol 41:1639–1642
54. Kordes C, Sawitza I, Häussinger D (2009) Hepatic and pancreatic stellate cells in focus. Biol Chem 390:1003–1012
55. Novo E, di Bonzo LV, Cannito S, Colombatto S, Parola M (2009) Hepatic myofibroblasts: a heterogeneous population of multifunctional cells in liver fibrogenesis. Int J Biochem Cell Biol 41:2089–2093
56. Xia Y, Chen R, Song Z et al (2010) Gene expression profiles during activation of cultured rat hepatic stellate cells by tumoral hepatocytes and fetal bovine serum. J Cancer Res Clin Oncol 136:309–321
57. Olaso E, Salado C, Egilegor E et al (2003) Proangiogenic role of tumor-activated hepatic stellate cells in experimental melanoma metastasis. Hepatology 37:674–685
58. Matsusue R, Kubo H, Hisamori S et al (2009) Hepatic stellate cells promote liver metastasis of colon cancer cells by the action of SDF-1/CXCR4 axis. Ann Surg Oncol 16: 2645–2653
59. Vidal-Vanaclocha F, Rocha MA, Asumendi A, Barberá-Guillem E (1993) Role of periportal and perivenous sinusoidal endothelial cells in hepatic homing of blood and metastatic cancer cells. Semin Liver Dis 13:60–71
60. Vidal-Vanaclocha F (2008) The prometastatic microenvironment of the liver. Cancer Microenviron 1:113–129
61. Qi K, Qiu H, Rutherford J, Zhao Y, Nance DM, Orr FW (2004) Direct visualization of nitric oxide release by liver cells after the arrest of metastatic tumor cells in the hepatic microvasculature. J Surg Res 119:29–35
62. Kamiyama H, Toyama N, Mori Y et al (2002) Resection of hepatocellular carcinoma with tumor thrombus of the portal vein after neoadjuvant regional chemotherapy. J Hepatobiliary Pancreat Surg 9:759–763
63. Mendoza L, Carrascal T, De Luca M et al (2001) Hydrogen peroxide mediates vascular cell adhesion molecule-1 expression from interleukin-18-activated hepatic sinusoidal endothelium: implications for circulating cancer cell arrest in the murine liver. Hepatology 34:298–310
64. Inokuma T, Haraguchi M, Fujita F, Tajima Y, Kanematsu T (2009) Oxidative stress and tumor progression in colorectal cancer. Hepatogastroenterology 56:343–347
65. Enns A, Gassmann P, Schlüter K et al (2004) Integrins can directly mediate metastatic tumor cell adhesion within the liver sinusoids. J Gastrointest Surg 8:1049–1059
66. Gout S, Tremblay PL, Huot J (2008) Selectins and selectin ligands in extravasation of cancer cells and organ selectivity of metastasis. Clin Exp Metastasis 25:335–344
67. Dymicka-Piekarska V, Kemona H (2009) Does colorectal cancer clinical advancement affect adhesion molecules (sP-selectin, sE-selectin and ICAM-1) concentration? Thromb Res 124:80–83
68. St Hill CA, Farooqui M, Mitcheltree G (2009) The high affinity selectin glycan ligand C2-O-sLex and mRNA transcripts of the core 2 beta-1,6-N-acetylglucosaminyltransferase (C2GnT1) gene are highly expressed in human colorectal adenocarcinomas. BMC Cancer 9:79
69. Khatib AM, Auguste P, Fallavollita L et al (2005) Characterization of the host proinflammatory response to tumor cells during the initial stages of liver metastasis. Am J Pathol 167:749–759
70. Rudmik LR, Magliocco AM (2005) Molecular mechanisms of hepatic metastasis in colorectal cancer. J Surg Oncol 92:347–359
71. Ashizawa T, Okada R, Suzuki Y et al (2006) Study of interleukin-6 in the spread of colorectal cancer: the diagnostic significance of IL-6. Acta Med Okayama 60:325–330

72. Auguste P, Fallavollita L, Wang N, Burnier J, Bikfalvi A, Brodt P (2007) The host inflammatory response promotes liver metastasis by increasing tumor cell arrest and extravasation. Am J Pathol 170:1781–1792
73. Gulubova M, Manolova I, Cirovski G, Sivrev D (2008) Recruitment of dendritic cells in human liver with metastases. Clin Exp Metastasis 25:777–785
74. Wang HH, Nance DM, Orr FW (1999) Murine hepatic microvascular adhesion molecule expression is inducible and has a zonal distribution. Clin Exp Metastasis 17:149–155
75. Mendoza L, Valcárcel M, Carrascal T et al (2004) Inhibition of cytokine-induced microvascular arrest of tumor cells by recombinant endostatin prevents experimental hepatic melanoma metastasis. Cancer Res 64:304–310
76. Shimizu S, Yamada N, Sawada T et al (2000) Ultrastructure of early phase hepatic metastasis of human colon carcinoma cells with special reference to desmosomal junctions with hepatocytes. Pathol Int 50:953–959
77. Friedman SL (2008) Hepatic stellate cells: protean, multifunctional, and enigmatic cells of the liver. Physiol Rev 88:125–172
78. Corpechot C, Barbu V, Wendum D et al (2002) Hypoxia-induced VEGF and collagen I expressions are associated with angiogenesis and fibrogenesis in experimental cirrhosis. Hepatology 35:1010–1021
79. Gonda TA, Varro A, Wang TC, Tycko B (2010) Molecular biology of cancer-associated fibroblasts: can these cells be targeted in anti-cancer therapy? Semin Cell Dev Biol 21:2–10
80. Mani SA, Guo W, Liao MJ et al (2008) The epithelial-mesenchymal transition generates cells with properties of stem cells. Cell 133:704–715
81. Polyak K, Haviv I, Campbell IG (2009) Co-evolution of tumor cells and their microenvironment. Trends Genet 25:30–38
82. Lunevicius R, Nakanishi H, Ito S et al (2001) Clinicopathological significance of fibrotic capsule formation around liver metastasis from colorectal cancer. J Cancer Res Clin Oncol 127:193–199
83. Yang YM, Chang JW (2008) Current status and issues in cancer stem cell study. Cancer Invest 26:741–755
84. Li F, Tiede B, Massague J, Kang Y (2007) Beyond tumorigenesis: cancer stem cells in metastasis. Cell Res 17:3–14
85. Lobo NA, Shimono Y, Qian D, Clarke MF (2007) The biology of cancer stem cells. Annu Rev Cell Dev Biol 23:675–688
86. Allan AL, Vantyghem SA, Tuck AB, Chambers AF (2006-2007) Tumor dormancy and cancer stem cells: implications for the biology and treatment of breast cancer metastasis. Breast Dis 26:87–98
87. Ricci-Vitiani L, Fabrizi E, Palio E, De Maria R (2009) Colon cancer stem cells. J Mol Med 87:1097–1104
88. Kalluri R (2009) EMT: when epithelial cells decide to become mesenchymal-like cells. J Clin Invest 119:1417–1419
89. Scopelliti A, Cammareri P, Catalano V, Saladino V, Todaro M, Stassi G (2009) Therapeutic implications of Cancer initiating cells. Expert Opin Biol Ther 9:1005–1016
90. Papathanasiou P, Attema JL, Karsunky H et al (2009) Self-renewal of the long-term reconstituting subset of hematopoietic stem cells is regulated by Ikaros. Stem Cells 27:3082–3092
91. Marhaba R, Klingbeil P, Nübel T, Nazarenko I, Büchler MW, Zöller M (2008) CD44 and EpCAM, cancer-initiating cell markers. Curr Mol Med 8:784–804
92. Clarke MF, Dick JE, Dirks PB et al (2006) Cancer stem cells – perspectives on current status and future directions: AACR Workshop on cancer stem cells. Cancer Res 66:9339–9344
93. Huang EH, Hynes MJ, Zhang T et al (2009) Aldehyde dehydrogenase 1 is a marker for normal and malignant human colonic stem cells (SC) and tracks SC overpopulation during colon tumorigenesis. Cancer Res 69:3382–3389
94. Telford WG, Bradford J, Godfrey W, Robey RW, Bates SE (2007) Side population analysis using a violet-excited cell-permeable DNA binding dye. Stem Cells 25:1029–1036

95. Stewart MH, Bendall SC, Bhatia M (2008) Deconstructing human embryonic stem cell cultures: niche regulation of self-renewal and pluripotency. J Mol Med 86:875–886
96. van den Brink GR, Offerhaus GJ (2007) The morphogenetic code and colon cancer development. Cancer Cell 11:109–117
97. Saini V, Shoemaker RH (2010) Potential for therapeutic targeting of tumor stem cells. Cancer Sci 101:16–21
98. Yin T, Li L (2006) The stem cell niches in bone. J Clin Invest 116:1195–1201
99. Selleri C, Ragno P, Ricci P et al (2006) The metastasis-associated 67-kDa laminin receptor is involved in G-CSF-induced hematopoietic stem cell mobilization. Blood 108:2476–2484
100. Kucia M, Reca R, Miekus K et al (2005) Trafficking of normal stem cells and metastasis of cancer stem cells involve similar mechanisms: pivotal role of the SDF-1-CXCR4 axis. Stem Cells 23:879–894
101. Ara T, Nakamura Y, Egawa T et al (2003) Impaired colonization of the gonads by primordial germ cells in mice lacking a chemokine, stromal cell-derived factor-1 (SDF-1). Proc Natl Acad Sci USA 100:5319–5323
102. Askari AT, Unzek S, Popovic ZB et al (2003) Effect of stromal-cell-derived factor 1 on stem-cell homing and tissue regeneration in ischaemic cardiomyopathy. Lancet 362:697–703
103. Balkwill F, Coussens LM (2004) Cancer: an inflammatory link. Nature 431:405–406
104. Jung Y, Wang J, Schneider A et al (2006) Regulation of SDF-1 (CXCL12) production by osteoblasts; a possible mechanism for stem cell homing. Bone 38:497–508
105. Yilmaz OH, Valdez R, Theisen BK et al (2006) Pten dependence distinguishes haematopoietic stem cells from leukaemia-initiating cells. Nature 441:475–482
106. Polyak K, Hahn WC (2006) Roots and stems: stem cells in cancer. Nat Med 12: 296–300
107. Clarke MF, Fuller M (2006) Stem cells and cancer: two faces of eve. Cell 124:1111–1115
108. Mueller MM, Fusenig NE (2004) Tumor-stroma interactions directing phenotype and progression of epithelial. Nat Rev Cancer 4:839–849
109. Forte G, Minieri M, Cossa P et al (2006) Hepatocyte growth factor effects on mesenchymal stem cells: proliferation, migration, and differentiation. Stem Cells 24:23–33
110. Boccaccio C, Comoglio PM (2006) Invasive growth: a MET-driven genetic programme for cancer and stem cells. Nat Rev Cancer 6:637–645
111. Ratajczak MZ, Zuba-Surma E, Kucia M, Reca R, Wojakowski W, Ratajczak J (2006) The pleiotropic effects of the SDF-1-CXCR4 axis in organogenesis, regeneration and tumorigenesis. Leukemia 20:1915–1924
112. Deshpande AJ, Buske C (2007) Knocking the Wnt out of the sails of leukemia stem cell development. Cell Stem Cell 1:597–598
113. Vescovi AL, Galli R, Reynolds BA (2006) Brain tumour stem cells. Nat Rev Cancer 6: 425–436
114. Dalerba P, Dylla SJ, Park IK et al (2008) Phenotypic characterization of human colorectal cancer stem cells. Gastroenterology 134:1262–1264
115. O'Brien CA, Pollett A, Gallinger S, Dick JE (2007) A human colon cancer cell capable of initiating tumour growth in immunodeficient mice. Nature 445:106–110
116. Ricci-Vitiani L, Lombardi DG, Pilozzi E et al (2007) Identification and expansion of human colon-cancer-initiating cells. Nature 445:111–115
117. Artells R, Moreno I, Díaz T et al (2010) Tumour CD133 mRNA expression and clinical outcome in surgically resected colorectal cancer patients. Eur J Cancer 46:642–649
118. Swart GW, Lunter PC, Kilsdonk JW, Kempen LC (2005) Activated leukocyte cell adhesion molecule (ALCAM/CD166): signaling at the divide of melanoma cell clustering and cell migration? Cancer Metastasis Rev 24:223–236
119. Ohneda O, Ohneda K, Arai F et al (2001) ALCAM (CD166): its role in hematopoietic and endothelial development. Blood 98:2134–2142
120. Oswald J, Boxberger S, Jorgensen B et al (2004) Mesenchymal stem cells can be differentiated into endothelial cells in vitro. Stem Cells 22:377–384

121. Li C, Heidt DG, Dalerba P et al (2007) Identification of pancreatic cancer stem cells. Cancer Res 67:1030–1037
122. Yamashita T, Ji J, Budhu A et al (2009) EpCAM-positive hepatocellular carcinoma cells are tumor-initiating cells with stem/progenitor cell features. Gastroenterology 136: 1012–1024
123. Tárnok A, Ulrich H, Bocsi J (2010) Phenotypes of stem cells from diverse origin. Cytometry A 77:6–10
124. Zou GM (2008) Cancer initiating cells or cancer stem cells in the gastrointestinal tract and liver. J Cell Physiol 217:598–604
125. Yeung TM, Mortensen NJ (2009) Colorectal cancer stem cells. Dis Colon Rectum 52: 1788–1796
126. Er O (2009) Cancer stem cells in solid tumors. Onkologie 32:605–609
127. Momburg F, Moldenhauer G, Hämmerling GJ, Möller P (1987) Immunohistochemical study of the expression of a Mr 34,000 human epithelium-specific surface glycoprotein in normal and malignant tissues. Cancer Res 47:2883–2891
128. Bergsagel PL, Victor-Kobrin C, Brents LA, Mushinski JF, Kühl WM (1992) Genes expressed selectively in plasmacytomas: markers of differentiation and transformation. Curr Top Microbiol Immunol 182:223–238
129. Balzar M, Winter MJ, de Boer CJ, Litvinov SV (1999) The biology of the 17-1A antigen (Ep-CAM). J Mol Med 77:699–712
130. Gastl G, Spizzo G, Obrist P, Dünser M, Mikuz G (2000) Ep-CAM overexpression in breast cancer as a predictor of survival. Lancet 356:1981–1982
131. Braun S, Pantel K (1998) Prognostic significance of micrometastatic bone marrow involvement. Breast Cancer Res Treat 52:201–216
132. Litvinov SV, van Driel W, van Rhijn CM et al (1996) Expression of Ep-CAM in cervical squamous epithelia correlates with an increased proliferation and the disappearance of markers for terminal differentiation. Am J Pathol 148:865–875
133. Went PT, Lugli A, Meier S et al (2004) Frequent EpCam protein expression in human carcinomas. Hum Pathol 35:122–128
134. Chong JM, Speicher DW (2001) Determination of disulfide bond assignments and N-glycosylation sites of the human gastrointestinal carcinoma antigen GA733-2 (CO17-1A, EGP, KS1-4, KSA, and EpCAM). J Biol Chem 276:5804–5813
135. Trebak M, Begg GE, Chong JM, Kanazireva EV, Herlyn D, Speicher DW (2001) Oligomeric state of the colon carcinoma-associated glycoprotein GA733-2 (Ep-CAM/EGP40) and its role in GA733-mediated homotypic cell-cell adhesion. J Biol Chem 276:2299–2309
136. Balzar M, Briaire-de Bruijn IH, Rees-Bakker HA et al (2001) Epidermal growth factor-like repeats mediate lateral and reciprocal interactions of Ep-CAM molecules in homophilic adhesions. Mol Cell Biol 21:2570–2580
137. Behrens J (1994) Cell contacts, differentiation, and invasiveness of epithelial cells. Invasion Metastasis 14:61–70
138. Winter MJ, Nagelkerken B, Mertens AE, Rees-Bakker HA, Briaire-de Bruijn IH, Litvinov SV (2003) Expression of Ep-CAM shifts the state of cadherin-mediated adhesions from strong to weak. Exp Cell Res 285:50–8
139. Mohan A, Nalini V, Mallikarjuna K, Jyotirmay B, Krishnakumar S (2007) Expression of motility-related protein MRP1/CD9, N-cadherin, E-cadherin, alpha-catenin and beta-catenin in retinoblastoma. Exp Eye Res 84:781–789
140. Yamashita T, Budhu A, Forgues M, Wang XW (2007) Activation of hepatic stem cell marker EpCAM by Wnt-beta-catenin signaling in hepatocellular carcinoma. Cancer Res 67: 10831–10839
141. Guillemot JC, Naspetti M, Malergue F, Montcourrier P, Galland F, Naquet P (2001) Ep-CAM transfection in thymic epithelial cell lines triggers the formation of dynamic actin-rich protrusions involved in the organization of epithelial cell layers. Histochem Cell Biol 116:371–378

142. Münz M, Kieu C, Mack B, Schmitt B, Zeidler R, Gires O (2004) The carcinoma-associated antigen EpCAM upregulates c-myc and induces cell proliferation. Oncogene 23: 5748–5758
143. Osta WA, Chen Y, Mikhitarian K et al (2004) EpCAM is overexpressed in breast cancer and is a potential target for breast cancer gene therapy. Cancer Res 64:5818–5824
144. Münz M, Zeidler R, Gires O (2005) The tumour-associated antigen EpCAM upregulates the fatty acid binding protein E-FABP. Cancer Lett 225:151–157
145. Hussain S, Pluckthun A, Allen TM, Zangemeister-Wittke U (2006) Chemosensitization of carcinoma cells using epithelial cell adhesion molecule-targeted liposomal antisense against bcl-2/bcl-xL. Mol Cancer Ther 5:3170–3180
146. Maetzel D, Denzel S, Mack B et al (2009) Nuclear signalling by tumour-associated antigen EpCAM. Nat Cell Biol 11:162–171
147. Morita K, Furuse M, Fujimoto K, Tsukita S (1999) Claudin multigene family encoding four-transmembrane domain protein components of tight junction strands. Proc Natl Acad Sci USA 96:511–516
148. Balda MS, Matter K (1998) Tight junctions. J Cell Sci 111:541–547
149. Schneeberger, EE, Lynch RD (2004) The tight junction: a multifunctional complex. Am J Physiol Cell Physiol 286:1213–1228
150. Tsukita S, Yamazaki Y, Katsuno T, Tamura A, Tsukita S (2008) Tight junction-based epithelial microenvironment and cell proliferation. Oncogene 27:6930–6938
151. Furuse M, Hata M, Furuse K et al (2002) Claudin-based tight junctions are crucial for the mammalian epidermal barrier: a lesson from claudin-1-deficient mice. J Cell Biol 156: 1099–11111
152. Al Moustafa AE, Alaoui-Jamali MA, Batist G et al (2002) Identification of genes associated with head and neck carcinogenesis by cDNA microarray comparison between matched primary normal epithelial and squamous carcinoma cells. Oncogene 21: 2634–2640
153. Sheehan GM, Kallakury BV, Sheehan CE, Fisher HA, Kaufman RP Jr, Ross JS (2007) Loss of claudins-1 and -7 and expression of claudins-3 and -4 correlate with prognostic variables in prostatic adenocarcinomas. Hum Pathol 38:564–569
154. Park D, Kåresen R, Noren T, Sauer T (2007) Expression pattern of adhesion molecules (E-cadherin, alpha-, beta-, gamma-catenin and claudin-7), their influence on survival in primary breast carcinoma, and their corresponding axillary lymph node metastasis. APMIS 115:52–65
155. Gonzalez-Mariscal L, Namorado Mdel C, Martin D, Sierra G, Reyes JL (2006) The tight junction proteins claudin-7 and -8 display a different subcellular localization at Henle's loops and collecting ducts of rabbit kidney. Nephrol Dial Transplant 21:2391–2398
156. Fujita H, Chiba H, Yokozaki H et al (2006) Differential expression and subcellular localization of claudin-7, -8, -12, -13, and -15 along the mouse intestine. J Histochem Cytochem 54:933–944
157. Darido C, Buchert M, Pannequin J et al (2008) Defective claudin-7 regulation by Tcf-4 and Sox-9 disrupts the polarity and increases the tumorigenicity of colorectal cancer cells. Cancer Res 68:4258–4268
158. Van Itallie CM, Gambling TM, Carson JL, Anderson JM (2005) Palmitoylation of claudins is required for efficient tight-junction localization. J Cell Sci 118:1427–1436
159. Yeaman C, Grindstaff KK, Hansen MD, Nelson WJ (1999) Cell polarity: versatile scaffolds keep things in place. Curr Biol 9:515–517
160. Sasaki H, Matsui C, Furuse K, Mimori-Kiyosue Y, Furuse M, Tsukita S (2003) Dynamic behavior of paired claudin strands within apposing plasma membranes. Proc Natl Acad Sci USA 100:3971–3976
161. Ivanov AI, Nusrat A, Parkos CA (2004) The epithelium in inflammatory bowel disease: potential role of endocytosis of junctional proteins in barrier disruption. Novartis Found Symp 263:115–124

162. D'Souza T, Agarwal R, Morin PJ (2005) Phosphorylation of claudin-3 at threonine 192 by cAMP-dependent protein kinase regulates tight junction barrier function in ovarian cancer cells. J Biol Chem 280:26233–26240

163. Nunbhakdi-Craig V, Machleidt T, Ogris E, Bellotto D, White CL 3rd, Sontag E (2002) Protein phosphatase 2A associates with and regulates atypical PKC and the epithelial tight junction complex. J Cell Biol 158:967–978

164. Ikenouchi J, Matsuda M, Furuse M, Tsukita S (2003) Regulation of tight junctions during the epithelium-mesenchyme transition: direct repression of the gene expression of claudins/occludin by Snail. J Cell Sci 116:1959–1967

165. Carrozzino F, Soulie P, Huber D et al (2005) Inducible expression of Snail selectively increases paracellular ion permeability and differentially modulates tight junction proteins. Am J Physiol Cell Physiol 289:1002–1014

166. Okamoto R, Irie K, Yamada A, Katata T, Fukuhara A, Takai Y (2005) Recruitment of E-cadherin associated with alpha- and beta-catenins and p120ctn to the nectin-based cell-cell adhesion sites by the action of 12-O-tetradecanoylphorbol-13-acetate in MDCK cells. Genes Cells 10:435–445

167. Kuhn S, Koch M, Klingbeil P et al (2007) Complex formation between CD44 variant isoforms with EpCAM and Claudin-7 in tetraspanin-enriched membrane microdomains promotes colorectal cancer progression. Mol Cancer Res 5:553–567

168. Le Naour F, André M, Boucheix C, Rubinstein E (2006) Membrane microdomains and proteomics: lessons from tetraspanin microdomains and comparison with lipid rafts. Proteomics 6:6447–6454

169. Hemler ME (2005) Tetraspanin functions and associated microdomains. Nat Rev Mol Cell Biol 6:801–811

170. Nübel T, Preobraschenski J, Tuncay H et al (2009) Claudin-7 regulates EpCAM-mediated functions in tumor progression. Mol Cancer Res 7:285–299

171. Günthert U, Hofmann M, Rudy W et al (1991) A new variant of glycoprotein CD44 confers metastatic potential to rat carcinoma cells. Cell 65:13–24

172. Ponta H, Sherman L, Herrlich PA (2003) CD44: from adhesion molecules to signalling regulators. Nat Rev Mol Cell Biol 4:33–45

173. Naor D, Sionov RV, Ish-Shalom D (1997) CD44: structure, function, and association with the malignant process. Adv Cancer Res 71:241–319

174. Lapidot T, Sirard C, Vormoor J et al (1994) A cell initiating human acute myeloid leukaemia after transplantation into SCID mice. Nature 367:645–648

175. Collins AT, Berry PA, Hyde C, Stower MJ, Maitland NJ (2005) Prospective identification of tumorigenic prostate cancer stem cells. Cancer Res 65:10946–10951

176. Ponti D, Zaffaroni N, Capelli C, Daidone MG (2006) Breast cancer stem cells: an overview. Eur J Cancer 42:1219–1224

177. Stingl J, Eirew P, Ricketson I et al (2006) Purification and unique properties of mammary epithelial stem cells. Nature 439:993–997

178. Ratajczak MZ (2005) Cancer stem cells – normal stem cells "Jedi" that went over to the "dark side". Folia Histochem Cytobiol 43:175–181

179. Screaton GR, Bell MV, Jackson DG, Cornelis FB, Gerth U, Bell JI (1992) Genomic structure of DNA encoding the lymphocyte homing receptor CD44 reveals at least 12 alternatively spliced exons. Proc Natl Acad Sci USA 89:12160–12164

180. Lynch KW (2004) Consequences of regulated pre-mRNA splicing in the immune system. Nat Rev Immunol 4:931–940

181. Ruiz P, Schwärzler C, Günthert U (1995) CD44 isoforms during differentiation and development. Bioessays 17:17–24

182. Labarrière N, Piau JP, Otry C et al (1994) H blood group antigen carried by CD44V modulates tumorigenicity of rat colon carcinoma cells. Cancer Res 54:6275–6281

183. Wielenga VJ, Heider KH, Offerhaus GJ et al (1993) Expression of CD44 variant proteins in human colorectal cancer is related to tumor progression. Cancer Res 53:4754–4756

184. Lakshman M, Subramaniam V, Wong S, Jothy S (2005) CD44 promotes resistance to apoptosis in murine colonic epithelium. J Cell Physiol 203:583–588
185. Harada N, Mizoi T, Kinouchi M et al (2001) Introduction of antisense CD44S CDNA down-regulates expression of overall CD44 isoforms and inhibits tumor growth and metastasis in highly metastatic colon carcinoma cells. Int J Cancer 91:67–75
186. Reeder JA, Gotley DC, Walsh MD, Fawcett J, Antalis TM (1998) Expression of anti-sense CD44 variant 6 inhibits colorectal tumor metastasis and tumor growth in a wound environment. Cancer Res 58:3719–3726
187. Kim H, Yang XL, Rosada C, Hamilton SR, August JT (1994) CD44 expression in colorectal adenomas is an early event occurring prior to K-ras and p53 gene mutation. Arch Biochem Biophys 310:504–507
188. Wielenga VJ, Smits R, Korinek V et al (1999) Expression of CD44 in Apc and Tcf mutant mice implies regulation by the WNT pathway. Am J Pathol 154:515–523
189. Konstantopoulos K, Thomas SN (2009) Cancer cells in transit: the vascular interactions of tumor cells. Annu Rev Biomed Eng 11:177–202
190. Almond A (2007) Hyaluronan. Cell Mol Life Sci 64:1591–1596
191. Aruffo A, Stamenkovic I, Melnick M, Underhill CB, Seed B (1990) CD44 is the principle cell surface receptor for hyaluronate. Cell 61:1303–1313
192. Toole BP (2004) Hyaluronan: from extracellular glue to pericellular cue. Nat Rev Cancer 4:528–539
193. Ropponen K, Tammi M, Parkkinen J et al (1998) Tumor cell-associated hyaluronan as an unfavorable prognostic factor in colorectal cancer. Cancer Res 58:342–347
194. Kim HR, Wheeler MA, Wilson CM et al (2004) Hyaluronan facilitates invasion of colon carcinoma cells in vitro via interaction with CD44. Cancer Res 64:4569–4576
195. Ratajczak MZ, Reca R, Wysoczynski M et al (2004) Transplantation studies in C3-deficient animals reveal a novel role of the third complement component (C3) in engraftment of bone marrow cells. Leukemia 18:1482–1490
196. Avigdor A, Goichberg P, Shivtiel S et al (2004) CD44 and hyaluronic acid cooperate with SDF-1 in the trafficking of human CD34+ stem/progenitor cells to bone marrow. Blood 103:2981–2989
197. Jin L, Hope KJ, Zhai Q, Smadja-Joffe F, Dick JE (2006) Targeting of CD44 eradicates human acute myeloid leukemic stem cells. Nat Med 12:1167–1174
198. Krause DS, Lazarides K, von Andrian UH, van Etten RA (2006) Requirement for CD44 in homing and engraftment of BCR-ABL-expressing leukemic stem cells. Nat Med 12: 1175–1180
199. Bourguignon LY (2001) CD44-mediated oncogenic signaling and cytoskeleton activation during mammary tumor progression. J Mammary Gland Biol Neoplasia 6:287–297
200. Tsukita S, Yonemura S, Tsukita S (1997) ERM proteins: head-to-tail regulation of actin-plasma membrane interaction. Trends Biochem Sci 22:53–58
201. Legg JW, Isacke CM (1998) Identification and functional analysis of the ezrin-binding site in the hyaluronan receptor, CD44. Curr Biol 8:705–708
202. Ng T, Parsons M, Hughes WE et al (2001) Ezrin is a downstream effector of trafficking PKC-integrin complexes involved in the control of cell motility. EMBO J 20:2723–2741
203. Lamontagne CA, Grandbois M (2008) PKC-induced stiffening of hyaluronan/CD44 linkage; local force measurements on glioma cells. Exp Cell Res 314:227–236
204. Pierini LM, Eddy RJ, Fuortes M, Seveau S, Casulo C, Maxfield FR (2003) Membrane lipid organization is critical for human neutrophil polarization. J Biol Chem 278:10831–10841
205. Nandi A, Estess P, Siegelman MH (2000) Hyaluronan anchoring and regulation on the sur-face of vascular endothelial cells is mediated through the functionally active form of CD44. J Biol Chem 275:14939–14948
206. Lesley J, English NM, Gál I, Mikecz K, Day AJ, Hyman R (2002) Hyaluronan binding properties of a CD44 chimera containing the link module of TSG-6. J Biol Chem 277: 26600–26608

207. Mohamadzadeh M, DeGrendele H, Arizpe H et al (1998) Proinflammatory stimuli regulate endothelial hyaluronan expression and CD44/HA-dependent primary adhesion. J Clin Invest 101:97–108
208. Baronas-Lowell D, Lauer-Fields JL, Borgia JA et al (2004) Differential modulation of human melanoma cell metalloproteinase expression by alpha2beta1 integrin and CD44 triple-helical ligands derived from type IV collagen. J Biol Chem 279:43503–43513
209. Yu Q, Stamenkovic I (2004) Transforming growth factor-beta facilitates breast carcinoma metastasis by promoting tumor cell survival. Clin Exp Metastasis 21:235–242
210. Yu WH, Woessner JF Jr, McNeish JD, Stamenkovic I (2002) CD44 anchors the assembly of matrilysin/MMP-7 with heparin-binding epidermal growth factor precursor and ErbB4 and regulates female reproductive organ remodeling. Genes Dev 16:307–323
211. Lynch CC, Vargo-Gogola T, Martin MD, Fingleton B, Crawford HC, Matrisian LM (2007) Matrix metalloproteinase 7 mediates mammary epithelial cell tumorigenesis through the ErbB4 receptor. Cancer Res 67:6760–6767
212. Fjeldstad K, Kolset SO (2005) Decreasing the metastatic potential in cancers – targeting the heparan sulfate proteoglycans. Curr Drug Targets 6:665–682
213. Taylor KR, Gallo RL (2006) Glycosaminoglycans and their proteoglycans: host-associated molecular patterns for initiation and modulation of inflammation. FASEB J 20:9–22
214. Levesque MC, Haynes BF (2001) Activated T lymphocytes regulate hyaluronan binding to monocyte CD44 via production of IL-2 and IFN-gamma. J Immunol 166:188–196
215. Kazanecki CC, Uzwiak DJ, Denhardt DT (2007) Control of osteopontin signaling and function by post-translational phosphorylation and protein folding. J Cell Biochem 102:912–924
216. Corso S, Comoglio PM, Giordano S (2005) Cancer therapy: can the challenge be MET? Trends Mol Med 11:284–292
217. Diehn M, Clarke MF (2006) Cancer stem cells and radiotherapy: new insights into tumor radioresistance. J Natl Cancer Inst 98:1755–1757
218. Garcea G, Neal CP, Pattenden CJ, Steward WP, Berry DP (2005) Molecular prognostic markers in pancreatic cancer: a systematic review. Eur J Cancer 41:2213–2236
219. Tuck AB, Chambers AF, Allan AL (2007) Osteopontin overexpression in breast cancer: knowledge gained and possible implications for clinical management. J Cell Biochem 102:859–868
220. Aziz KA, Till KJ, Zuzel M, Cawley JC (2000) Involvement of CD44-hyaluronan interaction in malignant cell homing and fibronectin synthesis in hairy cell leukemia. Blood 96: 3161–3167
221. Charnaux N, Brule S, Chaigneau T et al (2005) RANTES (CCL5) induces a CCR5-dependent accelerated shedding of syndecan-1 (CD138) and syndecan-4 from HeLa cells and forms complexes with the shed ectodomains of these proteoglycans as well as with those of CD44. Glycobiology 15:119–130
222. Sherman L, Wainwright D, Ponta H, Herrlich P (1998) A splice variant of CD44 expressed in the apical ectodermal ridge presents fibroblast growth factors to limb mesenchyme and is required for limb outgrowth. Genes Dev 12:1058–1071
223. Kim MS, Park MJ, Moon EJ et al (2005) Hyaluronic acid induces osteopontin via the phosphatidylinositol 3-kinase/Akt pathway to enhance the motility of human glioma cells. Cancer Res 65:686–691
224. Orian-Rousseau V, Chen L, Sleeman JP, Herrlich P, Ponta H (2002) CD44 is required for two consecutive steps in HGF/c-Met signaling. Genes Dev 16:3074–3086
225. Recio JA, Merlino G (2003) Hepatocyte growth factor/scatter factor induces feedback up-regulation of CD44v6 in melanoma cells through Egr-1. Cancer Res 63:1576–1582
226. Stern R, Asari AA, Sugahara KN (2006) Hyaluronan fragments: an information-rich system. Eur J Cell Biol 85:699–715
227. Bourguignon LY, Gilad E, Peyrollier K (2007) Heregulin-mediated ErbB2-ERK signaling activates hyaluronan synthases leading to CD44-dependent ovarian tumor cell growth and migration. J Biol Chem 282:19426–19441

228. Marhaba R, Freyschmidt-Paul P, Zöller M (2006) In vivo CD44-CD49d complex formation in autoimmune disease has consequences on T cell activation and apoptosis resistance. Eur J Immunol 36:3017–3032

229. Wakahara K, Kobayashi H, Yagyu T et al (2005) Bikunin down-regulates heterodimerization between CD44 and growth factor receptors and subsequently suppresses agonist-mediated signaling. J Cell Biochem 94:995–1009

230. Wielenga VJ, van der Voort R, Taher TE et al (2000) Expression of c-Met and heparan-sulfate proteoglycan forms of CD44 in colorectal cancer. Am J Pathol 157:1563–1573

231. Orian-Rousseau V, Morrison H, Matzke A et al (2007) Hepatocyte growth factor-induced Ras activation requires ERM proteins linked to both CD44v6 and F-actin. Mol Biol Cell 18:76–83

232. Matzke A, Sargsyan V, Holtmann B et al (2007) Haploinsufficiency of c-Met in cd44-/- mice identifies a collaboration of CD44 and c-Met in vivo. Mol Cell Biol 27:8797–8806

233. Ghatak S, Misra S, Toole BP (2005) Hyaluronan constitutively regulates ErbB2 phosphorylation and signaling complex formation in carcinoma cells. J Biol Chem 280: 8875–8883

234. Turley EA, Noble PW, Bourguignon LY (2002) Signaling properties of hyaluronan receptors. J Biol Chem 277:4589–4592

235. Föger N, Marhaba R, Zöller M (2000) CD44 supports T cell proliferation and apoptosis by apposition of protein kinases. Eur J Immunol 30:2888–2899

236. Ingley E (2008) Src family kinases: regulation of their activities, levels and identification of new pathways. Biochim Biophys Acta 1784:56–65

237. Mitsuda T, Furukawa K, Fukumoto S, Miyazaki H, Urano T, Furukawa K (2002) Overexpression of ganglioside GM1 results in the dispersion of platelet-derived growth factor receptor from glycolipid-enriched microdomains and in the suppression of cell growth signals. J Biol Chem 277:11239–11246

238. Prag S, Parsons M, Keppler MD et al (2007) Activated ezrin promotes cell migration through recruitment of the GEF Dbl to lipid rafts and preferential downstream activation of Cdc42. Mol Biol Cell 18:2935–2948

239. Föger N, Marhaba R, Zöller M (2001) Involvement of CD44 in cytoskeleton rearrangement and raft reorganization in T cells. J Cell Sci 114:1169–1178

240. Marhaba R, Bourouba M, Zöller M (2003) CD44v7 interferes with activation-induced cell death by up-regulation of anti-apoptotic gene expression. J Leukoc Biol 74:135–148

241. Delon J, Kaibuchi K, Germain RN (2001) Exclusion of CD43 from the immunological synapse is mediated by phosphorylation-regulated relocation of the cytoskeletal adaptor moesin. Immunity 15:691–701

242. Köbel M, Weichert W, Crüwell K, Schmitt WD, Lautenschläger C, Hauptmann S (2004) Epithelial hyaluronic acid and CD44v6 are mutually involved in invasion of colorectal adenocarcinomas and linked to patient prognosis. Virchows Arch 445:456–464

243. Peng J, Lu JJ, Zhu J et al (2008) Prediction of treatment outcome by CD44v6 after total mesorectal excision in locally advanced rectal cancer. Cancer J 14:54–61

244. Zlobec I, Günthert U, Tornillo L et al (2009) Systematic assessment of the prognostic impact of membranous CD44v6 protein expression in colorectal cancer. Histopathology 55: 564–575

245. Schofield R (1978) The relationship between the spleen colony-forming cell and the haemopoietic stem cell. Blood Cells 4:7–25

246. Morrison SJ, Spradling AC (2008) Stem cells and niches: mechanisms that promote stem cell maintenance throughout life. Cell 132:598–611

247. Kuhn NZ, Tuan RS (2010) Regulation of stemness and stem cell niche of mesenchymal stem cells: implications in tumorigenesis and metastasis. J Cell Physiol 222:268–277

248. Khaldoyanidi S (2008) Directing stem cell homing. Cell Stem Cell 2:198–200

249. Ghotra VP, Puigvert JC, Danen EH (2009) The cancer stem cell microenvironment and anti-cancer therapy. Int J Radiat Biol 85:955–962

250. Wang N, Tytell JD, Ingber DE (2009) Mechanotransduction at a distance: mechanically coupling the extracellular matrix with the nucleus. Nat Rev Mol Cell Biol 10:75–82
251. Johnston LA (2009) Competitive interactions between cells: death, growth, and geography. Science 324:1679–1682
252. Bhowmick NA, Chytil A, Plieth D et al (2004) TGF-beta signaling in fibroblasts modulates the oncogenic potential of adjacent epithelia. Science 303:848–851
253. Bissell MJ, Labarge MA (2005) Context, tissue plasticity, and cancer: are tumor stem cells also regulated by the microenvironment? Cancer Cell 7:17–23
254. Kaplan RN, Riba RD, Zacharoulis S et al (2005) VEGFR1-positive haematopoietic bone marrow progenitors initiate the pre-metastatic niche. Nature 438:820–827
255. Erler JT, Bennewith KL, Cox TR et al (2009) Hypoxia-induced lysyl oxidase is a critical mediator of bone marrow cell recruitment to form the premetastatic niche. Cancer Cell 15:35–44
256. He S, Nakada D, Morrison SJ (2009) Mechanisms of stem cell self-renewal. Rev Cell Dev Biol 25:377–406
257. Jung T, Castellana D, Klingbeil P et al (2009) CD44v6 dependence of premetastatic niche preparation by exosomes. Neoplasia 11:1093–1105
258. Janowska-Wieczorek A, Wysoczynski M, Kijowski J et al (2005) Microvesicles derived from activated platelets induce metastasis and angiogenesis in lung cancer. Int J Cancer 113:752–760
259. Hao S, Ye Z, Li F et al (2006) Epigenetic transfer of metastatic activity by uptake of highly metastatic B16 melanoma cell-released exosomes. Exp Oncol 28:126–131
260. Zöller M (2006) Gastrointestinal tumors, metastasis and tetraspanins. Z Gastroenterologie 44:573–586
261. Zöller M (2009) Tetraspanins: push and pull in suppressing and promoting metastasis. Nat Rev Cancer 9:40–55
262. Gesierich S, Berezovkiy I, Ryschich E, Zöller M (2006) Systemic angiogenesis induction by the tetraspanin D6.1A. Cancer Res 66:7083–7094
263. Nazarenko I, Rana S, Baumann A et al (2010) Cell surface tetraspanin Tspan8 contributes to molecular pathways of exosome-induced endothelial cell activation. Cancer Res 70:1668–1678
264. Adamia S, Maxwell CA, Pilarski LM (2005) Hyaluronan and hyaluronan synthases: potential therapeutic targets in cancer. Curr Drug Targets Cardiovasc Haematol Disord 5:3–14
265. Comoglio PM, Giordano S, Trusolino L (2008) Drug development of MET inhibitors: targeting oncogene addiction and expedience. Nat Rev Drug Discov 7:504–516
266. Lee KH, Choi EY, Hyun MS et al (2008) Role of hepatocyte growth factor/c-Met signaling in regulating urokinase plasminogen activator on invasiveness in human hepatocellular carcinoma: a potential therapeutic target. Clin Exp Metastasis 25:89–96
267. Kobayashi H, Suzuki M, Kanayama N, Nishida T, Takigawa M, Terao T (2002) CD44 stimulation by fragmented hyaluronic acid induces upregulation of urokinase-type plasminogen activator and its receptor and subsequently facilitates invasion of human chondrosarcoma cells. Int J Cancer 102:379–389
268. Mazar AP (2008) Urokinase plasminogen activator receptor choreographs multiple ligand interactions: implications for tumor progression and therapy. Clin Cancer Res 14:5649–5655
269. Zhang J, Ren H, Yuan P, Lang W, Zhang L, Mao L (2006) Down-regulation of hepatoma-derived growth factor inhibits anchorage-independent growth and invasion of non-small cell lung cancer cells. Cancer Res 66:18–23
270. Uyama H, Tomita Y, Nakamura H et al (2006) Hepatoma-derived growth factor is a novel prognostic factor for patients with pancreatic cancer. Clin Cancer Res 12:6043–6048
271. Tsang TY, Tang WY, Tsang WP, Co NN, Kong SK, Kwok TT (2008) Downregulation of hepatoma-derived growth factor activates the Bad-mediated apoptotic pathway in human cancer cells. Apoptosis 13:1135–1147

272. Pucci S, Mazzarelli P, Nucci C, Ricci F, Spagnoli LG (2009) CLU "in and out": looking for a link. Adv Cancer Res 105:93–113
273. Sercu S, Zhang L, Merregaert J (2008) The extracellular matrix protein 1: its molecular interaction and implication in tumor progression. Cancer Invest 26:375–384
274. da Costa CA (2007) DJ-1: a newcomer in Parkinson's disease pathology. Curr Mol Med 7:650–657
275. Wysoczynski M, Ratajczak J, Reca R et al (2007) A pivotal role of activation of complement cascade (CC) in mobilization of hematopoietic stem/progenitor cells (HSPC). Adv Exp Med Biol 598:226–239
276. Liszewski MK, Kemper C, Price JD, Atkinson JP (2005) Emerging roles and new functions of CD46. Springer Semin Immunopathol 27:345–358
277. Marzesco AM, Janich P, Wilsch-Bräuninger M et al (2005) Release of extracellular membrane particles carrying the stem cell marker pro-minin-1 (CD133) from neural progenitors and other epithelial cells. J Cell Sci 118:2849–2858
278. Février B, Raposo G (2004) Exosomes: endosomal-derived vesicles shipping extracellular messages. Curr Opin Cell Biol 16:415–421
279. Keller S, Sanderson MP, Stoeck A, Altevogt P (2006) Exosomes: from biogenesis and secretion to biological function. Immunol Lett 107:102–108
280. Hood JL, Pan H, Lanza GM, Wickline SA (2009) Consortium for translational research in advanced imaging and nanomedicine (C-TRAIN). Paracrine induction of endothelium by tumor exosomes. Lab Invest 89:1317–1328
281. Park JE, Tan HS, Datta A et al (2010) Hypoxia modulates tumor microenvironment to enhance angiogenic and metastatic potential by secretion of proteins and exosomes. Mol Cell Proteomics 9:1085–1099
282. Johnstone RM (2006) Exosomes biological significance: a concise review. Blood Cells Mol Dis 36:315–321
283. Lakkaraju A, Rodriguez-Boulan E (2008) Itinerant exosomes: emerging roles in cell and tissue polarity. Trends Cell Biol 18:199–209
284. Gruenberg J, Stenmark H (2004) The biogenesis of multivesicular endosomes. Nat Rev Mol Cell Biol 5:317–323
285. Schorey JS, Bhatnagar S (2008) Exosome function: from tumor immunology to pathogen biology. Traffic 9:871–881
286. Théry C, Ostrowski M, Segura E (2009) Membrane vesicles as conveyors of immune responses. Nat Rev Immunol 9:581–593
287. Valenti R, Huber V, Iero M, Filipazzi P, Parmiani G, Rivoltini L (2007) Tumor-released microvesicles as vehicles of immunosuppression. Cancer Res 67:2912–2915
288. Valadi, H., Ekström K, Bossios A, Sjöstrand M, Lee JJ, Lötvall JO (2007) Exosome-mediated transfer of mRNAs and microRNAs is a novel mechanism of genetic exchange between cells. Nat Cell Biol 9:654–659
289. Baj-Krzyworzeka M, Szatanek R, Weglarczyk K et al (2006) Tumour-derived microvesicles carry several surface determinants and mRNA of tumour cells and transfer some of these determinants to monocytes. Cancer Immunol Immunother 55:808–818
290. Ratajczak J, Wysoczynski M, Hayek F, Janowska-Wieczorek A, Ratajczak MZ (2006) Membrane-derived microvesicles: important and underappreciated mediators of cell-to-cell communication. Leukemia 20:1487–1495
291. Deregibus MC, Cantaluppi V, Calogero R et al (2007) Endothelial progenitor cell derived microvesicles activate an angiogenic program in endothelial cells by a horizontal transfer of mRNA. Blood 110:2440–2448
292. Skog J, Würdinger T, van Rijn S et al (2008) Glioblastoma microvesicles transport RNA and proteins that promote tumour growth and provide diagnostic biomarkers. Nat Cell Biol 10:1470–1476
293. Zakharova L, Svetlova M, Fomina AF (2007) T cell exosomes induce cholesterol accumulation in human monocytes via phosphatidylserine receptor. J Cell Physiol 212:174–181

294. Hurley JH (2008) ESCRT complexes and the biogenesis of multivesicular bodies. Curr Opin Cell Biol 20:4–11
295. Pilzer D, Gasser O, Moskovich O, Schifferli JA, Fishelson Z (2005) Emission of membrane vesicles: roles in complement resistance, immunity and cancer. Springer Semin Immunopathol 27:375–387
296. Tran JH, Chen CJ, Emr S, Schekman R (2009) Cargo sorting into multivesicular bodies in vitro. Proc Natl Acad Sci USA 106:17395–17400
297. Simons M, Raposo G (2009) Exosomes – vesicular carriers for intercellular communication. Curr Opin Cell Biol 21:575–581
298. Simpson RJ, Lim JW, Moritz RL, Mathivanan S (2009) Exosomes: proteomic insights and diagnostic potential. Expert Rev Proteomics 6:267–283
299. Ahmed KA, Xiang J (2010) Mechanisms of cellular communication through intercellular protein transfer. J Cell Mol Med Jan 11 (Epub ahead of print)
300. Levy S, Shoham T (2005) The tetraspanin web modulates immune-signalling complexes. Nat Rev Immunol 5:136–148
301. Boucheix C, Rubinstein E (2001) Tetraspanins. Cell Mol Life Sci 58:1189–1205
302. Le Naour F, André M, Boucheix C, Rubinstein E (2006) Membrane microdomains and proteomics: lessons from tetraspanin microdomains and comparison with lipid rafts. Proteomics 6:6447–6454
303. Levy S, Shoham T (2005) Protein-protein interactions in the tetraspanin web. Physiology 20:218–224
304. Berditchevski F, Odintsova E (2007) Tetraspanins as regulators of protein trafficking. Traffic 8:89–96
305. Berditchevski F (2001) Complexes of tetraspanins with integrins: more than meets the eye. J Cell Sci 114:4143–4151
306. Murayama Y, Shinomura Y, Oritani K et al (2008) The tetraspanin CD9 modulates epidermal growth factor receptor signaling in cancer cells. J Cell Physiol 216:135–143
307. Sridhar SC, Miranti CK (2006) Tetraspanin KAI1/CD82 suppresses invasion by inhibiting integrin-dependent crosstalk with c-Met receptor and Src kinases. Oncogene 25:2367–2378
308. Little KD, Hemler ME, Stipp CS (2004) Dynamic regulation of a GPCR-tetraspanin-G protein complex on intact cells: central role of CD81 in facilitating GPR56-Galpha q/11 association. Mol Biol Cell 15:2375–2387
309. André M, Le Caer JP, Greco C et al (2006) Proteomic analysis of the tetraspanin web using LC-ESI-MS/MS and MALDI-FTICR-MS. Proteomics 6:1437–1449
310. Claas C, Wahl J, Orlicky DJ et al (2005) The tetraspanin D6.1A and its molecular partners on rat carcinoma cells. Biochem J 389:99–110
311. Zhang J, Lu SH, Liu YJ, Feng Y, Han ZC (2004) Platelet factor 4 enhances the adhesion of normal and leukemic hematopoietic stem/progenitor cells to endothelial cells. Leuk Res 28:631–638
312. Todeschini AR, Dos Santos JN, Handa K, Hakomori SI (2008) Ganglioside GM2/GM3 complex affixed on silica nanospheres strongly inhibits cell motility through CD82/cMet-mediated pathway. Proc Natl Acad Sci USA 105:1925–1930
313. Xu C, Zhang YH, Thangavel M et al (2009) CD82 endocytosis and cholesterol-dependent reorganization of tetraspanin webs and lipid rafts. FASEB J. 23:3273–3288
314. Marks MS, Ohno H, Kirchnausen T, Bonracino JS (1997) Protein sorting by tyrosine-based signals: adapting to the Ys and wherefores. Trends Cell Biol 7:124–128
315. Stipp CS, Kolesnikova TV, Hemler ME (2003) Functional domains in tetraspanin proteins. Trends Biochem Sci 28:106–112
316. Winterwood NE, Varzavand A, Meland MN, Ashman LK, Stipp CS (2006) A critical role for tetraspanin CD151 in alpha3beta1 and alpha6beta4 integrin-dependent tumor cell functions on laminin-5. Mol Biol Cell 17:2707–2721
317. Kaji K, Oda S, Shikano T et al (2000) The gamete fusion process is defective in eggs of Cd9-deficient mice. Nat Genet 24:279–282

318. Zhang XA, Kazarov AR, Yang X, Bontrager AL, Stipp CS, Hemler ME (2002) Function of the tetraspanin CD151-alpha6beta1 integrin complex during cellular morphogenesis. Mol Biol Cell 13:1–11

319. Takeda Y, Kazarov AR, Butterfield CE et al (2007) Deletion of tetraspanin Cd151 results in decreased pathologic angiogenesis in vivo and in vitro. Blood 109:1524–1532

320. Yanez-Mo M, Barreiro O, Gonzalo P, Sala-Valdés M, Sánchez-Madrid F (2008) MT1-MMP collagenolytic activity is regulated through association with tetraspanin CD151 in primary endothelial cells. Blood 112:3217–3226

321. Acker T, Plate KH (2003) Role of hypoxia in tumor angiogenesis-molecular and cellular angiogenic crosstalk. Cell Tissue Res 314:145–155

322. Kerbel RS (2008) Tumor angiogenesis. N Engl J Med 358:2039–2049

323. Roskoski R Jr (2007) Vascular endothelial growth factor (VEGF) signaling in tumor progression. Crit Rev Oncol Hematol 62:179–213

324. Zwicker JI, Furie BC, Furie B (2007) Cancer-associated thrombosis. Crit Rev Oncol Hematol 62:126–136

325. Re RN, Cook JL (2006) An intracrine view of angiogenesis. Bioessays 28:943–953

326. Sood SL (2009) Cancer-associated thrombosis. Curr Opin Hematol 16:378–385

327. Ahmed KA, Xiang J (2009) Microparticles, thrombosis and cancer. Best Pract Res Clin Haematol 22:61–69

328. Kim CW, Lee HM, Lee TH, Kang C, Kleinman HK, Gho YS (2002) Extracellular membrane vesicles from tumor cells promote angiogenesis via sphingomyelin. Cancer Res 62: 6312–6317

329. Millimaggi D, Mari M, D'Ascenzo S et al (2007) Tumor vesicle-associated CD147 modulates the angiogenic capability of endothelial cells. Neoplasia 9:349–357

330. Choi DS, Lee JM, Park GW et al (2007) Proteomic analysis of microvesicles derived from human colorectal cancer cells. J Proteome Res 6:4646–4655

331. van Niel G, Raposo G, Candalh C et al (2001) Intestinal epithelial cells secrete exosome-like vesicles. Gastroenterology 121:337–349

332. Rosi A, Guidoni L, Luciani AM, Mariutti G, Viti V (1988) RNA-lipid complexes released from the plasma membrane of human colon carcinoma cells. Cancer Lett 39: 153–160

333. Fleischhacker M, Schmidt B (2007) Circulating nucleic acids (CNAs) and cancer – a survey. Biochim Biophys Acta 1775:181–232

334. Akao Y, Nakagawa Y, Naoe T (2007) MicroRNA-143 and -145 in colon cancer. DNA Cell Biol 26:311–320

335. Xi Y, Edwards JR, Ju J (2007) Investigation of miRNA biology by bioinformatic tools and impact of miRNAs in colorectal cancer-regulatory relationship of c-Myc and p53 with miRNAs. Cancer Inform 3:245–253

336. Yang L, Belaguli N, Berger DH (2009) MicroRNA and colorectal cancer. World J Surg 33:638–646

337. Faber C, Kirchner T, Hlubek F (2009) The impact of microRNAs on colorectal cancer. Virchows Arch 454:359–367

338. Rossi S, Kopetz S, Davuluri R, Hamilton SR, Calin GA (2010) MicroRNAs, ultraconserved genes and colorectal cancers. Int J Biochem Cell Biol 42:1291–1297

339. Tang JT, Fang JY (2009) MicroRNA regulatory network in human colorectal cancer. Mini Rev Med Chem 9:921–926

340. Valeri N, Croce CM, Fabbri M (2009) Pathogenetic and clinical relevance of microRNAs in colorectal cancer. Cancer Genomics Proteomics 6:195–204

341. Zhang W, Dahlberg JE, Tam W (2007) MicroRNAs in tumorigenesis: a primer. Am J Pathol 171:728–738

342. Gramantieri L, Ferracin M, Fornari F et al (2007) Cyclin G1 is a target of miR-122a, a microRNA frequently down-regulated in human hepatocellular carcinoma. Cancer Res 67:6092–6099

343. Mitomo S, Maesawa C, Ogasawara S et al (2008) Downregulation of miR-138 is associated with overexpression of human telomerase reverse transcriptase protein in human anaplastic thyroid carcinoma cell lines. Cancer Sci 99:280–286

344. Barbarotto E, Schmittgen TD, Calin GA (2008) MicroRNAs and cancer: profile, profile, profile. Int J Cancer 122:969–977

345. Schetter AJ, Leung SY, Sohn JJ et al (2008) MicroRNA expression profiles associated with prognosis and therapeutic outcome in colon adenocarcinoma. JAMA 299:425–436

346. Tazawa H, Tsuchiya N, Izumiya M, Nakagama H (2007) Tumor-suppressive miR-34a induces senescence-like growth arrest through modulation of the E2F pathway in human colon cancer cells. Proc Natl Acad Sci USA 104:15472–15477

347. Guo C, Sah JF, Beard L, Willson JK, Markowitz SD, Guda K (2008) The noncoding RNA, miR-126, suppresses the growth of neoplastic cells by targeting phosphatidylinositol 3-kinase signaling and is frequently lost in colon cancers. Genes Chromosomes Cancer 47:939–946

348. Michael MZ, O'Connor SM, van Holst Pellekaan NG, Young GP, James RJ (2003) Reduced accumulation of specific microRNAs in colorectal neoplasia. Mol Cancer Res 1:882–891

349. Grady WM, Carethers JM (2008) Genomic and epigenetic instability in colorectal cancer pathogenesis. Gastroenterology 135:1079–1099

350. Si ML, Zhu S, Wu H, Lu Z, Wu F, Mo YY (2007) miR-21-mediated tumor growth. Oncogene 26:2799–2803

351. Zhu S, Si ML, Wu H, Mo YY (2007) MicroRNA-21 targets the tumor suppressor gene tropomyosin 1 (TPM1). J Biol Chem 282:14328–14336

352. Cummins JM, He Y, Leary RJ, Pagliarini R et al (2006) The colorectal microRNAome. Proc Natl Acad Sci USA 103:3687–3692

353. Xi Y, Formentini A, Chien M et al (2006) Prognostic values of microRNAs in colorectal cancer. Biomark Insights 2:113–121

354. Asangani IA, Rasheed SA, Nikolova DA et al (2008) MicroRNA-21 (miR-21) post-transcriptionally downregulates tumor suppressor Pdcd4 and stimulates invasion, intravasation and metastasis in colorectal cancer. Oncogene 27:2128–2136

355. Chen X, Ba Y, Ma L et al (2008) Characterization of microRNAs in serum: a novel class of biomarkers for diagnosis of cancer and other diseases. Cell Res 18:997–1006

356. Birchler JA, Kavi HH (2008) Molecular biology. Slicing and dicing for small RNAs. Science 320:1023–1024

357. Shi B, Sepp-Lorenzino L, Prisco M, Linsley P, deAngelis T, Baserga R (2007) Micro RNA 145 targets the insulin receptor substrate-1 and inhibits the growth of colon cancer cells. J Biol Chem 282:32582–32590

358. Taylor DD, Gercel-Taylor C (2008) MicroRNA signatures of tumor-derived exosomes as diagnostic biomarkers of ovarian cancer. Gynecol Oncol 110:13–21

Chapter 5
Role of CXC Chemokines and Receptors in Liver Metastasis – Impact on Liver Resection-Induced Engraftment and Tumor Growth

Otto Kollmar, Michael D. Menger, and Martin K. Schilling

Abstract Chemokines are inflammatory cytokines that stimulate the migration of distinct subsets of cells including tumor cells. The chemokines MIP (macrophage inflammatory protein)-2 and SDF (stromal cell-derived factor)-1 that are both members of the CXC chemokine superfamily have an important impact on tumor progression and metastasis of colorectal cancer. Our experimental studies demonstrate that chemotactic signaling does not only contribute to the metastatic spread of tumor cells, but is also essential for tumor engraftment and progression. These studies on chemokines have exceeded the previous expectations in elucidating homing mechanisms directing colorectal cancer metastasis and have given us a deeper insight into the mechanisms that regulate tumor growth. Chemotactic signaling is necessary for a variety of physiological and pathological processes including inflammatory response, leukocyte traffic, angiogenesis and programmed cell death. Therefore, it seems very unlikely that targeting one single chemokine will be sufficient as a single modality therapy for cancer treatment. The complex network of chemokines and chemokine receptors could provide compensatory mechanisms to overcome permanent deprivation of a specific chemokine, as we already demonstrated for MIP-2 and SDF-1. Our findings thus far encourage further investigation. The chemotactic signaling in cancer is a new and promising target/perspective for anti-tumor therapy.

Keywords Chemokines · Chemokine receptors · Colorectal cancer · Liver metastasis · Hepatectomy

Abbreviations

ENA-78	epithelial neutrophil-activating protein-78
GCP-2	granulocyte chemotactic protein-2
GFP	green fluorescent protein

O. Kollmar (✉)
Department of General, Visceral, Vascular and Pediatric Surgery, University of Saarland, D-66421 Homburg/Saar, Germany
e-mail: otto.kollmar@uks.eu

P. Brodt (ed.), *Liver Metastasis: Biology and Clinical Management*, Cancer Metastasis – Biology and Treatment 16, DOI 10.1007/978-94-007-0292-9_5, © Springer Science+Business Media B.V. 2011

GRO-α/-β/-γ	growth-related oncogene-α/-β/-γ
HCC	hepatocellular carcinoma
IL-8	interleukin-8
I-TAC	interferon-inducible T-cell alpha chemoattractant
MCP-1	monocyte chemotactic protein-1
MIP-2	macrophage inflammatory protein-2
PF-4	platelet factor-4
SDF-1	stromal cell-derived factor-1
TGF-α/-β	transforming growth factor-α/-β
TNF-α	tumour necrosis factor-α
VEGF	vascular endothelial growth factor

Contents

5.1 Liver and Extrahepatic Metastasis of Colorectal Cancer

Colorectal cancer is the second leading cause of cancer-related death in the Western World [1, 2]. The death of the patients is usually the result of the uncontrolled metastatic spread of the tumor. Therapeutic options in case of unresectable metastases are confined to non-curative chemotherapeutic treatment. As patients often present with advanced primary tumors, more than 50% of them suffer from synchronous or metachronous metastases [1–3]. The metastatic process consists of several steps all of which must be successfully completed until a metastatic tumor becomes clinically detectable [4]. Therefore, only a small subset of metastatic tumor cells will survive, proliferate and finally form a solid tumor [5]. Although much research effort has been made during the last decades, we are far from understanding the metastatic process as a whole.

The liver is the most common site of hematogenous metastasis for colorectal cancer. There is some evidence that this metastatic pattern is not only a result of hemodynamic factors and accessibility to the portal circulation but is also directed by "homing" mechanisms [6]. This hypothesis is not new. It is mainly based on the so called "seed and soil"-theory that was first published by Stephen Paget in 1889. Paget postulated that metastatic tumor growth ("seed") in host tissues ("soil") can only occur under appropriate, tissue specific conditions [7].

The benefit of curative resection of colorectal liver metastases with a 5-year overall survival rate of up to 58% is well recognized [1, 8–10]. Furthermore, anatomic resections reduce the rate of positive margins and improve overall survival [11]. In terms of radical tumor excision, modern surgical strategies from major hepatobiliary centers have demonstrated that hepatectomy of as much as 70 percent of the liver can be performed with a surgically associated mortality rate of less than 5% [12–15]. Compared to minor segmental liver resections, major hepatectomy has a higher complication rate, including bile leaks, abscesses and hepatic failure [16–18]. The extent of liver resection and the degree of baseline functional impairment are the main independent risk factors for these postoperative complications [13]. (For a more extensive discussion on clinical management of colorectal carcinoma liver metastases, see Chapter 12).

For a long time, extrahepatic metastases have been considered a contraindication for hepatectomy. Over the last few years, however, 5-year survival rates of up to 30% have been reported after resection of liver and extrahepatic colorectal metastases in the lung, brain, bone and other sites [19]. In line with this, Elias et al. have demonstrated that complete resection of all metastases of colorectal cancer is more important for the overall patient survival than the location and the number of the metastases [19].

5.2 Tumor Growth and Angiogenesis – Role of Chemokines

Innate immune system processes can potentially promote tumor progression through inflammation-dependent mechanisms [20, 21]. Clinical and experimental studies indicate that CXC chemokines enhance immunity to tumor-associated antigens. These chemokines also regulate angiogenesis, promote proliferation, control tumor apoptosis and mediate tumor cell invasion and trafficking in an organ-specific manner, ultimately supporting the formation of metastases [22–24].

The progressive growth of a malignant solid tumor depends on the development of new blood vessels that provide oxygen and nutrients to the tumor cells [25]. The tumor vasculature has to be considered abnormal [26], inasmuch as tumor vessels are organized in a chaotic fashion and do not follow the hierarchical branching pattern of normal vascular networks [27]. In addition, the endothelial cells form an imperfect lining with wide junctions resulting in a large number of fenestrations that expose cancer cells to the lumen, thus forming so-called "mosaic blood vessels" [28]. As a result of this abnormal organization and ultrastructure, the diameters of those tumor vessels are irregular, the blood flow is chaotic and the endothelial lining is leaky [27].

It is widely accepted that tumor angiogenesis is initiated due to an imbalance between positive and negative-regulating molecules that are released by tumor cells and host cells into the tumor micro-environment [29–31]. In addition to cytokines of the vascular endothelial growth factor (VEGF) family that play a key role in angiogenesis, chemokines are also considered to be important and powerful inducers of this process. The chemokines are chemotactic cytokines of small molecular weight that stimulate migration of a variety of cells including leukocytes, lymphocytes and tumor cells. They are the ligands of the chemokine receptors which represent a family of seven transmembrane domains, G-protein-coupled receptors on the cell surface [6, 32, 33]. Chemokines and their receptors can be further divided into subfamilies according to their protein structure. Of particular interest is the CXC chemokine subfamily [33]. CXC chemokines with the three amino acids glutamic acid-leucine-arginine immediately amino-terminal to the CXC motif (ELR$^+$) are thought to be angiogenic, while (ELR$^-$) CXC chemokines are angiostatic [34].

5.3 CXC Receptor Expression in Colorectal Cancer Metastasis

Because chemokines can induce cell motility, their role in metastasis- a process dependent on tumor cell migration- has been of great interest [35]. Several studies have already demonstrated a close correlation between the chemokine receptors expressed on neoplastic cells and the chemokine ligands found in their organ sites of metastasis [36].

The ELR$^+$ CXC chemokines such as interleukin-8 (IL-8), growth-related oncogenes -α, -β, -γ (GRO-α, GRO-β, GRO-γ), granulocyte chemotactic protein-2 (GCP-2), neutrophil-activating protein-2 and epithelial neutrophil-activating protein-78 (ENA-78) are potent promoters of angiogenesis (see Table 5.1). To date, CXCR1 and 2 are the only receptors identified for ELR$^+$ chemokines. While GCP-2, ENA-78 and IL-8 bind to both receptors, all other ELR$^+$ chemokines interact with,

Table 5.1 CXC chemokine/receptor nomenclature

Systematic name	Human ligand	Mouse ligand	Receptor(s)
CXCL1	GRO-α/MGSA-α	GRO/MIP-2/KC	CXCR1, CXCR2
CXCL2	GRO-β/MGSA-v	GRO/MIP-2/KC	CXCR2
CXCL3	GRO-γ/MGSA-γ	GRO/MIP-2/KC	CXCR2
CXCL4	PF-4	PF-4	Unknown
CXCL5	ENA-78	GCP-2/LIX	CXCR2
CXCL6	GCP-2	GCP-2/LIX	CXCR1, CXCR2
CXCL7	NAP-2	Unknown	CXCR2
CXCL8	IL-8	Unknown	CXCR1, CXCR2
CXCL9	Mig	Mig	CXCR3
CXCL10	IP-10	IP-10/CRG-2	CXCR3
CXCL11	I-TAC	I-TAC	CXCR3, CXCR7
CXCL12	SDF-1	SDF-1	CXCR4, CXCR7
CXCL13	BCA-1	BLC	CXCR5
CXCL14	BRAK	BRAK	Unknown
CXCL15	Unknown	Lungkine/WECHE	Unknown
CXCL16			CXCR6

and activate CXCR2 selectively. The receptor that has been identified for (ELR$^-$) CXC chemokines is CXCR3. ELR$^-$ CXC chemokines such as platelet factor-4 (PF-4) and interferon-inducible CXC chemokines are potent angiostatic factors that can inhibit neovascularization mediated by ELR$^+$ chemokines and other angiogenic factors such as basic fibroblast growth factor and vascular endothelial growth factor. Angiostatic CXC chemokines mediate inhibition of angiogenesis exclusively through binding and activation of CXCR3 that was originally identified on murine endothelial cells. The homeostatic chemokine SDF-1 is a non-ELR chemokine that signals via CXCR4 and has also been implicated in promoting angiogenesis and metastasis [36].

The CC-chemokines CCL19 and CCL21 are highly expressed in lymph nodes and signal through a common receptor, the lymphocyte chemoattractant receptor CCR7 [37, 38]. While CCR7 was recently reported to predict lymph node metastasis in colorectal carcinoma and other cancer types [39, 40], the cognate SDF-1 receptor CXCR4 has been suggested as a risk factor for the outgrowth of colon carcinoma micrometastases [41] and the invasion and spreading of several other cancers [36, 42]. Also, CCL20/CCR6 involvement in the neoplastic progression and site-specific metastasis of several tumor types has been reported, with major focus on the amplification of the local necro-inflammatory response in the liver [43, 44], identifying CCR6 as an important factor in the recruitment of lymphocytes from peripheral blood to hepatocellular carcinoma [45].

Comparing the expression profiles for several chemokine/chemokine receptor pairs namely, SDF-1/CXCR4, CCL20/CCR6 and CCL19/CCL21/CCR7 in hepatocellular carcinoma (HCC) versus colorectal liver metastases our group demonstrated an association between the CCR6/CCL20 expression in colorectal cancer and the promotion of colorectal liver metastasis [23, 46]. Furthermore, a correlation between the CCL20/CCR6 expression levels in HCC and colorectal liver metastases with a marked over-expression of the CCL20 gene product in relation to HCC tissues could be observed [46]. No correlation between the CCR7 expression levels of HCC or colorectal liver metastases and CCL19/CCL21 expression could be found. Similarly, the corresponding ligands CCL19 and CCL21 showed no significant difference in their gene expression levels measured in the tumor and tumor-neighboring tissues in either cancer type. Investigating SDF-1/CXCR4 expression, our group showed that CXCR4 is significantly up-regulated in colorectal liver metastases as compared with the tumor-neighboring liver tissues, whereas no significant difference in gene expression was detected for CXCR4 in the HCC tissues, indicating a distinct difference in the CXCR4 expression pattern in HCC and colorectal liver metastases [46]. Unlike CXCR4, expression of the chemokine ligand SDF-1 was not significantly different in the tumor and tumor-neighboring tissue in HCC or colorectal liver metastasis, indicating that SDF-1 and CXCR4 are inversely expressed in colorectal liver metastases. In summary, our group could demonstrate an association between expression of the CCL20/CCR6 pair and the development and progression of hepatic malignancies. CCL20, as well as the chemokine receptor CXCR4 are therefore potential predictive markers for tumor grading and the existence of liver metastases [46].

Analyzing the expression profile of the ELR$^+$ CXC chemokines GRO-α, ENA-78 and GCP-2 and their corresponding CXCR2 receptor in colorectal adenomas, colorectal carcinomas and the corresponding colorectal carcinoma liver metastases, our group demonstrates a direct correlation between GRO-α and ENA-78 expression and diagnosis of colon cancer [47]. GRO-α and ENA-78 were significantly up-regulated in neoplastic colorectal tissue compared to tissue of colorectal adenomas. Since colorectal adenomas are a pre-malignant condition, we hypothesize that both chemokines have a potential role in the progression from colorectal adenoma to colorectal carcinoma and thus in the initiation of colorectal liver metastases [47].

Despite increasing knowledge about the involvement of CXC receptors in the invasion and dissemination of various cancer types, the precise mechanisms regulating the process of organ-selective metastasis of colorectal cancer remain unclear. Therefore, our group analyzed the RNA and protein expression profile of chemokine receptors CXCR1–4 in inflammatory and malignant colorectal diseases along with their corresponding hepatic metastases to elucidate a potential association with colorectal cancer progression and the development of liver metastases. As we reported, no significant change in the expression levels of these receptors could be found in nonmalignant colorectal diseases such as ulcerative colitis or colorectal adenomas, conditions often preceding the development of colorectal malignancies. CXCR1 and 2 expressions were significantly upregulated only in the primary tumors and found mainly in mesenchymal cells. No upregulation of CXCR1 and 2 were observed in colorectal liver metastases, corresponding to low staining intensities restricted to few leukocytes only. CXCR3 expression was significantly upregulated only in colorectal liver metastases as reflected in intense staining of mesenchymal and tumour cells within colorectal liver metastases specimens. No substantial CXCR3 immunostaining was detected within primary colorectal cancer specimens corresponding to RNA and protein levels, which showed no CXCR3 upregulation in primary tumors. However, CXCR4 was significantly upregulated in primary tumors as well as in colorectal liver metastases, although it was differentially localized in these sites. In primary tumors it was expressed mainly by tumour cells while in colorectal liver metastases, strong CXCR4 staining intensities were detected mainly in a streak of hepatocytes along the tumour invasion front. In summary, our data revealed a differential expression pattern of CXCR1-4 in colorectal carcinomas and their corresponding liver metastases, with prominent expression profiles indicating a potential role of CXC chemokine receptors in the pathogenesis of colorectal cancer [48].

5.4 Interleukin-8/Macrophage Inflammatory Protein-2 and Colorectal Cancer

The human IL-8 has been shown to act as potent neutrophil chemoattractant that contributes to healing processes, but also to pathological manifestation of inflammatory conditions, such as sepsis, inflammatory bowel disease, rheumatoid arthritis and cerebral and myocardial infarction [49].

IL-8 is also thought to be involved in tumor growth and metastasis. Recent studies have indicated that constitutive IL-8 expression levels in individual tumor cell lines in vitro strongly correlate with the in vivo growth and metastatic potential [50, 51]. IL-8 may stimulate tumor cell motility and migration [52, 53] and has been shown to act as an autocrine growth factor for tumor cell proliferation [54]. In addition, the progression of tumor growth mediated by IL-8 may not only be due to a direct action on tumor cells, but has been proposed to involve the induction of angiogenesis [55]. This view is based on studies that demonstrated a significant correlation between tumor microvessel density and IL-8 levels [56] and an inhibition of tumor angiogenesis by neutralization of IL-8 [57–59].

The biological relevance of IL-8 expression and its role in tumor progression and metastasis, however, are still a subject of controversy [51, 53]. There are metastatic tumor cell lines that do not produce IL-8 [60] and other studies have indicated that there is a lack of correlation between the level of IL-8 expression and the tumorigenic/metastatic potential of tumor cells [53]. Although in epithelial ovarian cancer, VEGF and IL-8 expression have been considered to indicate poor prognosis [61], other studies have shown that IL-8 production by ovarian cancer cells significantly reduce tumor growth [62]. In one study of colorectal cancer patients, serum levels of IL-8 have been shown to be significantly higher in patients with liver metastases than in those without metastases [51, 63], but it has also been demonstrated that IL-8 can induce an anti-tumoral effect that is associated with an enhanced infiltration of T-lymphocytes [64]. Analyzing the expression profile of IL-8 in inflammatory and malignant colorectal diseases, our group showed that IL-8 expression strongly correlates with induction and progression of colorectal carcinoma [65]. The magnitude of IL-8 expression in colorectal liver metastases directly correlated with colorectal cancer progression and the development of synchronous and metachronous liver metastases. Irrespective of the tumor stage, IL-8 expression was significantly higher in colorectal cancer tissues as compared to inflammatory colorectal conditions and adenomas of the colon/rectum [65]. Our analyses suggested a close correlation between IL-8 up-regulation and the development of colorectal cancer. Furthermore, IL-8 was over-expressed in colorectal liver metastases as compared to the respective primary colorectal tumors, indicating a strong association between IL-8 expression and the malignant status of colorectal cancer cells as well as between IL-8 expression and the development of colorectal liver metastases [65].

The murine CXC chemokine MIP-2 is a functional analogue of the human IL-8 [66–72]. In general, macrophages, but also granulocytic and monocytic leukocytes, as well as endothelial cells and fibroblasts can produce MIP-2 upon stimulation [73–75]. However, MIP-2 is also expressed by a variety of different tumors, including colorectal carcinoma [34]. Similarly to IL-8, MIP-2 acts through interaction with its receptor CXCR2 as a potent neutrophil chemoattractant, contributing to wound healing [76], but also mediating inflammatory injury [77].

Little is known, however, about the pro-angiogenic properties of MIP-2 and its ability to induce tumor growth and metastasis. MIP-2 is thought to act via VEGF in a paracrine angiogenic loop. Liss et al. [78] demonstrated that the secretion of monocyte chemotactic protein (MCP)-1 and transforming growth factor-beta1

(TGF-β1) by tumor cells activates tumor-associated macrophages that act in a paracrine fashion by producing and secreting tumor necrosis factor-alpha (TNF-α) and interleukin-1. This stimulates tumor cells to secrete IL-8, the functional human analogue of the murine MIP-2, and VEGF [78], which can both promote cell proliferation and tumor vascularization. The impact of MIP-2/CXCR2 signaling in colorectal malignancy seems to be clinically important because, as indicated above, studies on colorectal diseases have revealed an association between an increase in the expression of human IL-8 and the induction and progression of colorectal carcinoma [65].

Investigating the influence of MIP-2 on tumor growth and metastasis in colorectal cancer, our group used the well established colorectal cancer cell line CT26.WT for in vitro and in vivo experiments [79–85]. The CT26.WT cell line is a chemically induced, undifferentiated adenocarcinoma of the colon, syngeneic with the BALB/c mouse. When implanted into BALB/c mice, almost 100% of the animals develop solid tumors with highly aggressive and metastatic growth characteristics [79, 86]. Using flow cytometry, our group found that 98.8% of the CT26.WT cells derived from cell culture expressed the CXCR2 receptor on the cell surface [80]. Not surprisingly therefore, these cells migrated in response to a MIP-2 gradient in an in vitro chemotactic assay using 24-well chemotaxis chambers. MIP-2 induced an increase in cell adhesion to the polycarbonate filters at a dose as low as 0.1 nM with the most pronounced increase in adhesion as compared to controls occurring at doses of 10 and 100 nM (4- and 6-fold increases respectively). Interestingly, a further increase of the MIP-2 concentration (200 and 400 nM) markedly attenuated the adhesive response measured as increased cell spreading. In accordance with these results, MIP-2 stimulation increased the number of cells that migrated through the filter into the lower wells of the chemotaxis chamber by 2 to 4-fold in response to the lower doses (0.1–100 nM) but when challenged with higher doses (200–400 nM) the migration increased exponentially (9 and 18-fold) as compared to controls. Under control conditions only a few adherent and migrating cells could be detected [80].

Because of the strong chemotactic response of the tumor cells to MIP-2, our group further investigated the influence of MIP-2 on metastatic colorectal tumors [80] using a standardized in vivo liver metastasis model in mice [79]. MIP-2 at a concentration of 10 nM significantly increased the tumor volume by 14-fold when compared to control animals. At 100 nM, tumor volume was further increased up to 27-fold. Interestingly, higher doses of MIP-2 (1 μM) were less effective and led to tumor volumes comparable in size to those of animals treated with 10 nM of MIP-2. The physiological levels of MIP-2 have not been reported in the literature. Because it was previously shown that high doses of MIP-2 were capable of inducing programmed cell death, we and other groups concluded that the delay in tumor growth may have been due to an increase in tumor cell apoptosis [80, 87]. Indeed, using intravital microscopy, our group found a 4-fold increase in nuclear condensation and fragmentation after an injection of 1 μM MIP-2. Tumor cell proliferation was not however affected by this concentration of MIP-2. CXCR2 expression, especially at the tumor margin, significantly increased after exposure to MIP-2 as compared to control tumors. This effect was most pronounced after treatment with 10 nM MIP-2. In this context, an association between the magnitude of CXCR2 receptor expression and the metastatic potential of the colon carcinoma cells could be assumed [31, 65, 80]. The fact that almost 100% of the CT26.WT cells were CXCR2 positive in culture suggests that these cells had the potential to be highly aggressive based on the criteria of growth rate and cell spreading, depending on the exposure to MIP-2. In vivo, approximately 40% of the cells of non-treated CT26.WT tumors showed positive CXCR2 staining 7 days after tumor cell implantation. This reduction (relative to in vitro conditions) can probably be explained by the fact that solid tumors in vivo consist of various non-malignant cells including endothelia, fibroblasts and stromal cells that do not necessarily express CXCR2. Our results show that exposure to MIP-2 in vivo could increase CXCR2 expression levels in the first week post-implantation, possibly due to receptor recycling that increased the efficiency of MIP-2 signaling [88]. Because receptor expression appears to be required for the proliferative effect of chemokines on tumors as shown for CXCR4 [41], the increased in vivo expression of CXCR2 may represent the underlying mechanism for the MIP-2-associated increase in tumor growth.

As tumor progression and increased local tumor growth are usually associated with an angiogenic response, our group analyzed the angioarchitecture of the intrahepatic tumors using intravital microscopy [80]. Within the angiogenic front, a network of chaotically arranged, newly developed capillaries and large draining venules were found (see Fig. 5.1). MIP-2 at concentrations of 100 and 1000 nM, but not of 10 nM, significantly increased the size of the angiogenic front and the density of draining venules (2- and 4-fold, respectively) when compared to controls. Interestingly, MIP-2, at any of these concentrations, significantly increased capillary density within the tumors (5 to 6-fold). The stimulated angiogenic activity in MIP-2-treated tumors was also associated with a significant enlargement of tumor capillaries within the tumor margin after exposure to 100 and 1000 nM MIP-2. These observations clearly show that local exposure to MIP-2 induced persistent changes within the angioarchitecture with overall stimulation of angiogenic activity.

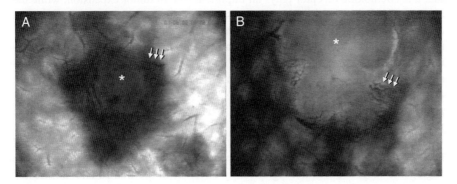

Fig. 5.1 Tumors locally treated with PBS (**a**; controls) and 1000 nM MIP-2 (**b**). The tumors (*asterisks*) are surrounded by an angiogenic front, which appears as a dark rim. Within this angiogenic front new tumor vessels could be observed (*triple arrows*)

Significantly, a single application of MIP-2 was sufficient to induce these effects identifying this chemokine as a potent pro-angiogenic factor. These findings were particularly interesting in view of the fact that there is still little information concerning the proangiogenic activity of MIP-2 in tumor growth [80]. Leukocytes are known to express VEGF, one of the most important angiogenic factors in malignant and non-malignant diseases. The angiogenic effect of MIP-2, as detected in our and others studies, may therefore be associated with an increased release of VEGF by the accumulated leukocytes within the tumor vasculature [80, 89]. This is supported by the finding that vasodilatation, which is also known to be associated with VEGF, was also found to increase after MIP-2 exposure.

As a further extension to these studies, we tested the effects of MIP-2 in a model of subcutaneously transplanted tumors. Using the dorsal skinfold chamber assay, we were able to study the early stages of tumor development, including early angiogenesis, repetitively over a period of 14 days using intravital microscopy [90]. To allow repetitive intravital microscopic analyses without additional application of fluorescent markers, CT26.WT cells had been transfected to express green fluorescent protein (GFP). Local application of MIP-2 was carried out 5 days after tumor cell implantation, when a small established tumor had grown in the dorsal skinfold chamber. As already observed in intrahepatic tumors, MIP-2 treatment provoked a significant acceleration of tumor growth [82]. This increased tumor growth was due to a stimulation of tumor cell proliferation. Whereas control tumors without MIP-2 treatment displayed a proliferation rate of ~40% at this time point, the proportion of proliferating tumor cells as assessed by proliferating cell nuclear antigen staining increased up to ~80% after exposure to MIP-2. It was further found that within the tumor margin, the majority of cells were CXCR2 positive whereas within the tumor center, only a minority of the cells expressed CXCR2. Local treatment with 100 nM MIP-2 did not affect CXCR2 expression in the tumor margin, but significantly increased the number of CXCR2-positive cells within the tumor center. Because tumor growth is usually highly pronounced in the tumor margin, but not in the center, the high CXCR2 expression levels seen in the margin may signify that this chemokine receptor plays an important role in tumor expansion, while the absence of a further increase in the expression in response to MIP-2 may have been due to the fact that it was already maximally upregulated in this region. In addition, histological examinations revealed a more pronounced muscle infiltration by tumors which had been exposed to MIP-2 suggesting that increased CXCR2 expression is associated with increased invasiveness and malignancy. Taken together, these results by our group demonstrate that MIP-2 can act autonomously to increase tumor growth by transcriptionally activating its own receptor and inducing an autocrine proliferative loop [82].

Contrary to the observations in hepatic metastases, MIP-2 administration did not stimulate angiogenesis of established extrahepatic metastases. The onset of the angiogenic response was not significantly different in the treated and non-treated groups, whereas the capillary density of newly formed tumor vessels was even lower in the MIP-2 treated than in the control group. These results indicate that in contrast to developing tumors, MIP-2 in established tumors does not provoke an increased release of VEGF. Accordingly, neither an increase of microvessel diameter nor an elevation of microvascular permeability that would have pointed towards a VEGF effect could be detected [82].

5.5 Stromal Cell-Derived Factor-1 and Colorectal Cancer

The findings described above showed that chemotactic signaling is of major importance during tumor engraftment and progression. They also suggested that MIP-2 is not the only chemotactic cytokine orchestrating tumor development. Another member of the CXC chemokine superfamiliy – SDF-1 – has become a subject of intense research. SDF-1 and its receptor CXCR4 were implicated in cell migration, proliferation, differentiation and survival of different subsets of cells [6, 88]. In the case of mammary carcinoma, Müller et al. who found CXCR4 expression on primary breast cancer cells, discovered elevated levels of SDF-1 in the first metastatic sites of breast cancer such as lymph nodes, lung, liver and bone marrow [36]. These results have been corroborated by several studies that demonstrated that elevated levels of plasma SDF-1 in patients with solid tumors, such as breast and gastric cancer, correlated with tumor progression and a poorer prognosis [91, 92].

Similar to the in vitro studies performed with MIP-2, our group showed that CT26.WT cells migrated towards a chemotactic gradient of SDF-1 in the chemotaxis chamber assay [83]. SDF-1 at a dose of 0.1 nM induced a 3.4-fold increase in cell adherence on the polycarbonate filters of the chamber. With 1 nM SDF-1, this effect was even more pronounced, as indicated by a 4.3-fold increase as compared to controls. Notably, a further increase in SDF-1 concentrations resulted in a markedly decreased number of adherent cells on the lower surface of the filters. Analysis of the number of tumor cells that had migrated through the filters to the lower wells indicated a 2 to 6-fold increase after low-dose stimulation with SDF-1 (0.1–100 nM), whereas higher doses of 200 and 400 nM resulted in an exponential increase (16 to 17-fold) when compared to controls [83]. These effects were also shown with non-small cell lung cancer cells and were similar to those described for MIP-2 [93].

Whereas many chemokines bind to more than one receptor and chemokine receptors generally bind more than one ligand, the SDF-1/CXCR4 interaction has long been considered "monogamous". Recently however, CXCR7 was identified as a second receptor for SDF-1 [94]. However, SDF-1 is still the only known ligand for CXCR4 [95]. SDF-1 induces the internalization of CXCR4, promoting calcium mobilization and activation of mitogen-activated protein kinase pathways, such as extracellular signal-regulated kinases 1 and 2, phosphatidylinositol 3-kinase and protein kinase B. These kinases are implicated in cell migration, proliferation, differentiation and survival [88]. CXCR4 is thought to facilitate the interaction between tumor cells and endothelial cells by activating rolling, integrin function, arrest and transendothelial migration of tumor cells [96, 97]. Although never proven in vivo, SDF-1 has been postulated to direct the intra-tissue localization of tumor cells and to induce metastasis through direct effects on tumor cell migration [32, 98].

As suggested by Zeelenberg et al. [41], SDF-1 also acts as a tissue specific growth factor which supports local tumor growth in vivo. Our group examined the effects of locally applied SDF-1 on colorectal metastases from CT26.WT-GFP cells in the dorsal skinfold chamber of BALB/c mice. Five days after implantation of the tumor cells into the chamber, we applied 100 nM SDF-1 onto the surface of the tumor and the surrounding tissue. We found that SDF-1 significantly induced progressive growth of the metastases. This enhanced tumor growth was associated with significantly increased tumor cell proliferation, whereas tumor cell apoptosis was significantly inhibited, as compared to controls [83]. In previous studies, it has been demonstrated that SDF-1 provokes activation of both the extracellular signal-regulated kinase-2, a known regulator of gene transcription, and protein kinase B [88, 99]. The SDF-1/CXCR4 pathway has also been shown to influence the growth of invasive and micrometastatic tumors reflecting downstream signaling through the anti-apoptotic Akt and the phosphatidylinositol 3-kinase [41, 100, 101]. Although all these studies have been performed using in vitro setups, our findings that SDF-1 increases tumor growth in vivo suggest that these mechanisms are also activated in vivo [83].

In the in vivo setting, the SDF-1 – mediated increase in neovascularization within the tumors was transient [83]. Immediately after a single application, microvessel densities within the tumors increased markedly relative to non-treated controls. But within nine days post treatment the capillary densities in both groups were comparable. However, microvessels in tumors that had been exposed to SDF-1 but not controls, showed a significant vasodilatation during the entire observation period. These results indicate that SDF-1 can promote intra-tumoral angiogenesis but that a sustained effect probably requires continuous stimulation. Interestingly, SDF-1 belongs to the group of ELR$^-$ CXC chemokines thought to be potent angiogenesis inhibitors [34], yet it was implicated in angiodevelopment during ontogenesis, suggesting that it may be an exception to the rule. Other studies also support the pro-angiogenic activities of the SDF-1/CXCR4 axis because they have shown a correlation between CXCR4 expression levels and microvessel density within tumors [96]. Furthermore, in vitro studies found increased VEGF mRNA and VEGF protein expression in colorectal cancer cells stimulated with SDF-1, suggesting that the pro-angiogenic effect of SDF-1 is VEGF-mediated [99]. This is also supported by our own findings of increased microvessel diameters, because VEGF is known to induce vasodilatation. In addition to the VEGF-dependent effect however, SDF-1 may also have VEGF-independent pro-angiogenic activity because it could increase vascular sprouting in vitro in an aortic ring model [102]. Moreover, it has been reported that carcinoma-associated fibroblasts secreting SDF-1, promote angiogenesis by recruiting endothelial precursor cells into growing tumors in vivo [103]. Consistent with the more aggressive nature of tumors with increased angiogenesis, we also observed that in SDF-1-treated tumors there was increased invasion of the underlying tissue at the base of the tumors relative to untreated controls [83].

Taken together, these data indicate that SDF-1 does not merely act as a chemotactic cytokine directing tumor cells to their metastatic sites, but is also a potent local growth factor supporting proliferation and angiogenesis on the one hand and inhibiting tumor cell apoptosis on the other. Thus it is an important component of the fertile "soil" that sustains the outgrowth of tumor metastases.

5.6 Liver Resection-Induced Tumor Growth

Major liver resection initiates rapid regeneration and growth of the remaining liver to restore the functional hepatic capacity [104]. The cellular changes that provoke liver regeneration are orchestrated by a complex network of different growth factors, cytokines [104–106] and chemokines [107–109]. The latter include MIP-2, ENA-78 and IL-8, which may all act through the CXCR2 receptor. The important role of this receptor has been confirmed by evidence that blockade with antibodies or gene-targeted deletions in transgenic animals significantly reduced regeneration after hepatectomy [107, 109]. There appears however, to be a redundancy in the role of individual chemokines in regeneration after hepatectomy. As already indicated above, the murine CXC chemokine MIP-2 is a functional analogue of human IL-8. While blockade of the chemokine receptor CXCR2 was found to decrease regeneration of the residual liver, neutralization of MIP-2 through the use of anti-MIP-2 antibodies did not affect the process of regeneration, as indicated by unchanged liver to body weight ratios [109]. These findings indicate that other chemokines may replace or act via the CXCR2 receptor to induce liver regeneration when MIP-2 is deleted [107, 109].

For patients with colorectal liver metastases, surgical resection is currently considered the only curative treatment. Modern surgical strategies from major hepatobiliary centers have demonstrated that hepatectomy of as much as 70% of the liver can be performed with a mortality rate of less than 5% [13, 14]. In addition to parenchymal regeneration, hepatectomy can also accelerate tumor growth in the remaining liver [110–114] as well as in remote organ sites [115]. Although it is well recognized that the liver completely regenerates after major hepatectomy, the effect of hepatic regeneration on intra- and extrahepatic tumor growth is still a matter of controversy with a considerable number of studies demonstrating an acceleration of intra- and extrahepatic tumor growth after liver resection [110, 112, 115–117] and others reporting no effects or even regression of tumor metastases after hepatectomy [117–119]. Slooter and coworkers showed that a 70% liver resection provoked excessive growth of liver metastases when compared to non-resected controls. Of interest, the intravenous application of TNF-α significantly reduced this outgrowth of tumor masses [114]. In fact, the magnitude of stimulation of tumor growth is thought to be proportional to the volume of the resected liver tissue [111, 113, 114]. The cause of enhanced tumor growth in the liver after hepatectomy is likely multifactorial. It has been suggested that in addition to mechanisms mediating liver regeneration e.g. rapid proliferation of all cellular elements within the liver, TGF-α and -β expression, residual "dormant" micrometastases or tumor cells in the remnant liver are stimulated through distinct pro-tumorigenic factors, e.g. increased growth factor expression, immunosuppression and Kupffer cell derangement after liver resection [112, 113]. In addition, a suppression of local defense mechanisms due to decreased tumoricidal activity of Kupffer cell and systemic immune paralysis may also contribute to the enhancement of tumor growth [120].

Because of these controversial results, our group analyzed the effect of minor (30%) and major (70%) hepatectomy on tumor engraftment, neovascularization and tumor cell migration using the dorsal skinfold chamber assay [121]. We found that the growth of CT26.WT-GFP tumors was stimulated proportionally to the extent of liver resection. Whereas after minor hepatectomy only a slight increase in extra-hepatic tumor growth could be observed, major hepatectomy resulted in a rapid acceleration of tumor growth. In Accordance, a massive increase in the angiogenic activity could also be observed after major hepatectomy. These findings are not surprising because a considerable number of different hepatotrophic factors, which regulate the restoration of the liver cell mass after hepatectomy, such as VEGF and hepatocyte growth factor display angiogenic properties [122–124]. Furthermore, in addition to the massive stimulation of tumor growth and angiogenesis, a signifi-cant increase in tumor cell migration, especially after major hepatectomy could be observed [121].

The findings that chemotactic cytokines such as ENA-78 and MIP-2 also par-ticipate in liver regeneration and that their blockade with antibodies or deletion in gene-targeted animals significantly impaired liver regeneration [107, 109] suggest that increased chemotactic signaling after liver resection contributes to an acceler-ation of tumor growth. The clinical implication of this observation is that patients with colorectal liver metastases who have undergone surgical resection may often present with recurrent intra- and extrahepatic metastases [9]. Possible source of recurrent colorectal metastases are nests of tumor cells or dormant micrometastases that are <5 mm in diameter, cannot be detected by pre- or intraoperative imaging devices and therefore are not removed [125]. If these tumor cells remained dormant, they would not be clinically relevant. However, during liver regeneration, they may be initiated and become macrometastases [112]. Keeping these micrometastases in the dormant state by targeting chemokines and/or their receptors may therefore be an effective strategy for prolonging disease or progression-free survival of cancer patients.

5.7 Role of MIP-2 in Hepatectomy-Associated Metastatic Growth in the Remnant Liver

Based on prior findings on the effect of chemokine MIP-2 on the outgrowth and progression of colorectal metastases, we tested the effect of an anti MIP-2 antibody on the liver resection-associated acceleration of tumor growth as reflected in the development of colorectal carcinoma liver metastases.

Consistent with previous results, we found that the intrahepatic tumor growth was markedly stimulated after a 50%-hepatectomy, as indicated by an 18-fold increase in tumor volume in comparison to non-resected controls [81]. Treatment with the anti-MIP-2 antibody significantly reduced the tumor growth-stimulating effect of liver resection by 3-fold. Angiogenic activity, which was also found to be stimulated after hepatectomy, was also reduced after anti-MIP-2 treatment. In addition, we found an increase in CXCR2 expression on the tumor cells after hepatectomy consistent with a role for the CXCR2/MIP-2 axis in liver resection-associated acceleration of tumor growth [81]. As previous results of the group indicated that elevated levels of MIP-2 enhance the expression of their own receptor, this may represent an autocrine mechanism that stimulates tumor growth [80]. In line with these results, blockade of MIP-2 significantly reduced tumor cell proliferation as well as CXCR2 expression on the tumor cells as compared to controls. Notably, tumors of animals treated with anti-MIP-2 antibody, but not of controls exhibited central necrotic areas. This increased necrosis may be due to several mechanisms: (1) the reduced vascularization within the tumors following anti-MIP-2 treatment may result in hypoxic conditions causing ischemia and necrotic cell death [126] and (2) the functional inhibition of MIP-2 may reduce the recruitment of inflammatory cells that could otherwise remove cell debris from the center of the tumor [81, 126, 127].

Notably, the administration of anti MIP-2 antibodies did not impair the proliferation of normal hepatocytes in the regenerating liver [81]. This is in line with reports by others, who did not observe a change in liver-to-body weight ratio in animals that underwent major hepatectomy and a simultaneous blockade of MIP-2 [109]. On the other hand, blockade of CXCR2 was shown to decrease regeneration of the liver parenchyma [107]. This suggests that in mice depleted of MIP-2, other chemokines may substitute its function and/or activate CXCR2 in liver regeneration [81].

5.8 MIP-2 and Growth of Extrahepatic Metastases After Liver Resection

After liver resection about 20% of patients develop extrahepatic metastases in the lung and 2–5% in the brain, bone and other sites [128, 129]. There is no information, however, on whether liver resection-associated MIP-2 or SDF-1 production also accelerates the engraftment of colorectal cancer cells in extrahepatic sites.

To elucidate the role of MIP-2 during early tumor engraftment post liver resection, our group used the dorsal skinfold chamber assay [84]. As reported above, anti-MIP-2 treatment initiated on the day of liver resection significantly decreased tumor size compared to untreated controls. The continued administration of anti-MIP-2 at later time points could not however prevent an acceleration of tumor growth, indicating that anti-MIP-2 treatment delayed early tumor cell engraftment but did not inhibit further tumor growth. Accordingly, treatment of established extrahepatic tumors with anti-MIP-2 antibodies did not affect tumor growth [84].

In contrast, treatment of mice with anti MIP-2 antibodies initiated on the day of tumor cell implantation induced a significant increase in capillary density that was evident during the later part of the observation period. This may indicate that a compensatory mechanism may exist in these mice to counteract the delay in engraftment during the early phase of tumor outgrowth. Interestingly, this compensatory stimulation of tumor growth was not due to an increase in tumor cell proliferation. More probably, it was the result of reduced apoptotic cell death after anti-MIP-2 administration [84]. Treatment of established tumors with anti MIP-2 did not change angiogenic activity within the tumors and this corresponded to a lack of effect on the growth of established metastases. Migrating tumor cells were detectable at the tumor margin during the observation period and could be recognized based on their spindle-shaped morphology. Interestingly, anti-MIP-2 treatment initiated on day 0 led to a significantly increased number of migrating tumor cells throughout the observation period as compared to either non-treated or day 5-treated animals [84]. This could be due to a compensatory stimulation of tumor growth after the initial suppression resulting in increased tumor cell susceptibility to other chemokines and chemoattractant factors released during liver regeneration [41, 130]. Of interest, anti-MIP-2 treatment initiated on day 5 inhibited rather than accelerated tumor cell migration. This was probably due to a direct effect of MIP-2 neutralization because neither an initial delay of tumor growth nor a compensatory stimulation could be observed in these animals [80, 84]. It should also be noted that CXCR2 expression in anti-MIP-2 treated animals was significantly decreased, supporting our conclusion that the enhanced tumor cell migration observed following anti-MIP-2 treatment was due to compensatory chemotactic signaling mediated independently of CXCR2. We also observed that the reduction in CXCR2 expression levels was associated with a decrease in tumor cell proliferation [84].

5.9 Balance Between Pro- and Anti-angiogenic Chemokine Signaling Regulates Angiogenesis and Tumor Growth

Recent studies have shown that the SDF-1/CXCR4 axis is involved in metastasis of different types of malignant tumors [36, 41, 83, 131, 132]. Although SDF-1 and CXCR4 have been implicated in liver regeneration after hepatectomy [133, 134], there was no information as to whether the SDF-1/CXCR4 interaction influences liver resection-induced acceleration of tumor growth. To determine whether the SDF-1/CXCR4 interaction plays a role in hepatectomy -induced acceleration of tumor growth, we used our established extrahepatic murine colon cancer model described above [85]. We found no specific effect of SDF-1 blockade on tumor growth in liver-resected or non-resected animals, indicating that liver resection does not induce a specific stimulation of SDF-1 activity. This is in line with the report by Mavier et al. [133], demonstrating that a two-third hepatectomy did not affect SDF-1 expression as compared to normal control livers. However, these results appear to contradict other findings demonstrating an inhibition of local tumor growth and tumor angiogenesis after blockade of the SDF-1/CXCR4 axis by CXCR4 neutralization. For example, in human CXCR4-overexpressing prostate tumors implanted in SCID mice, Darash-Yahana and coworkers found a decrease in the growth and vascularization following treatment with an anti-CXCR4 antibody [96]. Similar results were obtained by Guleng et al. [131] who found that after subcutaneous implantation of colon and pancreatic carcinoma cells, neutralization of CXCR4 suppressed tumor growth and angiogenesis. These results are in line with those obtained by our own group demonstrating reduced neovascularization and tumor growth after anti-CXCR4 treatment [85]. Of interest, however, when using a neutralizing anti-SDF-1 antibody, Phillips et al. found a reduction of metastatic spread but no significant effects on the vasculature and the size of non-small cell lung cancer tumors in SCID mice [93]. These seeming discrepancies further highlight the importance of distinguishing between the potential effect of blockade of the CXCR4 receptor and that of its ligand SDF-1. It is unlikely however, that signaling through CXCR4 can be sustained in the absence of SDF-1, because no other ligands for CXCR4 are presently known. Although the possibility that another, yet to be identified CXCR4 ligand is involved cannot be excluded, it is likely that the persistent tumor growth after SDF-1 blockade was mediated by an alternative pathway.

Recent studies have identified a novel receptor for SDF-1, i.e. CXCR7 that interacts not only with SDF-1 but also with the interferon-inducible T-cell alpha chemoattractant (I-TAC) chemokine [94]. I-TAC is constitutively expressed in a variety of healthy tissues, including liver, lymph nodes, spleen, thymus, kidney and brain, and in addition to CXCR7 can also bind to the CXCR3 receptor and act as a potent chemoattractant for T-lymphocytes [135]. This mechanism results in a strong anti-tumor activity in vivo, involving the attraction of CD8+ T-lymphocytes to the tumor site [136]. Romagnani et al. also demonstrated that signaling of I-TAC through CXCR3 exerts angiostatic activity by inhibition of endothelial cell proliferation [137]. The angiostatic activity of the I-TAC/CXCR3 axis was also confirmed by Burdick et al., demonstrating that application of I-TAC inhibited the angiogenic activity of IL-8. This effect could also be antagonized by an anti-CXCR3 antibody [138]. Contrary to the angiostatic activity of the I-TAC/CXCR3 axis, signaling through CXCR7 is most likely pro-angiogenic. Miao et al. [139] found a consistent expression of CXCR7 in the tumor-associated vasculature of mammary and lung carcinomas, but it was rarely detectable on blood vessels of normal mammary tissue. In addition, CXCR7 knockdown in zebrafish resulted in a phenotype similar to that of a VEGF knockdown with development of enlarged pericardium and major blood vessel deficiencies [139]. In line with these results, Burns and coworkers found that tumors of SCID mice treated with an anti-CXCR7 antibody were poorly organized and only minimally vascularized [94]. Consistent with these findings, our group also demonstrated a significant reduction of neovascularization and tumor growth upon blockade of CXCR7 [85].

It is generally accepted that the angiogenic switch which occurs during tumor progression is a result of a disturbed balance between pro-and anti-angiogenic signaling, favoring the pro-angiogenic pathway [29]. Under physiological conditions it seems very likely that the chemotactic axes, consisting of the ligands SDF-1 and I-TAC and the receptors CXCR3, CXCR4 and CXCR7 produce a steady-state balance between angiogenesis and angiostasis. Both SDF-1 and I-TAC bind to CXCR7 and mediate a pro-angiogenic response. Under steady-state conditions, this pathway is antagonized by the binding of I-TAC to its second receptor CXCR3, which is angiostatic. Disturbance of this balance can favor the angiogenic CXCR4- and CXCR7-dependent or the angiostatic CXCR3-dependent pathways. After blockade of SDF-1, I-TAC binding to CXCR7 increases and its availability for binding to the angiostatic CXCR3 diminishes so that the pro-angiogenic, CXCR7-dependent pathway dominates leading to increased angiogenesis. The strong stimulation of tumor angiogenesis and neovascularization with an earlier onset of bud and sprout formation after blockade of SDF-1, as observed by our group, may therefore be ascribed to an activation of the pro-angiogenic, CXCR7-dependent pathway and a relative inhibition of the angiostatic, CXCR3-dependent pathway [85]. As tumor vascularization is essential to maintain a sufficient supply of oxygen and nutrients to the tumor, as well as to remove harmful waste products [29, 140], it is likely that the late phase acceleration of tumor growth in the anti-SDF-1-treated animals is due to the preceding stimulation of tumor angiogenesis.

Because a strong angiogenic responses, as well as pronounced invasiveness are characteristic of an aggressive phenotype, a shift from CXCR4- to CXCR7-mediated signaling may represent a critical step in tumor progression. Interestingly, CXCR7 is rarely expressed on the surface of normal adult tissue, whereas transformed cells, different tumor cell lines and embryonic tissues express membrane CXCR7 protein [94, 139]. Accordingly, our group observed CXCR7 expression on the surface of 65% of CT26.WT colon carcinoma cells analyzed [85]. The expression pattern of this receptor suggests a possible role for CXCR7 during embryonic development and the reactivation of its surface expression when cells are malignantly transformed. In CXCR7-expressing tumor cells, signaling through this receptor promotes cell survival under suboptimal culture conditions, rather than cell proliferation. This effect is due to a reduction in apoptotic cell death [94]. Accordingly, our group found a significant decrease in apoptotic cell death in anti-SDF-1-treated tumors 14 days after tumor cell implantation, while tumor cell proliferation was not affected. These findings further support the hypothesis that an I-TAC/CXCR7-dependent pathway is activated under persistent SDF-1 neutralization [85]. In summary, the results show that a blockade of endogenous SDF-1 cannot inhibit the growth of extrahepatic colorectal tumors. Instead, neutralization of SDF-1 promotes tumor invasiveness and induces an increase in growth. The slight initial delay of tumor cell engraftment after SDF-1 blockade is compensated by an accelerated growth during the later phase, most probably due to enhanced VEGF-mediated angiogenesis and reduced apoptotic cell death. Blockade of SDF-1 during tumor engraftment promotes a shift towards a more aggressive phenotype, most likely due to the activation of an alternative I-TAC/CXCR7-related pathway.

5.10 Summary

During tumor progression, tumor cells interact with stromal cells and modulate both haemangio- as well as lymphangiogenesis. Subsequently, intravasation of tumor cells initiates a cascade leading to metastasis formation. These processes likely require bi-directional communication guiding sprouting microvessels to tumors and instructing tumor cells to intravasate. To date, the underlying chemoattractive signals remain elusive. Our studies provide insight into homing mechanisms directing colorectal carcinoma metastasis and regulating tumor growth. Chemotactic signaling is necessary for angiogenesis, metastasis and programmed cell death. Therefore, it seems very unlikely, that targeting one single chemokine will be sufficient for anti-tumor therapy. The complex network of chemokines and chemokine receptors also entails compensatory mechanisms that can overcome permanent deprivation of individual chemokines, as we demonstrated for MIP-2 and SDF-1. Nevertheless, anti-MIP-2 therapy was found to be experimentally effective or colorectal liver metastases, underlining the crucial role of this chemokine in the metastatic process. Additionally, the unique properties of the SDF-1/CXCR4 and I-TAC/CXCR7 axis merit further investigation of their potential role and targeting in liver metastasis.

References

1. Abdalla EK, Vauthey JN, Ellis LM, Ellis V, Pollock R, Broglio KR, Hess K, Curley SA (2004) Recurrence and outcomes following hepatic resection, radiofrequency ablation, and combined resection/ablation for colorectal liver metastases. Ann Surg 239:818–825
2. Jemal A, Siegel R, Ward E, Hao Y, Xu J, Thun MJ (2009) Cancer statistics, 2009. CA Cancer J Clin 59:225–249
3. Manfredi S, Lepage C, Hatem C, Coatmeur O, Faivre J, Bouvier AM (2006) Epidemiology and management of liver metastases from colorectal cancer. Ann Surg 244:108–113
4. Chambers AF, Groom AC, MacDonald IC (2002) Dissemination and growth of cancer cells in metastatic sites. Nat Rev Cancer 2:563–572
5. Luzzi KJ, MacDonald IC, Schmidt EE, Kerkvliet N, Morris VL, Chambers AF, Groom AC (1998) Multistep nature of metastatic inefficiency. AJP 153:865–873
6. Burger JA, Kipps TJ (2006) CXCR4: a key receptor in the crosstalk between tumor cells and their microenvironment. Blood 107:1761–1767
7. Paget S (1998) The distribution of secondary growths in cancer of the breast. 1889. Cancer Metast Rev 8:98–101
8. Choti MA, Sitzmann JV, Tiburi MF, Sumetchotimetha W, Rangsin R, Schulick RD, Lillemoe KD, Yeo CJ, Cameron JL (2002) Trends in long-term survival following liver resection for hepatic colorectal metastases. Ann Surg 235:759–766
9. Fong Y, Fortner J, Sun RL, Brennan MF, Blumgart LH (1999) Clinical score for predicting recurrence after hepatic resection for metastatic colorectal cancer: analysis of 1001 consecutive cases. Ann Surg 230:309–318
10. Yamamoto J, Shimada K, Kosuge T, Yamasaki S, Sakamoto M, Fukuda H (1999) Factors influencing survival of patients undergoing hepatectomy for colorectal metastases. Br J Surg 86:332–337
11. DeMatteo RP, Palese C, Jarnagin WR, Sun RL, Blumgart LH, Fong Y (2000) Anatomic segmental hepatic resection is superior to wedge resection as an oncologic operation for colorectal liver metastases. J Gastrointest Surg 4:178–184
12. Chang YC (2004) Low mortality major hepatectomy. Hepatogastroenterology 51: 1766–1770
13. Imamura H, Seyama Y, Kokudo N, Maema A, Sugawara Y, Sano K, Takayama T, Makuuchi M (2003) One thousand fifty-six hepatectomies without mortality in 8 years. Arch Surg 138:1198–1206
14. Jarnagin WR, Gonen M, Fong Y, DeMatteo RP, Ben-Porat L, Little S, Corvera C, Weber S, Blumgart LH (2002) Improvement in perioperative outcome after hepatic resection: analysis of 1803 consecutive cases over the past decade. Ann Surg 236:397–406
15. Seyama Y, Kubota K, Sano K, Noie T, Takayama T, Kosuge T, Makuuchi M (2003) Long-term outcome of extended hepatectomy for hilar bile duct cancer with no mortality and high survival rate. Ann Surg 238:73–83

16. Abdalla EK, Ribero D, Pawlik TM, Zorzi D, Curley SA, Muratore A, Andres A, Mentha G, Capussotti L, Vauthey JN (2007) Resection of hepatic colorectal metastases involving the caudate lobe: perioperative outcome and survival. J Gastrointest Surg 11:66–72

17. Lang BH, Poon RT, Fan ST, Wong J (2003) Perioperative and long-term outcome of major hepatic resection for small solitary hepatocellular carcinoma in patients with cirrhosis. Arch Surg 138:1207–1213

18. Stewart GD, O'Suilleabhain CB, Madhavan KK, Wigmore SJ, Parks RW, Garden OJ (2004) The extent of resection influences outcome following hepatectomy for colorectal liver metastases. Eur J Surg Oncol 30:370–376

19. Elias D, Liberale G, Vernerey D, Pocard M, Ducreux M, Boige V, Malka D, Pignon JP, Lasser P (2005) Hepatic and extrahepatic colorectal metastases: when resectable, their localization does not matter, but their total number has a prognostic effect. Ann Surg Oncol 12:900–909

20. Dong C, Slattery MJ, Liang S, Peng HH (2005) Melanoma cell extravasation under flow conditions is modulated by leukocytes and endogenously produced interleukin 8. Mol Cell Biomech 2:145–159

21. Noonan DM, Benelli R, Albini A (2007) Angiogenesis and cancer prevention: a vision. Recent Results Cancer Res 174:219–224

22. Gomperts BN, Strieter RM (2006) Chemokine-directed metastasis. Contrib Microbiol 13:170–190

23. Rubie C, Oliveira V, Kempf K, Wagner M, Tilton B, Rau B, Kruse B, Konig J, Schilling MK (2006) Involvement of chemokine receptor CCR6 in colorectal cancer metastasis. Tumour Biol 27:166–174

24. Zlotnik A (2004) Chemokines in neoplastic progression. Semin Cancer Biol 14:181–185

25. Liotta LA, Kohn EC (2001) The microenvironment of the tumour-host interface. Nature 411:375–379

26. Jain RK, Munn LL, Fukumura D (2002) Dissecting tumour pathophysiology using intravital microscopy. Nat Rev Cancer 2:266–276

27. Jain RK (2003) Molecular regulation of vessel maturation. Nat Med 9:685–693

28. Chang YS, di Tomaso E, McDonald DM, Jones R, Jain RK, Munn LL (2000) Mosaic blood vessels in tumors: frequency of cancer cells in contact with flowing blood. Proc Natl Acad Sci USA 97:14608–14613

29. Bergers G, Benjamin LE (2003) Tumorigenesis and the angiogenic switch. Nat Rev Cancer 3:401–410

30. Coussens LM, Werb Z (2002) Inflammation and cancer. Nature 420:860–867

31. Li A, Varney ML, Singh RK (2004) Constitutive expression of growth regulated oncogene (gro) in human colon carcinoma cells with different metastatic potential and its role in regulating their metastatic phenotype. Clin Exp Metastasis 21:571–579

32. Balkwill F (2003) Chemokine biology in cancer. Semin Immunol 15:49–55

33. Rollins BJ (1997) Chemokines. Blood 90:909–928

34. Homey B, Müller A, Zlotnik A (2002) Chemokines: agents for the immunotherapy of cancer? Nat Rev Immunol 2:175–184

35. Kassis J, Lauffenburger DA, Turner T, Wells A (2001) Tumor invasion as dysregulated cell motility. Semin Cancer Biol 11:105–117

36. Müller A, Homey B, Soto H, Ge N, Catron D, Buchanan ME, McClanahan T, Murphy E, Yuan W, Wagner SN (2001) Involvement of chemokine receptors in breast cancer metastasis. Nature 410:50–56

37. Campbell JJ, Bowman EP, Murphy K, Youngman KR, Siani MA, Thompson DA, Wu L, Zlotnik A, Butcher EC (1998) 6-C-kine (SLC), a lymphocyte adhesion-triggering chemokine expressed by high endothelium, is an agonist for the MIP-3beta receptor CCR7. J Cell Biol 141:1053–1059

38. Yoshida R, Imai T, Hieshima K, Kusuda J, Baba M, Kitaura M, Nishimura M, Kakizaki M, Nomiyama H, Yoshie O (1997) Molecular cloning of a novel human CC chemokine

EBI1-ligand chemokine that is a specific functional ligand for EBI1, CCR7. J Biol Chem 272:13803–13809

39. Gunther K, Leier J, Henning G, Dimmler A, Weissbach R, Hohenberger W, Forster R (2005) Prediction of lymph node metastasis in colorectal carcinoma by expression of chemokine receptor CCR7. Int J Cancer 116:726–733

40. Mashino K, Sadanaga N, Yamaguchi H, Tanaka F, Ohta M, Shibuta K, Inoue H, Mori M (2002) Expression of chemokine receptor CCR7 is associated with lymph node metastasis of gastric carcinoma. Cancer Res 62:2937–2941

41. Zeelenberg IS, Ruuls-Van Stalle L, Roos E (2003) The chemokine receptor CXCR4 is required for outgrowth of colon carcinoma micrometastases. Cancer Res 63: 3833–3839

42. Taichman RS, Cooper C, Keller ET, Pienta KJ, Taichman NS, McCauley LK (2002) Use of the stromal cell-derived factor-1/CXCR4 pathway in prostate cancer metastasis to bone. Cancer Res 62:1832–1837

43. Shimizu Y, Murata H, Kashii Y, Hirano K, Kunitani H, Higuchi K, Watanabe A (2001) CC-chemokine receptor 6 and its ligand macrophage inflammatory protein 3alpha might be involved in the amplification of local necroinflammatory response in the liver. Hepatology 34:311–319

44. Rubie C, Frick VO, Wagner M, Rau B, Weber C, Kruse B, Kempf K, Tilton B, Konig J, Schilling M (2006) Enhanced expression and clinical significance of CC-chemokine MIP-3 alpha in hepatocellular carcinoma. Scand J Immunol 63:468–477

45. Liu Y, Poon RT, Hughes J, Feng X, Yu WC, Fan ST (2005) Chemokine receptors support infiltration of lymphocyte subpopulations in human hepatocellular carcinoma. Clin Immunol 114:174–182

46. Rubie C, Frick VO, Wagner M, Weber C, Kruse B, Kempf K, König J, Rau B, Schilling M (2006) Chemokine expression in hepatocellular carcinoma versus colorectal liver metastases. World J Gastroenterol 12:6627–6633

47. Rubie C, Frick VO, Wagner M, Schuld J, Gräber S, Brittner B, Bohle RM, Schilling MK (2008) ELR+ CXC chemokine expression in benign and malignant colorectal conditions. BMC Cancer 8:178

48. Rubie C, Kollmar O, Frick VO, Wagner M, Brittner B, Gräber S, Schilling MK (2008) Differential CXC receptor expression in colorectal carcinomas. Scand J Immunol 68: 635–644

49. Tracey KJ (2002) The inflammatory reflex. Nature 420:853–859

50. Luca M, Huang S, Gershenwald JE, Singh RK, Reich R, Bar-Eli M (1997) Expression of interleukin-8 by human melanoma cells up-regulates MMP-2 activity and increases tumor growth and metastasis. Am J Pathol 151:1105–1113

51. Ueda T, Sakabe T, Oka M, Maeda Y, Nishida M, Murakami F, Maekawa T (2000) Levels of interleukin (IL)-6, IL-8, and IL-1 receptor antagonist in the hepatic vein following liver surgery. Hepatogastroenterology 47:1048–1051

52. Miller LJ, Kurtzman SH, Wang Y, Anderson KH, Lindquist RR, Kreutzer DL (1998) Expression of interleukin-8 receptors on tumor cells and vascular endothelial cells in human breast cancer tissue. Anticancer Res 18:77–81

53. Xie K (2001) Interleukin-8 and human cancer biology. Cytokine Growth Factor Rev 12: 375–391

54. Brew R, Erikson JS, West DC, Kinsella AR, Slavin J, Christmas SE (2000) Interleukin-8 as an autocrine growth factor for human colon carcinoma cells in vitro. Cytokine 12:78–85

55. Takeda A, Stoeltzing O, Ahmad SA, Reinmuth N, Liu W, Parikh A, Fan F, Akagi M, Ellis LM (2002) Role of angiogenesis in the development and growth of liver metastasis. Ann Surg Oncol 9:610–616

56. Haraguchi M, Komuta K, Akashi A, Matsuzaki S, Furui J, Kanematsu T (2002) Elevated IL-8 levels in the drainage vein of resectable Dukes' C colorectal cancer indicate high risk for developing hepatic metastasis. Oncol Rep 9:159–165

57. Arenberg DA, Kunkel SL, Polverini PJ, Glass M, Burdick MD, Strieter RM (1996) Inhibition of interleukin-8 reduces tumorigenesis of human non-small cell lung cancer in SCID mice. J Clin Invest 97:2792–2802

58. Huang S, Mills L, Mian B, Tellez C, McCarty M, Yang XD, Gudas JM, Bar-Eli M (2002) Fully humanized neutralizing antibodies to interleukin-8 (ABX-IL8) inhibit angiogenesis, tumor growth, and metastasis of human melanoma. Am J Pathol 161:125–134

59. Strieter RM, Polverini PJ, Arenberg DA, Walz A, Opdenakker G, Van Damme J, Kunkel SL (1995) Role of C-X-C chemokines as regulators of angiogenesis in lung cancer. J Leukoc Biol 57:752–762

60. Balbay MD, Pettaway CA, Kuniyasu H, Inoue K, Ramirez E, Li E, Fidler IJ, Dinney CP (1999) Highly metastatic human prostate cancer growing within the prostate of athymic mice overexpresses vascular endothelial growth factor. Clin Cancer Res 5:783–789

61. Kassim SK, El-Salahy EM, Fayed ST, Helal SA, Helal T, Azzam Eel-D, Khalifa A (2004) Vascular endothelial growth factor and interleukin-8 are associated with poor prognosis in epithelial ovarian cancer patients. Clin Biochem 37:363–369

62. Lee LF, Hellendall RP, Wang Y, Haskill JS, Mukaida N, Matsushima K, Ting JP (2000) IL-8 reduced tumorigenicity of human ovarian cancer in vivo due to neutrophil infiltration. J Immunol 164:2769–2775

63. Ueda T, Shimada E, Urakawa T (1994) Serum levels of cytokines in patients with colorectal cancer: possible involvement of interleukin-6 and interleukin-8 in hematogenous metastasis. J Gastroenterol 29:423–429

64. Reisser D, Lejeune P, Lagadec P, Onier N, Dasilva C, Lindley I, Jeannin JF (1994) Interleukin-8 antitumor effect is associated with a local infiltration but not with a systemic activation of T lymphocytes. Anticancer Res 14:977–979

65. Rubie C, Oliveira-Frick V, Pfeil S, Wagner M, Kollmar O, Kopp B, Gräber S, Rau B, Schilling MK (2007) Correlation of IL-8 with induction, progression and metastatic potential of colorectal cancer. World J Gastroenterol 13:4996–5002

66. Mosher B, Dean R, Harkema J, Remick D, Palma J, Crockett E (2001) Inhibition of Kupffer cells reduced CXC chemokine production and liver injury. J Surg Res 99:201–210

67. Ness TL, Hogaboam CM, Strieter RM, Kunkel SL (2003) Immunomodulatory role of CXCR2 during experimental septic peritonitis. J Immunol 171:3775–3784

68. Oppenheim JJ, Zachariae CO, Mukaida N, Matsushima K (1991) Properties of the novel proinflammatory supergene "intercrine" cytokine family. Annu Rev Immunol 9:617–648

69. Saijo Y, Tanaka M, Miki M, Usui K, Suzuki T, Maemondo M, Hong X, Tazawa R, Kikuchi T, Matsushima K, Nukiwa T (2002) Proinflammatory cytokine IL-1 beta promotes tumor growth of Lewis lung carcinoma by induction of angiogenic factors: in vivo analysis of tumor-stromal interaction. J Immunol 169:469–475

70. Schramm R, Liu Q, Thorlacius H (2000) Expression and function of MIP-2 are reduced by dexamethasone treatment in vivo. Br J Pharmacol 131:328–334

71. Schramm R, Thorlacius H (2003) Staphylococcal enterotoxin B-induced acute inflammation is inhibited by dexamethasone: important role of CXC chemokines KC and macrophage inflammatory protein 2. Infect Immun 71:2542–2547

72. Wang J, Mukaida N, Zhang Y, Ito T, Nakao S, Matsushima K (1997) Enhanced mobilization of haematopoietic progenitor cells by mouse MIP-2 and granulocyte colony-stimulating factor in mice. J Leukoc Biol 62:503–509

73. Armstrong DA, Major JA, Chudyk A, Hamilton TA (2004) Neutrophil chemoattractant genes KC and MIP-2 are expressed in different cell populations at sites of surgical injury. J Leukoc Biol 75:641–648

74. Otto VI, Heinzel-Pleines UE, Gloor SM, Trentz O, Kossmann T, Morganti-Kossmann MC (2000) A sICAM-1 and TNF-alpha induce MIP-2 with distinct kinetics in astrocytes and brain microvascular endothelial cells. J Neurosci Res 60:733–742

75. Xing Z, Jordana M, Kirpalani H, Driscoll KE, Schall TJ, Gauldie J (1995) Cytokine expression by neutrophils and macrophages in vivo: endotoxin induces tumor necrosis factor-alpha,

macrophage inflammatory protein-2, interleukin-1 beta, and interleukin-6 but not RANTES or transforming growth factor-beta 1 mRNA expression in acute lung inflammation. Am J Respir Cell Mol Biol 10:148–153

76. Fahey TJ 3rd, Sherry B, Tracey KJ, van Deventer S, Jones WG 2nd, Minei JP, Morgello S, Shires GT, Cerami A (1990) Cytokine production in a model of wound healing: the appearance of MIP-1, MIP-2, cachectin/TNF and IL-1. Cytokine 2:92–99

77. Schramm R, Thorlacius H (2004) Neutrophil recruitment in mast cell-dependent inflammation: inhibitory mechanisms of glucocorticoids. Inflamm Res 53:644–652

78. Liss C, Fekete MJ, Hasina R, Lam CD, Lingen MW (2001) Paracrine angiogenic loop between head-and-neck squamous-cell carcinomas and macrophages. Int J Cancer 93: 781–785

79. Kollmar O, Schilling MK, Menger MD (2004) Experimental liver metastasis: standards for local cell implantation to study isolated tumor growth in mice. Clin Exp Metastasis 21: 453–460

80. Kollmar O, Scheuer C, Menger MD, Schilling MK (2006) Macrophage inflammatory protein-2 promotes angiogenesis, cell migration, and tumor growth in hepatic metastasis. Ann Surg Oncol 13:263–275

81. Kollmar O, Menger MD, Schilling MK (2006) Macrophage inflammatory protein-2 contributes to liver resection-induced acceleration of hepatic metastatic tumor growth. World J Gastroenterol 12:858–867

82. Kollmar O, Junker B, Rupertus K, Menger MD, Schilling MK (2007) Studies on MIP-2 and CXCR2 expression in a mouse model of extrahepatic colorectal metastasis. EJSO 33: 803–811

83. Kollmar O, Rupertus K, Scheuer C, Junker B, Tilton B, Schilling MK, Menger MD (2007) Stromal cell-derived factor-1 promotes cell migration and tumor growth of colorectal metastasis. Neoplasia 9:862–870

84. Kollmar O, Junker B, Rupertus K, Scheuer C, Menger MD, Schilling MK (2008) Liver resection-associated macrophage inflammatory protein-2 stimulates engraftment but not growth of colorectal metastasis at extrahepatic sites. J Surg Res 145:295–302

85. Kollmar O, Rupertus K, Scheuer C, Nickels RM, Haberl GC, Tilton B, Menger MD, Schilling MK (2010) CXCR4 and CXCR7 regulate angiogenesis and CT26.WT tumor growth independent from SDF-1. Int J Cancer 126:1302–1315

86. Brattain MG, Strobel-Stevens J, Fine D, Webb M, Sarrif AM (1980) Establishment of mouse colonic carcinoma cell lines with different metastatic properties. Cancer Res 40:2142–2146

87. Li X, Klintman D, Liu Q, Sato T, Jeppsson B, Thorlacius H (2004) Critical role of CXC chemokines in endotoxemic liver injury in mice. J Leukoc Biol 75:443–452

88. Tilton B, Ho L, Oberlin E, Loetscher P, Baleux F, Clark-Lewis I, Thelen M (2000) Signal transduction by CXC chemokine receptor 4. Stromal cell-derived factor 1 stimulates prolonged protein kinase B and extracellular signal-regulated kinase 2 activation in T lymphocytes. J Exp Med 192:313–324

89. Scapini P, Morini M, Tecchio C, Minghelli S, Di Carlo E, Tanghetti E, Albini A, Lowell C, Berton G, Noonan DM, Cassatella MA (2004) CXCL1/macrophage inflammatory protein-2-induced angiogenesis in vivo is mediated by neutrophil-derived vascular endothelial growth factor-A. J Immunol 172:5034–5040

90. Menger MD, Laschke MW, Vollmar B (2002) Viewing the microcirculation through the window: some twenty years experience with the hamster dorsal skinfold chamber. Eur Surg Res 34:83–91

91. Potter SM, Dwyer RM, Curran CE, Hennessy E, Harrington KA, Griffin DG, Kerin MJ (2009) Systemic chemokine levels in breast cancer patients and their relationship with circulating menstrual hormones. Breast Cancer Res Treat 115:279–287

92. Woo IS, Hong SH, Byun JH, Kang JH, Jeon HM, Choi MG (2008) Circulating stromal cell derived factor-1alpha (SDF-1alpha) is predictive of distant metastasis in gastric carcinoma. Cancer Invest 26:256–261

93. Phillips RJ, Burdick MD, Lutz M, Belperio JA, Keane MP, Strieter RM (2003) The stromal derived factor-1/CXCL12-CXC chemokine receptor 4 biological axis in non-small cell lung cancer metastases. Am J Respir Crit Care Med 167:1676–1686

94. Burns JM, Summers BC, Wang Y, Melikian A, Berahovich R, Miao Z, Penfold MET, Sunshine MJ, Littman DR, Kuo CJ, Wei K, McMaster BE, Wright K, Howard MC, Schall TJ (2006) A novel chemokine receptor for SDF-1 and I-TAC involved in cell survival, cell adhesion, and tumor development. J Exp Med 203:201–213

95. Baggiolini M (1998) Chemokines and leukocyte traffic. Nature 392:565–568

96. Darash-Yahana M, Pikarsky E, Abramovitch R, Zeira E, Pal B, Karplus R, Beider K, Avniel S, Kasem S, Galun E, Peled A (2004) Role of high expression levels of CXCR4 in tumor growth, vascularization, and metastasis. FASEB J 18:1240–1242

97. Engl T, Relja B, Marian D, Blumenberg C, Muller I, Beecken WD, Jones J, Ringel EM, Bereiter-Hahn J, Jonas D, Blaheta RA (2006) CXCR4 chemokine receptor mediates prostate tumor cell adhesion through alpha5 and beta3 integrins. Neoplasia 8:290–301

98. Strieter RM, Belperio JA, Phillips RJ, Keane MP (2004) CXC chemokines in angiogenesis of cancer. Sem Cancer Biol 14:195–200

99. Brand S, Dambacher J, Beigel F, Olszak T, Diebold J, Otte JM, Goke B, Eichhorst ST (2005) CXCR4 and CXCL12 are inversely expressed in colorectal cancer cells and modulate cancer cell migration, invasion and MMP-9 activation. Exp Cell Res 310:117–130

100. Barbero S, Bonavia R, Bajetto A, Porcile C, Pirani P, Ravetti JL, Zona GL, Spaziante R, Florio T, Schettini G (2003) Stromal cell-derived factor 1alpha stimulates human glioblastoma cell growth through the activation of both extracellular signal-regulated kinases and Akt. Cancer Res 63:1969–1974

101. Lee BC, Lee TH, Avraham S, Avraham HK (2004) Involvement of the chemokine receptor CXCR4 and its ligand stromal cell-derived factor 1α in breast cancer cell migration through human brain microvascular endothelial cells. Mol Cancer Res 2:327–338

102. Carr AN, Howard BW, Yang HT, Eby-Wilkens E, Loos P, Varbanov A, Qu A, DeMuth JP, Davis MG, Proia A, Terjung RL, Peters KG (2006) Efficacy of systemic administration of SDF-1 in a model of vascular insufficiency: support for an endothelium-dependent mechanism. Cardiovasc Res 69:925–935

103. Orimo A, Gupta PB, Sgroi DC, Arenzana-Seisdedos F, Delaunay T, Naeem R, Carey VJ, Richardson AL, Weinberg RA (2005) Stromal fibroblasts present in invasive human breast carcinomas promote tumor growth and angiogenesis through elevated SDF-1/CXCL12 secretion. Cell 121:335–348

104. Fausto N (2000) Liver regeneration. J Hepatol 32:19–31

105. Kren BT, Trembley JH, Fan G, Steer CJ (1997) Molecular regulation of liver regeneration. Ann N Y Acad Sci 831:361–381

106. Sato Y, Farges O, Buffello D, Bismuth H (1999) Intra- and extrahepatic leukocytes and cytokine mRNA expression during liver regeneration after partial hepatectomy in rats. Dig Dis Sci 44:806–816

107. Colletti LM, Green M, Burdick MD, Kunkel SL, Strieter RM (1998) Proliferative effects of CXC chemokines in rat hepatocytes in vitro and in vivo. Shock 10:248–257

108. Hogaboam CM, Bone-Larson CL, Steinhauser ML, Lukacs NW, Colletti LM, Simpson KJ, Strieter RM, Kunkel SL (1999) Novel CXCR2-dependent liver regenerative qualities of ELR-containing CXC chemokines. FASEB J 13:1565–1574

109. Ren X, Carpenter A, Hogaboam C, Colletti L (2003) Mitogenic properties of endogenous and pharmacological doses of macrophage inflammatory protein-2 after 70% hepatectomy in the mouse. Am J Pathol 163:563–570

110. Drixler TA, Borel Rinkes IH, Ritchie ED, van Vroonhoven TJ, Gebbink MF, Voest EE (2000) Continuous administration of angiostatin inhibits accelerated growth of colorectal liver metastases after partial hepatectomy. Cancer Res 60:1761–1765

111. Mizutani J, Hiraoka T, Yamashita R, Miyauchi Y (1992) Promotion of hepatic metastases by liver resection in the rat. Br J Cancer 65:794–797

112. Panis Y, Ribeiro J, Chretien Y, Nordlinger B (1992) Dormant liver metastases: an experi- mental study. Br J Surg 79:221–223
113. Picardo A, Karpoff HM, Ng B, Lee J, Brennan MF, Fong Y (1998) Partial hepatectomy accelerates local tumor growth: potential roles of local cytokine activation. Surgery 124: 57–64
114. Slooter GD, Marquet RL, Jeekel J, Ijzermans JN (1995) Tumour growth stimulation after partial hepatectomy can be reduced by treatment with tumour necrosis factor alpha. Br J Surg 82:129–132
115. Schindel DT, Grosfeld JL (1997) Hepatic resection enhances growth of residual intra- hepatic and subcutaneous hepatoma, which is inhibited by octreotide. J Pediatr Surg 32: 995–997
116. Rashidi B, An Z, Sun FX, Sasson A, Gamagammi R, Moossa AR, Hoffmann RM (1999) Minimal liver resection strongly stimulates the growth of human colon cancer in the liver of nude mice. Clin Exp Metastasis 17:497–500
117. DeJong KP, Lont HE, Bijma AM, Brouwers MA, de Vries EG, van Veen ML, Marquet RL, Slooff MJ, Terpstra OT (1995) The effect of partial hepatectomy on tumor growth in rats: in vivo and in vitro studies. Hepatology 22:1263–1272
118. Ono M, Tanaka N, Orita K (1986) Complete regression of mouse hepatoma transplanted after partial hepatectomy and the immunological mechanisms of such regression. Cancer Res 46:5049–5053
119. Yokoyama H, Goto S, Chen CL, Pan TL, Kawano K, Kitano S (2000) Major hepatic resec- tion may suppress the growth of tumours remaining in the residual liver. Br J Cancer 83:1096–1101
120. Karpoff HM, Jarnagin W, Delman K, Fong Y (2000) Regional muramyl tripeptide phosphatidylethanolamine administration enhances hepatic immune function and tumor surveillance. Surgery 128:213–218
121. Rupertus K, Kollmar O, Scheuer C, Junker B, Menger MD, Schilling MK (2007) Major but not minor hepatectomy accelerates engraftment of extrahepatic tumor cells. Clin Exp Metastasis 24:39–48
122. Drixler TA, Vogten MJ, Ritchie ED, van Vroonhoven TJ, Gebbink MF, Voest EE, Borel Rinkes IH (2002) Liver regeneration is an angiogenesis- associated phenomenon. Ann Surg 236:703–711
123. Michalopoulos GK, DeFrances MC (1997) Liver regeneration. Science 276:60–66
124. Taub R (2004) Liver regeneration: from myth to mechanism. Nature Rev Mol Cell Biol 5:836–847
125. Stoeckli SJ, Steinert H, Pfaltz M, Schmid S (2002) Is there a role for positron emission tomography with 18F-fluorodeoxyglucose in the initial staging of nodal negative oral and oropharyngeal squamous cell carcinoma. Head Neck 24:345–349
126. Jaeschke H, Lemasters JJ (2003) Apoptosis versus oncotic necrosis in hepatic ischemia/reperfusion injury. Gastroenterology 125:1246–1257
127. Hohlbaum AM, Gregory MS, Ju ST, Marshak-Rothstein A (2001) Fas ligand engagement of resident peritoneal macrophages in vivo induces apoptosis and the production of neutrophil chemotactic factors. J Immunol 167:6217–6224
128. Labow DM, Buell JE, Yoshida A, Rosen S, Posner MC (2002) Isolated pulmonary recur- rence after resection of colorectal hepatic metastases – is resection indicated? Cancer J 8:342–347
129. Yoshidome H, Ito H, Kimura F, Ambiru S, Shimizu H, Togawa A, Ohtsuka M, Kato A, Nukui Y, Miyazaki M (2004) Surgical treatment for extrahepatic recurrence after hepatectomy for colorectal metastases. Hepatogastroenterology 51:1805–1809
130. Kimura F, Shimizu H, Yoshidome H, Ohtsuka M, Kato A, Yoshitomi H, Nozawa S, Furukawa K, Mitsuhashi N, Sawada S, Takeuchi D, Ambiru S, Miyazaki M (2006) Circulating cytokines, chemokines, and stress hormones are increased in patients with organ dysfunction following liver resection. J Surg Res 133:102–112

131. Guleng B, Tateishi K, Ohta M, Kanai F, Jazag A, Ijichi H, Tanaka Y, Washida M, Morikane K, Fukushima Y, Yamori T, Tsuruo T, Kawabe T, Miyagishi M, Taira K, Sata M, Omata M (2005) Blockade of the stromal cell-derived factor-1/CXCR4 axis attenuates in vivo tumor growth by inhibiting angiogenesis in a vascular endothelial growth factor-independent manner. Cancer Res 65:5864–5871

132. Ottaiano A, Franco R, Aiello Talamanca A, Liguori G, Tatangelo F, Delrio P, Nasti G, Barletta E, Facchini G, Daniele B, Di Blasi A, Napolitano M, Ierano C, Calemma R, Leonardi E, Albino V, De Angelis V, Falanga M, Boccia V, Capuozzo M, Parisi V, Botti G, Castello G, Vincenzo Iaffaioli R, Scala S (2006) Overexpression of both CXC chemokine receptor 4 and vascular endothelial growth factor proteins predicts early distant relapse in stage II-III colorectal cancer patients. Clin Cancer Res 12:2795–2803

133. Mavier P, Martin N, Couchie D, Preaux AM, Laperche Y, Zafrani ES (2004) Expression of stromal cell-derived factor-1 and of its receptor CXCR4 in liver regeneration from oval cells in rat. Am J Pathol 165:1969–1977

134. Zheng D, Oh SH, Jung Y, Petersen BE (2006) Oval cell response in 2-acetylaminofluorene/partial hepatectomy rat is attenuated by short interfering RNA targeted to stromal cell-derived factor-1. Am J Pathol 169:2066–2074

135. Meyer M, Hensbergen PJ, van der Raaij-Helmer EM, Brandacher G, Margreiter R, Heufler C, Koch F, Narumi S, Werner ER, Colvin R, Luster AD, Tensen CP, Werner-Felmayer G (2001) Cross reactivity of three T cell attracting murine chemokines stimulating the CXC chemokine receptor CXCR3 and their induction in cultured cells and during allograft rejection. Eur J Immunol 31:2521–2527

136. Hensbergen PJ, Wijnands PGJTB, Schreurs MWJ, Scheper RJ, Willemze R, Tensen CP (2005) The CXCR3 targeting chemokine CXCL11 has potent antitumor activity in vivo involving attraction of CD8+ T lymphocytes but not inhibition of angiogenesis. J Immunother 28:343–351

137. Romagnani P, Annunziato F, Lasagni L, Lazzeri E, Beltrame C, Francalanci M, Uguccioni M, Galli G, Cosmi L, Maurenzig L, Baggiolini M, Maggi E, Romagnani S, Serio M (2001) Cell cycle-dependent expression of CXC chemokine receptor 3 by endothelial cells mediates angiostatic activity. J Clin Invest 107:53–63

138. Burdick MD, Murray LA, Keane MP, Xue YY, Zisman DA, Belperio JA, Strieter RM (2005) CXCL11 attenuates bleomycin-induced pulmonary fibrosis via inhibition of vascular remodeling. Am J Respir Crit Care Med 171:261–268

139. Miao Z, Luker KE, Summers BC, Berahovich R, Bhojani MS, Rehemtulla A, Kleer CG, Essner JJ, Nasevicius A, Luker GD, Howard MC, Schall TJ (2007) CXCR7 (RCD1) promotes breast and lung tumor growth in vivo and is expressed on tumor-associated vasculature. PNAS 104:15735–15740

140. Carmeliet P, Jain RK (2000) Angiogenesis in cancer and other diseases. Nature 407:249–257

Chapter 6
Role of Inflammation in the Early Stages of Liver Metastasis

Jonathan Spicer, Pnina Brodt, and Lorenzo Ferri

Abstract Clinical investigations have revealed compelling data suggesting the presence of synergistic interactions between inflammatory processes and liver metastasis. A large body of evidence at the cellular and molecular levels corroborates these clinical findings. Indeed, the liver microenvironment has the capacity to generate and respond to inflammatory signals and cancer progression is characterized by inflammation. Inflammation can have a direct impact on the phenotype of circulating tumor cells, it can affect cell adhesion profiles within the liver's microvasculature and it can potentiate interactions between circulating cancer cells and circulating immune cells. This chapter outlines the major mechanisms by which the liver microenvironment responds to inflammatory cues and how this response affects the ability of circulating tumor cells to colonize the liver and generate metastases. This crossroad between inflammation and liver metastasis is an important avenue for therapeutic intervention.

Keywords Liver · Metastasis · Inflammation · Tumor necrosis factor · Neutrophils

Abbreviations

Generic abbreviations
BMDM   bone marrow derived macrophage
CAM   cell adhesion molecule
CTC   circulating tumor cell
HSC   hepatic stellate sell
IVM   intravital microscopy
SEC   sinusoidal endothelial cell
NKT   natural killer T cell

L. Ferri (✉)
The LD McLean Surgical Research Laboratories, Division of Surgical Research, Department of Surgery, The Montreal General Hospital, McGill University, Montreal, QC, Canada; Division of Thoracic Surgery, Department of Surgery, The Montreal General Hospital, McGill University, Room L9-112, 1650 Cedar Ave, Montreal, QC H3G 1A4, Canada
e-mail: lorenzo.ferri@muhc.mcgill.ca

P. Brodt (ed.), *Liver Metastasis: Biology and Clinical Management*, Cancer Metastasis – Biology and Treatment 16, DOI 10.1007/978-94-007-0292-9_6, © Springer Science+Business Media B.V. 2011

Adhesion molecules:

ICAM-1	intercellular adhesion molecule 1
LFA-1	lymphocyte function-associated antigen 1
PECAM-1	platelet endothelial cell adhesion molecule 1 or CD31
PSGL-1	P-selectin glycoprotein ligand 1
sLe^x	Sialyl Lewis X
sLe^a	Sialyl Lewis A
VLA-4	Very late antigen 4
ESL-1	E-selectin ligand 1

Cytokines, chemokines inflammatory mediators, and receptors:

CXCR2	CXCL1 and CXCL 7 receptor
IL-1	interleukin 1
IL-6	interleukin 6
IL-8	interleukin 8
IP-10	interferon-gamma-induced protein or CXCL10
IFN-γ	inteferon γ
KC/GRO	CXCL1
LPS	lipopolysaccharide
LTA	lipotechoic acid
Mac-1	macrophage-1 antigen. Composed of CD11b and CD18
MadCAM	mucosal vascular addressin cell adhesion molecule 1
MIP-1	macrophage Inflammatory Protein 1
MIP-2	macrophage Inflammatory Protein 2 or CXCL2
MIP-3	macrophage inflammatory protein 3 or CCL20
MCP-1	monocyte Chemotactic Protein 1 or CCL2 chemokine
RANTES	regulated upon Activation, Normal T-cell Expressed and Secreted. Also known as CCL-5 chemokine
TGF-β	transforming growth factor β
TLR	toll-like receptor
TNF-α	tumor necrosis factor α
TNFR1	tumor necrosis factor receptor 1
TNFR2	tumor necrosis factor receptor 2

Signalling molecules:

ERK	extracellular signal-regulated kinases
JNK	c-Jun N-terminal kinases
MAPK	mitogen activated protein kinase
MyD88	myeloid differentiation primary response gene 88
NF-κB	nuclear factor kappa-light-chain of activated B cells
PI3K	phosphoinositide 3-kinase

Cell lines:

H-59	murine Lewis lung carcinoma cell line, heavily metastatic to liver.
CX-1	human colon adenocarcinoma cell line metastatic to liver.

M-27   murine Lewis lung carcinoma cell line, poorly metastatic to liver.
MIP-101   human colon adenocarcinoma cell line poorly metastatic to liver.

Miscellaneous:
MMP   matrix metalloproteinase
TSU68   tyrosine kinase inhibitor

Growth factors
FGFR1   fibroblast growth factor receptor 1
PDGFR   platelet derived growth factor receptor
VEGFR2   vascular endothelial growth factor receptor 2
GFP   green fluorescent protein

Contents

6.1 Introduction

Liver metastasis is a source of significant morbidity for cancer patients and is frequently a harbinger of a patient's ultimate demise [1]. It is a favored site of metastasis for various malignancies such as colon, pancreatic and breast carcinomas and melanomas and one of the most common solid organs to host metastases [2]. The liver microenvironment is rich in inflammatory cells and mediators and emerging data now suggest that the liver's capacity to host metastases is intimately linked to this feature. This chapter will focus on the synergistic interactions between inflammation and the process of metastasis within this large and complex organ. Indeed, it will become clear that therapies aimed at the eradication of liver metastases must consider the impact of the local and systemic inflammatory environments on the progression of disease.

There are five lines of evidence that link cancer and inflammation: (1) Chronic inflammatory conditions of organs such as the bladder, cervix, esophagus, stomach, intestine, ovary, prostate and thyroid are associated with an increased risk of malignancy, (2) Patients who take non-steroidal anti-inflammatory medications are at decreased risk of developing certain malignancies and in fact have decreased mortality from these malignancies, (3) Signaling pathways involved in inflammation are activated following oncogenic mutations, (4) Inflammatory cells, chemokines and cytokines are present in the microenvironment of all tumors and targeting a number of these inflammatory mediators can decrease the incidence and spread of cancer in experimental models, (5) Adoptive transfer of inflammatory cells and over-expression of inflammatory cytokines promotes the development of tumors and conversely, in mice with targeted deletions in genes that regulate inflammation, the incidence of some cancers is reduced. These lines of evidence are the foundations for an entire field of research and provide numerous avenues of investigation that hold promise in the treatment of malignant disease [3]. Although there is a clear and well-accepted role for chronic inflammation in the pathogenesis of cancer, this chapter will deal primarily with the synergistic relationship between inflammation and cancer metastasis to the liver.

To date, there have been multiple clinical studies that have linked infectious and inflammatory complications from oncologic surgery to poor long-term survival. Several studies have shown that patients who develop complications from surgery for esophageal, head and neck, hepatic, colon and breast malignancies have reduced overall survival compared to those with an uneventful post-operative course [4–12]. Furthermore, some studies have begun to show that minimally invasive surgical techniques can improve long-term survival, potentially by reducing surgical trauma [13]. These studies raise the intriguing possibility that acute inflammatory stimuli produced either by surgical trauma and/or by infectious agents may promote the implantation and growth of circulating tumor cells (CTCs). It is possible that these inflammatory triggers prepare the stroma and microvasculature of solid organs such as the liver to receive these CTCs and engage a number of survival and angiogenic signals necessary for tumor growth. In addition, such external inflammatory stimuli have the potential to alter the CTC, increasing its ability to adhere and survive in the target organ. Similarly, evidence that the primary tumor itself can act as an inflammatory agent is emerging [14]. Indeed, most malignancies have been linked to increased levels of inflammatory cytokines. These cytokines and other factors are likely to help prepare the metastatic niche in the liver for the dissemination and growth of the CTCs.

The interest in the interplay between cancer and inflammation has led to a wealth of studies linking inflammation and liver metastasis. The concept that local, systemic, acute, and chronic inflammation can all affect the ability of certain malignancies to metastasize to the liver has gained much experimental and clinical support. It is now widely accepted that there exists a causal relationship between inflammation, innate immunity and many malignancies [15]. Indeed, cancer cells are not only a potential source of inflammation, but can also commandeer the molecular machinery utilized by immune cells to promote their dissemination throughout the host. This interplay between inflammation and cancer cells attempting to colonize the liver is becoming a central theme in liver metastasis research. Our aim is to summarize the literature on this area of investigation and highlight some of the potential future avenues for research and therapeutic innovation.

The liver is a site of hematogenous metastasis. Thus, following the classical paradigm, a cancer cell must detach from the primary tumor, enter into the circulation (intravasate), survive the harsh circulatory environment, adhere within a host organ's vasculature, extravasate into the virgin parenchyma and proliferate within it (Fig. 6.1) in order to establish a liver metastasis [16]. The focus of this chapter are the steps that occur after intravasation – that is, the role of inflammation in the recruitment of cancer cells to the liver's microvasculature and ultimate growth and progression of metastases within this organ. However, prior to tackling these complex oncologic events, it is essential to provide a broad overview of the pathophysiological processes that underlie inflammation in general, and specifically within the liver.

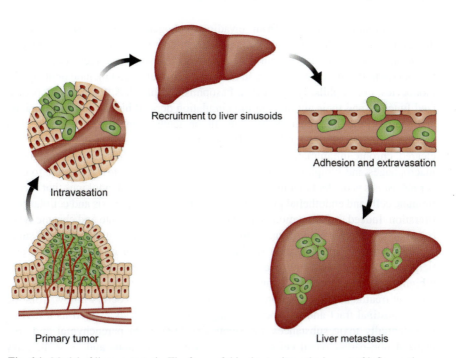

Fig. 6.1 Model of liver metastasis. The focus of this chapter is on the impact of inflammation on CTC adhesion and extravasation within the liver

6.2 Inflammation and the Liver

For centuries, cancers have been likened to non-healing wounds and in fact can frequently present as such [17]. This observation provides an interesting clue to understanding the interplay between malignant progression and inflammation and the similarities in the molecular pathways that underlie each process. Inflammation is a physiological process by which the innate immune system responds to allow for tissue repair following infection or trauma. The traditional pathological definition of inflammation describes it as a complex reaction to injurious agents, such as microbes and damaged cells, that consists of vascular responses, migration and activation of leukocytes, and systemic reactions [2]. Inflammation is therefore a process of repair that necessarily involves molecular cues for cellular growth, proliferation, survival and angiogenesis. Cancer cells usurp these signals for their own survival and this leads to pathological states of inflammation and the paradoxical situation of a non-healing but rapidly proliferating "wound". Host immune cells and soluble mediators drive the inflammatory cascade and as such, our discussion will be divided along these lines

6.2.1 Cellular Mediators of Inflammation

Noxious inflammatory cues from invading pathogens or traumatic injury are detected by the resident immune cells of a given host tissue. Tissue macrophages, dendritic cells and mast cells can trigger a series of events that recruit circulating leukocytes to the afflicted area. These circulating immune cells include neutrophils, monocytes, eosinophils, lymphocytes, basophils and platelets. Each has a specialized function and their numbers in the circulation depend highly on the chronicity and nature of the inflammatory stimulus. In the acute setting (6–24 h), neutrophils are the primary cellular mediators. If the initial acute insult is not successfully cleared, chronic inflammation ensues. In the chronic setting (usually beyond 48 h), macrophages and lymphocytes predominate. Perhaps of greatest relevance to cancer metastasis is the fact that macrophages produce the bulk of cytokines that recruit immune cells and endothelial progenitors to stimulate angiogenesis and cellular proliferation. Indeed, inflammation is most often classified into acute and chronic types based on the relative proportions of these different leukocytes at the inflamed site.

An interesting specialization of the liver is that most of its resident cells participate in the detection and execution of the inflammatory cascade. The liver is a highly specialized organ. It functions as a "power plant" on one hand and as a "sewage treatment and recycling facility" on the other. It receives inflow from the gastrointestinal tract and is exposed to high nutritional loads as well as a myriad of potentially toxic substances and organisms [18]. Both parenchymal and specialized non-parenchymal cells participate in these functions and as such, carry several immune properties. Thus, hepatocytes, Kupffer cells, sinusoidal endothelial cells (SECs), hepatic stellate cells (HSCs) and pit cells all participate in the unique inflammatory responses of the liver [19].

Kupffer cells are resident macrophages of the liver. They are the central actor in liver inflammation and have a particularly important role in metastasis [20]. Under physiologic conditions, they are responsible for the phagocytosis of expired erythrocytes as part of the reticuloendothelial system. They originate in the bone marrow and are of the monocyte lineage. Beyond their hematologic function, Kupffer cells are potent participants in the inflammatory processes of the liver. They are the focal point where toxic cues are processed and the mediators of inflammation are orchestrated. In response to hepatotoxins and microbial pathogens like bacterial lipopolysaccharide (LPS), Kupffer cells express an array of cytokines (IL-1, IL-6, IL-8 and TNF-α) and chemokines (MIP-2, IP-10, KC/GRO, MIP-1α, MCP-1 and RANTES). The released cytokines have a paracrine effect on neighboring SECs and HSCs resulting in important gene expression changes that favor the attraction of circulating immune cells like neutrophils and lymphocytes [19].

A key component of the inflammatory cascade is the specialized microvasculature in which cancer cells must arrest in order to extravasate into the parenchyma. The liver is composed of a network of sinusoids lined by a fenestrated endothelium. Unlike capillaries, the ante-luminal side of these fenestrated SECs does not rest upon an organized basement membrane, but on a delicate extracellular matrix that contains fibronectin and several collagens such as collagen I, III, and IV and forms the space of Disse [2]. These histological particularities are important because they enable potential interactions between circulating cancer cells and extracellular matrix components within these fenestrations as well hepatocytes and other non-parenchymal cells such as stellate and Kupffer cells. In addition to their architecture, SECs play an active role in the inflammatory cascade. While they express low levels of chemotactic factors (RANTES, MCP-1, IL-8 and MIP-1α) under normal conditions, inflammatory activation causes high levels of expression of these factors as well as important changes in cell adhesion molecule expression. Much like other endothelial cells in the body, SECs express high levels of VCAM-1, ICAM-1, E- and P-selectins in response to inflammation and down-regulate their expression of PECAM-1 [20]. These changes in chemokine production and cell adhesion molecule (CAM) expression promote leukocyte adhesion and there is significant evidence that they may serve as a basis for inflammation-facilitated cancer cell recruitment to the liver.

Acute inflammation ensures rapid delivery of plasma and leukocytes to a site of injury or infection through an ordered process of increased blood flow, enhanced microvascular permeability and increased endothelial cell activation. The molecular events that regulate leukocyte trafficking to an inflamed site have been studied extensively [21, 22]. These events share obvious similarities with the classical paradigm of hematogenous metastasis [23, 24]. It should therefore not be a surprise that many of the hypotheses generated to explain how cancer cells metastasize were derived from what was known about leukocytes migration to sites of inflammation. Leukocytes typically follow a multi-step process to reach their destination within sites of tissue injury or infection. Initially their flow in the blood vessel is slowed through adhesion to cytokine- inducible selectins [25], a family of C-type lectins expressed in response to inflammatory stimuli on endothelial cells

(E- and P-selectin), platelets (P-selectin) and leukocytes (L-selectin)[26] . This adhesion is mediated by selectin ligands expressed on the leukocyte cell surface such as glycoproteins decorated by oligosaccharides including sialyl Lewis X and the P-Selectin Glycoprotein Ligand-1 (PSGL-1). The bonds formed between inflammation-inducible selectins and mucin-like glycoproteins are short lived and of low-affinity but allow for a slower rolling to occur. Leukocyte tethering along the endothelial surface triggers signals that up-regulate integrins (VLA-4, MadCAM, Mac-1 and LFA-1) and immunoglobulin super-family CAMs (ICAM-1, VCAM-1 and PECAM) on leukocytes and endothelial cells, respectively. These homo- and heterotypic intercellular bonds allow for firm adhesion, which precedes trans-migration beyond the endothelial layer and basement membrane into the site of the inflammatory stimulus where the leukocytes will perform their effector functions [21].

In addition to Kupffer cells, SECs and the circulating leukocytes recruited to the liver under inflamed conditions, several other cell types within the liver can participate in the inflammatory cascade. Hepatocytes constitute approximately 70–80% of the liver's mass and are responsible for the majority of the specific functions of the liver. Although their primary functions are synthetic and metabolic, hepatocytes can also produce important cytokines such as Interleukin 8 (IL-8) and C reactive protein in response to acute phase mediators of inflammation including IL-6 [27, 28]. In addition to IL-8, stressed or damaged hepatocytes express other leukocyte attract-ing chemokines such as cytokine-induced chemoattractant (KC) and macrophage attractant proteins (MIP-1, 2 and 3) [29, 30].

Hepatic stellate cells (HSCs or Ito cells) have a modulatory effect on the inflammatory response. These cells are located in the space of Disse, between the sinusoidal endothelium and hepatocytes where lymph drains to the portal tract lymphatics. HSCs express ICAM-1 and VCAM-1 that are downregulated by the transforming growth factor (TGF) pathway and induced by the TNF-α pathway [31]. HSCs also secrete several cytokines and chemokines including IL-8, RANTES and MCP-1 [32, 33] and were recently shown to express the E-selectin ligand 1 (ESL-1) [34]. The presence of ESL-1 along the sinusoidal endothelium has implications for both leukocyte and tumor cell recruitment to the liver. Although the role of HSCs in liver fibrosis has been well established, their contribution to the process of liver metastasis has not been extensively studied. It appears that their main function is to trigger a wound-repair response that promotes collagen I and IV production and angiogenesis in response to tumor infiltration of the liver [35]. (The reader is referred to Chapter 3 in this volume for a more detailed discussion of the role of HSC in liver metastasis).

Macrophage and lymphocyte infiltration into primary tumors and metastases are common [3]. Lymphocytes are attracted to sites of chronic inflammation by mediators similar to those involved in neutrophil recruitment (i.e. via selectins, inte-grins and chemokines) and are activated by local tissue macrophages. Activated T lymphocytes can, in turn produce cytokines including Interferon γ (IFN-γ) that reciprocally further activate macrophages and can modulate the expression patterns of HSCs. Another lymphocyte subpopulation in the liver, i.e. the Pit cells or Natural

Killer T cells (NKT cells) mediates Natural Killer cell functions and is dependent on the presence of Kupffer cells for their survival [36]. These cells are known to express IFN-γ in response to liver injury but their main role (under physiological conditions) is to survey the liver for the presence of malignant or virus-infected cells. They interact with Kupffer cells as they patrol the liver sinusoids for foreign antigens [37]. While activated by IL-2, they have the capacity to destroy target cells even without prior activation [38].

Together, these cell populations all have the capacity to alter the metastatic microenvironment within the liver. Although the role of NKT cells, HSCs and hepatocytes in the process of liver metastasis remains to be fully elucidated, their physiologic functions, as well as their ability to influence the inflammatory microenvironment of the liver strongly support their potential involvement in this process. Indeed, further studies are required to better understand how these cell populations contribute to the natural history of liver metastasis. To date, Kupffer cells and SECs are the most studied local inflammatory cells in liver metastasis. They are the central actors of the inflammatory cascade in the liver and, as described below are intimately linked to the metastatic process.

6.2.2 Soluble Mediators of Inflammation

Endothelial cell activation greatly increases the adhesion of molecules required to optimally recruit leukocytes, and as detailed below, cancer cells [39]. Cytokines and chemokines released by local inflammatory cells such as tissue macrophages and activated lymphocytes are essential to trigger the acute phase response that allows the cellular mediators of inflammation to be recruited to an affected organ site. Two early and central cytokines in this process are Tumor Necrosis Factor alpha (TNF-α) and Interleukin-1 (IL-1). They are both produced by tissue macrophages, though other cells including tumor cells can secrete these cytokines. The trigger for TNF-α and IL-1 production by tissue macrophages includes microbial products such as endotoxin, immune complexes, physical injury and products of cellular necrosis. One of the primary effects of these cytokines is to induce alterations in the endothelial cell adhesion molecule profile, notably, increase surface expression of selectins (E and P) as well as integrin ligands such as ICAM-1 and VCAM-1. Furthermore, both TNF-α and IL-1 cause systemic effects such as fever, loss of appetite, release of primed neutrophils into the circulation, release of corticosteroids and specifically for TNF-α, the hemodynamic changes seen with septic shock, namely hypotension, decreased vascular resistance and increased heart rate. Interestingly, such syndromes as cancer cachexia may be related to ongoing TNF-α production, potentially by the tumor itself, and this may set the stage for a highly inflammatory metastatic microenvironment.

Resident immune cells of organs such as the liver are equipped with receptors specific for microbial insult or tissue injury [40]. Perhaps one of the more important families of molecules responsible for these sensor functions is the highly conserved Toll-like receptor family (TLR) [41]. Toll-like receptors are expressed on resident immune cells such as dendritic cells and macrophages and act as sentinels for the presence of pathogens. To date, 13 mammalian TLRs have been identified, each with distinct specificities that include pathogen-derived antigens such as lipoproteins, lipopolysaccharides (LPS), bacterial DNA and viral RNA. A number of endogenous ligands released by necrotic cells or tumor cells can also bind and activate TLRs [42]. TLRs signal primarily via the MyD88-dependent pathway resulting in the nuclear translocation of Nuclear Factor κB (NF-κB). NF-κB is a transcriptional activator of approximately 200 genes whose products control the immune system, growth, and inflammation [43]. In addition to immune cells, TLRs can also be expressed on epithelial tissues and the role that this plays in the cancer/inflammation crosstalk is increasingly being recognized [44–46]. Indeed, many human malignancies and cancer cell lines are now known to express a variety of TLRs raising the possibility that tumor cells themselves can respond to, and be affected by infectious pathogens [42, 47]. Thus, infectious agents and products of cellular necrosis or tissue trauma can affect signaling within the cancer cell as well as within stromal and inflammatory cells of the tumor microenvironment.

6.2.3 Chronic Inflammation and Termination of Inflammation

While the inflammatory process is geared towards tissue repair, healing and disposal of infectious agents, its effects are widespread and potentially harmful. It is this conflicting aspect of inflammation that is frequently referred to as a "double-edged sword" or the "friend or foe?" nature of inflammation. As we shall discuss, this duality is equally applicable to the role of inflammation in cancer progression [3, 15, 43, 48–50]. In an attempt to limit the potential deleterious effects of inflammation, the immune system can use several molecular switches to bring the inflammatory cascade to an end. Lipoxins are produced after the aggregation of platelets and neutrophils at sites of inflammation and inhibit further leukocyte recruitment. Anti-inflammatory cytokines including IL-10 and Transforming Growth Factor β (TGF-β) are produced by activated local macrophages. Lipid anti-inflammatory mediators known as resolvins and protectins act primarily by limiting neutrophil recruitment and are produced after the initiation of the inflammatory cascade [51, 52]. Indeed, these molecular "off" switches may be useful therapeutically to limit the cancer-promoting effects of inflammation. However, their potential role in inhibition of liver metastasis has not, to date, been elucidated.

Chronic inflammation can exist as a result of the failure of host mechanisms to terminate an acute inflammation or it can present insidiously as a smoldering condition without the presence of an acute insult. It is characterized by a series of events aimed at repairing traumatized or infected tissue or an inappropriate, immune-mediated form of tissue damage [2]. While these responses are designed to resolve the insult, the effects of chronic inflammation, much like acute inflammation, can be deleterious to host tissues. Unlike the acute setting, where the cellular players are predominantly neutrophils, chronic inflammatory infiltrates are typified by mononuclear cells such as macrophages, lymphocytes and plasma cells. The persistence of these cells can result in further tissue damage and trigger a wound-healing response in the form of angiogenesis and fibrosis [2]. The molecular cues for angiogenesis and proliferation of stromal cells that affect the fibrotic reactions are intimately linked with the growth requirements for metastases, particularly in the liver [53–55].

6.3 Tumor Cell Arrest and Inflammation

6.3.1 Cytokines and the Circulating Tumor Cell

There is a well-accepted association between malignancy and a systemic pro-inflammatory state. Indeed, numerous clinical studies have shown increased levels of circulating cytokines in patients bearing tumors [56]. Furthermore, there is emerging evidence to suggest that cancer patients with altered cytokine profiles or with elevated markers of systemic inflammation are more likely to develop metastases and succumb to their disease. However, it remains to be seen whether these increased cytokine profiles are a cause or consequence of cancer progression and metastasis. Increased circulating IL-1, IL-6 and IL-8 levels have all been shown to be predictive of liver metastasis and long term survival for patients with different primary solid malignancies including breast, lung, gastric, colorectal and urogenital carcinomas [57–61]. Similarly, markers of a systemic inflammatory response including C-reactive protein and an elevated neutrophil:lymphocyte ratio are predictors of poor prognosis for cancer specific outcomes [62–66]. Studies examining the relationship between serum TNF-α levels and cancer-related outcomes in patients with various malignancies have yielded inconsistent results. This may be related to a number of technical factors pertaining to the half-life of this cytokine and its potential dual function with respect to tumorigenesis and cancer progression. However, serum levels of the solubilized TNF receptor 1 (sTNFR1) were found to be elevated in a great proportion of patients with colorectal carcinoma and these levels were closely correlated with tumor grade and depth of invasion and were an independent predictor of survival [64]. Nevertheless, interpretation of such a finding remains difficult in terms of tumor biology without experimental evidence to corroborate either a tumor promoting or inhibiting effect. Certainly, the same molecular mediators may have varying effects depending on the source, stage or location of metastases.

True to its name, TNF-α is known to cause hemorrhagic necrosis of tumors following high dose intra-tumoral injection as a result of specific T cell mediated destruction of tumor blood vessels and direct cytotoxic effects upon cancer cells [67–70]. However, the data supporting TNF-α mediated cancer growth and progression is undeniable. Many malignancies produce TNF-α and its expression in the tumor microenvironment can act as a tumor promoter [48]. This discrepancy is partially related to the fact that TNF-α has two receptors, each with varying signaling pathways depending on context and cell type. The p55/p60 TNFR1 that is expressed on nearly all cells can activate transcription of genes involved in inflammation and cell survival; however, in a stressed cell where NF-κB induction fails or due to high levels of TNF-α, TNFR1 signaling induces cell death through its TNFR1-associated death domain (TRADD) [71, 72]. The p75/p80 TNFR2 is expressed in a more restricted manner on immune cells and a few other cell types. It can activate a number of pathways including NF-κB, ERK, JNK, p38, MAPK and PI3K and plays a major role in T-cell survival. However, its biological activity is still under study. One difference between these receptor systems is that TNFR1 is activated by soluble ligand, while TNFR2 primarily binds transmembrane TNF. Moreover, in contrast to TNFR1, TNFR2 lacks a death domain and its role in apoptosis is therefore likely limited. Recent evidence suggests that one of its functions may be to modulate and enhance the activities of TNFR1 on immune and endothelial cells. These receptors can also solubilize and act to bind TNF-α, thus prolonging its half-life but also potentially inhibiting its activity [73, 74].

In a recent study, treatment of mice with recombinant TNF-α resulted in both larger primary tumors and increased numbers of liver metastases in a xenograft, orthotopic implantation model of pancreatic cancer metastasis. Conversely, blockade of TNF-α using a TNF-trap or monoclonal antibodies (etanercept or infliximab, respectively) resulted in a significant reduction in both tumor volume and the number of metastases. Importantly, while there was a significant effect on tumor growth and metastasis in mice bearing local tumors, the inhibitory effect of both compounds was even more notable in the adjuvant setting when TNF-α blockade was initiated after resection of the primary tumors resulting in a marked reduction in the number of liver metastases. Because these reagents target the human TNF-α specifically, these data strongly suggest that TNF-α produced by the cancer cells can contribute to the metastatic process [75]. In a parallel study, the use of the glucocorticoid anti-inflammatory agent dexamethasone had very similar effects to TNF-α blockade [76]. Together, these results suggest that anti-inflammatory therapy in a peri-operative setting has the potential to reduce liver implantation of circulating cancer cells, thereby reducing the occurrence of metastases.

In the liver, Kupffer cells are the predominant source of TNF-α. Hence, reagents that suppress its function or block its action form a potential therapeutic strategy. By preventing local inflammatory changes in the liver, one may reduce CTC arrest. Indeed, molecules like bacterial endotoxin (lipopolysaccharide-LPS) are capable of activating endothelial cells directly via TLR4 or indirectly through Kupffer cells, resulting in a significant inflammatory cascade within the liver and systemically. Studies have previously demonstrated a pro-metastatic action of LPS in a number of experimental models of lung metastasis [77, 78]. The hypothesis that LPS may promote cancer progression clinically is supported by a combination of observations. Firstly, patients with clinically, non-metastatic solid cancers have CTCs [79] whose numbers increase as a result of surgical intervention, biopsy or tumor-associated complications [80–83]. Secondly, surgically curative therapy is associated with complications such as gram-negative sepsis with massive release of LPS. Together, these findings describe a fertile soil for the implantation of CTCs as a result of LPS-mediated CAM changes on SECs and on CTCs themselves. Indeed, there is a long history of clinical observations that have linked rapid metastatic progression in patients who have suffered severe infectious complications following resection for cancer [4–8, 10–12]. Employing a clinically relevant model of bacterial endotoxemia, we have recently attempted to investigate the mechanism by which LPS promotes the formation of metastases in the liver [84]. By using intra-vital microscopy of the liver, GFP-tagged H-59 murine Lewis lung carcinoma cells that are highly metastatic to the liver were visualized within the liver sinusoids following intra-arterial injection (Fig. 6.2a). We found a significant increase in the number of cells that arrested within the liver sinusoids in mice that were pre-treated with LPS 4 h prior to injection (Fig. 6.2b). Thus, circulating tumor cells are more likely to implant within the liver of a systemically inflamed animal.

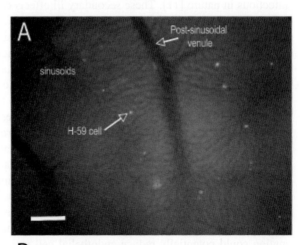

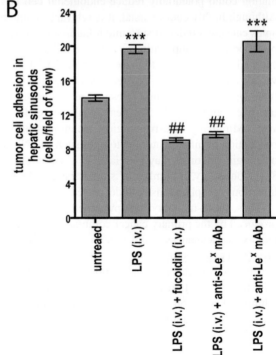

Fig. 6.2 Systemic inflammation increases tumor cell adhesion within the liver sinusoids and is attenuated by selectin/sialyl-Lewis X blockade. Liver sinusoids of mice were visualized by fluorescence intravital microscopy to assess the adhesion of H-59 cells in untreated or systemically inflamed (i.v. LPS) mice per field of view ($\times 200$) in five experimental groups (representative image in (**a**)). (**b**) Untreated mice (14.00 ± 0.40) and mice treated intravenously with 0.5 mg/kg LPS (19.7 ± 0.48) were injected with H-59 cells. Pre-treatment of tumor cells with neutralizing anti-sialyl Lewis X antibodies (9.71 ± 0.35) or anti-Le^X mAb (as control) (20.6 ± 1.21), or pre-treatment of mice with fucoidin (20 mg/kg) (9.08 ± 0.28) were employed in some LPS treated mice. Data are expressed as the means $\pm$ SEM of at least five animals per group. ***$p < 0.05$ relative to untreated controls; ## $p < 0.05$ relative to LPS-treated controls. Reproduced with permission from [84]

Together, these studies strongly suggest that inflammatory mediators including LPS TNF-α, IL-1, IL-6 and IL-8 can help prepare the liver to accept CTCs. It is likely that these cytokines, produced or stimulated by the primary tumor or released in response to treatment, participate in the establishment of a pro-metastatic niche with localized changes in cell-adhesion molecule expression and leukocyte margination that facilitate the implantation of CTCs [85, 86]. Indeed, patients treated for solid organ metastases frequently require surgery and systemic chemotherapy. Though highly effective for loco-regional disease control, surgical resection is associated with significant tissue trauma and complications, many of which are infectious in nature [11]. These secondary ill effects can trigger a significant acute inflammatory response that is likely to up-regulate the expression of inducible cell adhesion molecules in the liver and other metastatic sites. Decreasing the capacity of cancer cells to arrest within liver sinusoids may therefore be a promising treatment strategy for patients with cancers prone to metastasize to the liver and limiting the impact of inflammation-promoted arrest is of particular interest.

With the advent of minimally invasive techniques for cancer surgery, there are emerging data to suggest that the inflammatory process may be influenced by the manner in which a tumor is resected, and this, in turn, may impact cancer recurrence. This makes teleological sense since traditional open resection of cancers may result in markedly increased systemic inflammation due to surgical trauma and, concomitantly, in an increase in circulating tumor cells. The combination of increased systemic inflammation on one hand and the presence of surgically induced CTCs on the other [80–83] represents a fertile ground for the development of metastases. Attempts to reduce surgical trauma and therefore systemic inflammation could potentially reduce endothelial cell activation and cancer metastasis. Although highly controversial, it is relevant to note that less invasive surgical therapies causing a reduced systemic inflammatory response and associated with fewer post-operative complications have been linked to improved overall and disease-free survival [65]. In a randomized controlled trial of curative intent, in which open versus laparoscopically-assisted colectomy for colon carcinoma were compared, there was a 25% reduction in cancer recurrence for patients treated by a minimally invasive approach [13]. The benefits also extended to overall and disease-free survival. Minimally invasive surgical techniques have been associated with reduced production of inflammatory cytokines such as TNF-α, suggesting that the improved oncologic outcomes may be related to a reduction in systemic inflammation [9, 87, 88]. Conversely, a number of studies have linked the presence of post-operative infectious complications with decreased survival or early recurrence [5, 7, 89].

Thus, multi-modality therapy aimed at reducing the pro-inflammatory cascade produced by the primary cancer combined with therapies that have minimal inflammatory consequences could potentially limit the spread of metastases. However, given that cytokine production and the ability to respond to triggers such as LPS are essential to host defense against infection, and their impairment may have deleterious effects in a clinical setting, a more targeted approach that aims to specifically inhibit cell adhesion molecules that promote metastasis may be a preferred strategy. Indeed, a significant body of literature supports the role of inflammation-inducible cell adhesion molecules in the formation of liver metastases and identifies them as potential targets.

6.3.2 Inflammation-Inducible Cell-Adhesion Molecules

To survive, circulating cancer cells must perform many of the same "maneuvers" as leukocytes at sites of inflammation. Cancer cells that have survived the circulatory environment must arrest within the sinusoids, penetrate through the sinusoidal layer and survive within the liver's parenchyma. As described above, many studies have investigated the role of the selectin/selectin ligand axis in cancer metastasis, and more specifically in liver metastasis. Several in vitro studies have shown that inflammatory cytokines including TNF-α and IL-1β promote cancer cell rolling on an activated endothelium in a selectin dependent manner (Fig. 6.3) [90]. In addition, antibody-mediated blockade or enzymatic reduction of selectin ligands in the form of sialylated carbohydrate moieties inhibited cancer cell adhesion to cytokine-activated endothelial cells [91].

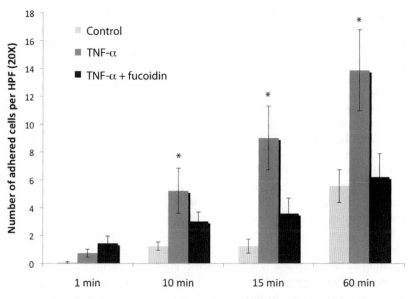

Fig. 6.3 Endothelial cell activation by TNF-α causes increased cancer cell adhesion in vitro that is reversed by selectin blockade. A flow chamber was used to demonstrate the effect of TNF-α-mediated activation of human umbilical vein endothelial cells (HUVECs) on cancer cell (H-59) adhesion. H-59 cells were flowed over HUVECs and adhesion was quantified at 1, 10, 15 and 60 min. Endothelial cells were either pre-treated with TNF-α for 4 h or not and in a third experiment the flowing media was treated with fucoidin. TNF-α treatment significantly increased adhesion at 10, 15 and 60 min, while fucoidin treatment almost completely reversed the TNF-α effect, suggesting that systemic inflammatory cues increase endothelial adhesion in a selectin-dependent manner. (*$p < 0.05$ as compared to control and TNF-α + fucoidin groups). HPF-High Power Field. Reproduced with permission from [84]

Concurrently, our studies and many others have shown that blockade of inflammation-inducible cell adhesion molecules reduces the arrest of circulating cancer cells within the liver and ultimately the development of gross metastases. Indeed, treatment of mice with the non-specific selectin small molecule blocker fucoidin attenuated the increased cancer cell adhesion mediated by LPS treatment (Fig. 6.2). In addition, treatment of the cancer cells with a blocking monoclonal antibody to the selectin ligand sLe^x also reversed the effects of LPS treatment [84]. The importance of the selectin/sLe^x axis in cancer metastasis is also highlighted by the fact that treatment of mice with a blocking monoclonal antibody to E-selectin reduced median number of liver metastases by 97% using a model of intrasplenic/portal injection of the metastatic H-59 cells [92]. Conversely, in another study, colorectal carcinoma cells with high mucin carbohydrate expression (and therefore rich in sLe^x moieties) metastasized to the liver more readily than cells with poor mucin expression [91]. Together, these results show that inflammation-inducible sinusoidal endothelial cell adhesion molecules such as E-selectin and their ligands are highly important for the development of gross metastases and that these interactions occur very early in the metastatic process. Indeed, E-selectin ligands such as sLe^x and sLe^a (an isomer of sLe^x) have been linked to clinical progression of cancer for many malignancies [93–96]. sLe^a, otherwise known as CA 19-9 is one of the most commonly used tumor markers and has been shown to be predictive of metastasis in a number of patient populations [97–101]. These findings suggest that high expression of E-selectin ligands on cancer cells correlate with metastatic potential and may explain why some malignancies are more prone to the effects of inflammatory signals.

The results described above identified E-selectin as important to liver metastasis. Yet under normal physiological conditions, E-selectin expression on endothelial cells is low. To address this discrepancy, the Brodt group analyzed the ability of metastatic cancer cells to induce a local inflammatory reaction within the liver and found that tumor cells themselves could induce the expression of E-selectin following their entry into the liver. In fact, within an hour of their intrasplenic/portal injection, a significant rise in cytokine expression was observed and this was followed by a rise in E-selectin expression on sinusoidal endothelial cells that peaked at 6–8 h post tumor cell inoculation [102]. Interestingly, a number of cell lines known to be poorly metastatic to the liver failed to induce a similar inflammatory reaction suggesting that this response is tumor-specific. Further characterization revealed that the source of TNF-α production originated in large part from Kupffer cells. Firstly, Kupffer cells were found to produce TNF-α in response to cells that are highly metastatic to the liver (H-59/CX-1) and not by those that are poorly metastasizing (M-27/MIP-101). Secondly, Kupffer cells co-culture with highly metastasizing cells resulted in a significant increase in TNF-α production almost comparable to LPS stimulation. Once again, these findings were not reproduced in the presence of poorly metastasizing cells. Thirdly, increases in TNF-α production were correlated with subsequent increases in a number of cell adhesion molecules known to be relevant to cancer cell metastasis including E-selectin, P-selectin, ICAM-1, VCAM-1 and PECAM. These changes in cell adhesion molecule expression were implicated in cancer cell extravasation and ultimate growth [90, 103, 104]. Further corroborating evidence for the role of TNF-α inducible-endothelial cell adhesion molecules in liver metastasis was obtained using murine C-raf antisense oligonucleotides that inhibited TNFR signaling via the Raf/ERK pathway and thereby endothelial E-selectin induction. Treatment with this antisense oligonucleotide inhibited human colon carcinoma CX-1 cell adhesion to cultured hepatic sinusoidal cells and reduced liver metastasis of these cells by 86% following their intrasplenic/portal injection [105], confirming the role of this pathway in vivo.

In a parallel series of investigations using the Lewis lung carcinoma model of site-specific liver metastasis, the type 1 insulin growth factor receptor (IGF-1R) was identified as a key regulator of liver metastasis. Interestingly, it was found that IGF-1R was a negative regulator of the anti-inflammatory factor, secretory leukocyte protease inhibitor (SLPI) in this model. SLPI can protect cells against the inflammation-induced damage of neutrophils and macrophages by inhibiting the activity of enzymes such as elastase, cathepsin G, trypsin and chymotrypsin [106], it can increase host resistance to certain bacterial and viral infections [107, 108], down-regulate prostaglandin E2 and matrix metalloproteinases 1 and 9 [109] and can attenuate the response of macrophages to LPS [110, 111] by inhibiting NF-κB signaling. When SLPI was over-expressed in liver-metastasizing H-59 highly metastatic cells, there was an 80% reduction in liver metastases following their intrasplenic/portal injection [112]. This correlated with a decrease in E-selectin up-regulation normally seen after H-59 injection but was not associated with a reduction in tumor cell invasion per se. These experiments lend further support to the concept that anti-inflammatory cues in the early phases of cancer cell metastasis to the liver can help reduce metastatic burden. It should be noted that while these studies highlight the ability of the cancer cell itself to trigger the inflammatory cascade when it enters the liver, the evidence when taken together suggests that both systemic activators of inflammation and cancer cell-induced inflammatory mediators play a role and their targeting is likely to affect the metastatic burden.

6.3.3 Circulating Inflammatory Cells

Circulating cytokines such as IL-1, IL-6 and TNF-α can affect different host cell populations. They can cause changes to endothelial cell CAM profile [39], affect neutrophil adhesion and transmigration into the parenchyma of organs such as the liver [37, 113] and activate platelets leading to their increased interaction with neutrophils [114] and the endothelium [39]. It is therefore possible that cancer cells and neutrophils may interact through these adhesive proteins. Indeed, there is mounting evidence that inflammatory cells and cancer cells interact at multiple time points throughout the metastatic cascade. One crucial and rate limiting event during liver metastasis is that of tumor cell adhesion and transmigration. Advanced imaging techniques utilizing intravital microscopy have identified the sinusoids as the predominant site of adhesion for most cancer cells analyzed [84, 115, 116]. If (as suggested by the evidence) cancer cells preferentially adhere to activated

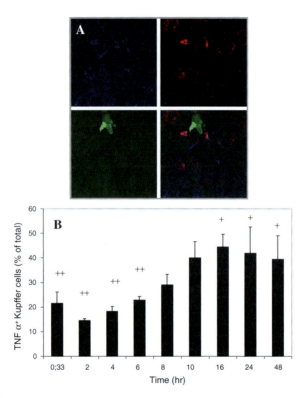

Fig. 6.4 Kupffer cells produce TNF-α in response to intrasplenic/portal injection of human colon carcinoma CX-1 cells. Cryostat sections were prepared following the injection of 10^6 tumour cells and immunolabeled with the macrophage-specific mAb F4/80 and an anti-TNF-a antibody. Shown in (**a**) are representative images of Kupffer cells (*blue*), TNF-a (*red*), CX-1 cells (*green*), and a merged confocal image. Shown in (**b**) are the percentages of TNF-a+ Kupffer cells at different time intervals after tumour injection. (+) $P < 0.05$ as compared to 20 min post tumour cell inoculation. (++) $P < 0.05$ as compared to percentage of TNF-a+ Kupffer cells at 16 h. Original magnifications, ×630. Reproduced with permission from: Khatib et al. (2005) Am J Pathol 167:749–759

endothelial cells and in proximity to activated Kupffer cells (Fig. 6.4), or even as a result of their self-induced microenvironmental activation, it is quite likely that circulating leukocytes and platelets would also be recruited and participate in the adhesion and transmigration process. Indeed, the potential for interactions between cancer cells and neutrophils is well documented in vitro. A series of studies using a physiologically relevant model of cancer cell adhesion have demonstrated dynamic interactions betweens neutrophils and melanoma cells under flow [117]. In addition, the presence of neutrophils has been shown to increase the invasiveness of melanoma cells under conditions of flow [118–121]. Finally, neutrophil-induced endothelial injury has previously been correlated with the pattern of cancer cell recruitment to the lung [122].

Our recent results have shown that neutrophils can co-localize with attached cancer cells within the liver sinusoids. Indeed, as many as 78% of H-59 cells were co-localized with a neutrophil following intra-carotid injection. However, neutrophils are not mere passive bystanders in the process and can actually promote the adhesion of circulating cancer cells in vivo (Fig. 6.5) [84]. When mice were treated with a neutrophil depleting monoclonal antibody prior to injection of H-59 cells, a significant reduction in cancer cell adhesion was noted in both LPS inflamed and non-inflamed mice. These results suggest that neutrophils have the capacity to interact with circulating cancer cells or perhaps prime the metastatic niche to receive a circulating cancer cell. Therefore, if neutrophils promote cancer cell adhesion within the liver and have the capacity to increase tumor cell invasiveness, strategies to limit this alliance may be beneficial in reducing the metastatic burden (Figs. 6.5 and 6.6).

The notion that leukocytes and particularly neutrophils may be involved in these early adhesive events is corroborated by a number of other studies. L-selectin is expressed exclusively on the surface of leukocytes and this expression is important for leukocyte rolling and adhesion. When L-selectin- deficient mice were inoculated intravenously with murine colon carcinoma MC-38 cells , a reduction in cancer cell arrest relative to control mice was noted as of 24 h. Furthermore, mice with a targeted L-selectin deletion had a great reduction in the number of tumor cells that co-localized with CD11b (Mac-1, a marker for granulocyte and monocyte linages)-positive leukocytes in the lung. Importantly, administration of a function-blocking antibody to L-selectin also reduced lung metastases [123]. In addition to a direct interaction with the tumor cells, it is possible that L-selectin allows leukocytes to interact with the pulmonary microvasculature to prepare the metastatic site for incoming CTCs, thereby facilitating metastasis to that organ. Though these mechanics have yet to be demonstrated in the liver, they remain an attractive subject of investigation and a potential therapeutic target.

Recently, a fascinating study linked neutrophils to the establishment of the pre-metastatic niche in the liver using an orthotopic model of colon carcinoma [124]. In tumor-bearing mice, there was a significant increase in the number of neutrophils present within liver sinusoids. This increased number of neutrophils was associated with a four-fold increase in the expression of the chemokine CXCL1 within the liver. The tyrosine kinase inhibitor TSU68 inhibits vascular endothelial growth factor receptor 2 (VEGFR2), platelet-derived growth factor receptor β (PDGFRβ) and fibroblast growth factor receptor 1 (FGFR1) and was shown to block metastasis in an experimental model. When it was used in this orthotopic colon carcinoma model before metastases were established, the level of CXCL1 mRNA and the number of neutrophils recruited to the liver were both reduced and this correlated with a reduction in liver metastasis suggesting that TSU68 affected chemokine expression. Moreover, when the CXCL1 receptor CXCR2 was inhibited with a function blocking monoclonal antibody in the same orthotopic model, liver metastasis was also inhibited. Therefore, neutrophils are clearly associated with the establishment of a pro-metastatic niche. Tumor-derived cues can lead to up-regulated expression of chemokines such as CXCL1 in the liver and this can

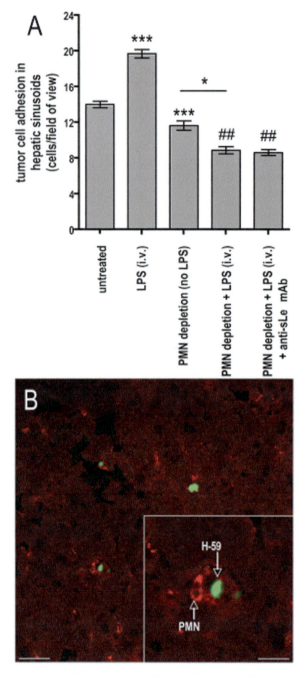

Fig. 6.5 Leukocyte-tumor cell interactions contribute to the arrest of circulating tumor cells in the liver sinusoids. (a) Fluorescence hepatic intravital microscopy was utilized to quantify the number of adherent H-59 cells per field of view (×200) within the liver sinusoids of untreated control mice

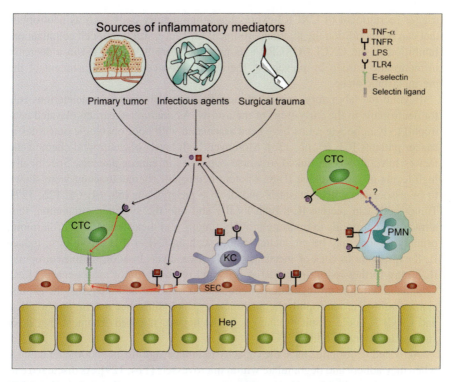

Fig. 6.6 The inflammatory microenvironment of the liver and its impact on metastasis. This simplified model highlights the potential sources of inflammatory mediators like LPS and TNF-α that include the primary tumor itself, infectious agents, surgical trauma, circulating tumor cells (CTC), circulating immune cells such as neutrophils (PMN) and resident immune cells such as Kupffer cells (KC). *Red arrows* indicate the presence of intracellular signaling events that lead to changes in expression of CAMs that may mediate CTC recruitment to the liver. This model does not take into account potential differences in TNFR1 versus TNFR2 signaling, nor is it an exhaustive representation of all potential inflammatory cytokines and inflammation inducible CAMs that could affect liver metastasis

Fig. 6.5 (continued) (14.0 ± 0.37), LPS-treated control mice (19.68 ± 0.48), control (no LPS) mice that were depleted of circulating PMN by a 24-h treatment with RB6-8C5 (11.65 ± 0.52; $p = 0.0041$), LPS-treated mice that were depleted of circulating PMN (8.9 ± 0.40; $p < 0.0001$), and LPS-treated mice that were depleted of circulating PMN that receive H-59 cells pre-treated with sLe^x blocking mAb (8.63 ± 0.33). Data are presented as the mean ± SEM of at least five livers per group. $^*p = 0.0037$ for PMN depleted mice compared to LPS-treated PMN depleted mice, $^{***}p < 0.05$ relative to untreated mice, ## $p < 0.05$ relative to LPS-treated mice. (b) Liver tissue sections obtained from LPS-treated mice that were inoculated by the intra-arterial route with 1.5×10^6 GFP-expressing H-59 cells (*green*) were stained with anti-neutrophil Ab and an Alexa 568 secondary Ab (*red*) and imaged using confocal microscopy. Images were acquired at ×400 magnification (*left scale bar* represents 25 μm, *right insert scale bar* represents 10 μm). Reproduced with permission from [84]

trigger recruitment of CXCR2-expressing inflammatory cells such as neutrophils that can pre-condition the microenvironment for successful tumor cell colonization. Inhibition of the CXCL1/CXCR2 axis may therefore have resulted in a decrease in metastatic burden by preventing the neutrophil-mediated establishment of the pre-metastatic niche.

Beyond the laboratory, several clinical findings also suggest a deleterious role for neutrophils in the early steps of metastasis. As mentioned earlier, elevated neutrophil to lymphocyte ratios have been associated with poor oncologic outcomes in cancer patients [63, 65, 66, 125]. Moreover, high levels of neutrophil chemotactic factors have also been linked to worse outcomes in cancer patients. Specifically, high levels of the cytokine IL-8, a potent neutrophil chemoattractant were shown to be associated with metastasis and disease progression [58, 61, 64, 126, 127]. Tumor cells can secrete IL-8 both locally and into the systemic circulation, thus attracting neutrophils to infiltrate primary tumors and metastatic foci. Furthermore, primary tumors may be producing factors such as TNF-α that can in turn, induce IL-8 expression in sites of metastasis such as the liver. In addition to neutrophils, IL-8 may further recruit endothelial cells and promote tumor angiogenesis [128]. Combined with the up-regulation of endothelial selectins and integrins, the expression of multiple neutrophil chemoattractants, including, but not limited to, IL-8 and CXCL1, could result in changes to the hepatic microenvironment that favor successful colonization by CTCs.

Activated neutrophils have the capacity to induce significant endothelial damage when they adhere and degranulate within microvessels [114, 129]. As discussed earlier, they release highly toxic reactive oxygen species, as well as matrix degrading enzymes such as matrix metalloproteinases (MMPs) and elastase. Thus, neutrophils co-localizing with adhering cancer cells may facilitate their transmigration and survival provided that the cancer cells can themselves resist the "harsh" environment created by neutrophils. A few studies have suggested that neutrophils may have a cytotoxic effect on cancer cells [130]. Nevertheless, the majority of in vitro and in vivo data suggest that the impact of neutrophils is mostly favorable to tumor cell dissemination and growth [84, 131].

Neutrophils are not the only circulating cells that participate in the inflammatory cascade. Platelets are important contributors and cooperate with neutrophils in the early phases of acute inflammation [132]. Both pharmacological and genetic depletion of platelets have been shown to reduce metastasis, while reinfusion of platelets in these models has restored the metastatic potential of cancer cells [133–135]. Platelets that become activated as a result of tumor-derived factors such as the tumor-associated tissue factor and subsequent thrombin production or inflammatory cues like LPS can release inflammatory mediators and cytokines from their α and dense granules. Moreover, platelets can bind both neutrophils (attached and circulating) [136] and tumor cells [137] via several receptor/ligand interactions including the P-selectin/P-selectin glycoprotein ligand 1 (PSGL-1) axis or integrin mediated binding. Thus, platelets may serve as a stabilizer of CTC adhesion by preventing immune destruction of circulating CTCs and by interacting with adhering neutrophils and CTCs along the sinusoidal endothelium.

6.4 Beyond Adhesion

The interactions between cancer cells and neutrophils or other myeloid cells can occur both directly or remotely. While our understanding of these interactions is still in its infancy, investigations are beginning to yield important information on these interactions. Recently, Kim et al. [138] found that Lewis lung carcinoma – conditioned media could induce significant IL-1β, IL-6 and TNF-α expression in bone marrow derived macrophages (BMDM). Multiple studies have also shown that tumor-educated macrophages are a key component of the tumor microenvironment in lung metastases and are required for lung metastases formation in experimental models [3]. Thus, when Lewis lung carcinoma cells were administered intravenously into TNF-α deficient mice, the occurrence of lung metastases was markedly reduced.

As discussed earlier, TNF-α production can result from the activation of a number of receptor signaling pathways. TLRs are important molecules for sensing the presence of infectious or potentially harmful substances and they signal for the production of numerous inflammatory cytokines. To determine whether they may be involved in sensing cues secreted by Lewis lung carcinoma cells, BMDMs from mice lacking different TLRs and intracellular mediators of TLR signaling (Myd88) were exposed to tumor-conditioned media and their cytokine expression then analyzed. TLR2 $^{-/-}$ BMDMs had the most marked reduction in cytokine expression relative to controls. When TLR2$^{-/-}$ mice were inoculated with Lewis lung carcinoma cells, they displayed greatly reduced numbers of lung, adrenal and liver metastases. These data strongly suggest that tumors are capable of inducing inflammatory reactions through receptors such as TLR2 and that the ensuing signal and downstream production of TNF-α are essential for the progression of metastases. In addition, this study also demonstrates the importance of inflammatory cells as part of the tumor microenvironment. This study supports the concept that infectious antigens such as LPS or the TLR2 bacterial antigen ligand lipotechoic acid (LTA) produced by gram positive bacteria could potentiate metastatic outgrowth by signaling via TLR4 or TLR2, respectively [139, 140].

While a systemic inflammatory response may promote the initial recruitment of cancer cells to the liver, persistence of these inflammatory signals in a more chronic fashion appears to be necessary for continued tumor growth. When tissue damage occurs, angiogenesis is required for the healing response to take place and this response is, in turn initiated by inflammatory cues. Likewise, neovascularization requires signals from inflammatory cells such as macrophages [141]. Similarly, proliferative cues are necessary for wound healing and inflammatory cells within wounds provide these signals, as well as trophic factors for proliferation of fibroblasts. These cues are delivered in the microenvironment of liver metastases by macrophages and HSC that promote the growth and proliferation of metastatic cancer cells [49, 142].

Although the details of these processes are beyond the scope of this chapter, they remain highly important avenues of research with significant promise for the development of anti-metastatic therapy (The reader is referred to Chapters 3, 5 and 7 in this volume, as well as excellent reviews in the literature [3, 143] for additional information). In addition, the inflammatory process is part of a spectrum of host reactivity that also includes acquired immune responses as mediated by dendritic cells, lymphocytes and natural killer cells. Several studies have documented the ability of the acquired immune system to attack and destroy implanted liver metastases [144–146]. The potential benefits of commandeering these mercenary cells of the acquired immune system in the fight against liver metastases are the subject of numerous previous and ongoing studies that have promising clinical implications [144, 146–156].

6.5 Conclusion

The metastatic cascade is a complex, highly orchestrated process. The liver is a frequent site of metastatic growth and this is largely due to its microvascular structure and the cells that compose it. The liver can produce a powerful inflammatory reaction in response to both systemic cues resulting from infectious or traumatic insults or tumor-derived signals. The interactions of the primary tumor and circulating tumor cells with the components of the inflammatory cascade are essential for the development of metastases within the liver (summarized in Fig. 6.6). Cytokines such as TNF-α or IL-1 produced due to infectious complications, surgical treatments or tumor complications such as a perforated colon carcinoma could potentially contribute to the establishment of a metastatic niche in the liver. They do so by rendering the sinusoidal endothelium highly adherent and suitable to the arrest of circulating tumor cells. Cytokines also prepare the niche by attracting neutrophils and platelets to putative metastatic sites within the liver and this can contribute to recruitment of cancer cells to the liver. In parallel, tumor cells within the primary and metastatic sites can further exacerbate the inflammatory cascade through production of cytokines and other tumor-derived soluble factors such as chemokines. This alliance that is created between cancer and inflammatory cells during the metastatic cascade continues beyond implantation and actually acts as a fuel for angiogenesis and proliferation. In this context, macrophages are the primary effectors, only to be followed by the potentially cytotoxic natural killer cells or the activated T lymphocytes of the acquired immune response. Thus, the essential message is that liver metastasis cannot be understood without considering the critical role that inflammation plays in its progression. Hence, strategies aimed at reducing the burden of liver metastases for cancer patients will have to include therapies that also target this "unholy" alliance between inflammation and cancer cells.

References

1. Townsend CM, Beauchamp RD, Evers BM, Mattox KL (2008) Townsend: Sabiston textbook of surgery, 18th edn. Saunders Elsevier, Philadelphia, PA
2. Kumar V, Abbas A, Fausto N, Aster JC (2009) Robbins and Cotran pathologic basis of disease, 8th edn. Saunders Elsevier, Philidelphia, PA

3. Mantovani A, Allavena P, Sica A, Balkwill F (2008) Cancer related inflammation. Nature 454:436–444
4. Rizk NP et al (2004) The impact of complications on outcomes after resection for esophageal and gastroesophageal junction carcinoma. J Am Coll Surg 198:42–50
5. Murthy BL et al (2007) Postoperative wound complications and systemic recurrence in breast cancer. Br J Cancer 97:1211–1217
6. Laurent C et al (2003) Influence of postoperative morbidity on long-term survival following liver resection for colorectal metastases. Br J Surg 90:1131–1136
7. Lagarde SM et al (2008) Postoperative complications after esophagectomy for adenocarcinoma of the esophagus are related to timing of death due to recurrence. Ann Surg 247:71–76
8. Hirai T et al (1998) Poor prognosis in esophageal cancer patients with postoperative complications. Surg Today 28:576–579
9. Hirai T, Matsumoto H, Yamashita K, Urakami A, Iki K, Yamamura M, Tsunoda T (2005) Surgical oncotaxis – excessive surgical stress and postoperative complications contribute to enhanced metastasis, resulting in a poor prognosis for cancer patients. Ann Thorac Cardiovasc Surg 11:4–6
10. Fujita S et al (1993) Anastomotic leakage after colorectal cancer surgery: a risk factor for recurrence and poor prognosis. Jpn J Clin Oncol 23:299–302
11. Ferri LE et al (2006) The influence of technical complications on postoperative outcome and survival after esophagectomy. Ann Surg Oncol 13:557–564
12. de Melo GM et al (2001) Risk factors for postoperative complications in oral cancer and their prognostic implications. Arch Otolaryngol Head Neck Surg 127:828–833
13. Lacy AM, Delgado S, Castells A, Prins HA, Arroyo V, Ibarzabal A, Pique JM (2008) The long-term results of a randomized clinical trial of laparoscopy-assisted versus open surgery for colon cancer. Ann Surg 248:1–7
14. Mantovani A (2009) Cancer: inflaming metastasis. Nature 457:36–37
15. Coussens LM, Werb Z (2002) Inflammation and cancer. Nature 420:860–867
16. Oppenheimer SB (2006) Cellular basis of cancer metastasis: a review of fundamentals and new advances. Acta Histochemica 108:327–334
17. Dvorak HF (1986) Tumors: wounds that do not heal. Similarities between tumor stroma generation and wound healing. N Engl J Med 315:1650–1659
18. Adams DH, Eksteen B, Curbishley SM (2008) Immunology of the gut and liver: a love/hate relationship. Gut 57:838–848
19. Ramadori G, Moriconi F, Malik I, Dudas J (2008) Physiology and pathophysiology of liver inflammation, damage and repair. J Physiol Pharmacol 59:107–117
20. Afford SC and Lalor PF (2006) Cell and molecular mechanisms in the development of chronic liver inflammation. In: Ali S, Friedman SL, Mann DA (eds) Liver diseases biochemical mechanisms and new therapeutic insights, pp 147–163. Science Publishers, Enfield, NH
21. Miles FL, Pruitt FL, van Golen KL, Cooper CR (2007) Stepping out of the flow: capillary extravasation in cancer metastasis. Clin Exp Metast 25:305–324
22. Tonnensen MG, Anderson DC, Springer TA et al (1989) Adherence of neutrophils to cultured human microvascular endothelial cells. Stimulation by chemotactic peptides and lipid mediators and dependence upon Mac-1, LFA-1, p150,95 glycoprotein family. J Clin Invest 83:637–646
23. Fidler IJ (2003) The pathogenesis of cancer metastasis: the 'seed and soil' hypothesis revisited. Nat Rev Cancer 3:453–458
24. Chambers AF, Groom AC, MacDonald IC (2002) Dissemination and growth of cancer cells in metastatic sites. Nat Rev Cancer 2:563–572
25. Brunk DK, Goetz DJ, Hammer DA (1996) Sialyl Lewis(x)/E-selectin-mediated rolling in a cell-free system. Biophys J 71:2902–2907
26. Simon SI, Green CE (2005) Molecular mechanics and dynamics of leukocyte recruitment during inflammation. Annu Rev Biomed Eng 7:151–185

27. Sheikh N, Tron K., Dudas J, Ramadori G (2006) Cytokine-induced neutrophil chemoattractant-1 is released by the noninjured liver in a rat acute-phase model. Lab Invest 86:800–814

28. Sambasivam H, Rassouli M, Murray RK et al (1993) Studies on the carbohydrate moiety and on the biosynthesis of rat C-reactive protein. J Biol Chem 26:10007–10016

29. Ren X, Kennedy A, Colletti LM (2002) CXC chemokine expression after stimulation with interferon-gamma in primary rat hepatocytes in culture. Shock 17:513–520

30. Li X, Klintman D, Liu Q, Sato T, Jeppson B, Thorlacius H (2004) Critical role of CXC chemokines in endotoxemic liver injury in mice. J Leukoc Biol 75:443–452

31. Knittel T, Dinter C, Kobold D et al (1999) Expression and regulation of cell adhesion molecules by hepatic stellate cells (HSC) of rat liver: involvement of HSC in recruitment of inflammatory cells during hepatic tissue repair. Am J Pathol 154:153–167

32. Schwabe RF, Bataller R, Brenner DA (2003) Human hepatic stellate cells express CCR5 and RANTES to induce proliferation and migration. Am J Physiol 285:G949–G958

33. Maher JJ, Lozier JS, Scott MK (1998) Rat hepatic stellate cells produce cytokine-induced neutrophil chemoattractant in culture and in vivo. Am J Physiol 275:G847–G853

34. Antoine M et al (2009) Expression of E-selectin ligand-1 (CFR/ESL-1) on hepatic stellate cells: implications for leukocyte extravasation and liver metastasis. Oncol Rep 21: 357–362

35. Olaso E et al (2003) Proangiogenic role of tumor-activated hepatic stellate cells in experimental melanoma metastasis. Hepatology 37:674–685

36. Vanderkerten K, Bowens L, Van Rooijen N et al (1995) The role of Kupffer cells in the differentiation process of hepatic natural killer cells. Hepatology 22:283–290

37. Lee WY, Kubes P (2008) Leukocyte adhesion in the liver: distinct adhesion paradigm from other organs. J Hepatol 48:504–512

38. Ramadori G, Saile B (2004) Inflammation, damage and repari, immune cells and liver fibrosis: specific or non-specific, this is the question. Gastroenterology 127:997–1000

39. Mantovani A et al (1997) Endothelial activation by cytokines. Ann N Y Acad Sci 832:93

40. Akira S et al (2006) Pathogen recognition and innate immunity. Cell 124:783

41. Meylan E et al (2006) Intracellular patter recognition receptors in the host response. Nature 442:39

42. Huang B, Zhao J, Unkeless JC, Feng ZH, Xiong H (2008) TLR signaling by tumor and immune cells: a double-edged sword. Oncogene 27:218–224

43. Shishodia S, Aggarwal BB (2004) Nuclear factor-KB: a friend or a foe in cancer? Biochem Pharmacol 68:1071–1080

44. Li X, Jiang S, Tapping RI (2010) Toll-like receptor signaling in cell proliferation and survival. Cytokine 49:1–9

45. Chen R et al (2008) Cancers take their Toll–the function and regulation of Toll-like receptors in cancer cells. Oncogene 27:225–233

46. Chen K et al (2007) Toll-like receptors in inflammation, infection and cancer. Int Immunopharmacol 7:1271–1285

47. Tsan M-F (2005) Toll-like receptors, inflammation and cancer. Semin Cancer Biol 16: 32–37

48. Balkwill F (2002) Tumor necrosis factor or tumor promoting factor? Cytokine Growth Factor Rev 13:135–141

49. Aggarwal BB, Vijayalekshmi RV, Sung B (2009) Targeting inflammatory pathways for prevention and therapy of cancer: short-term friend, long-term foe. Clin Cancer Res 15:425–430

50. Wang X, Lin Y (2008) Tumor necrosis factor and cancer, buddies or foes? Acta Pharmacol Sin 29:1275–1288

51. Serhan CN, Savill J (2005) Resolution of inflammation: the beginning programs the end. Nat Immunol 6:1191–1197

52. Schwab JM et al (2007) Resolvin E1 and protectin D1 activate inflammation-resolution programmes. Nature 447:869–874
53. Tsushima H et al (2001) Circulating transforming growth factor beta 1 as a predictor of liver metastasis after resection in colorectal cancer. Clin Cancer Res 7:1258–1262
54. Vidal-Vanaclocha F (2008) The prometastatic microenvironment of the liver. Cancer Microenviron 1:113–129
55. Folkman J (1974) Tumor angiogenesis. Adv Cancer Res 19:331–358
56. Colotta F et al (2009) Cancer-related inflammation, the seventh hallmark of cancer: links to genetic instability. Carcinogenesis 30:1073–1081
57. Matzaraki V et al (2007) Evaluation of serum procalcitonin and interleukin-6 levels as markers of liver metastasis. Clin Biochem 40:336–342
58. Ueda T, Shimada E, Urakawa T (1994) Serum levels of cytokines in patients with colorectal cancer: possible involvement of interleukin-6 and interleukin-8 in hematogenous metastasis. J Gastroenterol 29:423–429
59. Furuya Y, Ichikura T, Mochizuki H (1999) Interleukin-1alpha concentration in tumors as a risk factor for liver metastasis in gastric cancer. Surg Today 29:288–289
60. Salgado R et al (2003) Circulating interleukin-6 predicts survival in patients with metastatic breast cancer. Int J Cancer 103:642–646
61. Kaminska J, Kowalska M, Nowacki MP, Chwalinski MG, Ryinska A, Fuksiewicz M (2000) CRP, TNF1, IL-1ra, IL-6, IL-8 and IL-10 in blood serum of colorectal cancer patients. Pathol Oncol Res 6:38–41
62. Walsh SR, Cook EJ, Goulder F, Justin TA, Keeling NJ (2005) Neutrophil-lymphocyte ratio as a prognostic factor in colorectal cancer. J Surg Oncol 91:181–184
63. Halazun KJ et al (2008) Elevated preoperative neutrophil to lymphocyte ratio predicts survival following hepatic resection for colorectal liver metastases. Eur J Surg Oncol 34:55–60
64. Kaminska J et al (2005) Clinical significance of serum cytokine measurements in untreated colorectal cancer patients: soluble tumor necrosis factor receptor type I – an independent prognostic factor. Tumor Biol 26:186–194
65. Gomez D et al (2008) Surgical technique and systemic inflammation influences long-term disease-free survival following hepatic resection for colorectal metastasis. J Surg Oncol 98:371–376
66. Neal CP et al (2009) Evaluation of the prognostic value of systemic inflammation and socioeconomic deprivation in patients with resectable colorectal liver metastases. Eur J Cancer 45:56–64
67. Helson L et al (1975) Effect of tumour necrosis factor on cultured human melanoma cells. Nature 258:731–732
68. Carswell EA et al (1975) An endotoxin-induced serum factor that causes necrosis of tumors. Proc Natl Acad Sci USA 72:3666–3670
69. Curnis F, Sacchi A, Corti A (2002) Improving chemotherapeutic drug penetration in tumors by vascular targeting and barrier alteration. J Clin Invest 110:475–482
70. Lejeune FJ (2002) Clinical use of TNF revisited: improving penetration of anti-cancer agents by increasing vascular permeability. J Clin Invest 110:433–435
71. Faustman D, Davis M (2010) TNF receptor 2 pathway: drug target for autoimmune diseases. Nat Rev Drug Discov 9:482–493
72. Ha H, Han D, Choi Y (2009) TRAF-mediated TNFR-family signaling. Curr Protoc Immunol Chapter 11:Unit11 9D
73. Aggarwal BB et al (2006) TNF blockade: an inflammatory issue. Ernst Schering Res Found Workshop, 161–186
74. Balkwill F (2006) TNF-alpha in promotion and progression of cancer. Cancer Metastasis Rev 25:409–416
75. Egberts JH et al (2008) Anti-tumor necrosis factor therapy inhibits pancreatic tumor growth and metastasis. Cancer Res 68:1443–1450

76. Egberts JH et al (2008) Dexamethasone reduces tumor recurrence and metastasis after pancreatic tumor resection in SCID mice. Cancer Biol Ther 7:1044–1050

77. Harmey JH, Bucana C.D., Lu W, Byrne AM, McDonnell S, Lynch C, Bouchier-Hayes D, Dong Z (2002) Lipopolysaccharide-induced metastatic growth is associated with increased angiognensis, vascular permeability and tumor cell invasion. Int J Cancer 101:415–422

78. Pidgeon GP, Harmey JH, Kay E, Da Costa M, Redmond HP, Bouchier-Hayes DJ (1999) The role of endotoxin/lipopolysaccharide in surgically induced tumor growth in a murine model of metastatic disease. Br J Cancer 81:1311

79. Riethdorf S, Wikman H, Pantel K (2008) Review: biological relevance of disseminated tumor cells in cancer patients. Int J Cancer 123:1991–2006

80. Sawabata MD, Okumura M, Utsumi T, Inoue M, Shiono H, Minami M, Nishida T, Sawa Y (2007) Circulating tumor cells in peripheral blood caused by surgical manipulation of non-small-cell lung cancer: pilot study using an immunocytology method. Gen ThoracCardiovasc Surg 55:189–192

81. Sher W, Jin-Yuan S, Yang P, Roffler SR, Chu Y, Wu C, Yu C, Peck K (2005) Prognosis of non-small cell lung cancer patients by detecting circulating cancer cells in the peripheral blood with multiple marker genes. Clin Cancer Res 11:173–179

82. Liu A, Ming J, Zhao J, Huangxian J (2007) Circulating tumor cells in perioperative esophageal cancer patients: quantitative assay system and potential clinical utility. Clin Cancer Res 13:2992–2997

83. Dong Q, Huang J, Zhou Y, Li L, Guoliang B, Feng J, Sha H (2002) Hematogenous dissemination of lung cancer cells during surgery: quantitative detection by flow cytometry and prognostic significance. Lung Cancer 37:293–301

84. McDonald B et al (2009) Systemic inflammation increases cancer cell adhesion to hepatic sinusoids by neutrophil mediated mechanisms. Int J Cancer 125:1298–1305

85. Kaplan RN, Rafii S, Lyden D (2006) Preparing the "soil": the premetastatic niche. Cancer Res 66:11089–11093

86. Kaplan RN et al (2005) VEGFR1-positive haematopoietic bone marrow progenitors initiate the pre-metastatic niche. Nature 438:820–827

87. Boo YJ, Kim WB, Kim J, Song TJ, Choi SY, Kim YC, Suh SO (2007) Systemic immune response after open versus laparoscopic cholecystectomy in acute cholecystitis: a prospective randomized study. Scand J Clin Lab Invest 67:207–214

88. Shiromizu A, Suematsu T, Yamaguchi K, Shiraishi N, Adachi Y, Kitano S (2000) Effect of laparotomy and laparoscopy on the establishment of lung metastasis in a murine model. Surgery 128:799–805

89. Bell SW et al (2003) Anastomotic leakage after curative anterior resection results in a higher prevalence of local recurrence. Br J Surg 90:1261–1266

90. Witz IP (2008) The selectin-selectin ligand axis in tumor progression. Cancer Metast Rev 27:19–30

91. Bresalier RS et al (1998) Liver metastasis and adhesion to the sinusoidal endothelium by human colon cancer cells is related to mucin carbohydrate chain length. Int J Cancer 76:556–562

92. Brodt P et al (1997) Liver endothelial E-selectin mediates carcinoma cell adhesion and promotes liver metastasis. Int J Cancer 71:612–619

93. Sperti C et al (1993) CA 19-9 as a prognostic index after resection for pancreatic cancer. J Surg Oncol 52:137–141

94. Satoh H et al (1998) Elevated serum sialyl Lewis X-i antigen levels in non-small cell lung cancer with lung metastasis. Respiration 65:295–298

95. Duraker N, Celik AN (2001) The prognostic significance of preoperative serum CA 19-9 in patients with resectable gastric carcinoma: comparison with CEA. J Surg Oncol 76:266–271

96. Nakagoe T et al (2002) Difference in prognostic value between sialyl Lewis(a) and sialyl Lewis(x) antigen levels in the preoperative serum of gastric cancer patients. J Clin Gastroenterol 34:408–415

97. Yu CJ et al (2005) Sialyl Lewis antigens: association with MUC5AC protein and correlation with post-operative recurrence of non-small cell lung cancer. Lung Cancer 47:59–67

98. Lee IK et al (2009) Prognostic value of CEA and CA 19-9 tumor markers combined with cytology from peritoneal fluid in colorectal cancer. Ann Surg Oncol 16:861–870

99. Park IJ, Choi GS, Jun SH (2009) Prognostic value of serum tumor antigen CA19-9 after curative resection of colorectal cancer. Anticancer Res 29:4303–4308

100. Wang WS et al (2002) CA19-9 as the most significant prognostic indicator of metastatic colorectal cancer. Hepato-Gastroenterol 49:160–164

101. Nakagoe T et al (2001) Circulating sialyl Lewis(x), sialyl Lewis(a), and sialyl Tn antigens in colorectal cancer patients: multivariate analysis of predictive factors for serum antigen levels. J Gastroenterol 36:166–172

102. Khatib AM et al (1999) Rapid induction of cytokine and E-selectin expression in the liver in response to metastatic tumor cells. Cancer Res 59:1356–1361

103. Auguste P et al (2007) The host inflammatory response promotes liver metastasis by increasing tumor cell arrest and extravasation. Am J Pathol 170:1781–1792

104. Kim YJ, Borsig L, Varki NM, Varki A (1998) P-selectin deficiency attenuates tumor growth and metastasis. Proc Natl Acad Sci USA 95:9325–9330

105. Khatib AM et al (2002) Inhibition of hepatic endothelial E-selectin expression by C-raf antisense oligonucleotides blocks colorectal carcinoma liver metastasis. Cancer Res 62:5393–5398

106. Boudier C, Cadene M, Bieth JG (1999) Inhibition of neutrophil cathepsin G by oxidized mucus proteinase inhibitor. Effects of heparin. Biochemistry 38:451–457

107. McNeely TB, Dealy M, Dripps DJ, Orenstein JM, Eisenberg SP, Wahl SM (1995) Secretory leukocyte protease inhibitor: a human saliva protein exhibiting anti-human immunodeficiency virus 1 activity in vitro. J Clin Invest 96:456–464

108. Hiemstra PS, Maassen RJ, Sotlk J, Heinzel-Wieland R, Steffens GJ, Dijkman JH (1996) Antibacterial activity of antileukoprotease. Infect Immun 64:4520–4524

109. Zhang Y, DeWitt DL, McNeely TB, Wahl SM, Wahl LM (1997) Secretory leukocyte protease inhibitor suppresses the production of monocyte prostaglandin H synthase-2 prostaglandin E2, and matrix metalloproteinases. J Clin Invest 99:894–900

110. Jin F, Nathan CF, Radzioch D, Ding A (1998) Lipopolysaccharide-related stimuli induce expression of the secretory leukocyte protease inhibitor, a macrophage-derived lipopolysaccharide inhibitor. Infect Immun 66:2447–2452

111. Jin FY, Nathan C, Radzioch D, Dinag A (1997) Secretory leukocyte protease inhibitor: a macrophage product induced by and antagonistic to bacterial lipopolysaccharide. Cell 88:417–426

112. Wang N et al (2006) The secretory leukocyte protease inhibitor is a type 1 insulin-like growth factor receptor-regulated protein that protects against liver metastasis by attenuating the host proinflammatory response. Cancer Res 66:3062–3070

113. Fox-Robichaud A, Kubes P (2000) Molecular mechanisms of tumor necrosis factor alpha-stimulated leukocyte recruitment into the murine hepatic circulation. Hepatology 31:1123–1127

114. Clark SR et al (2007) Platelet TLR4 activates neutrophil extracellular traps to ensnare bacteria in septic blood.[see comment]. Nature Med 13:463–469

115. Chambers AF, MacDonald IC, Schmidt EE, Morris VL, Groom AC (2000) Clinical targets for anti-metastasis therapy. Adv Cancer Res 79:91–121

116. Kruskal JB et al (2007) Hepatic colorectal cancer metastases: imaging initial steps of formation in mice. Radiology 243:703–711

117. Liang S et al (2008) Hydrodynamic shear rate regulates melanoma-leukocyte aggregation, melanoma adhesion to the endothelium, and subsequent extravasation. Ann Biomed Eng 36:661–671

118. Slattery MJ, Dong C (2003) Neutrophils influence melanoma adhesion and migration under flow conditions. Int J Cancer 106:713–722

119. Slattery MJ, Liang S, Dong C (2005) Distinct role of hydrodynamic shear in leukocyte-facilitated tumor cell extravasation. Am J Physiol Cell Physiol 288:C831–839
120. Liang S, Slattery MJ, Dong C (2005) Shear stress and shear rate differentially affect the multi-step process of leukocyte-facilitated melanoma adhesion. Exp Cell Res 310: 282–292
121. Dong C et al (2005) Melanoma cell extravasation under flow conditions is modulated by leukocytes and endogenously produced interleukin 8. Mol Cell Biomech 2:145–159
122. Orr FW, Warner DJ (1987) Effects of neutrophil-mediated pulmonary endothelial injury on the localization and metastasis of circulating Walker carcinosarcoma cells. Inv Metast 7:183–196
123. Läubli H, Stevenson JL, Varki A, Varki NM, Borsig L (2006) L-selectin facilitation of metastasis involves temporal induction of Fut7-dependent ligands at sites of tumor cell arrest. Cancer Res 66:1536–1542
124. Yamamoto M et al (2008) TSU68 prevents liver metastasis of colon cancer xenografts by modulating the premetastatic niche. Cancer Res 68:9754–9762
125. Kishi Y et al (2009) Blood neutrophil-to-lymphocyte ratio predicts survival in patients with colorectal liver metastases treated with systemic chemotherapy. Ann Surg Oncol 16: 614–622
126. Terada H, Urano T, Konno H (2005) Association of interleukin-8 and plasminogen activator system in the progression of colorectal cancer. Eur Surg Res 37:166–172
127. De Larco JE, Wuertz BR, Furcht LT (2004) The potential role of neutrophils in promoting the metastatic phenotype of tumors releasing interleukin-8. Clin Cancer Res 10:4895–4900
128. Waugh DJ, Wilson C (2008) The interleukin-8 pathway in cancer. Clin Cancer Res 14: 6735–6741
129. Flierl MA et al (2009) Upregulation of phagocyte-derived catecholamines augments the acute inflammatory response. PLoS One 4:e4414
130. Di Carlo E et al (2001) The intriguing role of polymorphonuclear neutrophils in antitumor reactions. Blood 97:339–345
131. Konstantopoulos K, Thomas SN (2009) Cancer cells in transit: the vascular interactions of tumor cells. Annu Rev Biomed Eng 11:177–202
132. Weyrich AS, Zimmerman GA (2004) Platelets: signaling cells in the immune continuum. Trends Immunol 25:489–495
133. Gasic GJ, Gasic TB, Stewart CC (1968) Antimetastatic effects associated with platelet reduction. Proc Natl Acad Sci U S A 61:46–52
134. Camerer E et al (2004) Platelets, protease-activated receptors, and fibrinogen in hematogenous metastasis. Blood 104:397–401
135. Karpatkin S et al (1988) Role of adhesive proteins in platelet tumor interaction in vitro and metastasis formation in vivo. J Clin Invest 81:1012–1019
136. Ma AC, Kubes P (2008) Platelets, neutrophils, and neutrophil extracellular traps (NETs) in sepsis. J Thromb Haemost 6:415–420
137. Palumbo JS et al (2005) Platelets and fibrin(ogen) increase metastatic potential by impeding natural killer cell-mediated elimination of tumor cells. Blood 105:178–185
138. Kim S et al (2009) Carcinoma-produced factors activate myeloid cells through TLR2 to stimulate metastasis. Nature 457:102–106
139. Fitzgerald KA et al (2001) Mal (MyD88-adapter-like) is required for Toll-like receptor-4 signal transduction. Nature 413:78–83
140. Yang RB et al (1998) Toll-like receptor-2 mediates lipopolysaccharide-induced cellular signalling. Nature 395:284–288
141. Zumsteg A, Christofori G (2009) Corrupt policemen: inflammatory cells promote tumor angiogenesis. Curr Opin Oncol 21:60–70
142. Favaro E, Amadori A, Indraccolo S (2008) Cellular interactions in the vascular niche: implications in the regulation of tumor dormancy. APMIS 116:648–659

143. DeNardo DG, Johansson M, Coussens LM (2008) Immune cells as mediators of solid tumor metastasis. Cancer Metastasis Rev 27:11–18
144. Zabala M et al (2004) Optimization of the Tet-on system to regulate interleukin 12 expression in the liver for the treatment of hepatic tumors. Cancer Res 64:2799–2804
145. Pulaski BA, Smyth MJ, Ostrand-Rosenberg S (2002) Interferon-gamma-dependent phagocytic cells are a critical component of innate immunity against metastatic mammary carcinoma. Cancer Res 62:4406–4412
146. Tanji H et al (2002) Augmentation of local antitumor immunity in liver by interleukin-2 gene transfer via portal vein.[see comment]. Cancer Gene Ther 9:655–664
147. Demchak PA et al (1991) Interleukin-2 and high-dose cisplatin in patients with metastatic melanoma: a pilot study. J Clin Oncol 9:1821–1830
148. Chen SH et al (1995) Combination gene therapy for liver metastasis of colon carcinoma in vivo. Proc Natl Acad Sci USA 92:2577–2581
149. Okada K et al (1996) Elimination of established liver metastases by human interleukin 2-activated natural killer cells after locoregional or systemic adoptive transfer. Cancer Res 56:1599–1608
150. Hagenaars M et al (1998) Regional administration of natural killer cells in a rat hepatic metastasis model results in better tumor infiltration and anti-tumor response than systemic administration. Int J Cancer 75:233–238
151. Peron JM et al (1998) FLT3-ligand administration inhibits liver metastases: role of NK cells. J Immunol 161:6164–6170
152. Fuji N et al (1999) Augmentation of local antitumor immunity in the liver by tumor vaccine modified to secrete murine interleukin 12. Gene Ther 6:1120–1127
153. Iwazawa T et al (2001) Potent antitumor effects of intra-arterial injection of fibroblasts genetically engineered to express IL-12 in liver metastasis model of rat: no additional benefit of using retroviral producer cell. Cancer Gene Ther 8:17–22
154. Satoh Y et al (2002) Local administration of IL-12-transfected dendritic cells induces antitumor immune responses to colon adenocarcinoma in the liver in mice. J Exp Ther Oncol 2:337–349
155. Agarwala SS et al (2004) Immunotherapy with histamine and interleukin 2 in malignant melanoma with liver metastasis. Cancer Immunol Immunother 53:840–841
156. Kawaoka T et al (2008) Adoptive immunotherapy for pancreatic cancer: cytotoxic T lymphocytes stimulated by the MUC1-expressing human pancreatic cancer cell line YPK-1. Oncol Rep 20:155–163

Chapter 7
Signal Transduction in Tumor-Endothelial Cell Communication

Nicolas Porquet and Jacques Huot

Abstract Metastatic spread is a dreadful complication of neoplastic diseases that is responsible for most deaths due to cancer. It consists of the formation of secondary neoplasms from cancer cells that have detached from the primary site. The formation of these secondary foci is not random and several clinical observations indicate that the metastatic colonization exhibits organ selectivity. This organ tropism relies in part, on the complementary adhesive interactions between the cancer cells and their microenvironment. In particular, several lines of evidence suggest that the organ selectivity of colon cancer cells for the liver involves the attachment of circulating cancer cells to endothelial cell adhesion receptors. The aim of this review is to provide an integrative up-to-date review of the literature on the role of the endothelial-cancer cell interactions in liver colonization by metastatic cells.

Keywords Extravasation · Homing · Adhesion receptors · Liver colonization · Colorectal cancer · Metastasis

Abbreviations

APC	adenomatous polyposis coli
BM	basement membrane
CAMs	cell adhesion molecules
Cbl	Casitas B-lineage Lymphoma
CD44	cluster of differentiation 44
CEA	carcinoembryonic antigen
c-IAP2	cellular inhibitor of apoptosis 2
CRC	colorectal cancer
CRP	C-reactive protein

J. Huot (✉)
Le Centre de recherche en cancérologie de l'Université Laval et le Centre de recherche du CHUQ,
L'Hôtel-Dieu de Québec 9 rue McMahon, Québec, QC G1R 2J6, Canada
e-mail: Jacques.Huot@phc.ulaval.ca

P. Brodt (ed.), *Liver Metastasis: Biology and Clinical Management*, Cancer
Metastasis – Biology and Treatment 16, DOI 10.1007/978-94-007-0292-9_7,
© Springer Science+Business Media B.V. 2011

CXCR4	chemokine C-X-C motif receptor 4
DR3	death receptor-3
ECM	extracellular matrix
EGF	epidermal growth factor
EMT	epithelial mesenchymal transition
ERK	extracellular-signal regulated kinase
ESL-1	E-selectin ligand 1
FAK	focal adhesion kinase
FGF	fibroblast growth factor
FIP200	FAK-interacting protein 200
FOXC2	forkhead box C2
HUVEC	human umbilical vein endothelial cells
HMGB1	high-mobility group box 1
CAM-1	intercellular adhesion molecule-1
IgSFCAMs	the immunoglobulin superfamily of cell adhesion molecules
IL-3	interleukin-3
IMD	integrin-mediated death
IFN γ	interferon γ
ITAM	immunoreceptor tyrosine-based activation motif
ITIM	immunoreceptor tyrosine inhibitory motif
LAMP-1	lysosomal-associated membrane protein 1
LPS	lipopolysaccharides
NK cells	natural killer cells
PDGFR	platelet-derived growth factor receptor
PECAM-1	platelet endothelial cell adhesion molecule-1
PI3K	phosphatidyl inositol 3 kinase
p38 MAPK	p38 mitogen-activated protein kinase
RGD	arginine-Glycine-Aspartate
SECs	sinusoidal endothelial cells
SH2	Src Homology 2
TGFα	transforming growth factor alpha
TNF-α	tumor necrosis factor alpha
TNFR1	tumor necrosis factor receptor 1
VCAM	vascular cell adhesion molecule

Contents

7.1 Introduction

All portal area drainage flows to the liver, which explains why this organ is frequently involved as a site of haematogenous dissemination of cancer cells. Notably, the liver is the preferential homing organ for several types of metastatic cancer including colorectal cancer and uveal melanoma [1]. The metastatic colonization of the liver is characterized by four interrelated phases: (1) the microvascular phase of liver-invading cancer cells, comprising mechanisms of intravascular arrest, death and survival of cancer cells within the inflammatory micro-environment of tumour-activated sinusoidal cells; (2) the intralobular micrometastatic phase, comprising initiation of cancer cell growth and stromal cell recruitment; (3) the angiogenic/micrometastatic phase, including endothelial cell recruitment and blood vessel formation; and (4) the established hepatic metastasis phase [2]. In this chapter, we will review the mechanisms associated with the first phase of liver invasion by metastatic cancer cells. In particular, we will describe the adhesive interactions and the signaling mechanisms that are responsible for the arrest and extravasation of colon cancer cells as they colonize the liver. These interactions are associated with a forward and reverse signaling in endothelial cells and cancer cells, respectively, that culminate in diapedesis of the cancer cells across the endothelium [3, 4].

The cell-cell interactions associated with invasion and metastasis depend on several classes of cell adhesion molecules (CAMs) expressed at the surface of cancer cells and endothelial cells. They include: integrins, cadherins, members of the immunoglobulin superfamily of receptors, selectins and their respective ligands. CAMs are transmembrane receptors composed of three domains: an extracellular domain that interacts with the extracellular matrix (ECM) or with CAMs of the same (homotypic binding) or other (heterotypic binding) families of adhesion molecules present on the adhering cells, a transmembrane domain and an intracellular domain that interacts with specific cytoplasmic proteins. We will first briefly review the cell biology of these adhesion molecules and thereafter discuss their role in hepatic colonization by metastatic cancer cells.

7.2 The Integrins

7.2.1 Structure and Cell Biology of Integrins

Integrins are expressed on the surface of both normal and tumor cells. They are heterodimeric transmembrane glycoproteins consisting of non-covalently associated α and β subunits. Eight β subunits associate with one or more of 19 α subunits to form at least 25 distinct pairs of functional integrins. Both the α and β subunits have a large extracellular globular domain that contains the binding site, a single membrane-spanning region, and a short non-catalytic cytoplasmic tail that links the integrin to the actin cytoskeleton [5] (Fig. 7.1a, b). The integrins bind to small peptidic sequences such as Arginine-Glycine-Aspartate (RGD) contained within unique or shared sets of ECM ligands, including fibronectin, laminin and collagens [6]. The integrins are also involved in cell-cell interactions by binding to Ig-CAM, cadherins or oher integrins on the cell surface [5].

A

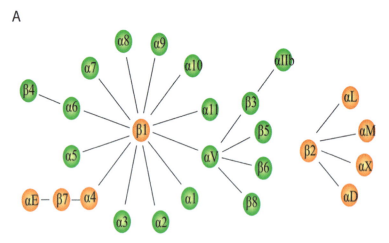

Fig. 7.1 The integrins. Shown in (**a**) are the known members of the integrin family. Integrins are expressed at the surface of both normal and tumor cells. They are heterodimeric transmembrane glycoproteins consisting of non-covalently associated α and β subunits. Eight β subunits associate with 19 α subunits to form at least 25 distinct pairs of functional integrins. The integrins bind to proteins of the extracellular matrix including collagens, vitronectin and fibronectin. They also serve as the entry port for several viruses and bacteria. Depicted in (**b**) are molecular interactions and signaling pathways mediated by integrins. Both the α and β subunits have a large extracellular globular domain that contains the binding site, a single membrane-spanning region and a short non-catalytic cytoplasmic tail. Both integrin subunits are involved in binding which requires a coordinated reaction with divalent ions. The integrins connect the extracellular matrix to the actin cytoskeleton mostly via the β subunit. The integrins are involved in a bi-directional outside-in and inside-out signaling. The outside-in signaling is initiated following their binding to ECM. It results in actin remodeling and governs functions such as cell adhesion, migration and survival. The inside-out signaling is initiated from inside the cells and is associated with actin remodeling. It regulates the affinity of the integrins for their ligands (adapted from [126])

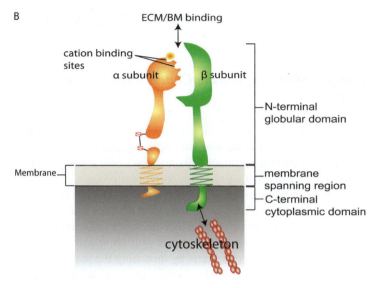

Fig. 7.1 (continued)

Integrins are bi-directional signaling receptors involved in outside-in and inside-out signaling. The inside-out signaling results from cytoskeletal remodelling that changes the integrin into its active conformation. In contrast, outside-in signaling refers to signals generated following the binding of integrins to their ligands. Integrin-dependent signaling events are complex and cell-specific, depending on which other signaling receptors and signaling systems are available in the cell. A major function of the integrins is to regulate cell migration. In this context, the integrins are implicated in two mechanisms by which cells alter their adhesive profiles to acquire a more migratory and invasive phenotype. First, tumor cells are characterized by important alterations in the expression profile and levels of integrins [7, 8]. For example, the expression of α6β4 is increased in thyroid carcinomas and papillomas whereas the expression of the α2 subunit is enhanced in liver-metastasing sub-line of B16 melanoma cells [9]. In contrast, the expression of α5β1 decreases during tumourigenesis [10]. Second, tumor cells may acquire a more invasive and migratory phenotype by modifying their affinity for ECM. For instance, the affinity of the integrin αvβ3 for its ligand is altered in a number of cancer cells. In particular, up-regulation of αvβ3 affinity was shown to increase cell adhesion and spreading, which is consistent with the fact that $\alpha_V\beta_3$ is subject to rapid, regulated changes in affinity that influence its biological functions [11]. Interestingly, the mechanical pressure imposed on the cancer cells is a major factor modulating integrin affinity and subsequently their binding to ligands and counter-receptors. In particular, it has been proposed that pressure-sensing involves cytoskeletal mechanosensors that regulate the association of β1-integrin heterodimers with focal adhesion kinase (FAK), a major mediator of integrin signaling, at the cell membrane. In turn, this modulates integrin binding affinity. This integrin-mediated signaling pathway represents a promising target for manipulations aimed at inhibiting metastatic cancer cell adhesion [12].

7.2.2 Integrin Signaling During Cancer Progression and Invasion

Integrins initiate outside-in and inside-out mechanical and chemical signals that regulate different processes associated with primary tumor growth and metastasis. After intravasation, circulating tumor cells associate with platelets and leukocytes to form small tumor emboli. This aggregation process protects cancer cells against shear stress and helps them remain in the circulation and adhere in the target organ. Selectins and integrins contribute to the formation of these microemboli [13]. For instance, integrin $\alpha_v\beta_3$ is often expressed by both tumor cells and platelets and can contribute to the co-aggregation of these cells with fibrin and fibrinogen. In turn, fibrin and fibrinogen facilitate metastasis by mediating the sustained adhesion and survival of tumor cells in the high shear environment of the circulation in target organs [14].

In addition to promoting the interaction between platelets, leukocytes and circulating cancer cells, integrins are also directly involved in the induction of survival pathways that protect tumor cell from apoptosis. Along these lines, malignant cells acquire a resistance to anoikis, a form of cell death that is characteristically associated with the loss of ECM adhesion in normal cells [15]. This resistance that results from-integrin-mediated activation of survival pathways is critical to metastasis-associated invasion [6]. Notably, any of the anti-apoptotic pathways activated downstream of integrins are also involved in regulating migration. For instance, ligation of integrins $\alpha5\beta1$ or $\alpha v\beta3$ under serum-free conditions leads to SHC (Src homology 2 domain-containing) transforming protein-1, phosphatidylinositol 3 kinase (PI3K)- and FAK-mediated survival and migration of CHO cells [6]. Moreover, FAK activation downstream of integrin may regulate tumor cell survival via different mechanisms. In particular, it is possible that the $\alpha2$ subunit can potentially limit p53-mediated apoptosis via a direct interaction between the FERM domain of FAK and the trans-activation region of p53 in the nucleus, thereby limiting p53 transcriptional activity. It is also possible that the association between FAK and the FAK-interacting protein 200 (FIP200) inhibits p53 functions. Moreover, the expression of the anti-apoptotic protein Bcl2 may be increased by integrin signaling. Along these lines, the inhibition of individual integrins is sufficient to induce apoptosis and block invasive events. For instance, the $\alpha_v\beta_3/\alpha_v\beta_5$ integrin antagonist S247 was shown to induce apoptosis and block angiogenesis and liver invasion by colon cancer cells [16]. This finding in is line with the fact that a form of apoptosis termed "integrin-mediated death" (IMD) is activated when adherent cells express specific integrin complexes in a microenvironment that lacks the corresponding activating ligand [6]. For example, expression of $\alpha_v\beta_3$ on cells that lack an $\alpha_v\beta_3$ ligand leads to the recruitment of caspase-8 to the membranes, and thereby to caspase-8 activation and cell death [6]. Overall, these findings indicate that integrins by regulating the survival/apoptosis balance are major regulators of metastasis.

Certain integrins also enable tumor cells to adhere to the vascular endothelium of the target organ and initiate signals allowing them to traverse the vessel wall to reach the interstitial matrix and form metastases. In this context, we have demonstrated that the adhesion of human colon carcinoma HT29 cells to activated endothelial cells follows at least two essential sequential steps involving the binding of E-selectin to its receptor on carcinoma cells and then the binding of $\beta 4$ integrin to its counter-receptor on endothelial cells [17]. Interestingly, the phosphorylation of integrin $\beta 4$ is important to this process because it contributes to enhancing the motile potential of the cancer cells and thereby increases their transendothelial migration. Other integrins also play a role in trans-endothelial migration. For example, another study has provided evidence that $\alpha_v\beta_3$ binds to the endothelial cell adhesion molecule L1, and that this adhesive interaction promotes migration of melanoma cells across the endothelium [13].

7.3 The Cadherins

7.3.1 Structure and Cell Biology of Cadherins

Cadherins are single pass transmembrane glycoproteins that constitute a family of more than 100 molecules among them classical and non-classical cadherins [18]. The classical cadherins that include epithelial (E), neuronal (N) and vascular endothelial (VE) cadherins are the main mediators of calcium-dependent, homotypic cell–cell adhesion whereas non-classical cadherins that include desmosomal cadherins and a large subfamily of protocadherins have been implicated in neuronal plasticity and other developmental processes. The extracellular domain of a classical cadherin consists of five cadherin monomers linked by calcium ions. Their binding domains, located at the N-terminus serve as dimerization site with other cadherins from the same cell (*cis*-dimerization) or from other cells (*trans*-dimerization) [19, 20]. A hydrophobic sequence anchors the cadherin to the cell membrane while a well-conserved cytoplasmic domain interacts with cytoskeletal elements via catenins. The association of classical cadherins with β-catenin and p120 catenin is important in the regulation of gene expression and cell migration in cancer cells [20, 21] (Fig. 7.2). The classical cadherins are important for the dynamic regulation of adhesive contacts associated with morphogenesis. In embryonic development, cadherins control the separation of distinct tissue layers or the fusion of tissues, the formation of tissue boundaries, changes in tissue ultrastructure, the long-range migration of cells and neuronal processes, the formation of synapses between neurons and the transition between histological cell states such the as epithelial-mesenchymal transition (EMT), a process that is key to neoplastic transformation and progression [20]. In this context, EMT is characterized by a switch between E-cadherin and N-cadherin expression [22, 23].

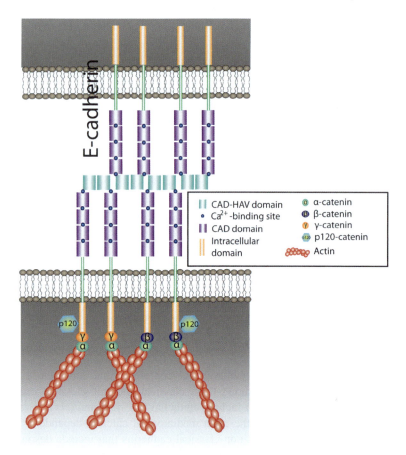

Fig. 7.2 The cadherin/catenin axis. Cadherins are single pass transmembrane glycoproteins that constitute a family of more than a hundred molecules of approximately 120 kDa consisting of classical and non-classical cadherins. The extracellular domain of a classical cadherin such as E-cadherin (epithelial cadherin) consists of five cadherin monomers (CAD) linked by calcium ions. Their binding domains located at the N-terminus serve as a dimerization site with other cadherins from the same cell (*cis*-dimerization) or from other cells (*trans*-dimerization). A hydrophobic sequence anchors the cadherin to the cell membrane while a well-conserved cytoplasmic domain interacts with cytoskeletal elements via catenins. The association of classical cadherins with β-catenin and p120 catenin plays an important role in regulating the expression of cancer-associated genes and cell migration (Adapted from [24])

7.3.2 Cadherin Signaling During Cancer Progression and Invasion

Loss of E-cadherins is a prerequisite for invasion and metastasis of several types of carcinomas [24]. This latter event results from mutations in the E-cadherin gene, proteolytic degradation of E-cadherin, IGF-1-mediated internalization of E-cadherin and disruption of the function of E-cadherin involving changes in its association with β-catenin [24]. Loss of E-cadherin can also result from promoter hypermethylation or the activation of transcriptional repressors such as Snail and FOXC2 [23, 25]. Interestingly, in melanoma, breast cancer and prostate cancer, the disruption of the E-cadherin-mediated cancer cell adhesion is associated with the so-called cadherin-switch in which the E-cadherin loss is accompanied by de novo expression of a mesenchymal cadherin, such as N-cadherin. This shift is important because the loss of E-cadherin is associated with loss of tumor cell adhesion to other tumor cells or to normal epithelial cells. Moreover, up-regulation of N-cadherin expression promotes cancer cells interaction with stromal cells, and favours the invasion of the surrounding stroma. In addition, N-cadherin confers a motile phenotype on the cancer cells thereby increasing their migration [22]. Hence, the cadherin switch is an important component of the EMT that characterizes early steps in the progression of cancer cells towards an invasive and metastatic phenotype (Fig. 7.2).

Several clinical studies have linked the cadherin–catenin system with colorectal cancer and liver metastasis. Notably, several studies indicate that the level of β-catenin may be a useful prognostic indicator for characterizing colorectal cancer types with different clinico-pathological features and outcomes, including primary vs metastatic tumors [8]. The level of α-catenin expression may also serve as a marker of colon cancer progression because a significant down-regulation of α-catenin expression in colorectal cancer is associated with poor differentiation, higher metastatic potential and poor prognosis. However, no definitive conclusion can be drawn concerning the impact of the level of α-catenin expression in CRC cells and their liver infiltration and metastasis [25].

7.4 The Immunoglobulin Superfamily of Cell Adhesion Molecules (IgSFCAMs)

7.4.1 Structure and Cell Biology of IgSFCAMs

The immunoglobulin superfamily of adhesion receptors is composed of numerous cell surface and soluble proteins involved in intercellular recognition and adhesion. In contrast to the cellular adhesion mediated by cadherins, the IgSFCAM-dependent adhesive interactions are independent of divalent cations such as Ca^{2+}. The structure of IgSFCAM is characterized by the presence of an immunoglobulin-like domain in their extracellular domain and by one or more copies of Ig fold, a compact structure containing two cysteine residues separated by 55–75 amino acids arranged as two antiparallel β sheets held together by hydrophobic bonds [21]. This large family of adhesion receptors includes antigens of tumor cells (e.g. carcinoembryonic antigen (CEA)), T-lymphocyte and natural killer (NK) cell receptors (e.g. CD4) and cellular adhesion molecules [8]. Among these latter, intercellular cell adhesion molecules 1 and 2 (ICAM-1, ICAM-2) and vascular cell adhesion molecules (VCAM) mediate heterophilic and homophilic cell-cell interactions and cell binding to ECM proteins.

The IgSFCAM receptors regulate different functions depending on the cells on which they are expressed. For example, neural cell adhesion molecule Holness Simmons (N-CAM) and ephrins mediate interactions between neurons [26]. Endothelial Ig-like cell adhesion molecules such as ICAM-1 and VCAM-1 play an important role, not only as ligands for leukocyte integrins, but also as signaling initiators. Clustering of these IgCAMs triggers a wide range of events inside endothelial cells. Among them, the activation of Rho-like GTPases, induction of cytoskeletal changes and the transient modulation of cell-cell contact are key events [27]. Platelet endothelial cell adhesion molecule-1 (PECAM-1) is expressed on all cells within the vascular compartment and may represent a prototype IgCAM signaling molecule. It is expressed to different degrees on most leukocyte sub-types, on platelets, and on endothelial cells where its expression is concentrated at junctions between adjacent cells. In addition to its adhesive properties, PECAM-1 is an efficient signaling molecule that has diverse roles in vascular biology including angiogenesis, platelet function, thrombosis, mechanosensing of endothelial cell response to fluid shear stress and regulation of various stages of leukocyte migration through venular walls [28]. PECAM has multiple ligands, which explains the wide spectrum of its effects including its role in transendothelial migration of neutrophils. These ligands include integrin $\alpha v\beta 3$, ADP-ribose cyclase and CD177 [29–31]. PECAM-1 is an efficient outside-in and inside-out signaling receptor. Its signaling properties rely on the presence of 2 immunoreceptor tyrosine inhibitory motifs (ITIMs) in its cytoplasmic domain. These ITIM domains serve as docking sites for signaling molecules such as protein tyrosine phosphatases. This event leads to recruitment of molecules including the SH2-containing phosphatases (SHP-1/2 and SHIP) and phospholipase C-1, which can lead to activation of other signaling pathways. Ligand-mediated phosphorylation of tyrosine residues within the PECAM-1 ITIM motif can also regulate actin remodeling via recruitment or direct interaction with β and α-catenin [32]. Current evidence strongly suggests that phosphorylation of the cytoplasmic domains of PECAM-1 can be triggered by numerous stimuli such as shear stress and exposure to cytokines, leading to altered and enhanced PECAM-1 functions [32].

CEA, another member of the IgCAM family is a soluble glycoprotein that contains significant levels of sialy-Lewis-a and sialyl-Lewis-x (sLe^a and sLe^x) carbohydrate antigens and is expressed at the cell surface of the majority of metastatic colon cancers [33]. The CEA family members do not contain cytoplasmic or transmembrane domains but are anchored to the external plasma membrane by a C-terminal glycophosphatidylinositol moiety. This glycoprotein is expressed in different cell types including columnar epithelial and goblet colon cells, mucousal cells of the stomach, squamous epithelia of the tongue, epithelia and ducts of sweat glands and prostate epithelia [8]. The levels of CEA expression in normal or malignant cells are determined by the degree of differentiation. In accordance, highly differentiated cells express the highest levels of CEA.

7.4.2 IgSFCAMs Signaling During Cancer Progression and Invasion

Several experimental studies suggest that CRC cells entering the liver activate Kupffer cells, which in turn produce inflammatory cytokines such as TNF-α within the hepatic sinusoids [34, 35]. These cytokines stimulate sinusoidal endothelial cells (SECs) to express important levels of Ig-CAMs including ICAM-1 and VCAM-1 or VCAM-1 and PECAM-1 that in turn can mediate cancer cell adhesion [8]. Further research on human liver tissue is needed in order to confirm the clinical relevance of this crosstalk between cancer cells, Kupffer cells and SECs in the hepatic sinusoids and to develop therapeutic strategies to block this process. In that regard, it has been shown that inhibition of HT29 colorectal cancer cell adhesion to endothelial cells via antisense oligonucleotides- and cimetidine-mediated inhibition of ICAM as well as of E-selectin reduces the adhesion between endothelial and cancer cells [36]. Reciprocally, celocoxib, a cyclooxygenase-2 inhibitor, downregulates ICAM-1 and VCAM-1 expression by colon cancer cells and this results in reduced tumor cell adhesion to the endothelium [37]. Hence, effective therapeutic strategies aimed at inhibiting cancer cell invasion may be expected from these findings.

The prototype member of the carcinoembryonic antigen family, CEA, is overproduced in various epithelial tumors such as colon carcinomas, stomach, lung, pancreas and bladder tumors, ovarian and breast carcinoma [8, 24]. Elevated serum levels of CEA (10- to 100-fold) indicate a poor prognosis in patients with adenocarcinomas of the colon, breast and lung. Accordingly, CEA is widely used as a clinical marker for tumor progression but its functional role in tumor development is not well defined. The use of CEA as a diagnostic tool is now controversial. However, in current clinical setting, recent studies suggest that it should be used for surveillance of colorectal cancer patients with stage II-III disease, before and after curative liver resection and for monitoring patients with advanced disease [38, 39]. CEA is an important player that regulates molecular interactions between CRC cells and Kupffer cells and thereby the secretion of large numbers of inflammatory cytokines including IL-1β, IL-6, IL-10 and TNF-α that, in turn can trigger CAM expression and promote the arrest and the subsequent extravasation of the CRC, as described earlier [40, 41]. More particularly, the induction of IL-10 release by Kupffer cells and the subsequent decrease in nitric oxide concentrations promote CRC cell survival [42].

7.5 The Selectins

7.5.1 Structure and Function of Selectins

The selectins are members of a family of three calcium-dependent adhesion receptors: L-, P- and E-selectin. L-selectin is expressed constitutively by lymphocytes, whereas E-selectin is expressed exclusively by endothelial cells that have been challenged by inflammatory stimuli. P-selectin is found in platelets and endothelial cells where it is stored in α-granules and Weibel-Palade bodies, respectively. In endothelial cells, P-selectin is transported to the plasma membrane in response to inflammatory cytokines such as IL-4 and IL-13 [43, 44]. The extracellular portion of each selectin consists of three different domains; a C-type lectin domain in the N-terminus, an EGF-type domain and short consensus repeats (∼60 amino acids) that are also found in complement regulatory proteins (CRP) (Fig. 7.2). The number of these CRP repeats is a major structural feature that distinguishes the extracellular domains of the selectins. In human, P-selectin contains nine repeats, E-selectin has six and L-selectin only two [45]. The selectins are anchored in the membrane through a single helicoidal transmembrane domain that is followed by a short cytoplasmic tail. The interaction of selectins with their ligands is mediated trough their N-terminus lectin domain and is Ca^{2+}-dependent. Three physicochemical parameters determine the function and specificity of each selectin in relation to a particular ligand: the length of the CRP repeats, the unique structure of the N-terminal, C-type calcium-dependent lectin-like domain and the particular post-translational carbohydrate modification displayed on the ligand that is recognized by the selectins [46]. The binding of cancer cells to E-selectin requires a molecular scaffold composed of oligosaccharides that are borne by a carrier protein or lipid on cancer cells. In particular, this group of cell surface adhesion receptors has a high affinity for sLe^a and sLe^x, among other molecules [33]. This complex macromolecular carbohydrate scaffold is known as selectin counter-receptor and is essential for cell binding [47]. The consensus repeats are important to assure the rolling of adhering cells whereas the cytoplasmic domains trigger signaling [4, 45, 48]. The normal physiological role of selectin is to assure the rolling of adhering leukocytes during inflammation. As described below circulating cancer cells usurp the normal function of selectin and use them to adhere to endothelium and then transmigrate to form metastases [49, 50].

7.5.2 Selectin Signaling During Cancer Progression and Invasion

E-selectin mediates the adhesion of tumor cells to endothelial cells and this interaction is associated with metastatic dissemination [34, 51–54]. For instance, the binding efficiency of clonal cancer cell lines to E-selectin on endothelial cells was shown to be directly proportional to their respective metastatic potential [55]. Moreover, when the expression of E-selectin was inhibited by cimetidine or c-Raf antisense oligonucleotides, metastasis was inhibited [56, 57]. Similarly, interfering with the binding of colon carcinoma cells to lung endothelium, by using an anti-E-selectin-immunoglobulin, impaired lung metastasis [58]. Most interestingly, the group of Dr Pnina Brodt (McGill University) showed that highly metastatic human colorectal and mouse lung carcinoma cells, on their entry into the hepatic microcirculation, triggered a rapid host pro-inflammatory response by inducing TNFα production in resident Kupffer cells. In turn, this triggered E-selectin expression by endothelial cells, presumably enhancing the binding and extravasation of the cancer cells [34, 35]. Along the same lines, this group recently reported that the host inflammatory response involving endothelial selectins and neutrophil-mediated mechanisms promoted liver metastasis by increasing tumor cell arrest and extravasation [59, 60]. Of note, E-selectin gene polymorphism is associated with poor prognosis in patients with stage II or III colorectal cancer [61]. Taken together, these studies point to a key role for E-selectin-mediated endothelial adhesion in cancer cell metastasis. Accordingly, attempts to inhibit colon cancer metastasis by inhibiting E-selectin may have therapeutic benefits [62].

7.5.2.1 E-Selectin Induces Forward Signaling in Endothelial Cells

The first evidence that E-selectin induces forward signaling came from Gimbrone's group who showed that cross-linking of E-selectin with activating antibodies or by adhesion of HL-60 cells triggered ERK activation in endothelial cells [63]. The same group reported that the activation of ERK by E-selectin required the phosphorylation of tyrosine 603 within E-selectin [64]. Another example of forward signaling induced by E-selectin is the observation that adhesion of leukocytes to IL-1ß-activated endothelial cells induces the clustering of E-selectin, initiating its association with actin and actin-associated proteins such as vinculin and paxillin [65]. The forward signaling that results from the adhesion of leukocytes to human umbilical vein endothelial cells (HUVEC) expressing E-selectin results in the clustering of E-selectin at the site of adhesion, an event that requires the rapid formation of focal adhesions and that depends, in part, upon Src-mediated phosphorylation of cortactin [66]. The cortactin-dependent formation of focal complexes serves to generate foci of contraction that contribute to the "pulling apart" of endothelial cells, increasing inter-endothelial spaces and permeability and allowing transendothelial migration and extravasation of the activated leukocytes, at their sites of adhesion [66]. In line with this model, we found that the activation on E-selectin, either by a cross-linking antibody or by addition of HT29 cells, triggered a disruption of the VE-cadherin/β-catenin complex in an ERK and c-Src-dependent manner. These processes facilitate transendothelial migration of colon cancer cells [48]. In particular, we identified three distinct mechanisms by which circulating cancer cells interact with E-selectin to initiate transendothelial migration: formation of a mosaic between cancer cells and endothelial cells, paracellular diapedesis at the junction of three endothelial cells and transcellular diapedesis. We also obtained evidence indicating that E-selectin-dependent paracellular extravasation (at least in vitro) is independent of ICAM and VCAM-1 and that it requires the activation of ERK downstream of E-selectin [4]. Taken together, these findings indicate that E-selectin activation on endothelial cells elicits forward signals in these cells that regulate inter-endothelial permeability and extravastion of circulating cells.

7.5.2.2 Reverse Signaling Induced in Cancer Cells Bound to E-Selectin

As mentioned above, the binding of cancer cells to E-selectin requires a molecular scaffold composed of oligosaccharides that are borne by a carrier protein expressed on the cancer cells [43, 67, 68]. This macromolecular scaffolding complex is known as the E-selectin counter-receptor and is essential for cell binding [43]. Furthermore, the expression of these glycosylated proteins correlates with tumor progression and a poor prognosis [69, 70]. In colorectal cancer cells, sLe^a and sLe^x are considered to be the representative oligosaccharides involved in E-selectin binding [54, 71–73]. The glycoprotein ESL-1, present on neutrophils and myeloid cells, was the first E-selectin counter-receptor to be described [74]. It is a variant of the tyrosine kinase FGF glycoreceptor, raising the possibility that its binding to E-selectin is involved in initiating signaling in the adhering cancer cells [74, 75]. In that regard, the binding of E-selectin to cancer cells triggers the tyrosine phosphorylation of several proteins including Src, c-Cbl, FAK and p38 [76–80]. Moreover, E-selectin when bound to counter-receptors on metastatic colon cancer cells alters the expression of several genes, including some that are involved in regulating apoptosis such as HMGB1[80]. LAMP-1, LAMP-2, cluster of differentiation 44 (CD44), CEA, podocalyxin-like protein and death receptor-3 (DR3) were also identified as E-selectin ligands present on colon cancer cells [3, 81–85]. With the exception of DR3 and CD44, relatively little is known about the signaling that these counter-receptors trigger in cancer cells upon their binding to E-selectin.

(i) *E-selectin signaling following binding to CD44*. The CD44 family of proteins is a polymorphic group of type I transmembrane proteins present on the surface of most vertebrate cells. The N-terminal extracellular domain interacts with hyaluronate, an acidic glycosaminoglycan present within the ECM. CD44 plays a role in cell motility and proliferation and contributes to the maintenance of polar orientation in epithelial cells by anchoring them to basement membranes. These two functions are associated with the glycosylation pattern of the molecule. The CD44 proteins are all encoded by a single, highly conserved gene comprising at least 20 exons [14]. The heterogeneity of the protein products is due to an alternative splicing of CD44 transcripts that affects predominantly the extracellular membrane-proximal stem structure of CD44 proteins. The qualitative and quantitative patterns of alternative CD44 splicing depend on the cell type and growth conditions. For instance, the standard isoform of CD44 generated by the splicing of exons 1–5, 16–18 and 20 is ubiquitously expressed in developing and adult vertebrates with a particularly strong expression on cells of the hematopoietic system [86]. In contrast, the larger variant isoforms are expressed in only a few types of proliferating epithelial cells and in several cancers [86, 87]. Of note, the degree of glycosylation of the CD44 variants has important effects on their binding to hyaluronate and on the local osmotic and electrical environment with consequent alterations in the adhesive properties of the cell [33, 34]. Several lines of evidence indicate that CD44 variants, and especially CD44v4, are counter-receptors for E/P-selectin that regulate transendothelial migration of several types of cancer cells including breast and colorectal cancer cells [83, 84]. In the case of colorectal carcinomas, the expression of CD44 variants containing exons 8-10 (CD44v8-10) predicts poor prognosis [88]. Moreover, CEA and CD44v synergistically contribute to E- and L-selectin adhesion at elevated shear stresses [83]. Interestingly, the upregulation of CD44 expression could be an early event in gastro-intestinal carcinogenesis and requires adenomatous polyposis coli (APC) gene inactivation. Whether this is related to the selectin binding function of CD44 remains to be ascertained. (For a more extensive review on the role of CD44 in liver metastasis, see Chapter 4 in this volume).

(ii) *E-selectin signaling following binding to DR3.* DR3 is a member of the TNF receptor superfamily. These receptors are characterized by the presence of a common homologous region in the cytoplasmic domain known as the death domain [89–95]. The signaling pathways induced by these receptors are similar and rely on oligomerization of the receptor by ligand binding, recruitment of death domain proteins through homophilic interaction between their death domains, and subsequent activation of the caspase-driven apoptotic cascade or the transcription factor NFκB [95]. DR3 shares a high homology with TNFR1 and its ectopic expression in mammalian cells induces signals that activate caspase-mediated apoptosis or NFκB, depending on the cellular context and on the cytoplasmic effectors engaged in the signaling complexes downstream of the death domain [89–92]. DR3 is expressed mainly by peripheral blood lymphocytes and to a lesser extent, in the small intestine and colon [90, 92–94]. DR3 exists in several splicing isoforms, some of which including isoforms 1, 2, 3, 4 and 7 contain a death domain, whereas others including isoform 12, have no death domain and are shorter [93]. Among these variants, DR3 isoform 2 is the major and prototypical member of the family and is referred to as DR3v2. The existence of these multiple variants raises the possibility that the splicing profile of DR3 may be altered in cancer and impact disease progression. Notably, a variant of DR3v2 (DR3β) differs from the described DR3 molecule by a 28 amino-acid stretch in the extracellular domain. Whereas DR3 is expressed in all cell lines and lymphoma samples tested, DR3β expression is restricted to lymphoid T-cell and immature B-cell lines and is found in some cases of follicular lymphoma. This suggests that several receptor isoforms can participate in lymphoid cell homeostasis [96]. Interestingly, the activation of DR3 by its cognate ligand TL1A is not followed by apoptosis in human erythroleukemic TF-1 cells, presumably because it is associated with an NFκB-dependent expression of c-IAP2 [97, 98]. Of note, the gene encoding DR3 is localized in position 1p36.3 on human chromosome 1. This chromosomal region is frequently altered in pathologies, including cancer [99–101].

Intriguingly, DR3 is expressed and binds E-selectin in uveal melanoma as well as colon cancer cells, both of which preferentially metastasizes to the liver [1, 102, 103]. In this context, we found that E-selectin-induces activation of DR3, present on HT29 and LoVo colon cancer cells, and this increases transendothelial migration and cancer cell survival through the activation of the MAP kinase p38 and ERK. However, although DR3 is a death receptor, E-selectin does not induce apoptosis in these cancer cells, suggesting that they have evolved to escape apoptosis to the benefit of pro-migratory (p38) and survival (ERK) signals [3]. DR3v2 contains four Tyr residues (Y285, Y336, Y376 and Y394) within its intracellular domain, two of which, Y376 and Y394 are within an ITAM motif [104]. Nothing is presently known concerning the signaling functions of Tyr residues within DR3 and we believe that they are involved as docking sites to initiate activation of kinase cascades in response to E-selectin binding. In this context, recent evidence indicates that Fas/CD95, a member of the TNFR family, induces PI3K signaling via phosphorylation of a Tyr residue present in its death domain [105].

7.6 Extravasation

For incoming tumor cells to grow and form metastases in a target organ, a permissive microenvironment is required [106]. As discussed above, the adhesive interactions between the cancer cells and target organ endothelial cells are crucial components of the metastatic process. These interactions determine the arrest of the circulatory cells in the capillaries and initiate the cascade of events that culminates in diapedesis of the cancer cells across the endothelium.

7.6.1 Adhesion to Endothelial Cells and the Homing Concept of Metastasis

Extravasation of circulating tumor cells in the host organ first requires successive adhesive interactions between endothelial cell receptors and their ligands or counter-receptors present on the cancer cells, and secondly, their passage across the endothelium [43, 107] (Fig. 7.3). Several types of cancers have an organ preference for metastases formation. For example, colorectal cancer metastasizes to liver and lung and uveal melanoma preferentially metastasizes to liver, but rarely to other organs. This organ selectivity was noted by Stephen Paget, over a century ago and led to his "seed and soil" hypothesis [108]. According to this postulate, the tumor cells (seed) are only able to grow if they are in a compatible environment (soil) conducive to their growth. Most likely, this requires specific adhesive interactions with cellular and matrix components of the target organ microenvironment. The Paget's "seed and soil" theory is supported by several clinical observations and experimental data. For example, the organ selectivity of B16 clonal melanoma cells that preferentially form metastases in the organ from which their parent cells have been isolated support the existence of genetic factors that predetermine the organ site

---

Fig. 7.3 The selectins and selectin ligands. The extracellular portion of the selectins is composed of a terminal C-type lectin domain that binds to counter-receptors or ligands on adhering cells. The lectin domain is followed by a single EGF-type repeat and various numbers of consensus repeats found in complement regulatory proteins (CRP). The selectins have a single transmembrane region and a short cytoplasmic tail. The selectin ligands on adhering cells consist of a scaffolding complex that contains various carbohydrates such as sialyl-Lewis a and x or other fucosylated oligosaccharides that are presented by carrier proteins and possibly lipid molecules. The best-known selectin ligands are GlyCAM-1 (glycosylation-dependent cell adhesion molecule-1) for l-selectin, ESL-1 (E-selectin ligand-1) and DR3 for E-Selectin and PSGL-1 (P-selectin glycoprotein ligand-1) for E- and P-selectin

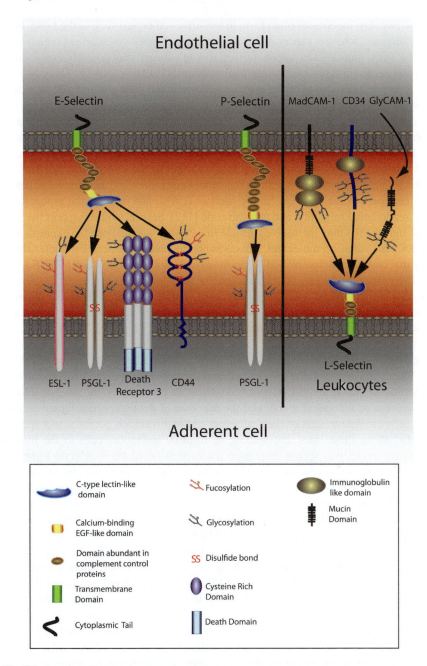

Fig. 7.3 (continued)

predilection of metastatic cells [109]. The "homing concept of metastasis" was challenged by James Ewing who suggested that organ-selectivity of metastasis merely results from mechanical factors involving the first circulatory bed encountered by the circulating cancer cells [110]. Several clinical observations do not support this view. Notably, metastases often form in low-irrigated organs such as the brain, bone and adrenals, whereas cancer cells rarely colonize highly-vascularized organs such as the heart, muscles and spleen. In fact, Ewing's theory may possibly explain only certain particular types of loco-regional metastasis [111].

Adhesive interactions between endothelial cells and their glycosylated ligands or counter-receptors present on cancer cells constitute an important mechanism that is consistent with the "seed and soil" theory [107]. In the case of liver metastasis, these interactions appear to rely on selectin-mediated initial attachment and rolling of the circulating cancer cells on the endothelium. Rolling cancer cells then become activated by locally released chemokines present at the endothelial cell surface. This triggers integrin activation on the cancer cells allowing their firmer adhesion via members of the Ig-CAM family such as ICAM, and initiates the processes of transendothelial migration and extravasation [112]. Several studies support the view that cancer cells may themselves initiate this cascade and activate the expression of endothelial adhesion molecules. This is supported, among others, by studies showing that cancer cell conditioned medium may contain cytokines such as TNFα, ILβ or INFγ that will directly activate endothelial cells to express E-selectin, P-selectin, ICAM-2 or VCAM-1 [47, 113]. Moreover, highly metastatic human colorectal and mouse lung carcinoma cells were shown to trigger a rapid host inflammatory response upon entry into the hepatic microcirculation by inducing TNFα production in resident Kupffer cells. In turn, this was shown to induce E-selectin expression by endothelial cells and enhance the binding and extravasation of the cancer cells [35].

Since tumor – endothelial cell adhesion requires the presence of endothelial selectins as well as sialyl-Lewis carbohydrates on cancer cells, the level of selectin expression on the vascular wall and the presence of the appropriate ligand on cancer cells are determinant of their adhesion and extravasation potential in a specific organ. Along these lines, the homing of B16F10 melanoma cells to the liver in a mouse model was shown to require the expression of the E-selectin ligand on the melanoma cells and correspondingly the expression of E-selectin in the liver [114]. Additionally, endothelial selectins are expressed differentially in blood vessels from different organs. For example, LPS and TNFα strongly induce expression of P-selectin on endothelial cells of the leptomeninges, but to a weaker level on blood vessels of the brain parenchyma [114]. Moreover, immunohistochemical studies performed on liver metastases show that the expression of E-selectin and other adhesion molecules is increased both in the sinusoidal endothelium surrounding metastases and in the tumor vessels [115]. On the other hand, we found that sialylated DR3-mediated tumor cell binding to endothelial E-selectin activated the invasive properties of colon cancer cells [3, 43]. Overall, these studies suggest that the DR3/E-selectin interaction may be an important contributor to the liver-preferential metastasis of colon cancer cells in the context of the inflammatory response induced by metastasizing tumor cells. Based on these findings, it can be proposed that the specific interactions that take place between selectins differentially expressed on endothelial cells of different target organs and the levels of expression of their ligands on cancer cells may be one of the factors that determine the organ – distribution of metastatic cells. As indicated above, it is noteworthy in this context that cancer cells that express DR3 such as uveal melanoma and colon carcinoma cells bind E-selectin and disseminate preferentially to the liver.

7.6.2 The Passage Across the Endothelium and the Colonization of Secondary Sites

Following their adhesion to endothelial cells of a target organ, cancer cells extend invadipodia into the endothelial cell junctions initiating their retraction and enabling transendothelial tumor migration. The mechanisms by which cancer cells regulate retraction of endothelial cells are not well-defined. In the case of Lewis lung carcinoma cells, it may rely on the release of 12(S)-hydroxyeicosatetraenoic acid by the cancer cells themselves [116]. On the other hand, we reported that retraction of endothelial cells following E-selectin-mediated adhesion of colon cancer cells results from an ERK-dependent dissociation of the VE-cadherin/β-catenin complex that is, in turn, associated with a p38-dependent actin filament retraction [4, 48]. In some cases, an irreversible retraction of the endothelial layer may be caused by cancer cell-induced apoptosis of endothelial cells. This for instance was shown to occur following the transcellular diapedesis of colon cancer cells across individual endothelial cells [4]. The extravasation process also involves the contribution of proteases (collagenases type I and IV) that are located at the invasive front of the cancer cells. These proteases degrade ECM components and can also trigger the release of growth factors, stored in the basement membrane (BM) that will induce retraction [117]. In both cases, extravasation is favoured. Following extravasation, cancer cells adhere to sub-endothelial ECM proteins, which in the case of the liver include mainly fibronectin and to a lesser extent types III, IV, V, and VI collagens, via cell adhesion receptors such as integrins and CD44 [117, 118]. Cancer cells will then grow and initiate the development of a secondary neoplasm. Alternatively, they will move across the ECM and grow at a further distance. Intriguingly, liver is devoid of basement membrane underneath the sinusoidal endothelium [119]. Nevertheless ECM components, such as laminin, and collagen type IV are present in the space of Disse between endothelial cells and hepatocytes [120]. Therefore, due to an incomplete layer of hepatic endothelial cells, these ECM components are directly accessible to circulating cells. This may explain why the interactions between these ECM components within the liver and tumor cells are crucial for the formation of hepatic metastases.

Following transendothelial migration, cancer cells that can escape apoptosis and initiate neo-vascularization will successfully colonize the target organ. In the case of colon cancer cells, it has been proposed that they release soluble CD44 which acts as a decoy receptor impairing interaction of cancer cells with their hyaluronate ligand within the ECM, thereby conferring resistance to apoptosis. This is supported by the findings that lysates from cells transfected with soluble CD44 were negative for cleaved PARP [121]. Several lines of evidence further indicate that the ECM, by altering the expression of growth factors and growth factor receptors in colon cancer cells, modulates their proliferation in the liver. For example, heparin proteoglycan stimulates colon cancer cell proliferation in the liver by inducing the expression of autocrine growth factors and their receptors [122]. Another factor that may limit the proliferation of all incoming cancer cells at secondary sites is the initial lack of adequate vascularization. This could result in dormant micrometastases that may eventually develop into macrometastases following appropriate remodelling of the microenvironment and angiogenesis. Notably, EGF receptor expression coupled to expression of growth factors such as TGFα are together among the well-known molecular factors that influence the ability of colon cancer cells to grow in the liver [123, 124]. Moreover, data suggest that the chemokine receptor CXCR4 is also required for outgrowth of colon carcinoma micrometastases in the liver [125].

In summary, the ability of cancer cells to grow at a specific site such as liver parenchyma depends on features inherent to the cancer cell and to the microenvironment of the invaded organ, as well as on the active interplay between these factors. Much remains to be learned about the detailed molecular interactions between cancer cells and the microenvironment of specific secondary sites. However, there is strong evidence indicating that these interactions are important in determining homing, survival potential and proliferation of cancer cells in a specific organ.

7.7 Concluding Remarks and Therapeutic Perspectives

Selective adhesion of circulating cancer cells to endothelial cells is a major mechanism that underlies metastasis. These adhesive interactions are characterized by an intense bi-directional signaling that contributes to extravasation of cancer in specific target organs such as the liver (e.g. for colon carcinoma cells). Nevertheless, much still remains to be done in order to better understand the homing process of metastatic cells. In particular, understanding the causal relationship between tumor-endothelial adhesion and metastasis in the clinical setting is mandatory, if this process is to be targeted therapeutically. Similarly, the signaling mechanisms that adhesion triggers in cancer and endothelial cells following their mutual binding should be better understood. A better understanding of these molecular processes will not only provide insight into the process of metastasis, but may also identify new targets for therapeutic intervention aimed at specifically inhibiting this major cause of cancer-related death. This effort has already begun and should be accelerating in the upcoming years.

Acknowledgements This work was supported by The Canadian Cancer Society Research Institute. Nicolas Porquet holds a studentship from le Centre de Recherche en Cancérologie de l'Université Laval.

References

1. Gout S, Huot J (2008) Role of cancer microenvironmentin metastasis: focus on colon cancer. Cancer Microenviron 1:69–83
2. Smedsrod B, Le Couteur D, Ikejima K et al (2009) Hepatic sinusoidal cells in health and disease: update from the 14th International Symposium. Liver Int 29:490–501

3. Gout S, Morin C, Houle F, Huot J (2006) Death receptor-3, a new E-Selectin counter-receptor that confers migration and survival advantages to colon carcinoma cells by triggering p38 and ERK MAPK activation. Cancer Res 66:9117–9124

4. Tremblay PL, Huot J, Auger FA (2008) Mechanisms by which E-selectin regulates diapedesis of colon cancer cells under flow conditions. Cancer Res 68:5167–5176

5. Barczyk M, Carracedo S, Gullberg D (2010) Integrins. Cell Tissue Res 339:269–280

6. Hood JD, Cheresh DA (2002) Role of integrins in cell invasion and migration. Nat Rev Cancer 2:91–100

7. Mizejewski GJ (1999) Role of integrins in cancer: survey of expression patterns. Proc Soc Exp Biol Med 222:124–138

8. Paschos KA, Canovas D, Bird NC (2009) The role of cell adhesion molecules in the progression of colorectal cancer and the development of liver metastasis. Cell Signal 21:665–674

9. Yoshimura K, Meckel KF, Laird LS et al (2009) Integrin alpha2 mediates selective metastasis to the liver. Cancer Res 69:7320–7328

10. Plantefaber LC, Hynes RO (1989) Changes in integrin receptors on oncogenically transformed cells. Cell 56:281–290

11. Pampori N, Hato T, Stupack DG et al (1999) Mechanisms and consequences of affinity modulation of integrin alpha(V)beta(3) detected with a novel patch-engineered monovalent ligand. J Biol Chem 274:21609–21616

12. Basson MD (2008) An intracellular signal pathway that regulates cancer cell adhesion in response to extracellular forces. Cancer Res 68:2–4

13. Guo W, Giancotti FG (2004) Integrin signalling during tumour progression. Nat Rev Mol Cell Biol 5:816–826

14. Konstantopoulos K, Thomas SN (2009) Cancer cells in transit: the vascular interactions of tumor cells. Annu Rev Biomed Eng 11:177–202

15. Chiarugi P, Giannoni E (2008) Anoikis: a necessary death program for anchorage-dependent cells. Biochem Pharmacol 76:1352–1364

16. Reinmuth N, Liu W, Ahmad SA et al (2003) Alphavbeta3 integrin antagonist S247 decreases colon cancer metastasis and angiogenesis and improves survival in mice. Cancer Res 63:2079–2087

17. Laferriere J, Houle F, Huot J (2004) Adhesion of HT-29 colon carcinoma cells to endothelial cells requires sequential events involving E-selectin and integrin beta4. Clin Exp Metastasis 21:257–264

18. Stemmler MP (2008) Cadherins in development and cancer. Mol Biosyst 4:835–850

19. Perez-Moreno M, Jamora C, Fuchs E (2003) Sticky business: orchestrating cellular signals at adherens junctions. Cell 112:535–548

20. Gumbiner BM (2005) Regulation of cadherin-mediated adhesion in morphogenesis. Nat Rev Mol Cell Biol 6:622–634

21. Juliano RL (2002) Signal transduction by cell adhesion receptors and the cytoskeleton: functions of integrins, cadherins, selectins, and immunoglobulin-superfamily members. Annu Rev Pharmacol Toxicol 42:283–323

22. Hazan RB, Phillips GR, Qiao RF, Norton L, Aaronson SA (2000) Exogenous expression of N-cadherin in breast cancer cells induces cell migration, invasion, and metastasis. J Cell Biol 148:779–790

23. Cano A, Perez-Moreno MA, Rodrigo I et al (2000) The transcription factor snail controls epithelial-mesenchymal transitions by repressing E-cadherin expression. Nat Cell Biol 2:76–83

24. Cavallaro U, Christofori G (2004) Cell adhesion and signalling by cadherins and Ig-CAMs in cancer. Nat Rev Cancer 4:118–132

25. Raftopoulos I, Davaris P, Karatzas G, Karayannacos P, Kouraklis G (1998) Level of alpha-catenin expression in colorectal cancer correlates with invasiveness, metastatic potential, and survival. J Surg Oncol 68:92–99

26. Huot J (2004) Ephrin signaling in axon guidance. Prog Neuropsychopharmacol Biol Psychiatry 28:813–818

27. van Buul JD, Kanters E, Hordijk PL (2007) Endothelial signaling by Ig-like cell adhesion molecules. Arterioscler Thromb Vasc Biol 27:1870–1876

28. Woodfin A, Voisin MB, Nourshargh S (2007) PECAM-1: a multi-functional molecule in inflammation and vascular biology. Arterioscler Thromb Vasc Biol 27:2514–2523

29. Sachs UJ, Andrei-Selmer CL, Maniar A et al (2007) The neutrophil-specific antigen CD177 is a counter-receptor for platelet endothelial cell adhesion molecule-1 (CD31). J Biol Chem 282:23603–23612

30. Deaglio S, Morra M, Mallone R et al (1998) Human CD38 (ADP-ribosyl cyclase) is a counter-receptor of CD31, an Ig superfamily member. J Immunol 160:395–402

31. Wong CW, Wiedle G, Ballestrem C et al (2000) PECAM-1/CD31 trans-homophilic binding at the intercellular junctions is independent of its cytoplasmic domain; evidence for heterophilic interaction with integrin alphavbeta3 in Cis. Mol Biol Cell 11:3109–3121

32. Ilan N, Madri JA (2003) PECAM-1: old friend, new partners. Curr Opin Cell Biol 15:515–524

33. Bird NC, Mangnall D, Majeed AW (2006) Biology of colorectal liver metastases: a review. J Surg Oncol 94:68–80

34. Khatib AM, Kontogiannea M, Fallavollita L, Jamison B, Meterissian S, Brodt P (1999) Rapid induction of cytokine and E-selectin expression in the liver in response to metastatic tumor cells. Cancer Res 59:1356–1361

35. Khatib AM, Auguste P, Fallavollita L et al (2005) Characterization of the host proinflammatory response to tumor cells during the initial stages of liver metastasis. Am J Pathol 167:749–759

36. Tang NH, Chen YL, Wang XQ, Li XJ, Yin FZ, Wang XZ (2004) Cooperative inhibitory effects of antisense oligonucleotide of cell adhesion molecules and cimetidine on cancer cell adhesion. World J Gastroenterol 10:62–66

37. Gallicchio M, Rosa AC, Dianzani C et al (2008) Celecoxib decreases expression of the adhesion molecules ICAM-1 and VCAM-1 in a colon cancer cell line (HT29). Br J Pharmacol 153:870–878

38. Locker GY, Hamilton S, Harris J et al (2006) ASCO 2006 update of recommendations for the use of tumor markers in gastrointestinal cancer. J Clin Oncol 24:5313–5327

39. Duffy MJ, van Dalen A, Haglund C et al (2007) Tumour markers in colorectal cancer: European Group on Tumour Markers (EGTM) guidelines for clinical use. Eur J Cancer 43:1348–1360

40. Thomas P, Gangopadhyay A, Steele G, Jr et al (1995) The effect of transfection of the CEA gene on the metastatic behavior of the human colorectal cancer cell line MIP-101. Cancer Lett 92:59–66

41. Gangopadhyay A, Lazure DA, Thomas P (1997) Carcinoembryonic antigen induces signal transduction in Kupffer cells. Cancer Lett 118:1–6

42. Jessup JM, Samara R, Battle P, Laguinge LM (2004) Carcinoembryonic antigen promotes tumor cell survival in liver through an IL-10-dependent pathway. Clin Exp Metastasis 21:709–717

43. Gout S, Tremblay PL, Huot J (2008) Selectins and selectin ligands in extravasation of cancer cells and organ selectivity of metastasis. Clin Exp Metastasis 25:335–344

44. Woltmann G, McNulty CA, Dewson G, Symon FA, Wardlaw AJ (2000) Interleukin-13 induces PSGL-1/P-selectin-dependent adhesion of eosinophils, but not neutrophils, to human umbilical vein endothelial cells under flow. Blood 95:3146–3152

45. Vestweber D, Blanks JE (1999) Mechanisms that regulate the function of the selectins and their ligands. Physiol Rev 79:181–213

46. Barthel SR, Gavino JD, Descheny L, Dimitroff CJ (2007) Targeting selectins and selectin ligands in inflammation and cancer. Expert Opin Ther Targets 11:1473–1491

47. Kannagi R, Izawa M, Koike T, Miyazaki K, Kimura N (2004) Carbohydrate-mediated cell adhesion in cancer metastasis and angiogenesis. Cancer Sci 95:377–384
48. Tremblay PL, Auger FA, Huot J (2006) Regulation of transendothelial migration of colon cancer cells by E-selectin-mediated activation of p38 and ERK MAP kinases. Oncogene 25:6563–6573
49. Smith CW (2008) Adhesion molecules and receptors. J Allergy Clin Immunol 121:S375–379; quiz S414
50. Langer HF, Chavakis T (2009) Leukocyte-endothelial interactions in inflammation. J Cell Mol Med 13:1211–1220
51. Brodt P, Fallavollita L, Bresalier RS, Meterissian S, Norton CR, Wolitzky BA (1997) Liver endothelial E-selectin mediates carcinoma cell adhesion and promotes liver metastasis. Int J Cancer 71:612–619
52. Gulubova MV (2002) Expression of cell adhesion molecules, their ligands and tumour necrosis factor alpha in the liver of patients with metastatic gastrointestinal carcinomas. Histochem J 34:67–77
53. Dimitroff CJ, Lechpammer M, Long-Woodward D, Kutok JL (2004) Rolling of human bone-metastatic prostate tumor cells on human bone marrow endothelium under shear flow is mediated by E-selectin. Cancer Res 64:5261–5269
54. Zipin A, Israeli-Amit M, Meshel T et al (2004) Tumor-microenvironment interactions: the fucose-generating FX enzyme controls adhesive properties of colorectal cancer cells. Cancer Res 64:6571–6578
55. Sawada R, Tsuboi S, Fukuda M (1994) Differential E-selectin-dependent adhesion efficiency in sublines of a human colon cancer exhibiting distinct metastatic potentials. J Biol Chem 269:1425–1431
56. Kobayashi K, Matsumoto S, Morishima T, Kawabe T, Okamoto T (2000) Cimetidine inhibits cancer cell adhesion to endothelial cells and prevents metastasis by blocking E-selectin expression. Cancer Res 60:3978–3984
57. Khatib AM, Fallavollita L, Wancewicz EV, Monia BP, Brodt P (2002) Inhibition of hepatic endothelial E-selectin expression by C-raf antisense oligonucleotides blocks colorectal carcinoma liver metastasis. Cancer Res 62:5393–5398
58. Mannori G, Santoro D, Carter L, Corless C, Nelson RM, Bevilacqua MP (1997) Inhibition of colon carcinoma cell lung colony formation by a soluble form of E-selectin. Am J Pathol 151:233–243
59. McDonald B, Spicer J, Giannais B, Fallavollita L, Brodt P, Ferri LE (2009) Systemic inflammation increases cancer cell adhesion to hepatic sinusoids by neutrophil mediated mechanisms. Int J Cancer 125:1298–1305
60. Auguste P, Fallavollita L, Wang N, Burnier J, Bikfalvi A, Brodt P (2007) The host inflammatory response promotes liver metastasis by increasing tumor cell arrest and extravasation. Am J Pathol 170:1781–1792
61. Hebbar M, Adenis A, Revillion F et al (2009) E-selectin gene S128R polymorphism is associated with poor prognosis in patients with stage II or III colorectal cancer. Eur J Cancer 45:1871–1876
62. Kneuer C, Ehrhardt C, Radomski MW, Bakowsky U (2006) Selectins – potential pharmacological targets? Drug Discov Today 11:1034–1040
63. Hu Y, Kiely JM, Szente BE, Rosenzweig A, Gimbrone MA Jr (2000) E-selectin-dependent signaling via the mitogen-activated protein kinase pathway in vascular endothelial cells. J Immunol 165:2142–2148
64. Hu Y, Szente B, Kiely JM, Gimbrone MA Jr (2001) Molecular events in transmembrane signaling via E-selectin. SHP2 association, adaptor protein complex formation and ERK1/2 activation. J Biol Chem 276:48549–48553
65. Yoshida M, Westlin WF, Wang N et al (1966) Leukocyte adhesion to vascular endothelium induces E-selectin linkage to the actin cytoskeleton. J Cell Biol 133:445–455

66. Tilghman RW, Hoover RL (2002) The Src-cortactin pathway is required for clustering of E-selectin and ICAM-1 in endothelial cells. Faseb J 16:1257–1259

67. Ben-David T, Sagi-Assif O, Meshel T, Lifshitz V, Yron I, Witz IP (2008) The involvement of the sLe-a selectin ligand in the extravasation of human colorectal carcinoma cells. Immunol Lett 116:218–224

68. Witz IP (2008) The selectin-selectin ligand axis in tumor progression. Cancer Metastasis Rev 27:19–30

69. Kannagi R (1997) Carbohydrate-mediated cell adhesion involved in hematogenous metastasis of cancer. Glycoconj J 14:577–584

70. Kim YJ, Varki A (1997) Perspectives on the significance of altered glycosylation of glycoproteins in cancer. Glycoconj J 14:569–576

71. Murata K, Miyoshi E, Ihara S et al (2004) Attachment of human colon cancer cells to vascular endothelium is enhanced by N-acetylglucosaminyltransferase V. Oncology 66:492–501

72. St Hill CA, Bullard KM, Walcheck B (2005) Expression of the high-affinity selectin glycan ligand C2-O-sLeX by colon carcinoma cells. Cancer Lett 217:105–113

73. Nakamori S, Kameyama M, Imaoka S et al (1993) Increased expression of sialyl Lewisx antigen correlates with poor survival in patients with colorectal carcinoma: clinicopathological and immunohistochemical study. Cancer Res 53:3632–3637

74. Lenter M, Levinovitz A, Isenmann S, Vestweber D (1994) Monospecific and common glycoprotein ligands for E- and P-selectin on myeloid cells. J Cell Biol 125:471–481

75. Steegmaier M, Levinovitz A, Isenmann S et al (1995) The E-selectin-ligand ESL-1 is a variant of a receptor for fibroblast growth factor. Nature 373:615–620

76. Soltesz SA, Powers EA, Geng JG, Fisher C (1997) Adhesion of HT-29 colon carcinoma cells to E-selectin results in increased tyrosine phosphorylation and decreased activity of c-src. Int J Cancer 71:645–653

77. Ohana-Malka O, Benharroch D, Isakov N et al (2003) Selectins and anti-CD15 (Lewis x/a) antibodies transmit activation signals in Hodgkin's lymphoma-derived cell lines. Exp Hematol 31:1057–1065

78. Di Bella MA, Flugy AM, Russo D, D'Amato M, De Leo G, Alessandro R (2003) Different phenotypes of colon carcinoma cells interacting with endothelial cells: role of E-selectin and ultrastructural data. Cell Tissue Res 312:55–64

79. Laferriere J, Houle F, Taher MM, Valerie K, Huot J (2001) Transendothelial migration of colon carcinoma cells requires expression of E-selectin by endothelial cells and activation of stress-activated protein kinase-2 (SAPK2/p38) in the tumor cells. J Biol Chem 276: 33762–33772

80. Aychek T, Miller K, Sagi-Assif O et al (2008) E-selectin regulates gene expression in metastatic colorectal carcinoma cells and enhances HMGB1 release. Int J Cancer 123: 1741–1750

81. Tomlinson J, Wang JL, Barsky SH, Lee MC, Bischoff J, Nguyen M (2000) Human colon cancer cells express multiple glycoprotein ligands for E-selectin. Int J Oncol 16:347–353

82. Hanley WD, Burdick MM, Konstantopoulos K, Sackstein R (2005) CD44 on LS174T colon carcinoma cells possesses E-selectin ligand activity. Cancer Res 65:5812–5817

83. Thomas SN, Zhu F, Schnaar RL, Alves CS, Konstantopoulos K (2008) Carcinoembryonic antigen and CD44 variant isoforms cooperate to mediate colon carcinoma cell adhesion to E- and L-selectin in shear flow. J Biol Chem 283:15647–15655

84. Zen K, Liu DQ, Guo YL et al (2008) CD44v4 is a major E-selectin ligand that mediates breast cancer cell transendothelial migration. PLoS One 3:e1826

85. Thomas SN, Schnaar RL, Konstantopoulos K (2009) Podocalyxin-like protein is an E-/L-selectin ligand on colon carcinoma cells: comparative biochemical properties of selectin ligands in host and tumor cells. Am J Physiol Cell Physiol 296:C505–513

86. Ponta H, Sherman L, Herrlich PA (2003) CD44: from adhesion molecules to signalling regulators. Nat Rev Mol Cell Biol 4:33–45

87. Milstone LM, Hough-Monroe L, Kugelman LC, Bender JR, Haggerty JG (1994) Epican, a heparan/chondroitin sulfate proteoglycan form of CD44, mediates cell-cell adhesion. J Cell Sci 107:3183–3190
88. Yamaguchi A, Urano T, Goi T et al (1996) Expression of a CD44 variant containing exons 8 to 10 is a useful independent factor for the prediction of prognosis in colorectal cancer patients. J Clin Oncol 14:1122–1127
89. Kitson J, Raven T, Jiang YP et al (1996) A death-domain-containing receptor that mediates apoptosis. Nature 384:372–375
90. Chinnaiyan AM, O'Rourke K, Yu GL et al (1996) Signal transduction by DR3, a death domain-containing receptor related to TNFR-1 and CD95. Science 274:990–992
91. Marsters SA, Sheridan JP, Donahue CJ et al (1996) Apo-3, a new member of the tumor necrosis factor receptor family, contains a death domain and activates apoptosis and NF-kappa B. Curr Biol 6:1669–1676
92. Bodmer JL, Burns K, Schneider P et al (1997) TRAMP, a novel apoptosis-mediating receptor with sequence homology to tumor necrosis factor receptor 1 and Fas(Apo-1/CD95). Immunity 6:79–88
93. Screaton GR, Xu XN, Olsen AL et al (1997) LARD: a new lymphoid-specific death domain containing receptor regulated by alternative pre-mRNA splicing. Proc Natl Acad Sci U S A 94:4615–4619
94. Tan KB, Harrop J, Reddy M et al (1997) Characterization of a novel TNF-like ligand and recently described TNF ligand and TNF receptor superfamily genes and their constitutive and inducible expression in hematopoietic and non-hematopoietic cells. Gene 204:35–46
95. Croft M (2009) The role of TNF superfamily members in T-cell function and diseases. Nat Rev Immunol 9:271–285
96. Warzocha K, Ribeiro P, Charlot C, Renard N, Coiffier B, Salles G (1998) A new death receptor 3 isoform: expression in human lymphoid cell lines and non-Hodgkin's lymphomas. Biochem Biophys Res Commun 242:376–379
97. Migone TS, Zhang J, Luo X et al (2002) TL1A is a TNF-like ligand for DR3 and TR6/DcR3 and functions as a T cell costimulator. Immunity 16:479–492
98. Wen L, Zhuang L, Luo X, Wei P (2003) TL1A-induced NF-kappaB activation and c-IAP2 production prevent DR3-mediated apoptosis in TF-1 cells. J Biol Chem 278:39251–39258 (Epub 2003 Jul 25)
99. Grenet J, Valentine V, Kitson J, Li H, Farrow SN, Kidd VJ (1998) Duplication of the DR3 gene on human chromosome 1p36 and its deletion in human neuroblastoma. Genomics 49:385–393
100. Osawa K, Takami N, Shiozawa K, Hashiramoto A, Shiozawa S (2004) Death receptor 3 (DR3) gene duplication in a chromosome region 1p36.3: gene duplication is more prevalent in rheumatoid arthritis. Genes Immun 5:439–443
101. Eggert A, Grotzer MA, Zuzak TJ, Ikegaki N, Zhao H, Brodeur GM (2002) Expression of Apo-3 and Apo-3L in primitive neuroectodermal tumours of the central and peripheral nervous system. Eur J Cancer 38:92–98
102. Damato B (2006) Treatment of primary intraocular melanoma. Expert Rev Anticancer Ther 6:493–506
103. Francken AB, Fulham MJ, Millward MJ, Thompson JF (2006) Detection of metastatic disease in patients with uveal melanoma using positron emission tomography. Eur J Surg Oncol 32:780–784
104. Lohi O, Lehto VP (1998) ITAM motif in an apoptosis-receptor. Apoptosis 3:335–336
105. Sancho-Martinez I, Martin-Villalba A (2009) Tyrosine phosphorylation and CD95: a FAScinating switch. Cell Cycle 8:838–842
106. Kaplan RN, Rafii S, Lyden D (2006) Preparing the "soil": the premetastatic niche. Cancer Res 66:11089–11093
107. Nicolson GL (1988) Cancer metastasis: tumor cell and host organ properties important in metastasis to specific secondary sites. Biochim Biophys Acta 948:175–224

108. Paget S (1889) The distribution of secondary growths in cancer of the breast. Lancet 133:571–573
109. Fidler IJ (1996) Critical determinants of melanoma metastasis. J Investig Dermatol Symp Proc 1:203–208
110. Ewing J (1928) Neoplastic diseases. A treatise on tumors, 3rd edn. WB Saunders Company, Philadelphia, PA, p 1127
111. Ribatti D, Mangialardi G, Vacca A (2006) Stephen Paget and the 'seed and soil' theory of metastatic dissemination. Clin Exp Med 6:145–149
112. Walzog B, Gaehtgens P (2000) Adhesion molecules: the path to a new understanding of acute inflammation. News Physiol Sci 15:107–113
113. Narita T, Kawakami-Kimura N, Kasai Y et al (1996) Induction of E-selectin expression on vascular endothelium by digestive system cancer cells. J Gastroenterol 31:299–301
114. Araki M, Araki K, Biancone L et al (1997) The role of E-selectin for neutrophil activation and tumor metastasis in vivo. Leukemia 11:209–212
115. Halacheva K, Gulubova MV, Manolova I, Petkov D (2002) Expression of ICAM-1, VCAM-1, E-selectin and TNF-alpha on the endothelium of femoral and iliac arteries in thromboangiitis obliterans. Acta Histochem 104:177–184
116. Honn KV, Tang DG, Grossi I et al (1994) Tumor cell-derived 12(S)-hydroxyeicosatetraenoic acid induces microvascular endothelial cell retraction. Cancer Res 54:565–574
117. Miles FL, Pruitt FL, van Golen KL, Cooper CR (2008) Stepping out of the flow: capillary extravasation in cancer metastasis. Clin Exp Metastasis 25:305–324
118. Martinez-Hernandez A, Amanta PS (1993) The hepatic extracellular matrix. I. Components and distribution in normal liver. Virchows Arch A Pathol Anat Histopathol 423:1–11
119. Enns A, Gassmann P, Schluter K et al (2004) Integrins can directly mediate metastatic tumor cell adhesion within the liver sinusoids. J Gastrointest Surg 8:1049–1059; discussion 60
120. Amenta PS, Harrison D (1997) Expression and potential role of the extracellular matrix in hepatic ontogenesis: a review. Microsc Res Tech 39:372–386
121. Subramaniam V, Gardner H, Jothy S (2007) Soluble CD44 secretion contributes to the acquisition of aggressive tumor phenotype in human colon cancer cells. Exp Mol Pathol 83:341–346
122. Zvibel I, Halpern Z, Papa M (1998) Extracellular matrix modulates expression of growth factors and growth-factor receptors in liver-colonizing colon-cancer cell lines. Int J Cancer 77:295–301
123. Radinsky R (1995) Molecular mechanisms for organ-specific colon carcinoma metastasis. Eur J Cancer 31A:1091–105
124. Radinsky R, Ellis LM (1996) Molecular determinants in the biology of liver metastasis. Surg Oncol Clin N Am 5:215–229
125. Zeelenberg IS, Ruuls-Van Stalle L, Roos E (2003) The chemokine receptor CXCR4 is required for outgrowth of colon carcinoma micrometastases. Cancer Res 63:3833–3839
126. Brooks SA, Lomax-Browne HJ, Carter TM, Kinch CE, Hall DM (2010) Molecular interactions in cancer cell metastasis. Acta Histochem 112:3–25

Chapter 8
Tumor Dormancy in Liver Metastasis: Clinical and Experimental Evidence and Implications for Treatment

Jason L. Townson and Ann F. Chambers

Abstract Cancer, and more specifically metastatic cancer, continues to be a leading cause of death worldwide. One of the most common organs in which metastatic cancer is diagnosed, and where it is often fatal, is the liver. This is not surprising given the large volume of nutrient-rich blood filtered through the fenestrated sinusoids of the liver. And while progress has been made in our understanding and treatment of metastatic disease, the majority of treatments are still ultimately unsuccessful in the metastatic setting. In the case of liver metastasis, even after apparently successful initial treatment, 5 year survival remains relatively low. Yet, although metastatic disease is associated with poor prognosis, the process of metastasis itself is known to be highly inefficient. The reasons for this inefficiency and the failure of cancer cells to form large vascularised metastases are, at least initially, twofold – cell death and dormancy. Dormant solitary metastatic cells and micrometastases have been proposed to be responsible, at least in part, for treatment failure and recurrence months to decades following initial treatment. Here we review experimental and clinical evidence regarding metastatic dormancy and discuss the implications of dormant cell populations for treatment of metastatic disease.

Keywords Metastasis · Liver · Dormancy · Solitary cell · Cancer treatment

Abbreviations

CDK	cyclin dependent kinase
CDKI	cyclin dependent kinase inhibitor
CMF	cyclophosphamide, methotrexate, fluorouracil
CSCs	cancer stem cells
CTCs	circulating tumor cells
DTCs	disseminated tumor cells

A.F. Chambers (✉)
London Regional Cancer Program, 790 Commissioners Road East, Office A4-903B, London, ON, Canada, N6A 4L6; Department of Oncology and Department of Medical Biophysics, University of Western Ontario, London, ON, Canada, N6A 4L6
e-mail: ann.chambers@Lhsc.on.ca

P. Brodt (ed.), *Liver Metastasis: Biology and Clinical Management*, Cancer Metastasis – Biology and Treatment 16, DOI 10.1007/978-94-007-0292-9_8, © Springer Science+Business Media B.V. 2011

FAK   focal adhesion kinase
MLCK   myosin light chain kinase
MRI   magnetic resonance imaging
uPAR   urokinase plasminogen activator receptor

Contents

8.1 The Process of Metastasis

Significant progress has been made in our understanding of cancer risk factors and cancer cell biology, as well as our ability to detect, localize and treat specific types of cancer. Indications that these advances are having an impact have recently been observed, including a 4.5% increase in 5-year relative survival for all cancers between 1992–1994 and 2002–2004 [1, 2]. However, despite considerable resources, dedicated research, knowledge generation and technological advancements, cancer remains a leading cause of death, responsible for approximately one in four deaths in North America [1, 2]. The majority of cancer-related deaths however are not due to primary tumors but to metastatic tumors arising from the spread of cancer from one site to another [3, 4]. Yet despite the associated lethality, metastasis is a highly inefficient process whereby only a small fraction of the cancer cells that leave a primary tumor successfully form a tumor in a secondary site [3–11]. This inefficiency is primarily due to cell death at one of the multiple steps a cell must successfully complete in order to form a large metastasis, including: detachment and migration from a primary tumor; intravasation into, and transit through,

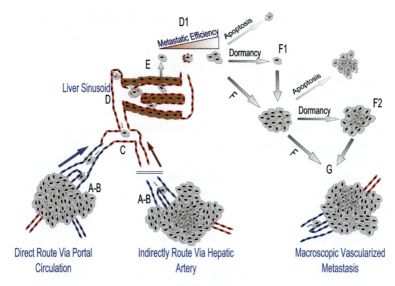

Fig. 8.1 The metastatic process. Metastasis is a multistep process in which all steps must be completed in order for a clinically apparent metastasis to be formed. The process of metastasis leading to a large vascularised secondary tumor starts with escape of a cell or group of cells from a primary tumor (**A**), intravasation into blood or lymph vasculature (**B**), transit in the vasculature (**C**), arrest in a secondary site (**D**), extravasation (**E**), proliferation and sustained growth (**F**) and angiogenesis (**G**). Metastatic dormancy is observed at two stages in the process, the solitary cell (F1) and micrometastasis (F2) stage. Arrest as a bolus of cells or a cell coated with platelets have been found to increase metastatic efficiency (D1). Liver metastases can develop from cancer cells that originate from primary tumors that drain directly into the portal system or indirectly after passing through an upstream organ and arriving via the hepatic artery

blood or lymph vessels; arrest in a secondary site; extravasation; and ultimately the initiation of proliferation, sustained growth and angiogenesis (Fig. 8.1). While cell death is often the primary reason for metastatic inefficiency, experimental metastasis models have revealed that metastatic inefficiency is also due, at least initially, to an often significant population of metastatic cells that remain in the tissue as solitary dormant cells [4–6, 8, 9, 12–16]. It has been proposed that this population of cells, in conjunction with dormant micrometastases, may be responsible for recurrence months to decades following apparently successful treatment [17–22]. However, the mechanisms regulating metastatic dormancy, and in fact the ultimate clinical significance of dormant metastatic disease, are incompletely understood.

8.1.1 Liver Metastasis

Liver is the second most common site of metastasis and metastasis to this site has been found to occur in approximately 41% of cancer patients with metastatic disease [23]. The frequency of metastasis to the liver is not unexpected given the significant volume of nutrient-rich blood that flows through the liver (portal vein and hepatic artery), the number of organs that drain directly into the portal system and the large number of fenestrated sinusoids within the liver. This large blood volume, filtered directly downstream of a number of organs, is significant, if the number of cells that may be shed into the venous circulation ($>3 \times 10^6$ per g of tumor/day) is considered [24]. While the majority of metastases observed in the liver originate from primary tumors in organs that drain directly into the portal system circulation, many, including from the eye, breast and lymph nodes, arrive in the liver via an arterial circulation path and thus do not arrive directly in the liver [3, 23, 25, 26]. The frequent incidence of liver metastasis from cells delivered via both the portal vein and hepatic artery indicate that the liver is a common site of metastasis due to both the incidence of cell arrest (first pass arrest from the portal system) and suitability of the microenvironment for growth (from the previously "filtered" arterial system). Yet despite the high incidence of liver metastasis from multiple primary tumors, the efficiency of metastases formation from cells that successfully arrive in the liver is very low [5, 6, 9, 15, 27]. In experimental models, the majority of cells have been shown to survive the process of cell arrest and extravasation in lung and liver, but most cells will subsequently either die or remain dormant [6, 8, 9, 16]. Liver resection techniques and chemotherapy treatment strategies have appreciably improved 5 year survival rates for patients with liver metastases, yet a large proportion of patients still do not survive that long [28]. In order to make substantial improvements to survival rates of patients with metastases to liver, as well as other organs, treatment strategies may need to be re-examined with increased consideration given to the entire cancer cell population, inclusive of the dormant metastatic cell population.

8.1.2 Treatment Failure and Recurrence

Cancer recurrence and the large number of deaths resulting from metastases are due to the failure of treatment to completely eradicate all cells responsible for the disease. Several plausible explanations for the often significant failure rates of treatment have been proposed including late stage of detection (i.e. number of metastases and extent of invasion), difficulty in accessing the tumor for treatment (barriers to physical and/or chemical intervention) and cancer cell drug or radiotherapy resistance. More recently, it has been proposed that failure to target distinct subpopulations of cancer cells with stem like properties (cancer stem cells [CSCs]) may in fact be responsible for treatment failure and recurrence [29, 30]. In any case, if treatment of all clinically apparent tumors is considered successful (i.e. no longer clinically detectable), recurrent disease is then due to occult or sub-clinical metastases, some of which may be dormant. As the dormant metastatic cell population has been shown to survive treatment that successfully inhibits growth of large vascularised metastases, treatment options will need to take into account the unique properties of this cancer cell population in order that it can be eradicated [5, 31]. Developing treatments that target specific subpopulations of cancer cells, and metastatic cells in particular, will require modifications to the way in which most

Table 8.1 Rational animal models for pre-clinical treatment development. Pre-clinical animal models of treatment efficacy should be chosen based on the clinical target. Patients can present with a primary tumor only, lymph node involvement and/or local metastases and/or distant metastases. The stage of disease in combination with other tumor properties (e.g. markers such as HER2, ER, PR receptors etc.) are used to determine the treatment regimen. Models that best mimic these clinical settings are available and treatment development should make use of experimental models that most closely mimic the stage of disease progression being targeted

Clinical target	Clinical treatment setting	Appropriate animal model
Primary tumor	Neoadjuvant and/or primary surgery	Orthotopic primary tumor model
Presumed micrometastatic disease	Adjuvant	Micrometastasis/dormancy models
Macroscopic metastatic disease	Metastatic	Metastasis models

treatments are developed and tested [32, 33]. There are multiple types of pre-clinical models of primary cancer and metastatic disease in which drug efficacy can be assessed (Table 8.1). Yet superficial orthotopic and ectopic injection sites, that are used to model primary tumor growth, are often chosen due to the relative ease of injection and quantification of treatment effects. However, recent evidence suggests that the focus on "primary tumor" models in drug efficacy studies may lead to the development of drugs that have minimal benefit, or may even be harmful, to patients with metastatic disease [32, 34, 35]. Moreover, it is unlikely that dormant metastases (either pre-angiogenic micrometastases or single cells) will respond to treatment in the same manner as primary tumors or large vascularised metastases. This has, in fact, been demonstrated in pre-clinical models and is supported by clinical data presented by Demicheli et al., showing that adjuvant systemic chemotherapy following surgery had no effect on a second peak (at around 60 months) of recurrence in breast cancer patients, a peak that was attributed to pre-existing dormant metastases [5, 36]. Given the differences in response of the various cancer cell subpopulations to treatment, it may be advantageous to choose pre-clinical models that better relate to the clinical setting in which the drug will be used, as outlined in Table 8.1. As such, a better understanding of metastatic dormancy and its therapeutic implications must also be considered in developing novel treatment strategies. In this chapter, we will review experimental and clinical data regarding metastatic dormancy and discuss the implications of the dormant metastatic population to cancer treatment.

8.2 Metastatic Dormancy in Experimental Models – Solitary Cells and Micrometastases

Dormancy has been used to describe two distinct subpopulations of metastatic cells, both of which have been observed to exist in multiple metastasis models [6, 12, 15, 17–19, 27, 37–39]. The two stages of metastatic progression at which dormancy has been observed and characterized are at the solitary cell stage and the pre-angiogenic micrometastasis stage (Fig. 8.1). However, although both are considered manifestations of metastatic dormancy, and often referred to as micrometastases, these distinct subpopulations of cells differ in several significant ways and will likely need to be dealt with as two distinct treatment targets. After arrival in a secondary site, the first stage at which dormant metastatic cells have been observed occurs at the solitary cell stage (Fig. 8.1 – F1). These cells are considered to be dormant due to the absence of markers of proliferation or apoptosis, as well as to retention of exogenous labels that are diluted below the threshold of detection following a few cell divisions [6, 8, 9, 12–14, 38]. However, the majority of solitary cells observed within a secondary site will not progress to form (micro or macro) metastases but will instead undergo apoptosis, even after initial survival and a variable period of dormancy [6, 8, 9, 16]. The small proportion of solitary cells that do initiate proliferation can give rise to a second category of metastatic dormancy at the micrometastasis stage (Fig. 8.1 – F2). These micrometastases are believed to be restricted in their ability to continue tumor growth, through balanced apoptosis and proliferation, due primarily to lack of their own vasculature or growth suppression by the immune system [17, 18, 39–41]. As these two dormant metastatic cell populations appear to be controlled by different mechanisms and will likely need to be treated as separate therapeutic targets, here we will distinguish between the two and refer to these distinct populations of cells as either solitary dormant metastatic cells or dormant micrometastases (or pre-angiogenic metastases). The understanding of mechanisms controlling dormancy of micrometastases is much further advanced than that of mechanisms controlling solitary cell dormancy [17–19]. Yet while distinct, these two metastatic cell populations do have multiple similarities that complicate both their study and treatment. Primary among these is the technical challenge involved in imaging these cell populations in their typical metastatic sites, that include non-superficial tissues such as liver, lung and bone. Additionally, metastatic efficiency from both of these metastatic cell populations is low as few solitary cells and/or micrometastases observed within an organ progress to form large vascularised metastases within the typical period of experimental observation [6, 8, 9, 42]. This means that even if an individual metastatic cell or micrometastasis is successfully monitored longitudinally, the likelihood that it will commence and continue proliferation within the observation period is low.

8.2.1 The Liver as a Model for Metastatic Dormancy

In addition to the frequency with which liver metastases are observed clinically, multiple properties of the liver make it a useful organ for experimental models of metastasis and in particular metastatic dormancy. First, in comparison to other common sites of metastasis including lung, bone and lymph nodes, the liver is relatively large and easy to access and image due to limited movement or obstruction by bone and/or air [9, 43–48]. Direct injection of cells to the liver via the portal vein system, along with the efficient entrapment of cells within the liver, allows for a relatively high degree of control over the number of cells that initially arrest in the liver. This is important because the number of cells initially present in an organ must be known in order to quantify the subsequent fate of the entire population [9, 48]. Because the majority of cells arrest in the liver following portal vein injection, no significant growth in other organs usually occurs. This ensures that the experiments do not terminate early due to non-specific morbidity [5, 6, 9]. The large number of sinusoids also provides an opportunity for cells to arrest as solitary cells or as small groups of cells. This is significant because the number of cells that arrest together is known to affect cell fate, with increased cell clump size leading to increase metastatic efficiency [49, 50]. By providing organ specific delivery in which the number of cells arresting can be controlled, while at the same time allowing for distribution of solitary cells throughout the entire organ, the liver provides advantages over injections in which cells arrive as a large fluid bolus of cells (i.e. mammary fat pat, subcutaneous, intradermal etc.) or through systemic injections (intracardiac, intravenous, etc.) for the study of metastatic dormancy.

8.2.2 Micrometastasis Dormancy

Dormant solitary cells and micrometastases have been observed in multiple organs, including liver, in a number of different metastasis models [6, 8, 9, 12–15, 18, 19, 27, 51]. Dormant micrometastases have long been recognized as a logical treatment target, with research yielding considerable advances in the understanding of mechanisms controlling pre-angiogenic dormancy [17, 39, 41, 52]. In addition, a number of anti-angiogenic therapies have been developed in order to inhibit growth of tumors beyond the stage of dormant micrometastases [17, 39, 41, 53]. Several recent reviews have discussed the mechanisms controlling tumor angiogenesis (and thereby maintenance of pre-angiogenic dormancy of micrometastases) and treatment strategies based on tumor angiogenesis (The reader is referred to references [17, 42, 54] herein as well to Chapter 15 in the present volume for comprehensive reviews on the subject). Dormant pre-angiogenic micrometastases will therefore be discussed here only in the context of their significance as a sub-population of metastatic cells that should be considered when planning treatment strategies to ensure that eradication of all cancer cells is achieved. To this end, it should be emphasized that micrometastasis dormancy is achieved by a state of balanced apoptosis and proliferation such that the tumor does not continue to expand beyond approximately 1 mm [42]. Thus, while "dormant" in terms of metastatic progression and tumor expansion, cells in pre-angiogenic micrometastases may not be dormant from a cell cycle perspective.

8.2.3 Models of Solitary Metastatic Cell Dormancy

Solitary dormant metastatic cells differ from dormant micrometastases in that solitary cell dormancy is defined by lack of proliferation and apoptosis (not balanced rates), and the cells are believed to be arrested in the G0–G1 phase of the cell cycle [6, 8, 9, 18, 19]. These cells have been observed to exist either alone or in the presence of actively proliferating and growing metastases [6, 8, 9, 12–15, 18,

19, 27, 51]. Despite their common presence, few of the solitary metastatic cells observed will ever begin proliferating or sustain growth to form the large vascularised metastases that are of primary clinical concern, at least within typical experimental observation periods. Most solitary metastatic cells will undergo apoptosis, or remain dormant for the duration of the observation [6, 8, 9]. Yet solitary dormant metastatic cells have been shown to maintain their ability to proliferate as they can form tumors in vivo or continue to grow in 2D cell cultures upon isolation even following treatment with cytotoxic chemotherapy [6, 14, 15]. Relatively few models of solitary cell dormancy, in which cells persist as solitary cells within an organ (without proliferating) for a prolonged period of time, have been identified due to the natural focus of research on cell lines which form metastases during a reasonably short experimental period. However, even in cell lines that are categorized as highly metastatic, a significant population of solitary dormant cells is often observed in the same organ that also harbors actively growing metastases [6, 8, 9]. In order to avoid the short experimental time frame often caused by the morbidity and mortality associated with rapidly growing metastatic cells lines, it may be better to choose "non-metastatic" or poorly metastatic cell lines to study solitary cell dormancy. Cells that persist within an organ for extended periods of time without commencing proliferation allow for a suitable period in which to modify and observe alterations to growth dynamics and fate. Studies of these cells may provide insight into mechanisms controlling dormancy. One of the better characterized and understood models of solitary metastatic cell dormancy is the D2.0R murine mammary carcinoma cell line in mouse liver [5, 6, 55–59]. When injected into mouse liver via the mesenteric vein, a large proportion of these cells initially remain dormant but maintain the capacity to form large macroscopic metastases approximately 11 weeks after injection [5, 6]. Additional cell lines have also been shown to preferentially survive in liver or lung for extended periods of time, yet the mechanisms controlling site-specific survival and dormancy remain to be fully understood [14, 15, 27].

8.2.4 Imaging and Mechanisms of Solitary Metastatic Cell Dormancy

Recent advances in imaging and diagnostic technology have increased the ability to detect and image solitary metastatic cells in vivo. Yet, while a number of imaging modalities now possess detailed μm (10–100 s) scale resolution (magnetic resonance imaging (MRI), computed tomography (CT), ultrasound and intravital microscopy), only MRI and intravital microscopy are currently capable of detecting, and only intravital microscopy is capable of resolving, at the scale of a single cell [60]. Additionally, optical microscopy continues to be the only imaging modality currently capable of the resolution necessary to visualize sub-cellular events. The ability to detect and image single cells has been enhanced by a number of improvements in fluorescent cell labels and molecular identification of human cells in mice [45, 60–66]. Both endogenous and exogenous fluorescent cell labels are continuing to improve, producing brighter, more specific (wavelengths and cellular localization) and stable cellular fluorescence options. Cellular MRI can also be used to provide a non-invasive mean by which the metastatic cell population can be monitored longitudinally, as solitary cells labelled with iron particles have been observed in brain and liver [12, 13, 38]. However, beyond single time point (or short observation times) imaging and detection, longitudinal in vivo cellular imaging remains a significant technical challenge. Barkan et al. [56], recently showed that while no significant period of dormancy is observed in metastatic cells lines in a 2D in vitro culture system, variable periods of solitary cell dormancy are observed with multiple cells lines in 3D cell culture conditions. This included the D2.0R cell line that remained dormant in the 3D cell culture model for the entire 14 day period of observation. In addition, a number of other cell lines were found to remain dormant in 3D cell cultures in a manner that correlated with their proliferative behavior in vivo [56]. It was reported that integrin β1 binding and myosin light chain kinase (MLCK) signalling were responsible for controlling solitary dormancy in this 3D cell culture model, and inhibition of MLCK led to enhanced solitary cell dormancy in a lung metastasis model. These results were subsequently confirmed using similar 3D cell culture and lung metastasis models in which integrin β1 signalling through focal adhesion kinase (FAK) was found to control solitary cell dormancy [55]. The results of these 3D cell culture models are in agreement with a number of in vivo experiments indicating that solitary metastatic cell dormancy is controlled by cell surface receptor binding (e.g. fibronectin, integrin β1, uPAR etc.), subsequent signal transduction (via MLCK, FAK, p38, ERK) and cell cycle control via cyclin dependent kinases (CDK) and cyclin dependent kinase inhibitors (CDKI) [55, 56, 67–76].

8.3 Clinical Dormancy and Recurrence

Improved screening techniques made possible by advances in medical imaging and diagnostic technology have allowed for detection and diagnosis of cancer while tumors are still relatively small (see Chapter 11 "Imaging of liver metastases"). Detection of single or small numbers of cancer cells in the bone marrow (disseminated tumor cells – DTCs) and blood (circulating tumor cells – CTCs) is possible using a variety of cytometric, immunological or molecular methods [77]. However, while it is possible to detect the presence of individual cancer cells in bone marrow, blood and other fluids, localization and longitudinal observation of individual solitary cells or pre-angiogenic micrometastases in patients over time is not yet feasible. As a result, the majority of clinical data regarding metastatic dormancy has been obtained primarily from studies of recurrence and/or death patterns following initial treatment or detailed examination of tissue at autopsy [7, 21–23, 36, 78–85]. However, several limitations exist regarding interpretation of these data with respect to metastatic dormancy. While analysis of recurrence patterns following initial treatment provides evidence for the existence of clinically undetectable disease, it does not yield any information regarding mechanisms and does not prove that recurrence is due to metastatic dormancy. In addition, much like in experimental models, only amplified by virtue of relative size and lack of cell labelling, the chances of "false negative" results during liver autopsy are high and autopsies can only provide information about the cells at a single point in time [79]. Despite these limitations, these two sources of clinical data when combined can yield significant information regarding a subpopulation of cells that is likely responsible for recurrence and ultimate treatment failure. Much of the data regarding recurrence and mortality following initial treatment have originated from patients with primary breast cancer, a tumor type that often metastasizes to the liver [3, 86, 87]. Interestingly, many of the findings regarding recurrence and mortality rates can probably be generalized to multiple sites of metastasis including the liver, as suggested by Demicheli et al. who recently found that breast cancer recurrence dynamics did not depend on the site of recurrence [88].

8.3.1 Patterns of Recurrence

While no definitive criteria for clinical classification of cancer as dormant have been established, it has been demonstrated that many cases of recurrence can be better explained by a kinetic growth model consistent with a period of dormancy followed by rapid growth than by a model of continuous tumor growth [21, 22, 78, 89]. Retrospective analysis of breast cancer patients treated by mastectomy, with or without adjuvant therapy has provided significant insight into the dynamics of recurrence and dormancy, revealing recurrence up to two decades following initial treatment [22, 36, 81, 84]. In 1173 patients treated by mastectomy alone between 1964 and 1980, two distinct peaks in recurrence (at any site) were observed at 18 and 60 months following surgery [21]. These peaks of recurrence following treatment were shown to be influenced by other factors including menopausal status, lymph node involvement, primary tumor size and adjuvant treatment [21, 36, 84, 90]. Interestingly, adjuvant treatment with a combination of cyclophosphamide, methotrexate, fluorouracil (CMF) was shown to reduce early recurrences (first 4 years) with little benefit for late recurrence or the overall recurrence rate [36, 82, 90, 91]. It was speculated that this was due to effective treatment of pre-existing micrometastases that would be sensitive to adjuvant therapy (and recur first) and inability to kill solitary dormant cells that may recur later [36, 82, 91]. Analysis of more recent data from patients treated with current standard therapy (combinations of surgery, radiation, chemotherapy and hormone and/or molecular targeted therapy, depending on tumor markers) have not consistently revealed the same dual peak recurrence pattern, although delayed recurrence was still observed and was suggestive of the presence of metastatic dormancy [92–94].

8.3.2 Circulating and Disseminated Tumor Cells

A number of recent studies have shown that circulating (CTCs) and disseminated (DTCs) tumor cells are present in many cancer patients [77]. While the significance of the presence of CTCs is still being evaluated, the presence of DTCs at the time of resection has been reported to correlate with poor prognosis in a variety of primary cancers [77]. Although able to show the presence of individual or small groups of cells, technologies for DTC and CTC detection are still subject to the limitation that while showing the presence of cells, they cannot discern if the cells are dormant metastases. Taken together, the clinical evidence discussed above strongly supports the clinical presence of dormant metastases. The detection of individual or small groups of cells (autopsy, CTCs and DTCs) that are associated with recurrence is better explained by kinetic models in which a period of dormancy exists. At a minimum, these findings support the idea that a heterogeneous population of cancer cells is present in most patients and that multiple treatment strategies will likely be required in order to eradicate all cells.

8.4 Therapeutic Implications

The presence of dormant metastases presents a number of therapeutic challenges ranging from the detection and localization of such inherently small events to treatment resistance of cells that can exhibit multiple passive and active defence mechanisms against traditional cancer treatments [5, 18, 19, 30, 95–97]. There is growing evidence that treatment that effectively inhibits growth of primary tumors may have little effect on metastases and may in some cases even enhance metastasis [32, 34, 35, 83]. This concept may be extended further to the different metastatic cell populations (i.e. solitary cells, micrometastases and large vascularised metastases) where treatment that effectively inhibits growing metastases has been shown to have no effect on viability or growth potential of solitary dormant cells [5, 97]. This is further complicated by the fact that not all occult metastases are dormant and not all dormant cells share the same fate or even metastatic potential. It is not currently feasible to determine if any given solitary dormant cell will eventually undergo apoptosis, continue to remain dormant or commence and continue proliferation and growth to form a clinically apparent large vascularized metastasis. Regardless of the fate of an individual cell, it is unlikely that these distinct populations of cells that differ in their vascularisation, proliferation status, drug resistance mechanisms and size will respond uniformly to treatment (Fig. 8.2). As such, the unique properties of the heterogeneous metastatic cell population, inclusive of dormant metastatic cell populations, should be considered in order to achieve the treatment goal of eradicating all cancer cells.

8.4.1 Direct Treatment Limitations Imposed by Size

At the most basic level, the first challenge associated with treatment of dormant metastatic cells is detection and localization of individual or small groups of cancer cells that can be as small as 10–20 μm. Advances in imaging technologies have successfully lowered the threshold of tumor detection to the millimetre range (see

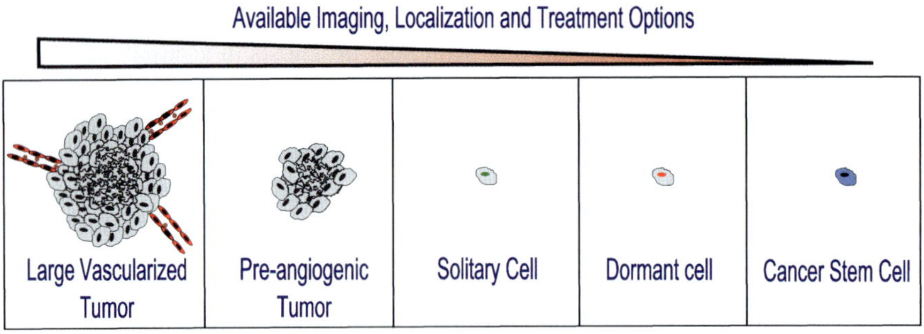

Available Imaging, Localization and Treatment Options

| Large Vascularized Tumor | Pre-angiogenic Tumor | Solitary Cell | Dormant cell | Cancer Stem Cell |

Fig. 8.2 Heterogeneity of cancer cell populations. The heterogeneous cancer cell subpopulations differ in their response to treatment, as well as their accessibility for detection clinically. Large, vascularized and localized tumors can often be successfully treated by loco-regional approaches (surgery, radiotherapy). However, the number of treatment options and the ability to image the cancer cell population decrease as a function of tumor size with individual cells and disseminated metastatic disease most difficult to image or treat. The gain of passive (dormancy) and active (drug resistance) defence mechanisms likely renders dormant cells and cells with stem-like properties a more difficult cell population to eradicate by treatment

Chapter 11), however this is insufficient to detect dormant solitary cells and in most cases, micrometastases. As such, these cancers are often referred to as "occult" or "clinically undetectable" metastases. And while it is possible to detect the presence of small numbers of cells in bone marrow and body fluids, this does not assist in localization of cells for direct treatment methods including surgery and radiation. Surgical resection of all visible liver metastases significantly improves survival, yet a considerable number of patients die from recurrence of metastases, not originally apparent (occult or sub-clinical) at the time of initial resection, even with the addition of adjuvant chemotherapy [98–100]. And while the addition of repeat resections, staged resections and portal vein embolization to treatments regimens have appreciably improved outcome (see Chapters 12 and 13 in this volume), a significant proportion of patients with metastatic liver cancer do not survive for 5 years [28, 101]. Surgical removal of tumors provides obvious and immediate clinical benefits; however, it has been proposed that surgery may also have a growth promoting effect on residual metastases by removing angiogenesis inhibition [102]. In addition, wound healing and immune suppression have both been shown (clinically and experimentally) to promote growth and recurrence of metastasis, raising the danger of unintended consequences of treatment [40, 103–105]. In any case, the inability to localize occult metastases seems to necessitate the use of adjuvant systemic therapy capable of targeting all occult cancer cells, including dormant metastatic cells, regardless of the ability to observe or localize them.

8.4.2 Systemic Therapy

The ideal systemic therapy would be delivered to and be effective against all target cells with limited effect and toxicity on non-target cells. This has long been a goal of cancer treatments. However, it is possible that the design of treatments that specifically target an individual cell when "scaled up" to target larger metastases will be more effective than most treatments that are "scaled down" from targeting larger tumors. A number of therapeutic strategies are now emerging that have the potential to treat all cells in the metastatic cell population, independently of their state of proliferation or the ability to clinically localize them. Targeting of individual metastatic cell populations may be achievable by increasing cell specific delivery and/or by enhancing the specific activity of a given treatment towards a particular cell type. These include a number of molecular targeting agents that exploit functional differences in cell surface receptor expression, kinase activity and signalling pathways between cancer and non-cancer cells [106–108]. In addition, targeted therapy that has the potential to deliver much higher doses of a drug to specific cell types has significant promise [109–111]. These types of therapies may be most advantageous as they would increase therapeutic ratio by increasing the amount and specificity of treatment delivered to cancer cells. A number of therapies that increase specific delivery and/or activity are now used in the clinic or being evaluated in pre-clinical models and clinical trials. Cancer vaccines have a number of obvious advantages, however notable challenges related to identification of cancer specific antigens and the associated danger of inducing an autoimmune reaction remain to been fully overcome [40, 112–114]. It is easier to cease an administered treatment to limit toxicity than to stop the activity of the immune system once it has been activated. A natural systemic approach that is showing promise is that of oncolytic viruses [115–119]. Their ability to preferentially infect and kill cancer cells (based on their dependency on aberrant pathway expression), as well as self-propagate and spread systemically to secondary tumors after inoculation are major advantages. Indeed, treatment with an oncolytic reovirus in patients (phase 1 clinical trial) with refractory primary or metastatic liver cancer resulted in stable disease or partial regression in nine of ten patients who had large tumors and were heavily pre-treated [116]. In addition, recent experimental evidence has demonstrated the ability of an oncolytic reovirus to target CSCs (CD44+/CD24- and Aldefluor +) as well as non-CSCs in an experimental mouse model of breast cancer [115]. This ability to target a number of specific cancer cell subpopulations, regardless of their differences will be essential for treatment to ultimately succeed and will likely require combination therapy.

8.4.3 Treatment Delivery and Combinations

Synthetic drug delivery systems have been developed which are now capable of delivering much higher drug concentrations with adjustable drug loading and release properties [109, 111, 120, 121]. Combining advanced drug delivery technology with cell membrane ligand identification techniques will allow for much more specific and concentrated drug delivery. A recent study of the membrane proteome of metastatic cells found that a number of unique surface markers exist, including many that were previously believed to be expressed only internally [122]. Targeting specific cell pathways, as well as rational drug combinations have also shown promise for treating solitary cells. Interestingly, in an experimental model of multiple myeloma, treatment with bortezomib induced dormancy in a subpopulation of cells, and the addition of salubrinal could eradicate this dormant cell fraction [123]. Given the heterogeneous nature of the cancer cell population, it is likely that a number of treatment approaches that can deliver high drug concentrations of molecular targeting agents to specific cells will be necessary in order to eradicate all cancer cells within the body.

8.5 Conclusion

Treatments that target primary tumors often do not effectively treat metastases and in some cases may actually enhance metastatic growth [32, 34, 35, 83]. Experimental evidence also suggests that treatment that successfully inhibits actively growing metastases does not target dormant metastatic cells [5]. As such, treatment failure and recurrence may therefore be the result of failure to target all cells in the heterogeneous metastatic cell population. Recent advances in cellular imaging and targeted therapies may assist in development of treatments capable of targeting the entire population of metastatic cells. However, appropriate experimental models that better mimic clinical disease progression should be used to develop effective treatments (Table 8.1). In order to target all cells within the cancer cell population, much remains to be learned about the mechanisms controlling this heterogeneity. This includes further elucidation of the intracellular and extracellular control mechanisms that regulate both solitary cell and micrometastatic dormancy. Indeed, the true clinical importance of these metastatic cell populations remains to be determined and many questions remained unanswered: Does the presence of these cell populations indeed cause poor outcome, or are they cancer cells that patients will die with, not from? Do different subpopulations exist within the dormant cell populations? Are surface receptors used to identify specific types of cancer expressed equally on all populations of cells such that they can be used for targeted therapy? Can treatment be used to maintain dormancy indefinitely? Is it possible to verify successful treatment against a population of individual cells distributed throughout the body? Clearly, until we have a better understanding of the significance and mechanisms controlling the heterogeneous metastatic cell populations, emphasis should be placed on treatment and eradication of all metastatic cells, inclusive of the clinically unobservable dormant cell populations.

Acknowledgements Supported by grant #42511 from the Canadian Institutes of Health Research (to AFC). JLT was supported by a doctoral research award from the Canadian Institutes of Health Research. AFC is Canada Research Chair in Oncology, and receives salary support from the Canada Research Chairs Program.

References

1. Canadian Cancer Society. Canadian Cancer Statistics 2009
2. American Cancer Society (2009) Cancer facts & figures 2009. American Cancer Society, Atlanta

3. Chambers AF, Groom AC, MacDonald IC (2002) Dissemination and growth of cancer cells in metastatic sites. Nat Rev Cancer 2:563–72

4. Ambrus JL, Ambrus CM, Mink IB, Pickren JW (1975) Causes of death in cancer patients. J Med 6:61–64

5. Naumov GN, Townson JL, MacDonald IC, Wilson SM, Bramwell VHC, Groom AC et al (2003) Ineffectiveness of doxorubicin treatment on solitary dormant mammary carcinoma cells or late-developing metastases. Breast Cancer Res Treat 82:199–206

6. Naumov GN, MacDonald IC, Weinmeister PM, Kerkvliet N, Nadkarni KV, Wilson SM et al (2002) Persistence of solitary mammary carcinoma cells in a secondary site: a possible contributor to dormancy. Cancer Res 62:2162–2168

7. Weiss L (2000) Metastasis of cancer: a conceptual history from antiquity to the 1990s. Cancer Metastasis Rev 19:I–XI, 193–383

8. Cameron MD, Schmidt EE, Kerkvliet N, Nadkarni KV, Morris VL, Groom AC et al (2000) Temporal progression of metastasis in lung: cell survival, dormancy, and location dependence of metastatic inefficiency. Cancer Res 60:2541–2546

9. Luzzi KJ, MacDonald IC, Schmidt EE, Kerkvliet N, Morris VL, Chambers AF et al (1998) Multistep nature of metastatic inefficiency: dormancy of solitary cells after successful extravasation and limited survival of early micrometastases. Am J Pathol 153:865–873

10. Weiss L (1996) Metastatic inefficiency: intravascular and intraperitoneal implantation of cancer cells. Cancer Treat Res 82:1–11

11. Tarin D, Price JE, Kettlewell MG, Souter RG, Vass AC, Crossley B (1984) Mechanisms of human tumor metastasis studied in patients with peritoneovenous shunts. Cancer Res 44:3584–3592

12. Shapiro EM, Sharer K, Skrtic S, Koretsky AP (2006) In vivo detection of single cells by MRI. Magn Reson Med 55:242–249

13. Heyn C, Ronald JA, Ramadan SS, Snir JA, Barry AM, MacKenzie LT et al (2006) In vivo MRI of cancer cell fate at the single-cell level in a mouse model of breast cancer metastasis to the brain. Magn Reson Med 56:1001–1010

14. Goodison S, Kawai K, Hihara J, Jiang P, Yang M, Urquidi V et al (2003) Prolonged dormancy and site-specific growth potential of cancer cells spontaneously disseminated from nonmetastatic breast tumors as revealed by labeling with green fluorescent protein. Clin Cancer Res 9:3808–3814

15. Guba M, Cernaianu G, Koehl G, Geissler EK, Jauch KW, Anthuber M et al (2001) A primary tumor promotes dormancy of solitary tumor cells before inhibiting angiogenesis. Cancer Res 61:5575–5579

16. Koop S, MacDonald IC, Luzzi K, Schmidt EE, Morris VL, Grattan M et al (1995) Fate of melanoma cells entering the microcirculation: over 80% survive and extravasate. Cancer Res 55:2520–2523

17. Naumov GN, Folkman J, Straume O, Akslen LA (2008) Tumor-vascular interactions and tumor dormancy. APMIS 116:569–585

18. Aguirre-Ghiso JA (2007) Models, mechanisms and clinical evidence for cancer dormancy. Nat Rev Cancer 7:834–846

19. Townson JL, Chambers AF (2006) Dormancy of solitary metastatic cells. Cell Cycle 5:1744–1750

20. Naumov GN, MacDonald IC, Chambers AF, Groom AC (2001) Solitary cancer cells as a possible source of tumour dormancy? Semin Cancer Biol 11:271–276

21. Demicheli R, Abbattista A, Miceli R, Valagussa P, Bonadonna G (1996) Time distribution of the recurrence risk for breast cancer patients undergoing mastectomy: further support about the concept of tumor dormancy. Breast Cancer Res Treat 41:177–185

22. Demicheli R, Terenziani M, Valagussa P, Moliterni A, Zambetti M, Bonadonna G (1994) Local recurrences following mastectomy: support for the concept of tumor dormancy. J Natl Cancer Inst 86:45–48

23. Pickren J, Tsukada Y, Lane W (1982) Liver metastasis. In: Weiss L, Gilbert L (eds) Liver Metastasis. G.K. Hall Medical Publishers, Boston, MA

24. Butler TP, Gullino PM (1975) Quantitation of cell shedding into efferent blood of mammary adenocarcinoma. Cancer Res 35:512–516

25. Diamond JR, Finlayson CA, Borges VF (2009) Hepatic complications of breast cancer. Lancet Oncol 10:615–621

26. Bakalian S, Marshall J, Logan P, Faingold D, Maloney S, Di Cesare S et al (2008) Molecular pathways mediating liver metastasis in patients with uveal melanoma. Clin Cancer Res 14:951–956

27. Logan PT, Fernandes BF, Di Cesare S, Marshall JA, Maloney SC, Burnier MNJ (2008) Single-cell tumor dormancy model of uveal melanoma. Clin Exp Metastasis 25:509–516

28. Sharma S, Camci C, Jabbour N (2008) Management of hepatic metastasis from colorectal cancers: an update. J Hepatobiliary Pancreat Surg 15:570–580

29. Goss P, Allan AL, Rodenhiser DI, Foster PJ, Chambers AF (2008) New clinical and experimental approaches for studying tumor dormancy: does tumor dormancy offer a therapeutic target?. APMIS 116:552–568

30. Croker A, Townson J, Allan A, Chambers A (2009) Tumor dormancy, metastasis, and cancer stem cells. In: Teicher B, Bagley R (eds) Stem Cells and Cancer. Humana Press, New York, NY

31. Eccles SA, Welch DR (2007) Metastasis: recent discoveries and novel treatment strategies. Lancet 369:1742–1757

32. Steeg PS, Anderson RL, Bar-Eli M, Chambers AF, Eccles SA, Hunter K et al (2009) Preclinical drug development must consider the impact on metastasis. Clin Cancer Res 15:4529–4530

33. Welch DR (2006) Do we need to redefine a cancer metastasis and staging definitions? Breast Dis 26:3–12

34. Pàez-Ribes M, Allen E, Hudock J, Takeda T, Okuyama H, Viñals F et al (2009) Antiangiogenic therapy elicits malignant progression of tumors to increased local invasion and distant metastasis. Cancer Cell 15:220–231

35. Ebos JML, Lee CR, Cruz-Munoz W, Bjarnason GA, Christensen JG, Kerbel RS (2009) Accelerated metastasis after short-term treatment with a potent inhibitor of tumor angiogenesis. Cancer Cell 15:232–239

36. Demicheli R, Miceli R, Moliterni A, Zambetti M, Hrushesky WJM, Retsky MW et al (2005) Breast cancer recurrence dynamics following adjuvant CMF is consistent with tumor dormancy and mastectomy-driven acceleration of the metastatic process. Ann Oncol 16:1449–1457

37. Naumov GN, Bender E, Zurakowski D, Kang S, Sampson D, Flynn E et al (2006) A model of human tumor dormancy: an angiogenic switch from the nonangiogenic phenotype. J Natl Cancer Inst 98:316–325

38. Heyn C, Ronald JA, Mackenzie LT, MacDonald IC, Chambers AF, Rutt BK et al (2006) In vivo magnetic resonance imaging of single cells in mouse brain with optical validation. Magn Reson Med 55:23–29

39. O'Reilly MS, Holmgren L, Shing Y, Chen C, Rosenthal RA, Moses M et al (1994) Angiostatin: a novel angiogenesis inhibitor that mediates the suppression of metastases by a Lewis lung carcinoma. Cell 79:315–328

40. Finn OJ (2006) Human tumor antigens, immunosurveillance, and cancer vaccines. Immunol Res 36:73–82

41. Holmgren L, O'Reilly MS, Folkman J (1995) Dormancy of micrometastases: balanced proliferation and apoptosis in the presence of angiogenesis suppression. Nat Med 1:149–153

42. Naumov GN, Akslen LA, Folkman J (2006) Role of angiogenesis in human tumor dormancy: animal models of the angiogenic switch. Cell Cycle 5:1779–1787

43. Graham KC, Ford NL, MacKenzie LT, Postenka CO, Groom AC, MacDonald IC et al (2008) Noninvasive quantification of tumor volume in preclinical liver metastasis models using contrast-enhanced x-ray computed tomography. Invest Radiol 43:92–99

44. Amoh Y, Nagakura C, Maitra A, Moossa AR, Katsuoka K, Hoffman RM et al (2006) Dual-color imaging of nascent angiogenesis and its inhibition in liver metastases of pancreatic cancer. Anticancer Res 26:3237–3242

45. Bouvet M, Tsuji K, Yang M, Jiang P, Moossa AR, Hoffman RM (2006) In vivo color-coded imaging of the interaction of colon cancer cells and splenocytes in the formation of liver metastases. Cancer Res 66:11293–11297

46. Wirtzfeld LA, Graham KC, Groom AC, Macdonald IC, Chambers AF, Fenster A et al (2006) Volume measurement variability in three-dimensional high-frequency ultrasound images of murine liver metastases. Phys Med Biol 51:2367–2381

47. Graham KC, Wirtzfeld LA, MacKenzie LT, Postenka CO, Groom AC, MacDonald IC et al (2005) Three-dimensional high-frequency ultrasound imaging for longitudinal evaluation of liver metastases in preclinical models. Cancer Res 65:5231–5237

48. MacDonald IC, Groom AC, Chambers AF (2002) Cancer spread and micrometastasis development: quantitative approaches for in vivo models. Bioessays 24:885–893

49. Enomoto T, Oda T, Aoyagi Y, Sugiura S, Nakajima M, Satake M et al (2006) Consistent liver metastases in a rat model by portal injection of microencapsulated cancer cells. Cancer Res 66:11131–11139

50. Liotta LA, Saidel MG, Kleinerman J (1976) The significance of hematogenous tumor cell clumps in the metastatic process. Cancer Res 36:889–894

51. Suzuki M, Mose ES, Montel V, Tarin D (2006) Dormant cancer cells retrieved from metastasis-free organs regain tumorigenic and metastatic potency. Am J Pathol 169:673–681

52. Folkman J, Merler E, Abernathy C, Williams G (1971) Isolation of a tumor factor responsible for angiogenesis. J Exp Med 133:275–288

53. O'Reilly MS, Holmgren L, Chen C, Folkman J (1996) Angiostatin induces and sustains dormancy of human primary tumors in mice. Nat Med 2:689–692

54. Favaro E, Amadori A, Indraccolo S (2008) Cellular interactions in the vascular niche: implications in the regulation of tumor dormancy. APMIS 116:648–659

55. Shibue T, Weinberg RA (2009) Integrin {beta}1-focal adhesion kinase signaling directs the proliferation of metastatic cancer cells disseminated in the lungs. Proc Natl Acad Sci USA 106:10290–10295

56. Barkan D, Kleinman H, Simmons JL, Asmussen H, Kamaraju AK, Hoenorhoff MJ et al (2008) Inhibition of metastatic outgrowth from single dormant tumor cells by targeting the cytoskeleton. Cancer Res 68:6241–6250

57. Morris VL, Koop S, MacDonald IC, Schmidt EE, Grattan M, Percy D et al (1994) Mammary carcinoma cell lines of high and low metastatic potential differ not in extravasation but in subsequent migration and growth. Clin Exp Metastasis 12:357–367

58. Morris VL, Tuck AB, Wilson SM, Percy D, Chambers AF (1993) Tumor progression and metastasis in murine D2 hyperplastic alveolar nodule mammary tumor cell lines. Clin Exp Metastasis 11:103–112

59. Rak JW, McEachern D, Miller FR (1992) Sequential alteration of peanut agglutinin binding-glycoprotein expression during progression of murine mammary neoplasia. Br J Cancer 65:641–648

60. Weissleder R, Pittet MJ (2008) Imaging in the era of molecular oncology. Nature 452:580–589

61. Yamamoto N, Jiang P, Yang M, Xu M, Yamauchi K, Tsuchiya H et al (2004) Cellular dynamics visualized in live cells in vitro and in vivo by differential dual-color nuclear-cytoplasmic fluorescent-protein expression. Cancer Res 64:4251–4256

62. Kobayashi H, Ogawa M, Kosaka N, Choyke PL, Urano Y (2009) Multicolor imaging of lymphatic function with two nanomaterials: quantum dot-labeled cancer cells and dendrimer-based optical agents. Nanomed 4:411–419

63. Shaner NC, Campbell RE, Steinbach PA, Giepmans BNG, Palmer AE, Tsien RY (2004) Improved monomeric red, orange and yellow fluorescent proteins derived from Discosoma sp. red fluorescent protein. Nat Biotechnol 22:1567–1572

64. Ikawa K, Terashima Y, Sasaki K, Tashiro S (2002) Genetic detection of liver micrometastases that are undetectable histologically. J Surg Res 106:124–130
65. Sakaue-Sawano A, Ohtawa K, Hama H, Kawano M, Ogawa M, Miyawaki A (2008) Tracing the silhouette of individual cells in S/G2/M phases with fluorescence. Chem Biol 15: 1243–1248
66. Sakaue-Sawano A, Kurokawa H, Morimura T, Hanyu A, Hama H, Osawa H et al (2008) Visualizing spatiotemporal dynamics of multicellular cell-cycle progression. Cell 132: 487–498
67. Allgayer H, Aguirre-Ghiso JA (2008) The urokinase receptor (u-PAR) – a link between tumor cell dormancy and minimal residual disease in bone marrow? APMIS 116:602–614
68. Schewe DM, Aguirre-Ghiso JA (2008) ATF6alpha-Rheb-mTOR signaling promotes survival of dormant tumor cells in vivo. Proc Natl Acad Sci USA 105:10519–10524
69. Aguirre-Ghiso JA, Ossowski L, Rosenbaum SK (2004) Green fluorescent protein tagging of extracellular signal-regulated kinase and p38 pathways reveals novel dynamics of pathway activation during primary and metastatic growth. Cancer Res 64:7336–7345
70. Aguirre-Ghiso JA, Estrada Y, Liu D, Ossowski L (2003) ERK(MAPK) activity as a determinant of tumor growth and dormancy; regulation by p38(SAPK). Cancer Res 63:1684–1695
71. Liu D, Aguirre Ghiso J, Estrada Y, Ossowski L (2002) EGFR is a transducer of the urokinase receptor initiated signal that is required for in vivo growth of a human carcinoma. Cancer Cell 1:445–457
72. Aguirre Ghiso JA (2002) Inhibition of FAK signaling activated by urokinase receptor induces dormancy in human carcinoma cells in vivo. Oncogene 21:2513–2524
73. Aguirre-Ghiso JA, Liu D, Mignatti A, Kovalski K, Ossowski L (2001) Urokinase receptor and fibronectin regulate the ERK(MAPK) to p38(MAPK) activity ratios that determine carcinoma cell proliferation or dormancy in vivo. Mol Biol Cell 12:863–879
74. Ossowski L, Aguirre-Ghiso JA (2000) Urokinase receptor and integrin partnership: coordination of signaling for cell adhesion, migration and growth. Curr Opin Cell Biol 12:613–620
75. Ossowski L, Aguirre Ghiso J, Liu D, Yu W, Kovalski K (1999) The role of plasminogen activator receptor in cancer invasion and dormancy. Medicina (B Aires) 59:547–552
76. Aguirre Ghiso JA, Kovalski K, Ossowski L (1999) Tumor dormancy induced by downregulation of urokinase receptor in human carcinoma involves integrin and MAPK signaling. J Cell Biol 147:89–104
77. Pantel K, Alix-Panabières C, Riethdorf S (2009) Cancer micrometastases. Nat Rev Clin Oncol 6:339–351
78. Demicheli R, Retsky MW, Swartzendruber DE, Bonadonna G (1997) Proposal for a new model of breast cancer metastatic development. Ann Oncol 8:1075–1080
79. Weiss L (1992) Comments on hematogenous metastatic patterns in humans as revealed by autopsy. Clin Exp Metastasis 10:191–199
80. Demicheli R, Terenziani M, Bonadonna G (1998) Estimate of tumor growth time for breast cancer local recurrences: rapid growth after wake-up? Breast Cancer Res Treat 51:133–137
81. Karrison TG, Ferguson DJ, Meier P (1999) Dormancy of mammary carcinoma after mastectomy. J Natl Cancer Inst 91:80–85
82. Demicheli R, Retsky MW, Hrushesky WJM, Baum M (2007) Tumor dormancy and surgery-driven interruption of dormancy in breast cancer: learning from failures. Nat Clin Pract Oncol 4:699–710
83. Retsky M, Bonadonna G, Demicheli R, Folkman J, Hrushesky W, Valagussa P (2004) Hypothesis: Induced angiogenesis after surgery in premenopausal node-positive breast cancer patients is a major underlying reason why adjuvant chemotherapy works particularly well for those patients. Breast Cancer Res 6:R372–374
84. Demicheli R, Bonadonna G, Hrushesky WJM, Retsky MW, Valagussa P (2004) Menopausal status dependence of the timing of breast cancer recurrence after surgical removal of the primary tumour. Breast Cancer Res 6:R689–696

85. Demicheli R (2001) Tumour dormancy: findings and hypotheses from clinical research on breast cancer. Semin Cancer Biol 11:297–306
86. Lee YT (1983) Breast carcinoma: pattern of metastasis at autopsy. J Surg Oncol 23:175–180
87. Cifuentes N, Pickren JW (1979) Metastases from carcinoma of mammary gland: an autopsy study. J Surg Oncol 11:193–205
88. Demicheli R, Biganzoli E, Boracchi P, Greco M, Retsky MW (2008) Recurrence dynamics does not depend on the recurrence site. Breast Cancer Res 10:R83
89. Norton L (2007) Tumor dormancy: separating observations from experimental science. Nat Clin Pract Oncol 4:671
90. Demicheli R, Miceli R, Brambilla C, Ferrari L, Moliterni A, Zambetti M et al (1999) Comparative analysis of breast cancer recurrence risk for patients receiving or not receiving adjuvant cyclophosphamide, methotrexate, fluorouracil (CMF). Data supporting the occurrence of 'cures'. Breast Cancer Res Treat 53:209–215
91. Retsky MW, Demicheli R, Swartzendruber DE, Bame PD, Wardwell RH, Bonadonna G et al (1997) Computer simulation of a breast cancer metastasis model. Breast Cancer Res Treat 45:193–202
92. Dignam JJ, Dukic VM (2009) Comments on: Yin W, Di G, Zhou L, Lu J, Liu G, Wu J, Shen K, Han Q, Shen Z, Shao Z. Time-varying pattern of recurrence risk for Chinese breast cancer patients. Breast Cancer Res Treat 116:209–210
93. Yin W, Di G, Zhou L, Lu J, Liu G, Wu J et al (2009) Time-varying pattern of recurrence risk for Chinese breast cancer patients. Breast Cancer Res Treat 114:527–535
94. Brackstone M, Townson JL, Chambers AF (2007) Tumour dormancy in breast cancer: an update. Breast Cancer Res 9:208
95. Dave B, Chang J (2009) Treatment resistance in stem cells and breast cancer. J Mammary Gland Biol Neoplasia 14:79–82
96. Zhou J, Zhang Y (2008) Cancer stem cells: models, mechanisms and implications for improved treatment. Cell Cycle 7:1360–1370
97. Trumpp A, Wiestler OD (2008) Mechanisms of disease: cancer stem cells–targeting the evil twin. Nat Clin Pract Oncol 5:337–347
98. Viganò L, Ferrero A, Lo Tesoriere R, Capussotti L (2008) Liver surgery for colorectal metastases: results after 10 years of follow-up. Long-term survivors, late recurrences, and prognostic role of morbidity. Ann Surg Oncol 15:2458–2464
99. Small R, Lubezky N, Ben-Haim M (2007) Current controversies in the surgical management of colorectal cancer metastases to the liver. Isr Med Assoc J 9:742–747
100. Adam R, Delvart V, Pascal G, Valeanu A, Castaing D, Azoulay D et al (2004) Rescue surgery for unresectable colorectal liver metastases downstaged by chemotherapy: a model to predict long-term survival. Ann Surg 240:644–657; discussion 657–658
101. Bismuth H, Adam R, Navarro F, Castaing D, Engerran L, Abascal A (1996) Re-resection for colorectal liver metastasis. Surg Oncol Clin N Am 5:353–364
102. Demicheli R, Valagussa P, Bonadonna G (2001) Does surgery modify growth kinetics of breast cancer micrometastases? Br J Cancer 85:490–492
103. von Breitenbuch P, Köhl G, Guba M, Geissler E, Jauch KW, Steinbauer M (2005) Thermoablation of colorectal liver metastases promotes proliferation of residual intrahepatic neoplastic cells. Surgery 138:882–887
104. Meredith K, Haemmerich D, Qi C, Mahvi D (2007) Hepatic resection but not radiofrequency ablation results in tumor growth and increased growth factor expression. Ann Surg 245:771–776
105. Ohsawa I, Murakami T, Uemoto S, Kobayashi E (2006) In vivo luminescent imaging of cyclosporin A-mediated cancer progression in rats. Transplantation 81:1558–1567
106. Collins I, Workman P (2006) New approaches to molecular cancer therapeutics. Nat Chem Biol 2:689–700
107. Petrelli A, Giordano S (2008) From single- to multi-target drugs in cancer therapy: when aspecificity becomes an advantage. Curr Med Chem 15:422–432

108. Press MF, Lenz H (2007) EGFR, HER2 and VEGF pathways: validated targets for cancer treatment. Drugs 67:2045–2075
109. Sajja HK, East MP, Mao H, Wang YA, Nie S, Yang L (2009) Development of multifunctional nanoparticles for targeted drug delivery and noninvasive imaging of therapeutic effect. Curr Drug Discov Technol 6:43–51
110. Farokhzad OC, Langer R (2009) Impact of nanotechnology on drug delivery. ACS Nano 3:16–20
111. Peer D, Karp JM, Hong S, Farokhzad OC, Margalit R, Langer R (2007) Nanocarriers as an emerging platform for cancer therapy. Nat Nanotechnol 2:751–760
112. Pittet MJ (2009) Behavior of immune players in the tumor microenvironment. Curr Opin Oncol 21:53–59
113. Aussilhou B, Panis Y, Alves A, Nicco C, Klatzmann D (2008) Tumor recurrence after partial hepatectomy for liver metastases in rats: prevention by in vivo injection of irradiated cancer cells expressing GMCSF and IL-12. J Surg Res 149:184–191
114. Pejawar-Gaddy S, Finn OJ (2008) Cancer vaccines: accomplishments and challenges. Crit Rev Oncol Hematol 2008;67:93–102
115. Marcato P, Dean CA, Giacomantonio CA, Lee PWK (2009) Oncolytic reovirus effectively targets breast cancer stem cells. Mol Ther 17:972–979
116. Park B, Hwang T, Liu T, Sze DY, Kim J, Kwon H et al (2008) Use of a targeted oncolytic poxvirus, JX-594, in patients with refractory primary or metastatic liver cancer: a phase I trial. Lancet Oncol 9:533–542
117. Bell JC (2007) Oncolytic viruses: what's next? Curr Cancer Drug Targets 7:127–131
118. Nguyên TL, Abdelbary H, Arguello M, Breitbach C, Leveille S, Diallo J et al (2008) Chemical targeting of the innate antiviral response by histone deacetylase inhibitors renders refractory cancers sensitive to viral oncolysis. Proc Natl Acad Sci USA 105:14981–14986
119. Muster T, Rajtarova J, Sachet M, Unger H, Fleischhacker R, Romirer I et al (2004) Interferon resistance promotes oncolysis by influenza virus NS1-deletion mutants. Int J Cancer 110:15–21
120. Liu J, Stace-Naughton A, Jiang X, Brinker CJ (2009) Porous nanoparticle supported lipid bilayers (protocells) as delivery vehicles. J Am Chem Soc 131:1354–1355
121. Liu J, Jiang X, Ashley C, Brinker CJ (2009) Electrostatically mediated liposome fusion and lipid exchange with a nanoparticle-supported bilayer for control of surface charge, drug containment, and delivery. J Am Chem Soc 131:7567–7569
122. Roesli C, Borgia B, Schliemann C, Gunthert M, Wunderli-Allenspach H, Giavazzi R et al (2009) Comparative analysis of the membrane proteome of closely related metastatic and nonmetastatic tumor cells. Cancer Res 69:5406–5414
123. Schewe DM, Aguirre-Ghiso JA (2009) Inhibition of eIF2alpha dephosphorylation maximizes bortezomib efficiency and eliminates quiescent multiple myeloma cells surviving proteasome inhibitor therapy. Cancer Res 69:1545–1552

Chapter 9
Role of the IGF-Axis in Liver Metastasis: Experimental and Clinical Evidence

Shun Li, Shoshana Yakar, and Pnina Brodt

Abstract The insulin-like growth factors (IGF)-I and -II and their receptor IGF-IR play a major role during embryogenesis, development and pre-pubertal growth and in the maintenance of tissue homeostasis. A large and compelling body of evidence that accumulated over the past 2 decades has implicated this axis in tumorigenesis and the progression of malignant diseases. Here we summarize the evidence, based on experimental and clinical data that collectively identify the IGF-I receptor/ligand system as an important mediator of tumor metastasis in general, and liver metastasis in particular. We show that the IGF axis can be involved in each of the critical steps of the metastatic process by regulating cell-cell connectivity, tumor cell migration and invasion, angiogenesis and lymphangiogenesis and tumor cell survival and growth in distant sites, particularly the liver. We summarize clinical data based on genomic/proteomic analyses of clinical specimens that identify the IGF axis proteins as potential tumor biomarkers and indicators of advanced disease and review the pharmacological strategies that have been developed to target the IGF axis for anti-cancer therapy and their translational status. Taken together, the data provide a compelling rationale for the use of IGF – targeting strategies as a single modality or in combination with other drugs for prevention and treatment of metastatic disease.

Keywords Metastasis · Liver · IGF · Therapy

Abbreviations

ADAM	a disintegrin and metalloprotease
ARNT	aryl hydrocarbon receptor nuclear translocator
Bcl	B-cell lymphoma -2 family member
bFGF	basic fibroblast growth factor
ECM	extracellular matrix

P. Brodt (✉)
Departments of Medicine and Surgery, The Montreal General Hospital, McGill University and the McGill University Health Center, Montreal, QC, Canada
e-mail: pnina.brodt@mcgill.ca

S. Li and S. Yakar contributed equally to this chapter

P. Brodt (ed.), *Liver Metastasis: Biology and Clinical Management*, Cancer
Metastasis – Biology and Treatment 16, DOI 10.1007/978-94-007-0292-9_9,
© Springer Science+Business Media B.V. 2011

EMT	epithelial-mesenchymal transition
eNOS	endothelial nitric oxide synthase
ERK	extracellular signal-regulated kinase
FAK	focal adhesion kinase
FAS	apoptosis stimulating fragment (CD95)
FASL	FAS ligand
GH	growth hormone
GHRH	GH release hormone
Grb2	growth factor receptor-bound protein 2
HGF	hepatocyte growth factor
HIF-1	hypoxia-inducible factor-1
HRE	hormone response element
HSP90	heat-shock protein 90
HCC	hepatocellular carcinoma
ICAM-1	inter-cellular adhesion molecule 1
IGF-I	type 1 insulin-like growth factor
IGF-II	type 2 insulin-like growth factor
IGF-IR	type 1 insulin-like growth factor receptor
IGF-IIR/M6P-R	type 2 insulin-like growth factor receptor/mannose 6 phosphate receptor
IGFBP	insulin-like growth factor binding protein
IL-1	interleukin 1
IR	insulin receptor
IRS	insulin receptor substrates
JAK	Janus kinase
LPS	lipopolysaccharides
MAPK	mitogen activated protein kinase
MEK	MAP kinase or ERK kinase
MMP	matrix metalloproteinase
MSC	marrow stromal cells
MT1-MMP	membrane type matrix metalloproteinase
mTOR	mammalian target of rapamycin
Np1	neuropilin-1
PDGF	platelet-derived growth factor
PECAM-1	platelet endothelial cell adhesion molecule
PI 3-K	phosphatidylinositol 3-kinase
PKC	protein kinase C
rhIGFBP-3	recombinant human IGFBP-3
Shc	Src homology 2 domain-containing
SLPI	secretory leukocyte proteinaseinhibitor
SOS	son of sevenless
SST-R-II	type II somatostatin receptor
STAT	signal transducers and activators of transcription
TGF	transforming growth factor
TKI	tyrosine kinase inhibitor(s)

TNF-α	tumor necrosis factor-α
TUNEL	terminal deoxynucleotidyl transferase dUTP nick end labeling
uPA	urokinase plasminogen activator
uPAR	uPA receptor
VCAM-1	vascular cell adhesion molecule -1
VEGF	vascular endothelial growth factor
ZEB1	Zinc finger E-box binding factor 1

Contents

9.1 Introduction

9.1.1 The IGF Axis and Its Role in Normal Physiology

The IGF axis consists of three ligands, IGF-I, IGF-II and insulin; five cell-membrane receptors, IGF-I receptor (IGF-IR), insulin receptor (IR), IGF-II receptor (IGF-IIR/mannose 6 phosphate receptor), Insulin receptor-related receptor, and the IGF-IR/IR hybrid heterotetramer; and at least six high affinity binding proteins, IGFBP-1 through -6 [1, 2].

9.1.1.1 The Ligands

IGF-I (70 amino acid residues) and IGF-II (67 amino acid residues) are single-chain polypeptides that are transcribed by two independently regulated genes. In contrast to the more specific secretion of insulin by pancreatic β cells, IGF-I and IGF-II are synthesized in virtually every tissue of the body. However, hepatocytes are the major source of serum IGF-I. Liver IGF-I is regulated mainly by pituitary gland-derived growth hormone (GH), although nutrition and insulin can also play a role [3, 4]. In turn, IGF-I regulates GH production through a tightly controlled feedback loop [5]. In extra-hepatic tissue *igf1* gene expression is regulated by GH as well as tissue-specific factors [6]. The *Igf2* gene is maternally imprinted in human and mice and its expression is GH – independent and regulated by hormones and tissue-specific growth factors [7, 8]. IGF-I and IGF-II share a 62% homology in amino acid sequence and there is a 40% homology between the IGFs and proinsulin [9]. In humans, IGF-I and IGF-II play a major role during embryogenesis and in growth and development. While circulating IGF-I levels decrease after puberty, IGF-II levels remain high throughout adulthood and are 3.5-fold higher than IGF-I levels [1]. In rodents, however, IGF-II is functional during fetal growth and development, but IGF-I is the major circulating ligand in post-natal and adult animals (reviewed in [2]). The endocrine, as well as the autocrine/paracrine growth promoting effects of IGF-I and IGF-II are mediated mainly through binding to, and activation of the IGF-I receptor that conveys survival and mitogenic signals to the cell through a complex network of signaling mechanisms (see below, reviewed in [1]).

9.1.2 The Receptors

The IGF-I receptor is a type 2 tyrosine kinase receptor that has a 60% homology to IR but differs in ligand specificity and the ability to convey growth and survival signals to the cells. The mature cell membrane-bound IGF-IR is a heterotetramer consisting of two 130–135 kDa α-chains and two 90–95-kDa β-chains with several α–α and α–β disulfide bridges. The extracellular α-chains form the ligand-binding domain that binds one ligand molecule, while receptor signaling is transmitted by the intracellular domains of the β subunit. These consist of a binding site for phosphorylated substrates at tyrosine residue 950, a tyrosine kinase domain that contains an ATP-binding site at lysine 1003, three critical tyrosines at positions 1131, 1135 and 1136 and a C-terminal region with several tyrosines and serines such as tyrosines 1250, 1251 and 1316 and serines 1280–1283 that are phosphorylated and play a role in IGF-IR signaling. The receptor binds IGF-I with the highest affinity and IGF-II and insulin with 10 and 100–fold lower affinities, respectively. The IGF-IR is expressed in virtually every tissue of the body except hepatocytes and T lymphocytes [1].

The IGF-IIR (the cation-independent mannose-6-phosphate receptor) is a 300 kDa multifunctional single transmembrane glycoprotein that consists of 15 extracellular repeats, a 23 amino acid transmembrane domain and a 163 amino acid intracellular domain. This receptor mediates the uptake and processing of M6P-containing cytokines and peptide hormones and is involved in diverse functions related to lysosome biogenesis [10]. The IGF-IIR binds IGF-II with high affinity,

IGF-I with very low affinity and does not bind insulin. Unlike IGF-IR, IGF-IIR has no intrinsic signal transduction capability and is not involved in IGF signaling. Its main function within the IGF-axis is to target IGF-II for lysosomal degradation, thereby reducing its bioavailability and mitogenic activity [11].

IGF-II can also bind with high affinity to IR-A, an insulin receptor isoform with mitogenic activity. IR-A enhances the effects of IGF-II during embryogenesis and fetal development. It is also expressed in adult tissues, such as the brain and its upregulated expression has been documented in various cancer cell types such as human breast, colon and lung tumors [12, 13]. In contrast, IR-B is predominantly involved in mediating the metabolic effects of insulin. Finally, hybrid heterodimeric receptors consisting each of an insulin and IGF-IR α-β dimer can also form and participate in IGF signaling. The role of the hybrid receptors in physiology and carcinogenesis is not fully understood and remains an area of active investigation [12]. (Please see diagram in Fig. 9.1)

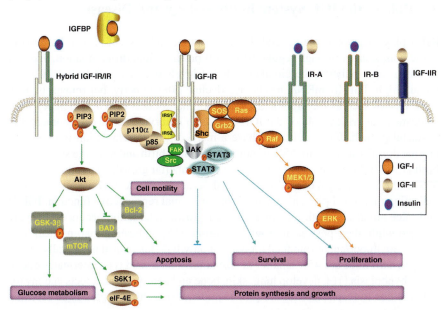

Fig. 9.1 The IGF axis components and signaling pathways downstream of IGF-IR. The IGF system consists of the ligands IGF-I, IGF-II, and insulin. The bioavailability of IGF-I and IGF-II is regulated by a family of IGF binding proteins (IGFBPs). IGF-I and IGF-II bind to IGF-IR-a transmembrane tyrosine kinase receptor that transmits survival and mitogenic signals. Insulin binds to the insulin receptor (IR) that mediates its metabolic effects. Two isoforms of IR can be found on the cell surface, IR-A and IR-B. IR-A is overexpressed in many cancers and can bind IGF-II with high affinity. In addition, hybrid receptors consisting of one α-β dimer of IGF-IR and one α–β dimer of IR-A or IR-B are also expressed on some cells and these can also bind IGF-I or IGF-II. IGF-II can also bind to IGF-IIR (the mannose-6-phosphate receptor) – a single transmembrane glycoprotein that targets IGF-II for lysosomal degradation, thereby regulating its bioavailability. Upon ligand binding, the intrinsic IGF-IR tyrosine kinase is activated and this initiates a phosphorylation/signaling cascade involving the ERK 1/2 of the MAPK pathway, the PI 3-K/Akt pathway and crosstalk with cytokine and integrin-mediated signaling via JAK/STAT and FAK activation, respectively leading to cell survival and proliferation, activation of transcription, increased protein synthesis, cells motility and growth. The ultimate outcome of IGF-IR signaling is cell context dependent

9.1.3 The IGF Binding Proteins

The physiological activities of the IGFs are modulated through their interaction with members of a family of at least six high affinity binding proteins known as the IGFBP-1-6. The IGFBP regulate the biological accessibility and activity of the IGFs and can inhibit or promote IGF functions. For example they can transport IGFs from the circulation to peripheral tissues, maintain a reservoir of IGFs in the circulation by stabilizing the peptides and increasing their half-life or block IGF receptor binding. Some IGFBP can also affect cell growth directly and either stimulate cell growth (e.g. IGFBP-5) or induce apoptosis (e.g. IGFBP-3) in a ligand-independent manner [14].

9.2 Role of the IGF System in Physiology and Disease

IGF-I plays a pivotal role in fetal development and adolescent growth but also in tissue homeostasis through regulation of cell proliferation, differentiation, and cell survival. After puberty, the circulating IGF-I levels decrease, while IGF-II levels remain high. IGF-IR mRNA levels also decline after puberty, but remain high in some tissues such as the brain and kidney. Animal models of IGF deficiency have confirmed the critical role of the IGF ligands in embryogenesis, development and postnatal growth. IGF-I null mice have a marked growth retardation in utero and postnatally. These mice are 65% of normal weight at birth and most die shortly after birth [15–17]. Survivors do not undergo a peri-pubertal growth spurt and have only 30% of the body weight of wild-type animals as adults. These mice are also infertile, indicating that IGF-I plays an essential role in normal reproductive function. IGF-II null mice are also growth impaired but their growth retardation occurs exclusively in utero while their post-natal growth is normal [16], indicating that in mice, both ligands are important during fetal growth but only IGF-I is critical postnatally. IGF-I receptor-null mice are 45% smaller in size at birth than wild type littermates due to organ hypoplasia [16], develop lung, skin, bone and neurological defects and invariably die due to respiratory failure [16, 17], identifying this receptor as an essential regulator of organogenesis.

During adult life, the IGF system continues to play a role in the maintenance of normal health. Together with the insulin system, it plays a role in regulating glucose and lipid metabolism and thereby maintaining muscle mass and function, and adiposity. The IGFs are also involved in the regulation of innate and acquired immunity, in wound healing and tissue repair and in cognitive functions (reviewed in [2, 8, 18]).

Because of the central role that the IGF axis plays in the regulation of cell survival, cell cycle progression, growth and differentiation, an imbalance in the expression of the IGF ligands and/or receptor can result in uncontrolled cell division and ultimately in malignant transformation. Indeed, increased levels of IGF-I,

IGF-II, IGF-IR, or combinations thereof have been documented in multiple human malignancies and high circulating IGF-I levels have been identified as a risk factor for several human malignancies including breast, prostate and colon carcinoma (reviewed extensively in [1, 19] and see further discussion below).

9.3 IGF Signaling

Binding of the IGF ligands to the IGF-IR, activates the intrinsic receptor tyrosine kinase, resulting in autophosphorylation of tyrosines on the intracellular portion of the β-subunit, including tyrosine residues in the juxtamembrane, kinase and C-terminal domains. Once phosphorylated, tyrosine 950 in the juxtamembrane domain serves as a docking site for several substrates, including the insulin receptor substrates (IRS) 1–4 and Shc that initiate phosphorylation cascades that serve to transmit the IGF-IR signal (see reviews in [1, 20]). Phosphorylated IRS-1 activates the p85 regulatory subunit of phosphatidylinositol 3-kinase (PI 3-K) and this results in activation of several downstream substrates, including the protein kinase B (Akt) and the p70 S6 kinase. Akt phosphorylation triggers the anti-apoptotic effects of IGF-IR through phosphorylation and inactivation of Bad and can increase protein synthesis through mTOR activation [21]. IRS-1 is also involved in crosstalk between the IGF axis and other signaling pathways including growth factor, cytokine and integrin – initiated signaling [22–24]. In parallel to PI-3K signaling, recruitment of Grb2/SOS by phosphorylated IRS-1 or Shc leads to activation of the Ras/Raf/MEK/ERK pathway, regulation of gene transcription, cell cycle progression and cell proliferation. IGF-1R can also inhibit the expression of the cell-cycle suppressor p27kip1 and may therefore promote cellular proliferation through multiple pathways.

In some cell types, the IGF-IR can also directly phosphorylate the Janus kinases (JAK)-1 and -2 that are involved in cytokine-mediated signaling, leading to phosphorylation/activation of signal transducers and activators of transcription (STAT) proteins [25]. STAT-3 activation has, in fact, been shown to play an essential role in the transforming activity of IGF-IR [26]. Other molecules activated downstream of IGF-IR are Src, focal adhesion kinase (FAK) and the proto-oncogenes c-Crk II and CrkL that link IGF-IR and integrin-mediated signaling and regulate cell shape and motility (see diagram in Fig. 9.1).

9.4 Role of the IGF Axis in Metastasis

The role of the IGF axis in tumor growth has been studied extensively in both in vitro and in vivo systems. Preclinical studies with numerous tumor cell-types, as well as clinical and epidemiological studies have implicated the IGF axis in the growth of various malignancies including carcinomas of the GI tract such as colorectal, hepatocellular and pancreatic carcinomas. It is important to note, however, that IGFs are not in themselves tumorigenic factors, but rather, activation of the IGF-IR appears to be required for oncogene activation and the resulting increase in cellular proliferation and tumorigenesis [27]. The compelling evidence for the critical role of the IGF axis in malignancy has in recent years led to the development of different strategies for targeting this system in cancer therapy and several therapeutic reagents are presently in clinical trials.

A review of the evidence for the causative/mechanistic role of the IGF axis in malignant disease is beyond the scope of this chapter. The reader is referred to several recent papers, including our own [1, 19, 28] for critical reviews of this subject. Here, we will focus on the evidence that implicates the IGF system in the process of cancer metastasis in general and liver metastasis in particular.

The metastatic process is complex and consists of multiple stages that can be tumor type–specific and depend on the location and molecular makeup of the cells. However, three major steps are commonly required for tumor cells to form distant metastases (1) they must detach from the primary site of growth and migrate; (2) they must access a venue for dissemination such as blood or lymphatic vessels, survive the transit through these venues and have the ability to exit into a secondary site and (3) once in a secondary site, they must survive local apoptosis-inducing mechanisms, proliferate and expand. Each of these steps depends, in turn on multiple molecular interactions between the disseminating tumor cells and their changing microenvironment. Herein, we review the evidence that implicates the IGF axis in each of these major steps and in this context, discuss the particular role of IGF-I, a factor abundant in the liver, in the process of liver metastasis.

9.4.1 Step 1 – Tumor Cell Detachment and Migration

In order for tumor cells to detach from a primary solid mass, cell-cell contacts must be severed. In the epithelium, tissue cohesion is maintained, in large part, by adherens junctions and the resident cadherin/catenin complex that is frequently altered in the tumorigenic process. In epithelial cells, β-catenin binds to the intracellular domain of E-cadherin, linking it to the actin cytoskeleton via α-catenin [29, 30]. Thus, deletion of the α-catenin gene in a human lung cancer [31] or ovarian carcinoma [32] was shown to correlate with loss of cell–cell adhesion. Alterations in the structure or expression of the cadherin-catenin complexes disrupt intercellular connectivity and are frequently a precursor to cell detachment and a key process in the epithelial-mesenchymal transition (EMT) associated with the acquisition of a migratory/invasive phenotype [33]. Indeed, the E-cadherin gene is inactivated in many diffuse-type cancers where the neoplastic cells have typically lost many of their epithelial characteristics and exhibit a highly invasive histological pattern throughout the tumor, as seen in breast lobular carcinoma and diffuse gastric carcinoma [34, 35]. In solid, non-diffuse type cancers, loss of E-cadherin has been observed at the tumor-stroma interface where solitary invading tumor cells can be seen, and the evidence suggests that this process may be regulated by the tumor microenvironment through mediators such as growth factors release by the stromal cells [36]. IGF-I is one factor secreted by different types of stromal cells [37] and in the liver, it is produced by the hepatocytes and can function in a paracrine manner to stimulate tumor cell growth [1, 38–40]. It may also increase the metastatic potential of tumor cells by participating in the EMT process. Indeed, Irie et al. have shown that in breast epithelial MCF-10A cells that were stably transfetced with IGF-IR, IGF-I induced a conversion from epithelial to spindle-shaped morphology and this was associated with E-cadherin repression and the induction of N-cadherin – a cadherin switch characteristic of EMT [41]. More recently, Graham et al. have shown that IGF-I could induce EMT in prostate cancer cells by upregulating ZEB1 – a transcription factor that suppresses E-cadherin expression in various cancer cells [42]. Moreover, tyrosine phosphorylation of the cadherin-associated β-catenin results in the loss of E-cadherin function and cell detachment and IGF-IR can trigger β-catenin phosphorylation through tyrosine phosphorylation of Src – a β-catenin kinase [43]. In α-catenin or E-cadherin-deficient colon cancer cells, IGF-IR signaling was essential for cellular migration and invasion, respectively [44]. In addition to modulating cell migration through regulation of E-cadherin function, the IGF-IR can also promote motility by crosstalk with integrins and molecular mediators of integrin signaling. Namely, IGF-IR can directly phosphorylate FAK and was implicated in paxillin phosphorylation and translocation to focal adhesions in a PI 3-K-dependent manner, resulting in activation of cell migration [45–47].

Several studies have implicated IGF-I induced motility in liver metastasis of different tumor types including human sarcoma [48] and uveal melanoma cells [49] and in the intra and extra-hepatic spread of hepatocarcinoma cells [50, 51].

9.4.2 Step 2 – Tissue Remodeling and Invasion

In order to detach from the primary mass and invade surrounding tissue barriers, tumor cells must also acquire the ability to degrade the extracellular matrix (ECM) and remodel their microenvironment, a process mediated by proteolytic enzymes that can be secreted directly by the tumor cells or by activated host cells residing within, or recruited into the surrounding tissue.

The major group of ECM–degrading proteinases to be implicated in tissue remodeling associated with invasion and metastasis are the matrix metalloproteinases (MMPs) [52]. These Zn^{++}-dependent proteinases play a major role in ECM remodeling and tissue homeostasis under normal physiological conditions and their increased expression/activity have been linked to the acquisition of an invasive/metastatic phenotype in human and animal tumors (see review in [28]). Prominent among the MMPs involved in metastasis are the type IV collagenases MMP-2 and MMP-9 and the membrane type matrix metalloproteinase 1 (MT1-MMP or MMP-14). The IGF system plays a role in the regulation of these MMPs and others and can, thereby, promote tumor invasion. Several groups, including our own, identified IGF-IR as an inducer of MMP-2 synthesis and tumor invasion, as measured in vitro in Matrigel [53–58] and in vivo in animal models [51, 59]. In previous studies by the Brodt group, down or up-modulation of IGF-IR expression was shown to alter MMP-2 expression levels, invasion and metastasis in a Lewis lung carcinoma model of liver metastasis [39, 55]. Using IGF-IR mutants with tyrosine-alanine substitutions in the kinase and C-terminal domains, it was found that signals from both regions of the receptor were required for MMP-2 induction and tumor invasion [60]. It was further shown that the IGF-IR can exert a dual regulatory effect on MMP-2 production, upregulating it when the PI 3-K signaling pathway is optimally activated, but reducing it under conditions that preferentially activate the MAPK pathway. This may partially explain an apparent dichotomy in the role of IGF in MMP-2 regulation, as both positive and negative regulatory effects have been reported [53]. The MMPs are generally produced as inactive proenzymes and require activation through proteolytic processing [52, 61]. MMP-14 is a major proteolytic activator of pro-MMP-2, and has recently been identified as another member of the MMP family that is subject to regulation by the IGF-IR, via PI 3-K/Akt/mTOR signaling [61, 62]. Thus, the IGF axis can optimize ECM degradation and invasion by coordinately modulating MMP-2 production and activation.

The involvement of the IGF axis in the regulation of MMP-9 has also been documented. The effect however, appears to be cell context-specific because IGF-IR activation can induce or block MMP-9 production and activity. For example, IGF-I could significantly increase human breast carcinoma MCF-7 cell surface-associated MMP-9 activity and MMP-9-mediated migration [63] and similarly, in human non-small cell lung carcinoma U-1810 cells, both IGF-I and IGF-II enhanced the expression of the latent forms of MMP-2 and MMP-9 and cell migration [64]. In contrast, we have shown that in murine Lewis lung carcinoma cells with an ectopic IGF-IR overexpression, MMP-9 levels were actually reduced and this was attributable to decreased PKC-α levels in these cells [65], suggesting that expression levels of co-regulators of MMP production may determine the ultimate effect of IGF on MMP-9 levels. Interestingly, a recent study suggests that the link between MMP-9 and the IGF axis may be reciprocal because MMP-9-induced ERK signaling in normal Schwann cells was completely ablated by inhibition of IGF-IR [66].

The MMPs can control IGF signaling through proteolytic cleavage of IGFBPs to releases IGFs and modulate their activity [67–69]. Recent studies have implicated the MMP-7 (also known as matrilysin), an enzyme frequently upregulated during malignant progression and implicated in invasion and metastasis [70] in proteolytic processing of all six IGFBPs, identifying it as an indirect activator of IGF-IR via increased IGF bioavailability [71, 72]. Indeed, MMP-7 and IGFs were coordinately upregulated in gene and protein arrays of various tumor types including head and neck, ovarian and gastric carcinomas, as well as in colon caner liver metastases [73–76]. Of particular interest to this review is the finding that in 205 colorectal specimens analyzed, both MMP-7 and IGF-IR gene expression levels were higher in the cancerous tissue than in adjacent normal mucosa and the expression of the IGF-IR correlated with venous invasion and liver metastasis [76]. Studies on gastrointestinal cancer cell lines identified IGF-IR as a regulator of MMP-7 production and MMP-7 mediated invasion and have shown that blockade of IGF-IR signaling by an IGF-IR dominant negative mutant or the inhibitor NVP-AEW541 reduced MMP-7 production and tumor invasiveness in three different GI cancers in vitro and in vivo [77].

In addition to contributing to invasion via proteolytic degradation of the ECM, MMPs can promote tumor growth and metastasis by other, indirect mechanisms. For example, MMP-7 was shown to release membrane-bound FASL, a transmembrane stimulator of the death receptor FAS and thereby induce apoptosis of neighboring epithelial cells [78] or protect tumor cells from chemotherapeutic-drug induced cytotoxicity [79]. Likewise, MMP-11 was shown to inhibit tumor cell apoptosis, likely via the release of IGFs [68]. The MMPs can also cause the release of growth and migration-stimulating factors sequestered in the ECM, contribute to the host inflammatory response induced by a growing tumor and regulate the process of angiogenesis through pro- and anti-angiogenic effects (reviewed extensively in [52]). IGF-I can therefore affect all of these processes indirectly, through its regulatory role in MMP synthesis.

Another proteinase that is critical in ECM remodeling and tumor invasion is the urokinase plasminogen activator (uPA). The uPA binds to a cell membrane-associated receptor (uPAR) and converts serum plasminogen to plasmin- a serine protease that can degrade basement membrane proteins and promote migration, invasion and metastasis of different cancer types including colon and breast carcinoma cells [80–82]. Plasmin can also contribute to ECM remodeling by activating latent MMPs [52]. In human breast cancer MDA-MB-231 cells, IGF-I was shown to induce uPA expression via PI3-K and MAPK-signaling [83, 84] and an IGF-I propeptide suppressed uPA expression and reduced invasion of these cells in vitro [85]. A reduction in uPA expression and in tumorigenesis was also noted in murine mammary carcinoma EMT6 cells expressing IGF-IR antisense RNA [86]. In human pancreatic carcinoma L3.6pl cells, IGF-IR was shown to regulate the expression of both uPA and uPAR and control cell migration and invasion [87]. In addition to direct transcriptional regulation of uPA via MAPK and PI3-K signaling [84], IGF-I and II can also increase the binding of single-chain uPA (scuPA) to cell-surface uPAR, possibly through post-transcriptional modification of uPAR and thereby trigger uPA activation, as was recently shown in a rhabdomyosarcoma cell line [88]. In addition to MMPs and the uPA/uPAR system, other proteases such as the cysteine protease cathepsin L [89], and the serine protease Matriptase-2 (TMPRSS6) [90] were implicated in cellular responsiveness to IGF and can thereby indirectly affect hepatic metastasis.

9.4.2.1   Step 2a – Angiogenesis

One of the major rate-limiting factors for tumor progression is the availability of nutrients and oxygen. Expanding tumors at the primary or secondary sites can overcome the lack of a nutrient supply and the hypoxic conditions by inducing a process of neo-vascularization, i.e. angiogenesis. The newly formed vessels can also provide the tumor cells with access to the circulation that is essential for hematogenous spread [91, 92].

The process of angiogenesis is triggered in parallel to the process of tumor invasion, and in part, as a response to tumor expansion and the local tissue breakdown and remodeling. Under normal physiological conditions, this is a tightly regulated, multi-step process involving new blood vessel formation from existing microvessels. This process is disregulated in the microenvironment of an invasive tumor, as a local tissue repair cascade is activated and the tumor microenvironment is altered by hypoxia and tumor derived pro-angiogenic factors such as vascular endothelial growth factor (VEGF) basic fibroblast growth factor (bFGF), hepatocyte growth factor (HGF), IGF-I and platelet derived growth factor (PDGF) (reviewed in [93]). These factors can activate endothelial cell migration and proliferation directly by binding to the respective cell surface receptors on the endothelium (e.g. VEGF and bFGF) or by contributing to the recruitment of smooth muscle cells and vessel maturation (e.g. PDGF) [94]. Among the endothelial cell receptors playing a major role in angiogenesis are the vascular endothelial growth factor receptors (VEGFR) -1 and -2 (VEGFR), and their co-receptors neuropilin (Np) -1 and 2. (see Chapter 15 for an overview on targeting angiogenesis in the treatment of hepatic metastases).

The IGF axis contributes to the process of angiogenesis in several ways. IGF-I can regulate VEGF production levels in tumor cells, as was shown in several tumor models. For example, in the thyroid carcinoma cell line SW579, IGF-1 was shown to upregulate VEGF mRNA expression and protein secretion and this was mediated by Akt signaling [95]. Another link between the IGF-IR and VEGFR pathways is via the hypoxia-inducible factors-HIF-1α and HIF-2α. These transcription factors are activated under reduced oxygen tension, and are involved in tumor progression/metastasis in various cancers. However, studies have shown that activation of the PI 3-K/Akt and MAPK pathways by growth factors can activate their expression independently of hypoxia [96–98]. The IGFs can induce the expression of HIF-1α [99], leading to the formation of the HIF-1α/aryl hydrocarbon receptor nuclear translocator (ARNT) complex that is involved in transcriptional regulation of hormone response element (HRE)-containing genes such as VEGF [100]. In contrast to hypoxia, which can induce HIF-1α expression by inhibiting its ubiquitination and degradation, IGF-I can induce HIF-1α and HIF-2α expression directly, via the MAPK and PI 3-K pathways as has been shown in several tumor types including prostate and colon carcinoma and Kaposi sarcoma [96, 101, 102]. This effect appears to depend on the involvement of the molecular chaperone heat-shock protein 90 (HSP90) because inhibition of HSP90 by the selective inhibitor SNX-2112 decreased IGF-I induced Akt and MAPK activation in multiple myeloma cells, blocked angiogenesis and overcame the growth advantage conferred by IGF-I [103]. HSP90 targeting by a geldanamycin derivative also impaired IGF-IR signaling and inhibited neovascularization in vivo in a human pancreatic cancer cell model [104]. In addition to VEGF, HIF-1α can also induce the expression of other genes that contribute to angiogenesis including IGFBPs [99], c-Met (the receptor for the hepatocyte growth factor -HGF) [105, 106], TGFα [107] as well as IGF-II [94, 108], suggesting that the IGF/HIF-1α regulatory link is reciprocal.

The IGF system can contribute to angiogenesis via other mechanisms. For example, IGF-I and II can induce endothelial cell migration [109–111] and IGF-I bound to the sub-endothelial ECM can act as an endothelial cell survival factor [112]. Accordingly, in mice with vascular endothelial cell-specific deletions in the insulin (VENIRKO) or IGF-I (VENIFARKO) receptors, a significant reduction in oxygen-induced retinal neovascularization relative to wild type mice was observed, implicating both insulin and IGF-I in neovascularization and regulation of the vascular mediators VEGF, eNOS, and endothelin-1 [113]. Furthermore, several in vivo studies have shown that IGF-IR inhibitors can reduce tumor-associated angiogenesis. For example, the small molecule IGF-IR kinase inhibitor NVP-AEW541, when administered in vivo, significantly reduced orthotopic pancreatic tumor growth, VEGF expression and tumor induced revascularization [111]. In addition, the IGF-IR tyrosine kinase inhibitor picropodophyllin (PPP) reduced angiogenesis in vivo in the murine multiple myeloma 5T33MM model, causing a significant increase in animal survival [114, 115] and, of particular relevance to this review, an anti-IGF-IR monoclonal antibody EM164, when administered alone or in combination with oxaliplatin, significantly inhibited tumor cell-induced angiogenesis and experimental liver metastasis of human colorectal carcinoma HT-29 cells [116]. Collectively, these studies identify the IGF-IR as a target for anti-angiogenic treatments with relevance to inhibition of liver metastasis.

In addition to angiogenesis, tumor cells can also induce the formation of new lymphatic vessels, a process known as lymphangiogenesis. The major lymphangiogenic factors are VEGF-C and VEGF-D and they bind and activate the receptor VEGFR-3 (also known as *fms*-like tyrosine kinase 4 (Flt-4)) that is specifically expressed on lymphatic endothelial cells. Overexpression of these lymphangiogenic factors in tumor cells leads to the outgrowth of new lymphatic vessels, lymphatic metastases and increased spread to different organ sites, including the liver [117–119]. Several studies, including our own, have identified IGF-IR as a positive regulator of lymphangiogenesis either by activation of VEGF-C production via PI 3-K signaling [120] or by direct stimulation of lymphatic endothelial cell proliferation and migration via IGF-I receptors expressed on these cells [121]. Supportive evidence for the coordinated roles of IGF and VEGF-C in the progression of human malignancies comes from genomic/proteomic analysis of human malignant specimens and serum samples. For example, in cervical cancer patients, a highly significant positive correlation between serum VEGF-C and IGF-II levels was found, with increased serum IGF-II levels indicative of tumor growth and VEGF-C upregulation identified as a unique marker for cervical cancer metastasis [122]. In another study, immunohistochemistry (IHC) performed on oral squamous cell carcinoma specimens identified a correlation between IGF-I expression levels and lymphatic microvessel density in these tumors [123].

Taken together, these results show that the IGF axis can impact angiogenesis and lymphangiogenesis by direct and indirect effects on vascular endothelial cells and through multiple pathways. The IGF system can thereby contribute to liver metastasis by increasing dissemination from the primary tumor, as well as by promoting tumor growth within the liver.

9.4.3 Step 3 – Extravasation and Activation of the Host Stroma in the Target Organ

The process of extravasation namely, tumor cell exit from the circulation into the extravascular space of the target organ is orchestrated by the endothelium and is triggered by tumor cell attachment to vascular endothelial cell adhesion molecules including selectins such as E- and P-selctins, Ig-like receptors such as VCAM-1 and PECAM-1 and integrins such as $\alpha_v\beta_3$. Adhesion to these receptors is mediated through the counter receptors on the tumor cell surface such as the sLew^x and sLew^a antigens (E-selctin ligands) and integrins such as $\alpha_4\beta_1$ (the VCAM-1 counter receptor). Integrins also facilitate tumor cells arrest and extravasation by mediating attachment to extracellular matrix proteins in the space of Disse that separates the endothelial and parenchymal compartments of the liver. Indeed, recent studies, including our own, have identified tumor cell ability to adhere to, and extravasate the hepatic microvasculature as a limiting step that defines the liver-metastasizing potential of colorectal carcinoma cells [124–128] (reviewed in [129]). Several integrins such as $\alpha_2\beta_1$, $\alpha_v\beta_3$ and $\alpha_v\beta_6$ were specifically implicated in adhesion and subsequent growth of colorectal carcinoma cells in the liver and identified as potential markers of liver metastasis and therapeutic targets in this malignancy [130, 131]. (For detailed reviews on the role of inflammation and tumor-endothelial cell adhesion receptors in liver metastasis, see Chapters 6 and 7 in this volume).

While the direct role of the IGF axis in tumor cell adhesion to the hepatic microvasculature and extravasation remains to be elucidated, IGF signaling has been implicated indirectly in these processes. For example, recent studies have shown that in patients with GH deficiency that were treated by GH replacement therapy, serum IGF-I as well as E-selectin and VCAM-1 levels were elevated. Furthermore, direct treatment of human endothelial cells with GH or IGF-I resulted in increased VCAM-1 expression in these cells [132, 133] and this may be due to the role of GH and IGF in regulating endothelial cell production of, and response to inflammatory mediators such as nitric oxide [134] and TNF-α [135].

The IGF axis can also affect the ability of tumor cells entering the liver to modulate the local microenvironment and induce an inflammatory response. Indeed, in a series of studies we have shown that tumor cells entering the liver trigger an inflammatory cascade that begins with a rapid release of TNF-α and IL-1β by resident Kupffer cells and neutrophils and leads to activation of E-selectin, VCAM-1 and ICAM-1 expression on hepatic endothelial cells, tumor cell adhesion and extravasation. Blockade of TNF-α-mediated E-selectin induction by mouse-specific c-Raf antisense oligonucleotides, or an inhibition of E-selectin function by specific neutralizing antibodies, markedly reduced the number of experimental liver metastases formed by human colorectal carcinoma CX-1 and mouse Lewis lung carcinoma-derived H-59 cells, respectively. Furthermore, the ability of tumor cells to activate this response was variable and correlated with the metastatic phenotype of the cells and with IGF-IR receptor levels on the tumor cells [125–128, 136, 137].

A subsequent study has shown that IGF-IR expression levels could regulate tumor cell potential to activate this response by controlling the levels of pro- and anti-inflammatory mediators such as the secretory leukocyte proteinase inhibitor (SLPI) that could modulate TNF-α production by macrophages [138]. The central role that the inflammatory response plays in the early stages of liver metastasis is supported by numerous other studies. For example, administration of LPS, IL-1β or TNF-α was shown to increase liver metastases formation in various tumor models [137, 139–142], whereas a blockade of the IL-1β receptor prior to tumor cell injection, significantly reduced hepatic metastases [143] and this was also observed in mice with a homozygous deletion in the *tnfr1* gene [144] (reviewed in [145]). Finally, we have recently identified hepatic IGF-I as a critical regulator of the local host inflammatory response in the liver. In a mouse model of liver IGF-I deficiency (LID), the metastatic burden following intrasplenic/portal inoculation of mouse colon 38 (MC-38) carcinoma cells was markedly reduced [146] and this was associated with reduced expression levels of multiple inflammatory cytokines such as TNF-α, IL-1β, IL-6 and IL-18, decreased P-selectin and VCAM-1 expression and reduced tumor cells retention in the hepatic microvasculature [146], suggesting that liver-derived IGF-I regulates the function of resident immune cell in the liver, thereby indirectly regulating the type and magnitude of the tumor-induced inflammatory reaction.

9.4.4 Step 4 – Survival and Growth in the Target Organ

Once tumor cells extravasate from the sinusoidal vessels into the space of Disse, several possible scenarios may occur. They may proliferate or migrate further into preferred sites of growth, possibly in response to local chemotactic or growth factors, to form macrometastases. Alternatively, they may initiate a short-lived process of proliferation that is aborted before a metastasis is established or enter a state of dormancy as solitary cells and never produce a metastasis [145, 147, 148]. While the factors that determine tumor cell fate have not been fully elucidated, the evidence suggests that growth factors produced in the liver microenvironment play a critical role.

The liver is the major site of IGF-I production and its role in promoting cancer survival and growth in secondary organs has been studied by several groups. Using variants of the Lewis lung carcinoma, our group identified IGF-I as the major paracrine factor promoting the growth of highly metastatic tumor cells in this organ [38, 39, 56]. Site-directed mutagenesis showed that tyrosines in the kinase and C-terminal domains of the IGF-IR were involved in promoting liver metastasis in this model [60]. Moreover, highly metastatic H-59 cells engineered to express a soluble IGF-IR molecule (IGF-IR^{933}) consisting of the entire extracellular domain of the receptor, had a significantly diminished potential to form liver metastases, directly implicating paracrine, hepatic IGF-I in liver metastasis in this model [149].

Supporting evidence for the role of the IGF axis in promoting cancer growth in the liver came from the LeRoith group using a mouse model of liver specific IGF-I-deficiency (LID) with a 75% reduction in serum IGF-I levels. This group has shown that in these mice, liver metastasis following orthotopic intra-cecal implantation of MC-38 colon adenocarcinoma fragments was inhibited. Moreover, injection of IGF-I into LID, as well as control mice significantly increased tumor development in the cecal wall, as well as liver metastasis, suggesting that liver-derived IGF-I played a role in primary tumor development and the formation of hepatic metastases.

Other studies also support the role of IGF-I as a survival and growth factor essential for colorectal carcinoma liver metastasis. Reinmuth et al. reported that human colon carcinoma KM12L4 and HT-29 cells expressing a dominant negative form of the IGF-IR failed to form metastases after direct injection into the liver [150, 151], likely as a consequence of increased tumor cell apoptosis and reduced angiogenesis. In a direct demonstration of the role of paracrine tumor growth stimulation by liver IGF-I, Miyamoto et al. have shown that blockade of the paracrine IGF-I supply in vivo with neutralizing antibodies suppressed liver metastasis of human colorectal carcinoma HT-29 cells [40]. Support for the role of IGF-IR in the clinical course of this disease was recently obtained in a gene profiling study performed using surgical specimens of cancerous tissue and adjacent normal mucosa obtained from 205 CRC patients. This study identified IGF-IR gene expression levels as a predictor of liver metastasis in this disease [76]. The PI 3-K/Akt/Bcl-xL pathway was identified as the survival pathway activated in colorectal carcinoma cells downstream of the IGF-IR [152].

IGF-IR blockade was also effective in inhibiting the growth of other malignancies that arise in, or are metastatic to the liver. For example, Girnita et al. have shown that the insulin-like growth factor-I receptor inhibitor picropodophyllin inhibited the growth of uveal melanoma cells in the liver [49, 153, 154] and a study by the same group found a significant association between high IGF-IR expression levels and death due to liver metastases of uveal melanoma [155]. This group has also shown that inhibition of the IGF-1R activity in vitro was associated with a drastic decrease in uveal melanoma cell viability [155], suggesting that liver metastasis in this malignancy is linked to the high dependence of these cells on IGF-I for survival and growth. Similar findings were reported for hepatocellular carcinoma where it was shown that IGF-IR antisense oligodeoxynucleotides could prevent the growth of these cells in the liver [156] and in fact, IGF-II was identified as a potential causative factor together with HIF-1α in a mouse hepatocarcinogenesis model [157].

Finally, a link between the IGF axis and liver metastasis was also identified in neuroendocrine tumors such as gastrinomas and in pancreatic carcinoma. A recent analysis of gastrinomas from 54 patients with Zollinger-Ellison syndrome revealed that increased IGF-IR mRNA levels correlated with increased aggressiveness and liver metastasis in this disease [158]. Similarly, an analysis of surgically resected and autopsy derived tissue revealed that expression of both IGF-IR and EGFR were increased in the hepatic metastases of ductal pancreatic carcinomas as compared to the primary tumors [159].

Taken together, the data show that the IGF axis can promote metastasis in general, and liver metastasis in particular, via diverse mechanisms that can be direct or indirect and can act at each phase of the metastatic process. They provide a compelling rationale for targeting this axis for prevention and treatment of liver metastases.

9.5   Gene and Protein Expression Profiling Identify IGF Axis Proteins as Potential Biomarkers

As the evidence summarized above indicates, the expression levels of the IGF-IR and/or its ligands have been identified as potential risk factor for liver metastasis in several tumor types. In this context, we review below evidence based on genomic and proteomic analysis of clinical specimens that collectively identifies the IGF-axis proteins as potential biomarkers and predictors of disease progression and outcome. This evidence also suggests that these proteins are often coordinately regulated with other molecular mediators of invasion and metastasis, suggesting that they may be functionally linked. For example, IGF ligands and MMP-7 were identified as biomarkers for several tumor types including head and neck squamous cell carcinoma, ovarian carcinoma and gastric cancer [73–75]. In hepatocellular carcinoma (HCC) specimens that were compared to corresponding normal liver, IGF-II and ADAM-9 (a disintegrin and metalloproteinase) expression in the tumor cells were coordinately upregulated [160]. As alluded to above, a recent study has shown that tumor-derived MMP-7 can cleave all six IGF binding proteins, thereby increasing IGF-I and IGF-II bioavailability in the tumor microenvironment [72]. Indeed, another study by the same group has shown that proteolysis of IGFBP-3 by MMP-7 increased IGF-I bioavailability and IGF-IR activation in cells of two human colon cancer cell lines [161] and could also degrade an ECM-bound IGF-II/IGFBP-2 complex, releasing bioactive IGF-II that could induce signal transduction in human colon cancer cells [162]. This provides a functional context for above cited findings that *mmp-7* and *igf-ir* gene expression were increased in colorectal cancer specimens and IGF-IR levels correlated with the incidence of liver metastases [76]. Interestingly, a recent study has shown that in colon cancer patients undergoing chemotherapy, there was a significant increase in serum concentrations of IGFBP-3 relative to basal levels during or after chemotherapy treatment with no progressive disease, whereas at disease progression, IGFBP-3 levels significantly declined while MMP-7 levels increased. This suggests that tumor-derived circulating MMP-7 may contribute to an acquired resistance to chemotherapy (and tumor cell growth) by degrading IGFBP-3 and increasing IGF bioavailability [163].

In an IHC-based analysis of prostate cancer specimens, IGF-IR and MMP-14 were found to be highly expressed in the carcinoma tissue relative to the adjacent normal epithelium and, based on mechanistic studies using human prostate cancer cell lines, the authors suggested that IGF-IR regulates MMP-14 expression in this malignancy [62].

In addition to MMPs, a coordinated upregulation of IGF-IR and the uPA/uPAR system has also been documented. For example, analysis of breast carcinoma tissue microarrays representing over 900 cases identified IGF-IR and uPA upregulation in over 50% of breast cancer cases. In this study, increased expression of either IGF-IR or uPA or both was associated with a worse disease outcome [82].

In addition to increased expression of IGF-IR and/or IGF that has been documented in microarray analyses performed on different tumor types including colorectal, gallbladder, prostate, hepatocellular, renal cell and ovarian carcinoma and meningioma [160, 164–169], significant increases in IGFBPs such as IGFBP-2 and IGFBP-3 were also identified in some screens [170, 171]. However, their role in tumor progression remains unclear. Taken together, these studies identify IGF axis proteins as potential biomarkers of disease progression in some malignancies and indicate that they may be most useful when measured together with other indicators of tumor aggressiveness such as MMPs and the uPA/uPAR proteins.

9.6 Targeting the IGF-I Axis in Cancer Therapy: the Experience to Date

The evidence outlined above and numerous other in vitro and in vivo studies have collectively identified the IGF axis as a target for cancer therapy. Indeed, various strategies have been used to target components of this axis in animal and human tumors, and they have been highly effective in inhibiting tumor cell growth and metastasis (reviewed in [1]). A recent report (published in April 2010) estimates that up to 30 agents that target the IGF axis are in clinical or preclinical developments and there were at least 58 clinical trials to evaluate IGF-IR inhibitors as single agents or in combination therapy, at the time of publication [172, 173]. However, targeting the IGF-I system in vivo poses several challenges; (A) Due to the high degree of homology between the IGF-I and insulin receptors, drugs that target the IGF axis may also affect the insulin receptor/insulin axis with undesirable effects on glucose and lipid metabolism [174–176]. Moreover, inhibition of IGF-I signaling may result in altered serum GH levels, leading to insulin insensitivity and could potentially cause a reduction in pancreatic insulin production and diabetes [172]; (B) The majority of tumor cells studied to date express the IGF-IR. However, no specific mutations in the receptor or its ligands have been identified in cancerous cells, and therefore specific biomarkers for pathway activation that will allow monitoring of the effects of candidate drugs have not been developed; (C) In some tumor systems, IGF-IR levels may actually decline as the tumors becomes more aggressive [1, 174] and their responsiveness to IGF-targeting drugs may therefore decrease. Careful selection of patients will therefore be critical for the success of any IGF-targeting strategies.

9.6.1 Strategies That Are in Development or Have Advanced from the Bench to the Bedside

Strategies that have been developed to date and already advanced to the clinic include targeting the IGF-I receptor and downstream signaling by humanized

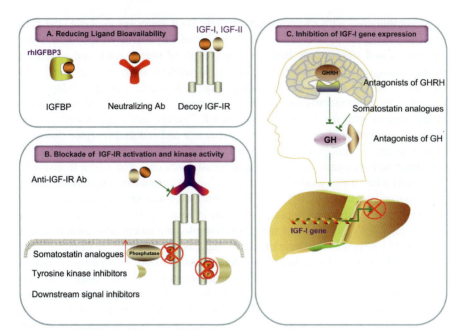

Fig. 9.2 Therapeutic strategies for targeting the IGF axis. Strategies for targeting the IGF axis include the use of reagents that bind and reduce ligand availability such as (**a**) – recombinant human IGFBP3, neutralizing antibody to IGF-I and soluble IGF-I receptors (**b**) – strategies for blockade of ligand binding and receptor activation including anti-IGF-IR antibodies, somatostatin analogues which enhance phosphatase activity and inactivate IGF-IR, tyrosine kinase inhibitors, and inhibitors of downstream transducers of the IGF-IR signal and (**c**) – strategies for inhibition of IGF-I production including antagonists of growth hormone (GH) and GH releasing hormone (GHRH)

monoclonal anti-IGF-IR antibodies or by small molecule tyrosine kinase inhibitors (TKI), respectively (see Fig. 9.2 for a summary of IGF targeting strategies). These two approaches require different exposure to the compound and therefore have diverse efficacy and toxicity profiles. While anti IGF-IR antibodies are more target-specific, TKI generally have a broader target profile, can cause nonspecific toxicity and may therefore not be well tolerated [176]. Moreover, tumors may develop drug-resistance during therapy by activating alternative survival mechanisms.

9.6.1.1 Antibodies Against the IGF-IR

Anti-IGF-IR antibodies can exert their inhibitory effect by blocking ligand binding and/or by triggering receptor internalization and degradation, thereby decreasing cell surface expression levels and reducing intracellular signaling, particularly through the PI 3-K/Akt pathway [172, 177–180]. An additional mechanism of action identified for humanized IgG1 antibodies is the initiation of an antibody-dependent cellular cytotoxicity (ADCC) response that could enhance the anti-tumorigenic effect but may also cause adverse lymphocytic toxicity [172]. In preclinical animal studies, several of these antibodies have shown efficacy either as monotherapy or in combination with chemotherapy. In one such study for example, the fully humanized Imclone monoclonal antibody A12 markedly increased apoptosis within the tumors and significantly inhibited the growth of breast, renal and pancreatic tumors xenografted into nude mice [181]. In another study, this antibody significantly blocked the growth of androgen-dependent and androgen-independent prostate cancer xenografts by inducing tumor cell apoptosis or G1 cycle arrest [182]. Studies with the Pfizer monoclonal CP-751,871 antibody showed that the antibody blocked binding of IGF-I to its receptor and induced receptor downregulation in tumor xenografts. Treatment with the antibody resulted in significant antitumor activity against colorectal and breast carcinoma and multiple myeloma xenografts when it was used as a single agent and in combination with Adriamycin, 5-fluorouracil or tamoxifen [183]. These antibodies and several other developed by Pharma have advanced into clinical trials in recent years and some trials have already recorded objective responses. For example, in a recent dose escalation trial with CP-751,871, 9/28, multiple myeloma patients had an objective response when the antibody was used together with dexamethasone [184]. In a phase 1 study of 53 patients with advanced solid malignancies treated with the Amgen antibody AMG-479, one durable complete response and one unconfirmed partial response were observed in two patients with Ewing/primitive neuroectodermal tumors and 2 partial-minor responses were seen in two patients with neuroendocrine tumors [185]. In this trial, adverse effects included thrombocytopenia and anorexia, the latter indicative of potential adverse metabolic effects (for a summary of current trials, see Table 9.1 and http://clinicaltrials.gov). In general, the clinical trials have shown that IGF-IR targeting is well tolerated as monotherapy, although mild toxicity has been documented. Typically, the adverse effects included increases in circulating IGF-1, insulin and GH. In some patients mild elevations in glucose levels have also been observed. In addition, hematological toxicities have been reported, particularly with IgG1 antibodies [172, 185, 186]. While metastatic liver disease has not been specifically targeted in these trials, the information obtained may nevertheless have implications for, and impact the design of future trials that evaluate the preventative and therapeutic benefit for hepatic metastases.

9.6.1.2 Blockade of the IGF-IR Kinase Activity

Another strategy for targeting the IGF-IR is the use of small molecule inhibitors that block the kinase domain of the receptor and thereby, receptor signaling (see Table 9.2). The main disadvantage of such drugs is their potential inhibitory activity against the highly homologous IR and potentially, other intracellular kinases. There are recent indications however, that simultaneous targeting of both the IGFIR and IR may, in fact be advantageous in some specific cases where both receptors and /or IGF-IR/IR hybrid receptors are involved in tumor growth and progression (e.g. in some breast cancers) [175, 187]. Additionally, because the IGF-IR crosstalks with other tyrosine kinases, combined strategies that target other cellular kinases implicated in tumor growth, such as Src or VEGFR together with the IGF-IR may result in synergistic therapeutic effects.

Table 9.1 Ongoing clinical trials with humanized anti-IGF-IR antibodies

Antibody	Description of clinical trials in progress
IMC-A12 (Imclone)	NCI selected 10 proposals for Phase I and II clinical trials of ImClone's IMC-A12 to explore the clinical activity, pharmacology and biological effects of IMC-A12 as a single agent or combined with other relevant anticancer agents, in a wide range of malignancies including breast, lung, pancreas and liver cancers, as well as both adult and pediatric sarcomas. In addition, Phase I/II studies will evaluate the safety, pharmacology, anticancer activity and biological effects of IMC-A12 in children and adolescents with cancer, as well as in combination with other novel targeting agents in which there is a specific rationale for combined use
R1507 (Roche)	Pase II trials of patients diagnosed with Ewing sarcoma, osteosarcoma, synovial sarcoma, rhabdomyosarcoma or other sarcomas that have recurred or spread despite previous treatment
AMG479 (Amgen)	A Phase 1b/2 trial of AMG 479 or AMG 102 with platinum-based chemotherapy as first-line treatment for advanced stage small-cell lung cancer (SCLC). Additionally, a phase 1b/2 open label, dose escalation study of AMG 655 in combination with AMG 479 in subjects with advanced, refractory solid tumors is ongoing in multiple centers
CP751-871 (Pfizer)	Randomized, open label, phase III trial of Erlotinib alone or in combination with Cp 751,871 in patients with advanced non small cell lung cancer of non adenocarcinoma histology
MK0646 (Merck/Pierre Fabre Medicament)	A phase I/randomized phase II study of gemcitabine plus erlotinib plus MK-0646, Gemcitabine plus MK-0646 and gemcitabine plus erlotinib for patients with advanced pancreatic cancer
SCH717454 (Schering-Plough)	A phase 1/1b dose-escalation study to determine the safety and tolerability of SCH 717454 administered in combination with chemotherapy in pediatric subjects with advanced solid tumors
AVE1642 (Sanofi-Aventis)	Dose-finding, safety, pharmacokinetic and pharmacodynamic study of AVE1642 administered as single agent and in combination with other anti cancer therapies (Sorafenib or Erlotinib) in patients with advanced liver carcinoma
BIIB022 (Biogen Idec)	A phase 1, open label, dose escalation study of BIIB022 in subjects with relapsed or refractory solid tumors

This table is based on information available in http://clinicaltrials.gov

9.6.1.3 Somatostatin Analogues

Somatostatin analogues have been used as a strategy to reduce circulating GH levels and thereby indirectly to downregulate hepatic IGF-I production. In addition, the type II somatostatin receptor (SST-R-II) is frequently expressed in human neoplasms and ligand binding to this receptor upregulates intracellular tyrosine phosphatase activity, reversing the phosphorylation events triggered by IGF-IR activation [188], thereby directly affecting IGF-IR-mediated signaling. Clinical trials with somatostatin analogues in the treatment of acromegaly and neuroendocrine

Table 9.2 Ongoing trials with (small molecule) protein kinase inhibitors

Small molecule	Description of the trial
INSM18 (Insmed/UCSF)	INSM-18 is a kinase inhibitor of the IGF-IR and the human epidermal growth factor receptor (Her2/Neu). Two single dose Phase I clinical studies in healthy volunteers have been previously completed with INSM-18. In both studies, INSM-18 was safe and well tolerated. The University of California, San Francisco, has completed a dose-escalating Phase I/II clinical study designed to define the maximum tolerated dose of INSM-18 in patients with relapsed prostate cancer
OSI906 (OSI pharmaceuticals)	A phase I dose escalation study of intermittent oral OSI-906 dosing in patients with advanced solid tumors
XL228 (Exelixis)	A phase 1 dose-escalation study of the safety, pharmacokinetics, and pharmacodynamics of XL228 administered intravenously to subjects with chronic myeloid leukemia (CML) or Philadelphia chromosome-positive acute lymphocytic leukemia (Ph+ ALL)
BMS-536924 (Bristol-Myers Squibb)	Preclinical [209–212]
BMS-554417 (Bristol-Myers Squibb)	Preclinical [212, 213]
NVP-ADW742 (Novartis Pharma)	Preclinical [213, 214]
NVP-AEW541 (Novartis Pharma)	Preclinical [111, 213, 215]
cyclolignan PPP	Preclinical [216, 217]
BVP-51004 (Biovitrum)	Preclinical [218, 219]
AG1024 (Merck)	Preclinical [213, 220, 221]

The information provided in this table is based on http://clinicaltrials.gov

tumors have already demonstrated efficacy [189, 190]. The preclinical data provides a rationale for controlled clinical trials in breast, prostate, and pancreatic cancer.

9.6.1.4 GH Releasing Hormone and GH Antagonists

Preclinical studies show that antagonists of GHRH block the GH/IGF-I axis and can inhibit proliferation of various cancers. Treatment with the GHRH antagonist JV-1-38 significantly inhibited the growth of non-small cell lung carcinoma xenografts in nude mice [191].

9.6.1.5 Use of Soluble Forms of the IGF-IR

The use of soluble receptor decoys to antagonize the activity of a soluble ligand in patients has become an accepted form of therapy. Examples include a soluble TNF receptor (Enbrel) now in routine clinical use for the treatment of some inflammatory conditions [192] and a VEGF–Trap that is currently in clinical trials for the treatment of cancer [193]. These reagents offer a few advantages to antibody-based therapy because they are highly specific, bind to the ligand with high affinity and bypass some of the undesirable effects of reagents with off-target activity. Several groups including our own, have engineered truncated, soluble forms of the IGF-I receptor and have shown that these molecules can act as decoys, reducing ligand bioavailability and inhibiting tumor growth. The Baserga group first reported in 1996 on the construction of an IGF-IR truncated at residue 486 (486/Stop) that is partially secreted into the medium and could induce apoptosis, inhibit tumor cell growth in soft agar and abrogate tumorigenesis of rat glioblastoma cells [194]. Similar results were subsequently reported for the human MDA-MB-435 breast carcinoma cells. These cells failed to form colonies in agar, had an increased sensitivity to taxol-induced cell death and their ability to metastasize to several organs, including the liver, was suppressed [195]. Human prostate, lung, ovarian and colon carcinoma cells expressing this soluble form of the receptor also had reduced growth when implanted into nude mice [196]. Hongo et al. used the same recombinant 486/stop protein partially purified from conditioned medium for direct injection in vivo in proximity to growing ovarian carcinoma xenografts and showed that this resulted in the inhibition of tumor growth [197], suggesting that recombinant soluble IGF-IR proteins may have translational applications. In a gene therapy-based approach, the transduction of lung carcinoma cells in vitro with an adenovirus vector expressing an IGF-IR truncated at amino acid residue 482 was shown to block IGF-I-induced signaling while the intra-tumoral injection of the Ad-IGF-IR/482 virus significantly suppressed the growth of established tumors [198]. The Brodt group engineered a soluble IGF-IR consisting of the first 933 amino acids that correspond to the entire extracellular domain of the receptor. We have shown that lung carcinoma cells producing this soluble receptor had suppressed IGF-I-induced signaling, lost all IGF-IR regulated functions including IGF-I induced VEGF-A and VEGF-C synthesis and survival and consequently failed to form liver metastases in 88% of injected animals, resulting in a markedly increased long term, disease free survival [149] (Fig. 9.3). Subsequently, autologous bone marrow stromal cells (MSC) were genetically engineered to produce this decoy receptor. When the MSC were embedded in Matrigel and implanted subcutaneously into syngeneic mice, plasma detectable levels of the decoy were produced for several weeks post implantation. We found that the circulating decoy receptor formed complexes with plasma IGF-I and this resulted in a marked inhibition of experimental liver metastases of several tumor cell types namely, syngeneic murine lung and colon carcinoma H-59 and MC-38 cells, respectively and human colorectal carcinoma KM12SM cells that were xenotransplanted into athymic nude mice (Fig. 9.4). Analysis of the underlying mechanisms revealed that in mice producing the soluble decoy, microvessel density within liver micrometastases, as measured 6 days post tumor injection was significantly reduced relative to controls, the number of apoptotic tumor cells increased and the proportion of proliferating cells declined, suggesting that in the treated mice, tumor-induced angiogenesis was inhibited and tumor cell death increased during the early stages of liver colonization (Fig. 9.5; [199]). Importantly, in the treated mice, we found no evidence of non-specific toxicity. Blood insulin and glucose levels were within the normal range and no adverse effects on the general health of the mice were observed. The results suggest that the soluble receptor acted

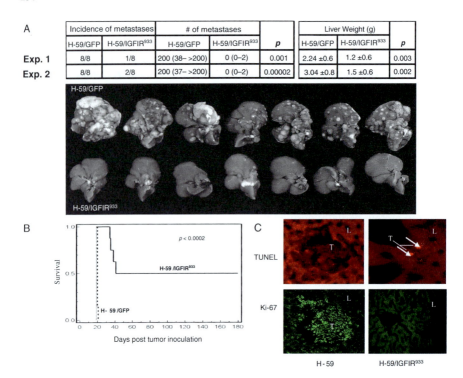

A	Incidence of metastases		# of metastases			Liver Weight (g)		
	H-59/GFP	H-59/IGFIR[933]	H-59/GFP	H-59/IGFIR[933]	p	H-59/GFP	H-59/IGFIR[933]	p
Exp. 1	8/8	1/8	200 (38– >200)	0 (0–2)	0.001	2.24 ±0.6	1.2 ±0.6	0.003
Exp. 2	8/8	2/8	200 (37– >200)	0 (0–2)	0.00002	3.04 ±0.8	1.5 ±0.6	0.002

Fig. 9.3 Loss of metastatic potential in tumor cells expressing a soluble IGF-I receptor. Highly metastatic H-59 cells were transduced with a retroviral vector expressing GFP and a soluble form of the IGF-IR (H-59/IGFIR[933]) or a control vector expressing GFP only (H-59/GFP). Mice were inoculated with 10^5 of these tumor cells by the intrasplenic/portal route and experimental liver metastases were enumerated 14 days later. Results (*top*) are expressed as the median and (range) of the number of metastases/liver in 2 experiments each based on 8 animals per group. Liver weights (means ± SD) are shown on the left and representative livers from experiment 2 are shown on the *bottom*. Shown in (**b**) are survival data for mice inoculated with tumor cells by the intrasplenic/portal route to generate experimental hepatic metastases. (**c**) TUNEL assay (for apoptotic cells – *top*) and Ki-67 staining (for proliferating cells – *bottom*) were performed on liver (L) cryostat sections prepared 5 days post tumor (T) injection (mag. ×135). Reproduced with permission from [149]

as an IGF-trap binding circulating IGF and reducing ligand bioavalability to the tumors.

Taken together, these results identify soluble IGF-IR proteins as potential anti-cancer drugs and provide a rationale for their development for clinical use.

9.6.1.6 IGFBP-3 Based Therapy

The rhIGFBP-3 has shown efficacy in preclinical studies with several cancer types including breast, prostate, liver, ovarian and colon carcinoma. Several lines

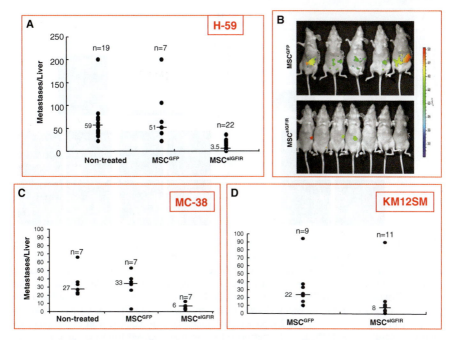

Fig. 9.4 Inhibition of experimental hepatic metastasis in mice implanted with bone marrow stromal cells that secrete plasma detectable levels of a soluble IGF-IR. Syngeneic female C57Bl/6 (**a, c**) or nude (**b, d**) mice were implanted with 10^7 genetically engineered marrow stromal cells producing the soluble IGFIR^{933} (MSC^{sIGFIR}) or control MSC (MSC^{GFP}) embedded in Matrigel. Fourteen days later, the mice were inoculated via the intrasplenic/portal route with 10^5 H-59 cells. Mice were sacrificed and liver metastases enumerated 14 days post tumor injection. Shown in (**a**) are the pooled data of 3 experiments performed with these tumor cells and in (**b**) results of live imaging performed on day 15 post inoculation of the same cells into nude mice. Shown in (**c**) are results of an experiment in which mice were inoculated via the intrasplenic route with 5×10^4 murine colon carcinoma MC-38 and in (**d**) with 2×10^5 human colon carcinoma KM12SM cells 14 days post MSC implantation. Mice were sacrificed and liver metastases enumerated 18 (**c**) or 21 (**d**) days post tumor injection. The p values were $p < 0.001$ (**a**), $p < 0.001$ (**c**) and $p < 0.01$ (**d**) when MSC^{sIGFIR}-treated mice were compared to each of the control groups. Reproduced with permission from [199]

of evidence have also suggested that rhIGFBP-3 may play an active, IGF-I-independent role in growth regulation of cancer cells by binding specifically and with high affinity to the surface of various cell types and directly inhibiting their growth. Recent independent studies have demonstrated that when IGFBP-3 is used in combination with other cancer therapies, it can augment the efficacy of standard cancer therapies [200]. For example paclitaxel-induced apoptosis was enhanced by the addition of rhIGFBP-3 [201]. This may be due to the ability of IGFBP-3 to sensitize tumor cells to apoptotic signals induced by pro-apoptotic agents as was shown for irradiation and ceramides [202, 203].

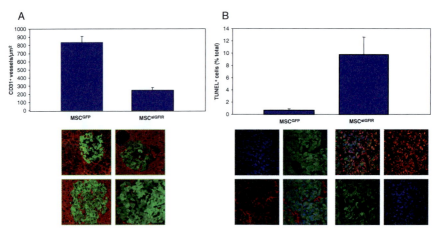

Fig. 9.5 Reduced angiogenesis and increased apoptosis in micrometastases of mice with plasma detectable levels of a soluble IGF-IR. Mice were implanted with MSC as described in the legend to Fig. 9.4 and 10^5 GFP-tagged H-59 cells were injected 14 days later. Livers were obtained on day 6 post tumor cell injection and processed for immunohistochemistry. Microvessels within micro-metastases were lebelled with a rat anti CD31 antibody followed by an Alexa Fluor 568 goat anti-rat IgG (*red fluorescence*). Shown in (**a**) are means (and SE) of CD31+ microvessels per μm (top, $p < 0.0001$) and 2 representative images/group acquired with a ×40 objective (*bottom*). Results of a TUNEL assay performed on sections derived from the same livers are seen in (**b**). Shown are means (and SE) of the proportions of TUNEL+ nuclei per total nuclei based on 12 individual images (top, $p = 0.0040$) and representative images showing GFP+ tumor cells (*green*), total nuclei (DAPI, *blue*), and apoptotic cells (*red*) and the merged images for each group acquired with a ×63 objective (*bottom*). Reproduced with permission from [199]

9.6.2 Combination Therapy – Evidence from Experimental Models

The clinical evidence accumulated to date on the use of targeted biological therapy such as growth factor receptor antagonists suggests that this family of therapeutics may be most efficacious when combined with other modalities, such as chemotherapy and radiation [204, 205] or with other biological drugs [206]. This may ultimately also prove to be the case with IGF-targeting drugs. Indeed, initial preclinical studies suggest that inhibition of the IGF-IR enhances the response to chemotherapy, radiation and siRNA therapy [205]. For example, the use of the mammalian target of rapamycin (mTOR) inhibitors CCI-779 and RAD001 leads to a negative feedback loop that results in the activation of Akt signaling, providing the tumor cells with an "escape mechanism" that renders them drug resistance. However, when these mTOR inhibitors were used in combination with the anti-IGF-IR antibody h7C10, a synergistic inhibition of cell survival and reduced tumor burden were observed [207]. Similarly, the use of IGF-IR inhibitors together with radiation enhanced tumor cell death [204]. In the H460 xenograft model, a combined treatment with radiation and the anti IGF-IR antibody A12, significantly enhanced antitumor efficacy, as compared with either modality alone [204]. Likewise, in a study with five human hepatoma cell lines, the use of the anti-IGF-IR antibody AVE1642 had moderate inhibitory effects on cell viability. However, in combination with the epidermal growth factor receptor (EGFR) inhibitor gefitinib or with rapamycin, a significant increase in the inhibition of cell cycle progression and Akt phosphorylation was seen [206]. In the human liver cancer cells, HEPG2 and Huh7, adriamycin-induced cell death was enhanced when combined with EGFR/IGF-IR inhibition, suggesting that targeting multiple pathways may improve efficacy [205]. Finally, treatment of nude mice xenografted with human breast cancer (MCF-7) or non small lung cancer (A549) cells with the anti IGF-IR antibodies h7C10 significantly inhibited tumor growth. However, an even greater effect was observed when these antibodies were combined either with the chemotherapeutic agent Vinorelbine or with an anti-EGFR antibody [208]. Since tumor cells activate distinct pro-survival and proliferation pathways, the therapeutic approaches ultimately used in the clinic may be most effective when individualized based on molecular profiling of the malignant cells.

9.7 Conclusion

The data reviewed above clearly show that the IGF axis can play a pivotal role in cancer dissemination by affecting different stages of the metastatic process. There is also compelling experimental evidence for the involvement of the IGF axis in the process of liver metastasis. However, the involvement of the IGF-IR may be tumor-type and tumor-stage specific. Emerging data from phase I and II clinical trials with novel IGF-targeting drugs, although encouraging, identify several challenges to the use of this family of drugs in the clinic. These include a variable effect when these drugs are used in single agent regimens and non-specific effects on the IR axis with undesirable metabolic consequences. Results thus far suggest that IGF-targeting agents may be most effective when combined with chemotherapeutic drugs. They also indicate that patient selection criteria will be crucial to optimize their successful utilization in the clinic.

Acknowledgement Pnina Brodt was supported by grant MOP-81201 from the Canadian Institute for Health Research. Shun Li was supported by a doctoral fellowship from the Research Institute of the McGill University Health Center.

References

1. Samani AA, Yakar S, LeRoith D, Brodt P (2007) The role of the IGF system in cancer growth and metastasis: overview and recent insights. Endocr Rev 8:20–47
2. Yakar S, Leroith D, Brodt P (2005) The role of the growth hormone/insulin-like growth factor axis in tumor growth and progression: Lessons from animal models. Cytokine Growth Factor Rev 16:407–420
3. Le Roith D, Bondy C, Yakar S, Liu JL, Butler A (2001) The somatomedin hypothesis: 2001. Endocr Rev 22:53–74
4. Sell C (2003) Caloric restriction and insulin-like growth factors in aging and cancer. Horm Metab Res 35:705–711

5. Tannenbaum GS, Guyda HJ, Posner BI (1983) Insulin-like growth factors: a role in growth hormone negative feedback and body weight regulation via brain. Science 220: 77–79

6. LeRoith D, Roberts CT Jr (2003) The insulin-like growth factor system and cancer. Cancer Lett 195:127–137

7. Haig D (2004) Genomic imprinting and kinship: how good is the evidence? Annu Rev Genet 38:553–585

8. Yakar S, Kim H, Zhao H et al (2005) The growth hormone-insulin like growth factor axis revisited: lessons from IGF-1 and IGF-1 receptor gene targeting. Pediatr Nephrol 20: 251–254

9. Furstenberger G, Senn HJ (2002) Insulin-like growth factors and cancer. Lancet Oncol 3:298–302

10. El-Shewy HM, Luttrell LM (2009) Insulin-like growth factor-2/mannose-6 phosphate receptors. Vitam Horm 80:667–697

11. Dupont J, Pierre A, Froment P, Moreau C (2003) The insulin-like growth factor axis in cell cycle progression. Horm Metab Res 35:740–750

12. Belfiore A, Frasca F, Pandini G, Sciacca L, Vigneri R (2009) Insulin receptor isoforms and insulin receptor/insulin-like growth factor receptor hybrids in physiology and disease. Endocr Rev 30:586–623

13. Avnet S, Sciacca L, Salerno M et al (2009) Insulin receptor isoform A and insulin-like growth factor II as additional treatment targets in human osteosarcoma. Cancer Res 69:2443–2452

14. Mohan S, Baylink DJ (2002) IGF-binding proteins are multifunctional and act via IGF-dependent and -independent mechanisms. J Endocrinol 175:19–31

15. Liu J-L, Grinberg A, Westphal H et al (1998) Insulin-like growth factor-I affects perinatal lethality and postnatal development in a gene dosage-dependent manner: manipulation using the Cre/loxP system in transgenic mice. Mol Endocrinol 12:1452–1462

16. Baker J, Liu J-P, Robertson EJ, Efstratiadis A (1993) Role of insulin-like growth factors in embryonic and postnatal growth. Cell 75:73–82

17. Powell-Braxton L, Hollingshead P, Warburton C et al (1993) IGF-I is required for normal embryonic growth in mice. Genes Dev 7:2609–2617

18. Yakar S, Wu Y, Setser J, Rosen CJ (2002) The role of circulating IGF-I: lessons from human and animal models. Endocrine 19:239–248

19. Pollak M (2008) Insulin and insulin-like growth factor signalling in neoplasia. Nat Rev Cancer 8:915–928

20. Butler AA, Yakar S, Gewolb IH, Karas M, Okubo Y, LeRoith D (1998) Insulin-like growth factor-I receptor signal transduction: at the interface between physiology and cell biology. Comp Biochem Physiol B Biochem Mol Biol 121:19–26

21. Petley T, Graff K, Jiang W, Yang H, Florini J (1999) Variation among cell types in the signaling pathways by which IGF-I stimulates specific cellular responses. Horm Metab Res 31:70–76

22. Argetsinger LS, Hsu GW, Myers MG Jr, Billestrup N, White MF, Carter-Su C (1995) Growth hormone, interferon-gamma, and leukemia inhibitory factor promoted tyrosyl phosphorylation of insulin receptor substrate-1. J Biol Chem 270:14685–14692

23. Myers MG Jr, Grammer TC, Wang LM et al (1994) Insulin receptor substrate-1 mediates phosphatidylinositol 3'-kinase and p70S6k signaling during insulin, insulin-like growth factor-1, and interleukin-4 stimulation. J Biol Chem 269:28783–28789

24. Vuori K, Ruoslahti E (1994) Association of insulin receptor substrate-1 with integrins. Science 266:1576–1578

25. Himpe E, Kooijman R (2009) Insulin-like growth factor-I receptor signal transduction and the Janus kinase/signal transducer and activator of transcription (JAK-STAT) pathway. Biofactors 35:76–81

26. Zong CS, Zeng L, Jiang Y, Sadowski HB, Wang LH (1998) Stat3 plays an important role in oncogenic Ros- and insulin-like growth factor I receptor-induced anchorage-independent growth. J Biol Chem 273:28065–28072
27. Sell C, Dumenil G, Deveaud C et al (1994) Effect of a null mutation of the insulin-like growth factor I receptor gene on growth and transformation of mouse embryo fibroblasts. Mol Cell Biol 14:3604–3612
28. Zhang D, Samani AA, Brodt P (2003) The role of the IGF-I receptor in the regulation of matrix metalloproteinases, tumor invasion and metastasis. Horm Metab Res 35:802–808
29. Benjamin JM, Nelson WJ (2008) Bench to bedside and back again: molecular mechanisms of alpha-catenin function and roles in tumorigenesis. Semin Cancer Biol 18:53–64
30. Kobielak A, Fuchs E (2004) Alpha-catenin: at the junction of intercellular adhesion and actin dynamics. Nat Rev Mol Cell Biol 5:614–625
31. Hirano S, Kimoto N, Shimoyama Y, Hirohashi S, Takeichi M (1992) Identification of a neural alpha-catenin as a key regulator of cadherin function and multicellular organization. Cell 70:293–301
32. Bullions LC, Notterman DA, Chung LS, Levine AJ (1997) Expression of wild-type alpha-catenin protein in cells with a mutant alpha-catenin gene restores both growth regulation and tumor suppressor activities. Mol Cell Biol 17:4501–4508
33. Thiery JP, Acloque H, Huang RYJ, Nieto MA (2009) Epithelial-mesenchymal transitions in development and disease. Cell 139:871–890
34. Guilford P, Humar B, Blair V (2010) Hereditary diffuse gastric cancer: translation of CDH1 germline mutations into clinical practice. Gastric Cancer 13:1–10
35. Fitzgerald RC, Hardwick R, Huntsman D et al (2010) Hereditary diffuse gastric cancer: updated consensus guidelines for clinical management and directions for future research. J Med Genet 47:436–444
36. Guarino M, Rubino B, Ballabio G (2007) The role of epithelial-mesenchymal transition in cancer pathology. Pathology 39:305–318
37. Kawada M, Inoue H, Masuda T, Ikeda D (2006) Insulin-like growth factor I secreted from prostate stromal cells mediates tumor-stromal cell interactions of prostate cancer. Cancer Res 66:4419–4425
38. Long L, Nip J, Brodt P (1994) Paracrine growth stimulation by hepatocyte-derived insulin-like growth factor-1: a regulatory mechanism for carcinoma cells metastatic to the liver. Cancer Res 54:3732–3737
39. Long L, Rubin R, Baserga R, Brodt P (1995) Loss of the metastatic phenotype in murine carcinoma cells expressing an antisense RNA to the insulin-like growth factor receptor. Cancer Res 55:1006–1009
40. Miyamoto Si, Nakamura M, Shitara K et al (2005) Blockade of paracrine supply of insulin-like growth factors using neutralizing antibodies suppresses the liver metastasis of human colorectal cancers. Clin Cancer Res 11:3494–3502
41. Irie HY, Pearline RV, Grueneberg D et al (2005) Distinct roles of Akt1 and Akt2 in regulating cell migration and epithelial-mesenchymal transition. J Cell Biol 171:1023–1034
42. Graham TR, Zhau HE, Odero-Marah VA et al (2008) Insulin-like growth factor-I-dependent up-regulation of ZEB1 drives epithelial-to-mesenchymal transition in human prostate cancer cells. Cancer Res 68:2479–2488
43. Playford MP, Bicknell D, Bodmer WF, Macaulay VM (2000) Insulin-like growth factor 1 regulates the location, stability, and transcriptional activity of beta-catenin. Proc Natl Acad Sci USA 97:12103–12108
44. Vermeulen SJ, Bruyneel EA, Bracke ME et al (1995) Transition from the noninvasive to the invasive phenotype and loss of alpha-catenin in human colon cancer cells. Cancer Res 55:4722–4728
45. Kiely PA, Baillie GS, Barrett R et al (2009) Phosphorylation of RACK1 on tyrosine 52 by c-Abl is required for insulin-like growth factor i-mediated regulation of focal adhesion kinase. J Biol Chem 284:20263–20274

46. Metalli D, Lovat F, Tripodi F et al (2010) The insulin-like growth factor receptor I promotes motility and invasion of bladder cancer cells through Akt- and mitogen-activated protein kinase-dependent activation of paxillin. Am J Pathol: ajpath.2010.090904

47. Furundzija V, Fritzsche J, Kaufmann J et al (2010) IGF-1 increases macrophage motility via PKC/p38-dependent [alpha]v[beta]3-integrin inside-out signaling. Biochem Biophys Res Commun 394:786–791

48. Patrizia N, Giordano N, Lorena L et al (1990) High metastatic efficiency of human sarcoma cells in Rag2/Î³c double knockout mice provides a powerful test system for antimetastatic targeted therapy. Eur J Cancer (Oxford, England) 46:659–668

49. Girnita A, All-Ericsson C, Economou MA et al (2006) The insulin-like growth factor-I receptor inhibitor picropodophyllin causes tumor regression and attenuates mechanisms involved in invasion of uveal melanoma cells. Clin Cancer Res 12:1383–1391

50. Nussbaum T, Samarin J, Ehemann V et al (2008) Autocrine insulin-like growth factor-II stimulation of tumor cell migration is a progression step in human hepatocarcinogenesis. Hepatology 48:146–156

51. Chen YW, Boyartchuk V, Lewis BC (2009) Differential roles of insulin-like growth factor receptor- and insulin receptor-mediated signaling in the phenotypes of hepatocellular carcinoma cells. Neoplasia 11:835–845

52. Kessenbrock K, Plaks V, Werb Z (2010) Matrix metalloproteinases: regulators of the tumor microenvironment. Cell 141:52–67

53. Zhang D, Bar-Eli M, Meloche S, Brodt P (2004) Dual regulation of MMP-2 expression by the type 1 insulin-like growth factor receptor: the phosphatidylinositol 3-kinase/Akt and Raf/ERK pathways transmit opposing signals. J Biol Chem 279:19683–19690

54. Yoon A, Hurta RA (2001) Insulin like growth factor-1 selectively regulates the expression of matrix metalloproteinase-2 in malignant H-ras transformed cells. Mol Cell Biochem 223:1–6

55. Long L, Navab R, Brodt P (1998) Regulation of the Mr 72,000 type IV collagenase by the type I insulin-like growth factor receptor. Cancer Res 58:3243–3247

56. Long L, Rubin R, Brodt P (1998) Enhanced invasion and liver colonization by lung carcinoma cells overexpressing the type 1 insulin-like growth factor receptor. Exp Cell Res 238:116–121

57. Grzmil M, Hemmerlein B, Thelen P, Schweyer S, Burfeind P (2004) Blockade of the type I IGF receptor expression in human prostate cancer cells inhibits proliferation and invasion, up-regulates IGF binding protein-3, and suppresses MMP-2 expression. J Pathol 202: 50–59

58. Ma Z, Dong A, Kong M, Qian J (2007) Silencing of the type 1 insulin-like growth factor receptor increases the sensitivity to apoptosis and inhibits invasion in human lung adenocarcinoma A549 cells. Cell Mol Biol Lett 12:556–572

59. Qian J, Dong A, Kong M, Ma Z, Fan J, Jiang G (2007) Suppression of type 1 Insulin-like growth factor receptor expression by small interfering RNA inhibits A549 human lung cancer cell invasion in vitro and metastasis in xenograft nude mice. Acta Biochim Biophys Sin (Shanghai) 39:137–147

60. Brodt P, Fallavollita L, Khatib AM, Samani AA, Zhang D (2001) Cooperative regulation of the invasive and metastatic phenotypes by different domains of the type I insulin-like growth factor receptor beta subunit. J Biol Chem 276:33608–33615

61. Zhang D, Brodt P (2003) Type 1 insulin-like growth factor regulates MT1-MMP synthesis and tumor invasion via PI 3-kinase/Akt signaling. Oncogene 22:974–982

62. Sroka IC, McDaniel K, Nagle RB, Bowden GT (2008) Differential localization of MT1-MMP in human prostate cancer tissue: role of IGF-1R in MT1-MMP expression. Prostate 68:463–476

63. Mira E, Manes S, Lacalle RA, Marquez G, Martinez AC (1999) Insulin-like growth factor-I-triggered cell migration and invasion are mediated by matrix metalloproteinase-9. Endocrinology 140:1657–1664

64. Bredin CG, Liu Z, Klominek J (2003) Growth factor-enhanced expression and activity of matrix metalloproteases in human non-small cell lung cancer cell lines. Anticancer Res 23:4877–4884

65. Li S, Zhang D, Yang L et al (2009) The IGF-I receptor can alter the matrix metalloproteinase repertoire of tumor cells through transcriptional regulation of PKC-{alpha}. Mol Endocrinol 23:2013–2025

66. Chattopadhyay S, Shubayev VI (2009) MMP-9 controls Schwann cell proliferation and phenotypic remodeling via IGF-1 and ErbB receptor-mediated activation of MEK/ERK pathway. Glia 57:1316–1325

67. Manes S, Llorente M, Lacalle RA et al (1999) The matrix metalloproteinase-9 regulates the insulin-like growth factor-triggered autocrine response in DU-145 carcinoma cells. J Biol Chem 274:6935–6945

68. Manes S, Mira E, Barbacid MM et al (1997) Identification of insulin-like growth factor-binding protein-1 as a potential physiological substrate for human stromelysin-3. J Biol Chem 272:25706–25712

69. Lee SE, Han BD, Park IS, Romero R, Yoon BH (2008) Evidence supporting proteolytic cleavage of insulin-like growth factor binding protein-1 (IGFBP-1) protein in amniotic fluid. J Perinat Med 36:316–323

70. Ii M, Yamamoto H, Adachi Y, Maruyama Y, Shinomura Y (2006) Role of matrix metalloproteinase-7 (matrilysin) in human cancer invasion, apoptosis, growth, and angiogenesis. Exp Biol Med (Maywood) 231:20–27

71. Hemers E, Duval C, McCaig C, Handley M, Dockray GJ, Varro A (2005) Insulin-like growth factor binding protein-5 is a target of matrix metalloproteinase-7: implications for epithelial-mesenchymal signaling. Cancer Res 65:7363–7369

72. Nakamura M, Miyamoto S, Maeda H et al (2005) Matrix metalloproteinase-7 degrades all insulin-like growth factor binding proteins and facilitates insulin-like growth factor bioavailability. Biochem Biophys Res Commun 333:1011–1016

73. Weber A, Hengge UR, Stricker I et al (2007) Protein microarrays for the detection of biomarkers in head and neck squamous cell carcinomas. Hum Pathol 38:228–238

74. Ajisaka H, Fushida S, Yonemura Y, Miwa K (2001) Expression of insulin-like growth factor-2, c-MET, matrix metalloproteinase-7 and MUC-1 in primary lesions and lymph node metastatic lesions of gastric cancer. Hepatogastroenterology 48:1788–1792

75. Davidson B, Zhang Z, Kleinberg L et al (2006) Gene expression signatures differentiate ovarian/peritoneal serous carcinoma from diffuse malignant peritoneal mesothelioma. Clin Cancer Res 12:5944–5950

76. Oshima T, Akaike M, Yoshihara K et al (2008) Clinicopathological significance of the gene expression of matrix metalloproteinase-7, insulin-like growth factor-1, insulin-like growth factor-2 and insulin-like growth factor-1 receptor in patients with colorectal cancer: insulin-like growth factor-1 receptor gene expression is a useful predictor of liver metastasis from colorectal cancer. Oncol Rep 20:359–364

77. Adachi Y, Li R, Yamamoto H et al (2009) Insulin-like growth factor-I receptor blockade reduces the invasiveness of gastrointestinal cancers via blocking production of matrilysin. Carcinogenesis 30:1305–1313

78. Powell WC, Fingleton B, Wilson CL, Boothby M, Matrisian LM (1999) The metalloproteinase matrilysin proteolytically generates active soluble Fas ligand and potentiates epithelial cell apoptosis Curr Biol 9:1441–1447

79. Mitsiades N, Yu WH, Poulaki V, Tsokos M, Stamenkovic I (2001) Matrix metalloproteinase-7-mediated cleavage of Fas ligand protects tumor cells from chemotherapeutic drug cytotoxicity. Cancer Res 61:577–581

80. Mekkawy AH, Morris DL, Pourgholami MH (2009) Urokinase plasminogen activator system as a potential target for cancer therapy. Future Oncol 5:1487–1499

81. Bauer TW, Fan F, Liu W et al (2005) Insulinlike growth factor-I-mediated migration and invasion of human colon carcinoma cells requires activation of c-Met and urokinase plasminogen activator receptor. Ann Surg 241:748–756; discussion 56–68

82. Nielsen TO, Andrews HN, Cheang M et al (2004) Expression of the insulin-like growth factor I receptor and urokinase plasminogen activator in breast cancer is associated with poor survival: potential for intervention with 17-allylamino geldanamycin. Cancer Res 64: 286–291

83. Dunn SE, Torres JV, Nihei N, Barrett JC (2000) The insulin-like growth factor-1 elevates urokinase-type plasminogen activator-1 in human breast cancer cells: a new avenue for breast cancer therapy. Mol Carcinog 27:10–17

84. Dunn SE, Torres JV, Oh JS, Cykert DM, Barrett JC (2001) Up-regulation of urokinase-type plasminogen activator by insulin-like growth factor-I depends upon phosphatidylinositol-3 kinase and mitogen-activated protein kinase kinase. Cancer Res 61:1367–1374

85. Siri S, Chen MJ, Chen TT (2006) Inhibition of human breast cancer cell (MBA-MD-231) invasion by the Ea4-peptide of rainbow trout pro-IGF-I. J Cell Biochem 99:1363–1373

86. Chernicky CL, Tan H, Yi L, Loret de Mola JR, Ilan J (2002) Treatment of murine breast cancer cells with antisense RNA to the type I insulin-like growth factor receptor decreases the level of plasminogen activator transcripts, inhibits cell growth in vitro, and reduces tumorigenesis in vivo. Mol Pathol 55:102–109

87. Bauer TW, Liu W, Fan F et al (2005) Targeting of urokinase plasminogen activator receptor in human pancreatic carcinoma cells inhibits c-Met- and insulin-like growth factor-I receptor-mediated migration and invasion and orthotopic tumor growth in mice. Cancer Res 65:7775–7781

88. Gallicchio MA, Kaun C, Wojta J, Binder B, Bach LA (2003) Urokinase type plasminogen activator receptor is involved in insulin-like growth factor-induced migration of rhabdomyosarcoma cells in vitro. J Cell Physiol 197:131–138

89. Navab R, Pedraza C, Fallavollita L et al (2008) Loss of responsiveness to IGF-I in cells with reduced cathepsin L expression levels. Oncogene 27:4973–4985

90. Tsai WC, Chao YC, Lee WH, Chen A, Sheu LF, Jin JS (2006) Increasing EMMPRIN and matriptase expression in hepatocellular carcinoma: tissue microarray analysis of immuno-histochemical scores with clinicopathological parameters. Histopathology 49:388–395

91. Otrock ZK, Mahfouz RAR, Makarem JA, Shamseddine AI (2007) Understanding the biology of angiogenesis: Review of the most important molecular mechanisms. Blood Cells Mol Dis 39:212–220

92. Nussenbaum F, Herman IM (2010) Tumor angiogenesis: insights and innovations. J Oncol:132641 (in press)

93. Samaranayake H, Maatta AM, Pikkarainen J, Yla-Herttuala S (2010) Future prospects and challenges of antiangiogenic cancer gene therapy. Hum Gene Ther 21:381–396

94. Nektaria M, Theodora L, Vassilia X, Ilias N, Kostas S (2009) The role of angiogenesis in solid tumours: an overview. Eur J Intern Med 20:663–671

95. Poulaki V, Mitsiades CS, McMullan C et al (2003) Regulation of vascular endothelial growth factor expression by insulin-like growth factor I in thyroid carcinomas. J Clin Endocrinol Metab 88:5392–5398

96. Fukuda R, Hirota K, Fan F, Jung YD, Ellis LM, Semenza GL (2002) Insulin-like growth factor 1 induces hypoxia-inducible factor 1-mediated vascular endothelial growth factor expression, which is dependent on MAP kinase and phosphatidylinositol 3-kinase signaling in colon cancer cells. J Biol Chem 277:38205–38211

97. Laughner E, Taghavi P, Chiles K, Mahon PC, Semenza GL (2001) HER2 (neu) signaling increases the rate of hypoxia-inducible factor 1alpha (HIF-1alpha) synthesis: novel mechanism for HIF-1-mediated vascular endothelial growth factor expression. Mol Cell Biol 21:3995–4004

98. Zhong H, Chiles K, Feldser D et al (2000) Modulation of hypoxia-inducible factor 1alpha expression by the epidermal growth factor/phosphatidylinositol 3-kinase/PTEN/AKT/FRAP

pathway in human prostate cancer cells: implications for tumor angiogenesis and therapeutics. Cancer Res 60:1541–1545

99. Feldser D, Agani F, Iyer NV, Pak B, Ferreira G, Semenza GL (1999) Reciprocal positive regulation of hypoxia-inducible factor 1alpha and insulin-like growth factor 2. Cancer Res 59:3915–3918

100. Zelzer E, Levy Y, Kahana C, Shilo BZ, Rubinstein M, Cohen B (1998) Insulin induces transcription of target genes through the hypoxia-inducible factor HIF-1alpha/ARNT. EMBO J 17:5085–5094

101. Burroughs KD, Oh J, Barrett JC, DiAugustine RP (2003) Phosphatidylinositol 3-kinase and mek1/2 are necessary for insulin-like growth factor-I-induced vascular endothelial growth factor synthesis in prostate epithelial cells: a role for hypoxia-inducible factor-1? Mol Cancer Res 1:312–322

102. Catrina SB, Botusan IR, Rantanen A et al (2006) Hypoxia-inducible factor-1alpha and hypoxia-inducible factor-2alpha are expressed in kaposi sarcoma and modulated by insulin-like growth factor-I. Clin Cancer Res 12:4506–4514

103. Okawa Y, Hideshima T, Steed P et al (2009) SNX-2112, a selective Hsp90 inhibitor, potently inhibits tumor cell growth, angiogenesis, and osteoclastogenesis in multiple myeloma and other hematologic tumors by abrogating signaling via Akt and ERK. Blood 113:846–855

104. Lang SA, Moser C, Gaumann A et al (2007) Targeting heat shock protein 90 in pancreatic cancer impairs insulin-like growth factor-I receptor signaling, disrupts an interleukin-6/signal-transducer and activator of transcription 3/hypoxia-inducible factor-1alpha autocrine loop, and reduces orthotopic tumor growth. Clin Cancer Res 13:6459–6468

105. Hayashi M, Sakata M, Takeda T et al (2005) Up-regulation of c-met protooncogene product expression through hypoxia-inducible factor-1alpha is involved in trophoblast invasion under low-oxygen tension. Endocrinology 146:4682–4689

106. Pennacchietti S, Michieli P, Galluzzo M, Mazzone M, Giordano S, Comoglio PM (2003) Hypoxia promotes invasive growth by transcriptional activation of the met protooncogene. Cancer Cell 3:347–361

107. Semenza GL (2000) Hypoxia, clonal selection, and the role of HIF-1 in tumor progression. Crit Rev Biochem Mol Biol 35:71–103

108. Sulpice E, Ding S, Muscatelli-groux Ba et al (2009) Cross-talk between the VEGF-A and HGF signalling pathways in endothelial cells. Biol Cell 101:525–539

109. Lee OH, Bae SK, Bae MH et al (2000) Identification of angiogenic properties of insulin-like growth factor II in in vitro angiogenesis models. Br J Cancer 82:385–391

110. Shigematsu S, Yamauchi K, Nakajima K, Iijima S, Aizawa T, Hashizume K (1999) IGF-1 regulates migration and angiogenesis of human endothelial cells. Endocr J 46:S59–S62

111. Moser C, Schachtschneider P, Lang SA et al (2008) Inhibition of insulin-like growth factor-I receptor (IGF-IR) using NVP-AEW541, a small molecule kinase inhibitor, reduces orthotopic pancreatic cancer growth and angiogenesis. Eur J Cancer 44:1577–1586

112. Grulich-Henn J, Ritter J, Mesewinkel S, Heinrich U, Bettendorf M, Preissner KT (2002) Transport of insulin-like growth factor-I across endothelial cell monolayers and its binding to the subendothelial matrix. Exp Clin Endocrinol Diabetes 110:67–73

113. Kondo T, Vicent D, Suzuma K et al (2003) Knockout of insulin and IGF-1 receptors on vascular endothelial cells protects against retinal neovascularization. J Clin Invest 111:1835–1842

114. Menu E, Jernberg-Wiklund H, Stromberg T et al (2006) Inhibiting the IGF-1 receptor tyrosine kinase with the cyclolignan PPP: an in vitro and in vivo study in the 5T33MM mouse model. Blood 107:655–660

115. Menu E, van Valckenborgh E, van Camp B, Vanderkerken K (2009) The role of the insulin-like growth factor 1 receptor axis in multiple myeloma. Arch Physiol Biochem 115:49–57

116. Bauer TW, Fan F, Liu W et al (2007) Targeting of insulin-like growth factor-I receptor with a monoclonal antibody inhibits growth of hepatic metastases from human colon carcinoma in mice. Ann Surg Oncol 14:2838–2846

117. Stacker SA, Achen MG (2008) From anti-angiogenesis to anti-lymphangiogenesis: emerging trends in cancer therapy. Lymphat Res Biol 6:165–172

118. Stacker SA, Baldwin ME, Achen MG (2002) The role of tumor lymphangiogenesis in metastatic spread. FASEB J 16:922–934

119. Stacker SA, Caesar C, Baldwin ME et al (2001) VEGF-D promotes the metastatic spread of tumor cells via the lymphatics. Nat Med 7:186–191

120. Tang Y, Zhang D, Fallavollita L, Brodt P (2003) Vascular endothelial growth factor C expression and lymph node metastasis are regulated by the type I insulin-like growth factor receptor. Cancer Res 63:1166–1171

121. Bjorndahl M, Cao R, Nissen LJ et al (2005) Insulin-like growth factors 1 and 2 induce lymphangiogenesis in vivo. Proc Natl Acad Sci USA 102:15593–15598

122. Mathur SP, Mathur RS, Gray EA et al (2005) Serum vascular endothelial growth factor C (VEGF-C) as a specific biomarker for advanced cervical cancer: relationship to insulin-like growth factor II (IGF-II), IGF binding protein 3 (IGF-BP3) and VEGF-A [corrected]. Gynecol Oncol 98:467–483

123. Ali MA (2008) Lymphatic microvessel density and the expression of lymphangiogenic factors in oral squamous cell carcinoma. Med Princ Pract 17:486–492

124. Schluter K, Gassmann P, Enns A et al (2006) Organ-specific metastatic tumor cell adhesion and extravasation of colon carcinoma cells with different metastatic potential. Am J Pathol 169:1064–1073

125. Auguste P, Fallavollita L, Wang N, Burnier J, Bikfalvi A, Brodt P (2007) The host inflammatory response promotes liver metastasis by increasing tumor cell arrest and extravasation. Am J Pathol 170:1781–1792

126. Brodt P, Fallavollita L, Bresalier RS, Meterissian S, Norton CR, Wolitzky BA (1997) Liver endothelial E-selectin mediates carcinoma cell adhesion and promotes liver metastasis. Int J Cancer 71:612–619

127. Khatib AM, Auguste P, Fallavollita L et al (2005) Characterization of the host proinflammatory response to tumor cells during the initial stages of liver metastasis. Am J Pathol 167:749–759

128. Khatib AM, Fallavollita L, Wancewicz EV, Monia BP, Brodt P (2002) Inhibition of hepatic endothelial E-selectin expression by C-raf antisense oligonucleotides blocks colorectal carcinoma liver metastasis. Cancer Res 62:5393–5398

129. Paschos KA, Canovas D, Bird NC (2009) The role of cell adhesion molecules in the progression of colorectal cancer and the development of liver metastasis. Cell Signal 21:665–674

130. Yoshimura K, Meckel KF, Laird LS et al (2009) Integrin {alpha}2 mediates selective metastasis to the liver. Cancer Res 69:7320–7328

131. Conti JA, Kendall TJ, Bateman A et al (2008) The desmoplastic reaction surrounding hepatic colorectal adenocarcinoma metastases aids tumor growth and survival via α_v integrin ligation. Clin Cancer Res 14:6405–6413

132. Gomez JM, Sahun M, Vila R et al (2007) Elevation of E-selectin concentrations may correlate with potential endothelial dysfunction in individuals with hypopituitarism during therapy with growth hormone. Curr Neurovasc Res 4:55–62

133. Hansen TK, Fisker S, Dall R, Ledet T, Jorgensen JOL, Rasmussen LM. Growth Hormone Increases Vascular Cell Adhesion Molecule 1 Expression: in Vivo and in Vitro Evidence. J Clin Endocrinol Metab 2004; 89:909–916

134. Thum T, Tsikas D, Frolich JC, Borlak J (2003) Growth hormone induces eNOS expression and nitric oxide release in a cultured human endothelial cell line. FEBS Lett 555:567–571

135. Che W, Lerner-Marmarosh N, Huang Q et al (2002) Insulin-like growth factor-1 enhances inflammatory responses in endothelial cells: role of Gab1 and MEKK3 in

TNF-{alpha}-induced c-Jun and NF-{kappa}B activation and adhesion molecule expression. Circ Res 90:1222–1230

136. Khatib AM, Kontogiannea M, Fallavollita L, Jamison B, Meterissian S, Brodt P (1999) Rapid induction of cytokine and E-selectin expression in the liver in response to metastatic tumor cells. Cancer Res 59:1356–1361

137. McDonald B, Spicer J, Giannais B, Fallavollita L, Brodt P, Ferri LE (2009) Systemic inflammation increases cancer cell adhesion to hepatic sinusoids by neutrophil mediated mechanisms. Int J Cancer 125:1298–1305

138. Wang N, Thuraisingam T, Fallavollita L, Ding A, Radzioch D, Brodt P (2006) The secretory leukocyte protease inhibitor is a type 1 insulin-like growth factor receptor-regulated protein that protects against liver metastasis by attenuating the host proinflammatory response. Cancer Res 66:3062–3070

139. Bani MR, Garofalo A, Scanziani E, Giavazzi R (1991) Effect of interleukin-1-beta on metastasis formation in different tumor systems. J Natl Cancer Inst 83:119–123

140. Read MA, Whitley MZ, Williams AJ, Collins T (1994) NF-kappa B and I kappa B alpha: an inducible regulatory system in endothelial activation. J Exp Med 179:503–512

141. Vidal-Vanaclocha F, Alvarez A, Asumendi A, Urcelay B, Tonino P, Dinarello CA (1996) Interleukin 1 (IL-1)-dependent melanoma hepatic metastasis in vivo; increased endothelial adherence by IL-1-induced mannose receptors and growth factor production in vitro. J Natl Cancer Inst 88:198–205

142. Vidal-Vanaclocha F, Fantuzzi G, Mendoza L et al (2000) IL-18 regulates IL-1beta-dependent hepatic melanoma metastasis via vascular cell adhesion molecule-1. Proc Natl Acad Sci USA 97:734–739

143. Vidal-Vanaclocha F, Amezaga C, Asumendi A, Kaplanski G, Dinarello CA (1994) Interleukin-1 receptor blockade reduces the number and size of murine B16 melanoma hepatic metastases. Cancer Res 54:2667–2672

144. Kitakata H, Nemoto-Sasaki Y, Takahashi Y, Kondo T, Mai M, Mukaida N (2002) Essential roles of tumor necrosis factor receptor p55 in liver metastasis of intrasplenic administration of colon 26 cells. Cancer Res 62:6682–6687

145. Vidal-Vanaclocha F (2008) The prometastatic microenvironment of the liver. Cancer Microenviron 1:113–129

146. Wu Y, Brodt P, Sun H et al (2010) Insulin-like growth factor-I regulates the liver microenvironment in obese mice and promotes liver metastasis. Cancer Res 70:57–67

147. Chambers AF, Groom AC, MacDonald IC (2002) Dissemination and growth of cancer cells in metastatic sites. Nat Rev Cancer 2:563–572

148. Groom AC, MacDonald IC, Schmidt EE, Morris VL, Chambers AF (1999) Tumour metastasis to the liver, and the roles of proteinases and adhesion molecules: new concepts from in vivo videomicroscopy. Can J Gastroenterol 13:733–743

149. Samani AA, Chevet E, Fallavollita L, Galipeau J, Brodt P (2004) Loss of tumorigenicity and metastatic potential in carcinoma cells expressing the extracellular domain of the type 1 insulin-like growth factor receptor. Cancer Res 64:3380–3385

150. Reinmuth N, Fan F, Liu W et al (2002) Impact of insulin-like growth factor receptor-I function on angiogenesis, growth, and metastasis of colon cancer. Lab Invest 82:1377–1389

151. Reinmuth N, Liu W, Fan F et al (2002) Blockade of insulin-like growth factor I receptor function inhibits growth and angiogenesis of colon cancer. Clin Cancer Res 8:3259–3269

152. Sulkowski S, Kanczuga-Koda L, Koda M, Wincewicz A, Sulkowska M (2006) Insulin-like growth factor-I receptor correlates with connexin 26 and Bcl-xL expression in human colorectal cancer. Ann N Y Acad Sci 1090:265–275

153. Girnita A, All-Ericsson C, Economou MA et al (2006) The insulin-like growth factor-I receptor inhibitor picropodophyllin causes tumor regression and attenuates mechanisms involved in invasion of uveal melanoma cells. Clin Cancer Res 12:1383–1391

154. Girnita A, All-Ericsson C, Economou MA et al (2008) The insulin-like growth factor-I receptor inhibitor picropodophyllin causes tumor regression and attenuates mechanisms involved in invasion of uveal melanoma cells. Acta Ophthalmol 86:26–34

155. All-Ericsson C, Girnita L, Seregard S, Bartolazzi A, Jager MJ, Larsson O (2002) Insulin-like growth factor-1 receptor in uveal melanoma: a predictor for metastatic disease and a potential therapeutic target. Invest Ophthalmol Vis Sci 43:1–8

156. Lin RX, Wang ZY, Zhang N et al (2007) Inhibition of hepatocellular carcinoma growth by antisense oligonucleotides to type I insulin-like growth factor receptor in vitro and in an orthotopic model. Hepatol Res 37:366–375

157. Tanaka H, Yamamoto M, Hashimoto N et al (2006) Hypoxia-independent overexpression of hypoxia-inducible factor 1{alpha} as an early change in mouse hepatocarcinogenesis. Cancer Res 66:11263–11270

158. Furukawa M, Raffeld M, Mateo C et al (2005) Increased expression of insulin-like growth factor I and/or its receptor in gastrinomas is associated with low curability, increased growth, and development of metastases. Clin Cancer Res 11:3233–3242

159. Ueda S, Hatsuse K, Tsuda H et al (2006) Potential crosstalk between insulin-like growth factor receptor type 1 and epidermal growth factor receptor in progression and metastasis of pancreatic cancer. Mod Pathol 19:788–796

160. Tannapfel A, Anhalt K, Hausermann P et al (2003) Identification of novel proteins associated with hepatocellular carcinomas using protein microarrays. J Pathol 201:238–249

161. Miyamoto S, Yano K, Sugimoto S et al (2004) Matrix metalloproteinase-7 facilitates insulin-like growth factor bioavailability through its proteinase activity on insulin-like growth factor binding protein 3. Cancer Res 64:665–671

162. Miyamoto S, Nakamura M, Yano K et al (2007) Matrix metalloproteinase-7 triggers the matricrine action of insulin-like growth factor-II via proteinase activity on insulin-like growth factor binding protein 2 in the extracellular matrix. Cancer Sci 98:685–691

163. Gallego R, Codony-Servat J, Garcia-Albeniz X et al (2009) Serum IGF-I, IGFBP-3, and matrix metalloproteinase-7 levels and acquired chemo-resistance in advanced colorectal cancer. Endocr Relat Cancer 16:311–317

164. Kornprat P, Rehak P, Ruschoff J, Langner C (2006) Expression of IGF-I, IGF-II, and IGF-IR in gallbladder carcinoma. A systematic analysis including primary and corresponding metastatic tumours. J Clin Pathol 59:202–206

165. Schips L, Zigeuner R, Ratschek M, Rehak P, Ruschoff J, Langner C (2004) Analysis of insulin-like growth factors and insulin-like growth factor I receptor expression in renal cell carcinoma. Am J Clin Pathol 122:931–937

166. Varghese S, Burness M, Xu H, Beresnev T, Pingpank J, Alexander HR (2007) Site-specific gene expression profiles and novel molecular prognostic factors in patients with lower gastrointestinal adenocarcinoma diffusely metastatic to liver or peritoneum. Ann Surg Oncol 14:3460–3471

167. Savli H, Szendroi A, Romics I, Nagy B (2008) Gene network and canonical pathway analysis in prostate cancer: a microarray study. Exp Mol Med 40:176–185

168. Wrobel G, Roerig P, Kokocinski F et al (2005) Microarray-based gene expression profiling of benign, atypical and anaplastic meningiomas identifies novel genes associated with meningioma progression. Int J Cancer 114:249–256

169. Sayer RA, Lancaster JM, Pittman J et al (2005) High insulin-like growth factor-2 (IGF-2) gene expression is an independent predictor of poor survival for patients with advanced stage serous epithelial ovarian cancer. Gynecol Oncol 96:355–361

170. So AI, Levitt RJ, Eigl B et al (2008) Insulin-like growth factor binding protein-2 is a novel therapeutic target associated with breast cancer. Clin Cancer Res 14:6944–6954

171. de Bont JM, van Doorn J, Reddingius RE et al (2008) Various components of the insulin-like growth factor system in tumor tissue, cerebrospinal fluid and peripheral blood of pediatric medulloblastoma and ependymoma patients. Int J Cancer 123:594–600

172. Zha J, Lackner MR (2010) Targeting the insulin-like growth factor receptor-1R pathway for cancer therapy. Clin Cancer Res 16:2512–2517

173. Gualberto A, Pollak M (2009) Emerging role of insulin-like growth factor receptor inhibitors in oncology: early clinical trial results and future directions. Oncogene 28:3009–3021

174. Bruchim I, Attias Z, Werner H (2009) Targeting the IGF1 axis in cancer proliferation. Expert Opin Ther Targets 13:1179–1192
175. Sachdev D, Yee D (2007) Disrupting insulin-like growth factor signaling as a potential cancer therapy. Mol Cancer Ther 6:1–12
176. Rodon J, DeSantos V, Ferry RJ, Kurzrock R (2008) Early drug development of inhibitors of the insulin-like growth factor-I receptor pathway: lessons from the first clinical trials. Mol Cancer Ther 7:2575–2588
177. Rowinsky EK, Youssoufian H, Tonra JR, Solomon P, Burtrum D, Ludwig DL (2007) IMC-A12, a human IgG1 monoclonal antibody to the insulin-like growth factor I receptor. Clin Cancer Res 13:5549s–5555s
178. Broussas M, Dupont J, Gonzalez A et al (2009) Molecular mechanisms involved in activity of h7C10, a humanized monoclonal antibody, to IGF-1 receptor. Int J Cancer 124: 2281–2293
179. Gualberto A, Karp D (2009) Development of the monoclonal antibody Figitumumab, targeting the insulin-like growth factor-1 receptor, for the treatment of patients with non–small-cell lung cancer. Clin Lung Cancer 10:273–280
180. Shang Y, Mao Y, Batson J et al (2008) Antixenograft tumor activity of a humanized anti-insulin-like growth factor-I receptor monoclonal antibody is associated with decreased AKT activation and glucose uptake. Mol Cancer Ther 7:2599–2608
181. Burtrum D, Zhu Z, Lu D et al (2003) A fully human monoclonal antibody to the insulin-like growth factor I receptor blocks ligand-dependent signaling and inhibits human tumor growth in vivo. Cancer Res 63:8912–8921
182. Wu JD, Odman A, Higgins LM et al (2005) In vivo effects of the human type I insulin-like growth factor receptor antibody A12 on androgen-dependent and androgen-independent xenograft human prostate tumors. Clin Cancer Res 11:3065–3074
183. Gualberto A (2010) Figitumumab (CP-751,871) for cancer therapy. Expert Opin Biol Ther 10:575–585
184. Lacy MQ, Alsina M, Fonseca R et al (2008) Phase I, pharmacokinetic and pharmacodynamic study of the anti-insulinlike growth factor type 1 receptor monoclonal antibody CP-751,871 in patients with multiple myeloma. J Clin Oncol 26:3196–3203
185. Tolcher AW, Sarantopoulos J, Patnaik A et al (2009) Phase I, pharmacokinetic, and pharmacodynamic study of AMG 479, a fully human monoclonal antibody to insulin-like growth factor receptor 1. J Clin Oncol 27:5800–5807
186. Haluska P, Shaw HM, Batzel GN et al (2007) Phase I dose escalation study of the anti insulin-like growth factor-I receptor monoclonal antibody CP-751,871 in patients with refractory solid tumors. Clin Cancer Res 13:5834–5840
187. Sachdev D, Zhang X, Matise I, Gaillard-Kelly M, Yee D (2010) The type I insulin-like growth factor receptor regulates cancer metastasis independently of primary tumor growth by promoting invasion and survival. Oncogene 29:251–262
188. Szereday Z, Schally AV, Szepeshazi K et al (2003) Effective treatment of H838 human non-small cell lung carcinoma with a targeted cytotoxic somatostatin analog, AN-238. Int J Oncol 22:1141–1146
189. Pollak MN, Schally AV (1998) Mechanisms of antineoplastic action of somatostatin analogs. Proc Soc Exp Biol Med 217:143–152
190. Hofland LJ, Lamberts SW (2004) Somatostatin receptors in pituitary function, diagnosis and therapy. Front Horm Res 32:235–252
191. Kiaris H, Koutsilieris M, Kalofoutis A, Schally AV (2003) Growth hormone-releasing hormone and extra-pituitary tumorigenesis: therapeutic and diagnostic applications of growth hormone-releasing hormone antagonists. Expert Opin Invest Drugs 12:1385–1394
192. Richard-Miceli C, Dougados M (2001) Tumour necrosis factor-[alpha] blockers in rheumatoid arthritis: review of the clinical experience. BioDrugs 15:251–259
193. Rudge JS, Thurston G, Davis S et al (2005) VEGF trap as a novel antiangiogenic treatment currently in clinical trials for cancer and eye diseases, and VelociGeneÂ®-based discovery

of the next generation of angiogenesis targets. Cold Spring Harbor Symp Quant Biol 70: 411–418

194. D'Ambrosio C, Ferber A, Resnicoff M, Baserga R (1996) A soluble insulin-like growth factor I receptor that induces apoptosis of tumor cells in vivo and inhibits tumorigenesis. Cancer Res 56:4013–4020

195. Dunn SE, Ehrlich M, Sharp NJH et al (1998) A dominant negative mutant of the insulin-like growth factor-I receptor inhibits the adhesion, invasion, and metastasis of breast cancer. Cancer Res 58:3353–3361

196. Reiss K, D'Ambrosio C, Tu X, Tu C, Baserga R (1998) Inhibition of tumor growth by a dominant negative mutant of the insulin-like growth factor I receptor with a bystander effect. Clin Cancer Res 4:2647–2655

197. Hongo A, Kuramoto H, Nakamura Y et al (2003) Antitumor effects of a soluble insulin-like growth factor I receptor in human ovarian cancer cells: advantage of recombinant protein administration in vivo. Cancer Res 63:7834–7839

198. Lee C-T, Park K-H, Adachi Y et al (2003) Recombinant adenoviruses expressing dominant negative insulin-like growth factor-I receptor demonstrate antitumor effects on lung cancer. Cancer Gene Ther 10:57–63

199. Wang N, Fallavollita L, Nguyen L et al (2009) Autologous bone marrow stromal cells genetically engineered to secrete an igf-I receptor decoy prevent the growth of liver metastases. Mol Ther 17:1241–1249

200. Lee DY, Yi HK, Hwang PH, Oh Y (2002) Enhanced expression of insulin-like growth factor binding protein-3 sensitizes the growth inhibitory effect of anticancer drugs in gastric cancer cells. Biochem Biophys Res Commun 294:480–486

201. Fowler CA, Perks CM, Newcomb PV, Savage PB, Farndon JR, Holly JM (2000) Insulin-like growth factor binding protein-3 (IGFBP-3) potentiates paclitaxel-induced apoptosis in human breast cancer cells. Int J Cancer 88:448–453

202. Granata R, Trovato L, Garbarino G et al (2004) Dual effects of IGFBP-3 on endothelial cell apoptosis and survival: involvement of the sphingolipid signaling pathways. FASEB J 18:1456–1458

203. Perks CM, McCaig C, Holly JM (2000) Differential insulin-like growth factor (IGF)-independent interactions of IGF binding protein-3 and IGF binding protein-5 on apoptosis in human breast cancer cells. Involvement of the mitochondria. J Cell Biochem 80: 248–258

204. Allen GW, Saba C, Armstrong EA et al (2007) Insulin-like growth factor-I receptor signaling blockade combined with radiation. Cancer Res 67:1155–1162

205. Niu J, Li XN, Qian H, Han Z (2008) siRNA mediated the type 1 insulin-like growth factor receptor and epidermal growth factor receptor silencing induces chemosensitization of liver cancer cells. J Cancer Res Clin Oncol 134:503–513

206. Desbois-Mouthon C, Baron A, Blivet-Van Eggelpoel MJ et al (2009) Insulin-like growth factor-1 receptor inhibition induces a resistance mechanism via the epidermal growth factor receptor/HER3/AKT signaling pathway: rational basis for cotargeting insulin-like growth factor-1 receptor and epidermal growth factor receptor in hepatocellular carcinoma. Clin Cancer Res 15:5445–5456

207. Wan X, Harkavy B, Shen N, Grohar P, Helman LJ (2007) Rapamycin induces feedback activation of Akt signaling through an IGF-1R-dependent mechanism. Oncogene 26: 1932–1940

208. Goetsch L, Gonzalez A, Leger O et al (2005) A recombinant humanized anti-insulin-like growth factor receptor type I antibody (h7C10) enhances the antitumor activity of vinorelbine and anti-epidermal growth factor receptor therapy against human cancer xenografts. Int J Cancer 113:316–328

209. Novosyadlyy R, Lann DE, Vijayakumar A et al (2010) Insulin-mediated acceleration of breast cancer development and progression in a nonobese model of type 2 diabetes. Cancer Res 70:741–751

210. Litzenburger BC, Kim HJ, Kuiatse I et al (2009) BMS-536924 reverses IGF-IR-induced transformation of mammary epithelial cells and causes growth inhibition and polarization of MCF7 cells. Clin Cancer Res 15:226–237

211. Law JH, Habibi G, Hu K et al (2008) Phosphorylated insulin-like growth factor-i/insulin receptor is present in all breast cancer subtypes and is related to poor survival. Cancer Res 68:10238–10246

212. Haluska P, Carboni JM, TenEyck C et al (2008) HER receptor signaling confers resistance to the insulin-like growth factor-I receptor inhibitor, BMS-536924. Mol Cancer Ther 7: 2589–2598

213. Hewish M, Chau I, Cunningham D (2009) Insulin-like growth factor 1 receptor targeted therapeutics: novel compounds and novel treatment strategies for cancer medicine. Recent Pat Anticancer Drug Discov 4:54–72

214. Morgan GJ, Krishnan B, Jenner M, Davies FE (2006) Advances in oral therapy for multiple myeloma. Lancet Oncol 7:316–325

215. Mukohara T, Shimada H, Ogasawara N et al (2009) Sensitivity of breast cancer cell lines to the novel insulin-like growth factor-1 receptor (IGF-1R) inhibitor NVP-AEW541 is dependent on the level of IRS-1 expression. Cancer Lett 282:14–24

216. Economou MA, Andersson S, Vasilcanu D et al (2008) Oral picropodophyllin (PPP) is well tolerated in vivo and inhibits IGF-1R expression and growth of uveal melanoma. Acta Ophthalmol 86:35–41

217. Klinakis A, Szabolcs M, Chen G, Xuan S, Hibshoosh H, Efstratiadis A (2009) Igf1r as a therapeutic target in a mouse model of basal-like breast cancer. Proc Natl Acad Sci USA 106:2359–2364

218. Weroha SJ, Haluska P (2008) IGF-1 receptor inhibitors in clinical trials – early lessons. J Mammary Gland Biol Neoplasia 13:471–483

219. Rodon J, DeSantos V, Ferry RJ, Jr, Kurzrock R (2008) Early drug development of inhibitors of the insulin-like growth factor-I receptor pathway: lessons from the first clinical trials. Mol Cancer Ther 7:2575–2588

220. Wen B, Deutsch E, Marangoni E et al (2001) Tyrphostin AG 1024 modulates radiosensitivity in human breast cancer cells. Br J Cancer 85:2017–2021

221. Deutsch E, Maggiorella L, Wen B et al (2004) Tyrosine kinase inhibitor AG1024 exerts antileukaemic effects on STI571-resistant Bcr-Abl expressing cells and decreases AKT phosphorylation. Br J Cancer 91:1735–1741

Chapter 10
Breast Cancer Liver Metastasis

Sébastien Tabariès and Peter M. Siegel

Abstract The emergence of metastatic breast cancer is the most deadly aspect of this disease and once it has spread from the primary site, it is largely incurable. Upon dissemination from the primary tumor, breast cancer cells display preferences for specific metastatic sites. The liver represents the third most frequent site for breast cancer metastasis, following the bone and lung. Despite the evidence that hepatic metastases are associated with poor clinical outcome in breast cancer patients, little is known about the molecular mechanisms governing the spread and growth of breast cancer cells in the liver. In recent years, researchers have utilized animal model systems to isolate breast cancer cells that weakly or aggressively metastasize to the liver and have utilized gene expression profiling to compare these populations. In this manner, genes whose expression is elevated or diminished in highly metastatic breast cancer cells have been identified. We highlight both tumor intrinsic factors as well as aspects of the metastatic microenvironment that contribute to the establishment and growth of breast cancer liver metastases.

Keywords Breast cancer · Liver metastasis · Tight junctions · Cell-cell adhesion

Abbreviations

ASC	adipocyte stem cell
BCLivM:	breast cancer liver metastasis
BMDC:	bone marrow derived cell
BMSC:	bone marrow stem cell
CRC	colorectal cancer
DCIS	ductal carcinoma in situ
DOX	doxycycline
ECM	extracellular matrix
ER	estrogen receptor

P.M. Siegel (✉)
Goodman Cancer Research Centre, McGill University, Montréal, QC, Canada H3A 1A3;
Departments of Medicine and Biochemistry, McGill University, 1160 Pine Avenue West, Room 513, Montréal, QC, Canada H3A 1A3
e-mail: peter.siegel@mcgill.ca

P. Brodt (ed.), *Liver Metastasis: Biology and Clinical Management*, Cancer Metastasis – Biology and Treatment 16, DOI 10.1007/978-94-007-0292-9_10,
© Springer Science+Business Media B.V. 2011

HPC	haematopoietic progenitor cell
IDC	invasive ductal carcinoma
ILC	invasive lobular carcinoma
LCIS	lobular carcinoma in situ
MMP	matrix metalloproteinase
MSC	mesenchymal stem cell
PR	progesterone receptor
SAGE	serial analysis of gene expression
SDPP	stroma-derived prognostic predictor
SIRT	selective internal radiotherapy
TACE	transcatheter arterial chemoembolization
TEM	tetraspanin-enriched membrane microdomains
TMN	tumor-node-metastasis system

Contents

10.1 Introduction

Breast cancer represents the most commonly diagnosed cancer affecting Canadian women and is the second leading cause of cancer deaths in women [1]. It is estimated that 1 in 9 women will develop breast cancer in their lifetime and that 1 in 27 will die from this disease (Canadian Cancer Statistics). While breast cancer is a disease that predominantly affects women, about 1% of breast cancer cases are detected in men [1].

Breast cancer is a heterogeneous disease that is characterized by diverse histopathologies and molecular features that are associated with distinct clinical outcomes. This disease is driven by the accumulation of genetic abnormalities and can be broadly divided into inherited or sporadic breast cancer. Hereditary breast cancer accounts for approximately 5–10% of all breast cancers, the majority of which are linked to mutations in breast cancer gene 1 (BRCA1) or breast cancer gene 2 (BRCA2). Patients harboring BRCA1 or BRCA2 alterations have a much greater risk of developing both breast and ovarian cancer [2]. The remaining cases of breast cancer cannot be associated with an inherited genetic predisposition, and are termed sporadic breast cancers.

10.1.1 Classification of Breast Cancer

Breast cancer staging is used to predict patient prognosis, guide treatment decisions and is based on the tumor-node-metastasis (TNM) system [3]. Based on the size of the primary tumor (T), the presence and degree of involvement of the regional lymph nodes (N) and the presence of distant metastases (M), breast cancers can be sub-divided into stage 0-IV disease. Stage 0 describes up to 20% of breast cancers, represents non invasive lesions that have not spread distally and includes both lobular carcinoma in situ (LCIS) and ductal carcinoma in situ (DCIS). Stage I refers to tumors that have not spread from the primary site and are smaller than 2 cm in diameter. Stage II breast cancer tumors range from 2 to 5 cm in diameter and have spread to 1–3 lymph nodes. Breast tumors that are larger than 5 cm in diameter and have spread to more than 3 axillary lymph nodes are categorized as Stage III breast cancer. By stage IV, cancer cells have spread through the bloodstream or lymphatic system to colonize other parts of the body. The 5 year survival rates diminish with increasing grade and stage III/IV breast cancers are characterized by a significantly poorer prognosis compared to stage I/II cancers [4]. It is the development of distal metastases that accounts for the majority of cancer-related deaths in patients with this disease.

10.1.2 Towards a Molecular Classification of Breast Cancer

Microarray-based profiling has led to the classification of primary human breast cancers based on distinct gene expression signatures [5–7]. The first major study utilized breast specimens obtained from 42 individuals, which included 36 invasive ductal carcinomas, two invasive lobular carcinomas, one ductal carcinoma in situ, one fibroadenoma and three normal breast tissue samples [5]. Genes that displayed little variance within repeat samples from the same tumor and a high variance across tumors formed an "intrinsic" gene set that was used to identify five subtypes of breast cancers. These subtypes include luminal A, luminal B, basal-like, HER2-positive and normal-like breast cancers and they have been subsequently identified in independent datasets [6–8]. In general, breast tumors belonging to the luminal A and B subtypes are estrogen receptor (ER) and/or progesterone receptor (PR) positive. The HER2 subgroup displays elevated HER2 expression, as a result of genomic amplification, and typically possesses low or negative hormone receptor expression, whereas basal breast cancers are characterized as ER-negative, PR-negative and HER2-negative. Signatures within the normal-like breast cancer subtype encompass genes known to be expressed by cell types within the normal breast, including genes associated with adipose tissue. This subtype remains under-studied at present and there is some concern as to whether it simply represents the degree of "normal"-tissue contamination present within tumor samples [9, 10].

Importantly, it has become clear that these breast cancer subtypes are linked to patient outcomes. The HER2 and basal-like subtypes are associated with the poorest patient prognosis, exhibiting the shortest overall survival and relapse-free survival times. In contrast, the luminal A subtype is associated with the best prognosis whereas patients with luminal B cancers have an intermediate prognosis [6–8, 11, 12]. At present, the identification of molecular subtypes affirms the selection of treatment strategies that are based on more traditional clinico-pathological characteristics of the disease. Luminal cancers, by virtue of their hormone receptor positive status, typically respond well to endocrine therapies such as Tamoxifen. On the other hand, HER2-driven breast tumors, which are usually hormone receptor negative, are resistant to Tamoxifen. However, Trastuzumab, a humanized monoclonal antibody against HER2 specifically inhibits cell growth of HER2-positive cancers. At present, there is a lack of targeted agents that can be effectively used against the basal subtype of breast cancer. However, epidermal growth factor receptor (EGFR) inhibitors are active in basal-like breast cancer with EGFR gene amplification [13]. Furthermore, it has been reported that the basal-like subtype is significantly associated with distant metastasis and displays a greater likelihood of developing visceral metastases [14]. By analyzing the expression data of 344 breast cancers, the preferential sites of relapse have been correlated with each molecular subtype [15]. Recurrence to the bone is most commonly found in patients with breast tumors from the Luminal B and A subtypes (36.6 and 31%, respectively); whereas recurrence to the lung is more frequent in patients with breast cancers belonging to the Luminal B and the HER2 subtypes (36.7 and 40%, respectively). Similarly, the HER2 and basal subtypes of breast cancer preferentially metastasize to the liver (33.3 and 22%, respectively), while brain metastases are mostly found in patients from the Luminal A or the basal subtypes (21.4 and 57.1%, respectively) [15].

The majority of these profiling studies have used RNA extracted from whole tumor samples, which include both the tumor component and elements of the infiltrating stroma. Growing interest in tumor – stromal interactions and their importance in breast cancer progression has led investigators to analyze gene expression changes, specifically in the stroma of breast cancers [16–18]. Initial studies relied on the isolation of specific cells types from normal breast tissues, DCIS and invasive breast cancers using cell surface markers and magnetic bead enrichment of epithelial cells, endothelial cells, fibroblasts and leukocytes [19]. SAGE analysis revealed gene expression changes in all cell types during breast cancer progression, with the most dramatic differences observed during the transition from normal breast epithelium to DCIS [19]. Recently, the question of stromal gene expression profiles has been examined through the use of laser capture microdissection of fresh frozen breast cancer specimens to selectively harvest the epithelial or stromal components of the tumor without the need for sorting techniques [20]. Using this approach, a 26-gene stromally derived signature was identified, termed the stroma-derived prognostic predictor (SDPP), which could predict outcome in datasets derived using whole tumor material [20]. Together, these studies indicate that gene expression data from both the tumor epithelium and tumor stroma can be informative in identifying breast cancers that are associated with poor patient prognosis and highlight the fact that different and complementary information may be gained from these cellular compartments.

10.1.3 The Clinical Promise of Molecular Profiling in Breast Cancer

Initial concerns regarding the clinical applicability of gene expression signatures included questions regarding quality control of the RNA isolated from samples, the reliability of DNA microarrays for measuring gene expression and the reproducibility of the results generated within a lab and between labs. Many of these issues have been systematically addressed through the microarray quality control project (MQCP consortium, 2006). To date, several molecular predictors for patient prognosis, such as Mammaprint and Oncotype DX, have been described. Mammaprint is a 70-gene signature that was developed by comparing tumors from patients free of metastatic relapse versus those taken from patients with relapse within 5 years [21]. Currently, Mammaprint is being tested in the MINDACT trial to determine whether this gene expression signature is capable of identifying good prognosis patients that could receive less aggressive adjuvant chemotherapy [22]. Another signature, termed Oncotype DX, consists of 21 genes and is being used to identify patients with ER-positive, lymph node negative breast cancer that are at risk for distant recurrence [23, 24]. The gene expression results from these 21 genes are converted into a recurrence score that indicates which patients may require only endocrine therapy versus those that would benefit from adjuvant chemotherapy. The utility of this test in clinical decision-making is being examined in an ongoing TAILORx trial [24]. In addition to these prognosis signatures, expression signatures designed to predict response to current therapies are now being developed and tested. In fact, the role of breast tumor stroma in predicting response to therapy has also been examined and it was found that, in patients with ER-negative breast cancer, an increase in stromal gene expression correlated with resistance to chemotherapy [25]. Thus, there is hope that these initial signatures and second generation predictors will have a great impact on the way breast cancer is managed and treated [26].

10.1.4 Breast Cancer Metastasis

Most patients that develop metastatic breast cancer will ultimately die of their disease, with a median overall survival of 18–24 months following diagnosis of metastases [27]. Metastatic tumor cells must overcome numerous barriers in order

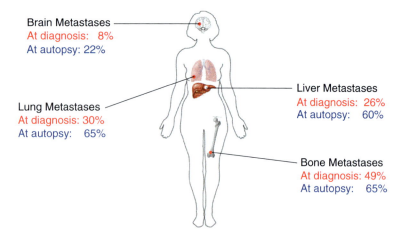

Brain Metastases
At diagnosis: 8%
At autopsy: 22%

Lung Metastases
At diagnosis: 30%
At autopsy: 65%

Liver Metastases
At diagnosis: 26%
At autopsy: 60%

Bone Metastases
At diagnosis: 49%
At autopsy: 65%

Fig. 10.1 Percentage of organ involvement in advanced breast cancer. Text in *red*: within 3 years of primary breast cancer diagnosis [29]; text in *blue*: at time of autopsy [30]

to disseminate. These include local invasion, migration and intravasation into the lymphatic system or bloodstream, survival in the circulation, immunosuppression, adhesion/extravasation at the metastatic site and tumor outgrowth in a foreign microenvironment [28]. Interestingly, breast cancer cells preferentially metastasize to specific organs and tissues including bone, lung, liver and brain (Fig. 10.1) [29, 30]. Communication between the tumor and host cells is likely to be the most important determinant contributing to the ability of cancer cells to metastasize to specific organs. This notion was first conceptualized over a century ago when Stephen Paget proposed that metastatic tumor cells were like "seeds" that would only grow in a suitable and compatible "soil" [31].

The bone represents the most frequent site for breast cancer metastasis. In approximately one quarter of all breast cancers, the bone will be the first site of metastasis and at the time of autopsy, about 65% of patients display bone metastases (Fig. 10.1) [29, 30]. Bone metastases are associated with significant morbidity in breast cancer patients, including complications such as bone pain, hypercalcemia or fractures [32–34]. When the bone is recorded as the first or the most significant metastatic site in patients with bone metastases, the 5-year overall survival rate is 16 % [35]. The lung is the second most common site for breast cancer relapse affecting about 60 % of patients with metastatic breast cancer as assessed at the time of autopsy (Fig. 10.1) [29, 30, 36]. In about 20 % of cases, the lung is the only site of metastasis. The prognosis for patients with breast cancer that has spread to the lungs is worse than for patients with bone metastases since the 5-year overall survival rate decreases to 12 % [35]. The brain is also considered a common site for breast cancer metastasis and is found in about 16 % of all metastatic breast cancers (Fig. 10.1). It is generally detected late in disease progression and the prognosis associated with brain metastasis is poor with a median survival times of less than 6 months [36].

10.2 Breast Cancer Metastasis to the Liver

Breast cancer liver metastases (BCLivM) are frequent in the clinical course of breast cancer and the liver represents the third most frequent site for breast cancer metastases [37, 38]. Within 3 years of primary tumor diagnosis, 49% of breast cancer patients have bone metastases, 30% have lung metastases and 26% have liver metastases (Fig. 10.1) [29]. At autopsy 65% of patients have bone or lung metastases while 60% of patients with metastatic breast cancers have liver involvement (Fig. 10.1) [30]. Breast cancer patients with hepatic metastases display a poor prognosis, with median survival times between 14–16 months and 5 year survival rates that reach only 5.5–8.5% [39, 40].

10.2.1 Treatment of Breast Cancer Liver Metastases

It is accepted that most patients with liver metastases also have extra hepatic lesions and the presentation of isolated liver metastases, with no evidence of metastatic disease in other sites, is only found in 1–5% of breast cancer patients [27, 41]. In patients with hormone positive breast cancer, systemic anti-endocrine therapy is warranted and the presence of hepatic breast cancer metastases is not contraindicating. However, since BCLivM are more likely to develop in patients with breast cancer belonging to the basal-like subtype, which are ER/PR-negative, hormonal therapy is rarely successful in these patients [42]. As a result, systemic chemotherapy is usually considered the standard therapeutic strategy [43]. BClivM are responsive to anthracyclines and taxane-based chemotherapy in 50–70% of the cases, with median survival times increasing to up to 24 months compared to less than 6 months in patients that have not received treatment [44]. Thus, chemotherapy in the setting of breast cancer that has spread to the liver serves to delay progression of the disease and prolongs patient survival, but is rarely curative.

While most of the blood supply in the liver originates from the hepatic portal vein, hepatic metastases generally derive their blood supply from the liver artery. This fact has been exploited by a procedure known as transcatheter arterial chemoembolization (TACE), in which catheters are inserted into branches of the hepatic artery that are supplying the metastases. Embolic particles in conjunction with chemotherapy, or particles laden with the chemotherapeutic agent, are injected into the catheter. Indeed, some breast cancer patients may benefit from TACE, which can result in a two fold increase in survival rates compared to patients treated with systemic chemotherapy [45]. Two factors contribute to the efficacy of TACE, the first being the focused administration and increased local concentration of the chemotherapeutic agent to the liver metastases and the second results from the embolization of the hepatic artery, which leads to necrosis of the developing liver metastases due to the reduction in blood flow.

Similarly to breast cancer patients, the liver is one of the most common sites for the spread of gastro-intestinal cancers and is the most frequent site for colorectal cancer (CRC) metastasis [29]. In CRC patients, surgical resection represents an important treatment modality and this approach is associated with 5 year survival rates ranging from 23 to 45% [41, 46, 47] (For more information on treatment options for CRC liver metastasis, see Chapter 12 in this volume). Based on these observations, liver resection as a treatment option for breast cancer patients with liver metastases is increasingly being explored. Indeed, breast cancer patients with BCLivM that have undergone liver resection have 5-year overall survival rates that range from 21 to 42% [41, 44, 46, 48–50]. This treatment option is only offered to those patients with low surgical risk, who present with an identifiable and low number of liver metastases in a location that permits resection and where the liver is the only site of distant metastases [51]. Unfortunately, only 1–5% of patients with hepatic metastases qualify under these criteria [27, 41].

Local ablation therapies have been developed and are beginning to be used in small case studies to directly kill tumor cells. This can be accomplished by cryotherapy (freezing cancer cells) or burning them through the use of radiofrequency ablation [52] or microwave coagulation therapy [53]. These loco-regional approaches are best applied to a small number of liver lesions, which are less than 5 cm, and are often used when surgical resection is not possible or following chemotherapy that has reduced the tumor burden in the liver [51].

For liver metastases that are too large to be treated with the above-mentioned local ablation therapies, localized radiation therapy such as selective internal radiotherapy (SIRT) and stereotactic body radiotherapy have been shown to be feasible and provide local control in breast cancer patients with liver metastases [54, 55] (for a more extensive discussion, see Chapter 13 in this volume). Despite these systemic and regional therapeutic strategies, a targeted reagent that could be employed in patients with breast cancer liver metastasis has not yet been developed.

10.2.2 The Liver as a Metastatic Site

Due to the numerous steps and barriers that constitute the metastatic cascade, the distal spread of cancer cells is considered to be an inefficient process [28]. The greatest hurdle that metastatic cancer cells must overcome is believed to be their early survival and growth once they have seeded the metastatic site [28] (For additional discussion, see Chapters 3 and 8 in this volume). Indeed, the ability of tumor cells to progress rapidly to macroscopic metastases depends on the compatibility of the tumor cell and the new microenvironment in which they now find themselves.

Although any malignancy can spread to the liver, the direct passage of blood from the gastrointestinal tract to the liver via the portal circulation results in a high rate of liver metastasis from gastrointestinal tract tumors. For example, liver metastases occur in 35–78% of patients with colorectal cancer [29, 56–60]. In fact, the liver represents the main target organ of gastrointestinal (GI) cancers such as carcinomas of the colon (35–78%), pancreas (85%), esophagus (52%) and the stomach (39%) [29, 57]. In other cancers such as the lung or the breast, the liver is rarely the only target organ (16 and 30%, respectively) and these cancers typically spread to other sites [29].

Most research on liver metastasis has been focused on CRC, in which cancer cells are directly delivered to the liver via the portal vein. However, observations made from the study of CRC liver metastasis may not be entirely applicable to BCLivM. While the underlying mechanisms that drive breast cancer liver metastasis may differ from those in CRC liver metastasis, it is likely that the nature of the liver architecture and microenvironment will impose specific constrains that select for unique characteristics within tumor cells that seed this organ, regardless of whether they originated from the breast or colon.

10.2.3 Architectural Features of the Liver

The liver is the largest gland in the body and its architecture is distinct from that of other organs. For example, blood delivery in the liver is provided by both the hepatic artery and the portal vein. Unlike what is observed in other organs, the majority of the liver's blood supply is venous blood. Indeed, the portal vein drains the blood from the GI tract and accounts for 70 % of the liver blood supply [61]. The first point of contact between metastatic cancer cells and cells within the liver microenvironment is with the endothelial cells lining the liver sinusoids. It has been shown that interactions between cancer cells and endothelial cells may be important in facilitating the arrest of tumor cells in the vessels, permitting the initiation of a cascade of events leading to the extravasation and colonization of distant organs by circulating cancer cells [62–64]. Liver sinusoids are lined by flat endothelial cells and also contain resident Kupffer cells. The Kupffer cells, which are liver-specific macrophages, anchor to the vessel walls and may partially obstruct the liver sinusoid, leading to the physical entrapment of tumor emboli [65]. In addition, the endothelial lining of the liver sinusoids possesses numerous fenestrae or small pores and the endothelial cells lack a well formed and substantial sub-endothelial basement membrane, two features which are uncharacteristic of blood vessels found in most other organs. These characteristics are likely to have important consequences for the early seeding and survival of cancer cells that invade the liver and may represent conditions that are conducive to the implantation of tumor cells in this organ (Fig. 10.2) [66] (for more on the unique architecture of the liver and the role of inflammation in liver metastasis, see Chapters 2, 3, 6 and 7 in this volume).

Following adhesion to endothelial cells in the liver sinusoids, tumor cells initially interact with underlying extracellular matrix (ECM) proteins rather than an organized, laminin-containing basement membrane such as exists in other organs. The space of Disse separates the sinusoidal endothelial cells from the hepatocytes. It contains extracellular matrix components that are deposited by hepatic stellate cells, which play an important role in cell differentiation and maintenance of cell function within the liver. In the adult liver, the sub-sinusoidal ECM is characterized predominantly by the presence of fibronectin and, to a lesser extent, collagen I [67]. Small quantities of collagen III, IV, V and VI are present, whereas the laminins are exceedingly low [67]. Nevertheless, it has recently been suggested that collagen IV and laminin-1, which are typical constituents of basement membranes, can

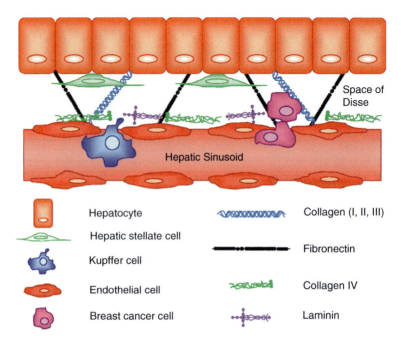

Fig. 10.2 The liver architecture. Four major cell types reside in the liver: the hepatocytes, the stellate cells, the Kupffer cells and the liver endothelial cells. The main cell types in the liver are the hepatocytes that perform vital and diverse metabolic functions such as the regulation of cholesterol levels, glucose storage and synthesis of albumin and bile. Liver sinusoidal endothelial cells separate the hepatocytes from the blood flowing through the sinusoids. These cells form a single layer with fenestrae that allow the efficient flow of essential materials from the blood to hepatocytes. The Space of Disse that separates sinusoidal endothelial cells from the hepatocytes, contains extracellular matrix (ECM) components that are deposited by hepatic stellate cells. In the adult liver, the sub-sinusoidal ECM is characterized predominantly by the presence of fibronectin and, to a lesser extent; collagen I. Small quantities of collagen III, IV, V and VI are present, whereas the laminins are exceedingly low. The fenestrated sinusoidal endothelium creates a unique situation where tumor cells have direct access to ECM components within the Space of Disse. Finally, Kupffer cells are the resident macrophages of the liver that adhere to the sinusoidal endothelium. These cells are responsible for clearing the blood of ingested bacterial pathogens and removing spent red blood cells from the circulation

also be detected in the Space of Disse (Fig. 10.2) [68]. The fenestrated sinusoidal endothelium provides a unique situation where tumor cells have direct access to ECM components within the Space of Disse. Such interactions with the underlying ECM components may provide attachment points for cancer cells and permit their early survival and growth in the liver. Cancer cell attachment to, and subsequent migration and invasion through the ECM requires interactions which are predominantly mediated by integrins. Indeed, metastatic CRC cells are characterized by specific expression patterns of adhesion molecules such as integrins [69]. Inhibition of certain integrins ($\alpha 2$, $\alpha 6$, $\beta 1$, $\beta 4$) results in a reduction in tumor cell adhesion within the sinusoid, suggesting that integrin-mediated adhesion to ECM plays an extremely important role in the ability of colon cancer cells to establish and grow in this organ [69]. Thus, tumor cells arresting in the liver sinusoids interact directly with the ECM, rather than basement membrane components, to facilitate their extravasation, survival and outgrowth [68, 70–72]. These distinctive features of the liver may require that diverse cancer cell types express similar mediators in order to successfully colonize this organ.

It is also conceivable that breast cancer cells may adopt unique strategies to metastasize to this organ that are distinct from other types of liver-metastatic cancers. For example, colorectal metastases to liver display three main types of growth. The "desmoplastic" growth pattern, where metastases are separated from the liver parenchyma by a layer of desmoplastic stroma is characterized by the prevention of direct interaction between tumor cells and hepatocytes. The second growth pattern is termed "pushing" type growth, with an absence of desmoplastic stroma and a thin layer of reticulin fibres separating the tumor cells from the hepatocytes. Finally, the minority of colorectal liver metastases exhibit a "replacement" type growth pattern, where tumor cells replace hepatocytes and co-opt the pre-existing sinusoidal blood vessels and this is characterized by minimal angiogenesis [73] (see Chapter 3 in this volume for a more extensive discussion on the different types of liver metastases) . In contrast to colorectal liver metastases that are predominantly of the "desmoplastic" (42%) or the "pushing" (46 %) growth types, breast cancer liver metastases are mostly of the replacement type (96%) [74]. In addition, it has been demonstrated that breast cancer cells interact directly with hepatocytes [75]. Remarkably, electron microscopy of metastatic breast cancer cells within the liver revealed that they form tight junctions with hepatocytes [76]. Together, these observations suggest that breast cancer cells may also evoke unique molecular mechanisms to facilitate their colonization, survival and growth in the liver.

10.3 Mediators of Breast Cancer Liver Metastasis

Organotropism of cancer cells may also be mediated by the expression of cell surface adhesion molecules or receptors that are specific for ligands (and counter receptors) found in the target organ. The expression of common genes may be found in different types of cancers that metastasize to the same organ. For instance, breast cancer cells expressing the chemokine receptor CXCR4 preferentially target organs with high levels of its natural ligand SDF-1 (CXCL12) such as the lung, bone and liver [19, 77]. Interestingly, CXCR4 has also been demonstrated to be involved in CRC liver metastasis [78]. Furthermore, hepatic stellate cells producing SDF-1 may facilitate the formation of liver metastases from CXCR4$^+$ CRC cells [79]. Similarly, elevated expression of PRL-3, a non-receptor protein tyrosine phosphatase, correlates with progression and metastasis of CRC, gastric and breast cancers [80–82]. These observations suggest that different cancers that metastasize to the liver may use common strategies. However, recent studies have highlighted the ability of breast cancer cells to adopt specific strategies to metastasize to the liver compared to other liver-metastatic cancers. Indeed, in vivo selection strategies, using xenograft or syngeneic breast cancer cell models, have allowed sub-populations of metastatic cells to be isolated from particular organs or tissues. Coupled with gene-expression profiling approaches, we and others have identified distinct genes which are characteristic of breast cancer cells that metastasize to several different organs [83–91]. While these studies have focused on metastatic sites such as the bone, lung and brain; relatively little work has been performed to identify functional mediators of breast cancer metastasis to the liver.

The identification of molecular mediators that govern organ-specific breast cancer metastasis has been largely achieved through the use of animal models of the disease. The most desirable models for investigating this process involve the orthotopic implantation of breast cancer cells into the mammary fat pad of syngeneic, immunocompetent mice, which permits spontaneous metastasis following primary tumor growth. The second approach utilizes immunodeficient mice in which human derived breast cancer cells (xenograft models) are introduced orthotopically to examine primary tumor growth and spontaneous metastasis or following injection directly into the bloodstream to study experimental metastasis to the bone, lung or liver [92].

Using these model systems, numerous genes involved in different pathways such as cell adhesion, apoptosis or TGF-β signaling have been identified. The importance of these genes in the liver metastatic phenotype will be described below.

10.3.1 Studies Using Xenograft Models

c-Jun: A potential role for c-Jun, a transcription factor, in promoting breast cancer liver metastasis has recently been suggested [93]. In this study, MCF-7 breast cancer cells were engineered to overexpress c-Jun and shown to possess enhanced proliferation, motility and adhesion in vitro and enhanced tumorigenicity in vivo, when compared to control cells. When c-Jun overexpressing cells were injected into the tail vein of mice, 50% of the animals developed macroscopic liver metastases while animals receiving the vector control cells failed to develop liver metastases. Interestingly, mice injected with c-Jun expressing MCF-7 cells failed to develop lung metastases suggesting that overexpression of c-Jun was sufficient to evoke a liver-specific metastatic phenotype. The same group subsequently demonstrated very similar results when c-Jun was expressed in SKBR3 human breast cancer cells. In this study, c-Jun overexpression was correlated with increased expression of VEGF, CXCR4 and eIF-4E as potential target genes; however, their functional involvement in promoting breast cancer metastasis to the liver was not demonstrated [94].

Galectin-3: Galectin-3 is a member of the lectin family and is involved in various biological processes, including tumorigenesis and metastasis [95, 96]. Galectin-3 overexpression in BT549 breast cancer cells, which do not normally express this protein, promotes their ability to form liver metastases following splenic injection [97]. It has been proposed that Galectin-3 expression can protect breast cancer cells from the toxicity associated with the formation of reactive oxygen species and nitric oxide production by hepatocytes or Kupffer cells during the arrest of tumor cells in the hepatic sinusoids. This protective effect is thought to be mediated by inhibition of apoptosis in Galectin-3 expressing cells [97, 98].

CD44: The adhesion molecule CD44, which is expressed at the surface of the cell, binds to hyaluronic acid as well as ECM components such as fibronectin or Collagen [99]. By alternative splicing, nine CD44 isoforms of different sizes are produced including the standard form of CD44 (CD44s), which corresponds to the shorter isoform and the one most frequently expressed in cells. Moreover, CD44 splice isoforms respond differently to post-translational modification and correlative evidence has linked CD44 expression, and specific splice variants, with the invasive and metastatic abilities of breast cancer cells [100]. Indeed, the CD44 variant v5 and v6 are the most frequently expressed in breast cancer tissues and elevated soluble CD44v6 levels in breast cancer patients correlates with the presence of liver or bone metastases [100]. Recently, experimental evidence based on the use of a Tet-Off regulatable system to control expression of CD44s has functionally implicated CD44s in promoting breast cancer liver metastasis. MCF-7 breast cancer cells became more motile and invasive in vitro when CD44 was expressed compared to the same cells in which CD44s expression was suppressed by the addition of doxycycline (DOX). When injected sub-cutaneously, the MCF-7 breast cancer cells formed tumors with the same penetrance and growth characteristics, irrespective of CD44s expression. However, 8/11 animals injected with MCF-7 cells that expressed CD44s (-DOX) developed liver metastases while 0/12 mice developed liver metastases when CD44s expression was suppressed by doxycycline treatment [101]. Interestingly, while MCF-7 cells have previously been reported to metastasize to different organs including the lung, bone and the liver; in this study CD44s expression resulted specifically in liver metastasis.

Smad7: Increases in TGF-β expression have been reported in several cancers, particularly breast cancers, and they have been correlated with increased invasiveness [102–104]. TGF-β signaling is transmitted through Smad proteins and among these, Smad7 functions as a dominant negative to inhibit TGF-β signaling by interacting with the TGF-β type I receptor [105, 106]. JygMC(A) cells, that were originally derived from a mouse mammary carcinoma and spontaneously metastasize to the lung and liver following subcutaneous injection in nude mice [107], have been used to demonstrate a negative role for Smad7 in breast cancer metastasis to the liver. Mice injected with JygMC(A) cells engineered to overexpress Smad7 displayed longer survival times and these animals displayed a decrease in metastasis to both the lung and the liver. Moreover, using a high-throughput Western blotting approach, protein expression changes were identified between parental or Smad7 expressing cells. In this way, several proteins involved in cell-cell adhesion were found to be upregulated in Smad7 expressing cells, including E-cadherin, α-catenin and β-catenin that are involved in the formation of adherens junctions or Occludin and ZO-2 that participate in the formation of tight junctions. The coordinated upregulation of these cell-cell adhesion proteins resulted in a decrease in the migratory and invasive abilities of the JygMC(A) cells, suggesting that Smad7 may function to inhibit breast cancer metastasis by stabilizing cell-cell adhesion complexes [108].

DEC1: More recently, the same group has compared the gene expression profiles of parental and Smad7 overexpressing JygMC(A) cells and reported that TGF-β may play a role in promoting breast cancer survival through the induction of DEC1 (*D*ifferentially *E*xpressed in *C*hondrocytes 1) expression in both JygMC(A) and 4T1 cells [109]. Moreover, inhibition of DEC1 function using a dominant-negative mutant resulted in a decrease in lung and liver metastasis through enhanced apoptosis, without affecting primary tumor growth. Finally, the authors showed that DEC1 expression is suppressed by a dominant negative mutant of the TGF-β receptor II or by Smad7 [109]. Taken together, these studies argue that autocrine TGF-β signaling induced in JygMC(A) breast cancer cells supports cell survival. Indeed, increased expression of Smad7 and decreased expression of DEC1, two molecules involved in TGF-β signaling, inhibited lung and liver metastasis [108, 109].

10.3.2 Studies Using Syngeneic Models

While the use of human-derived cell lines that can be xenografted into athymic mice has provided important insights into breast cancer metastasis in general and breast cancer liver metastasis in particular, there are a few caveats to this experimental system. First, injection of human-derived breast cancer cells requires the use of immuno-compromised mice. As a result, the metastatic process is modeled in the absence of a host anti-tumor adaptive immune response which undoubtedly has a significant impact on the dissemination of cancer cells. Second, the use of human tumor cells in a mouse host may result in the failure to detect important tumor/host cells interactions due to reduced affinities of receptor/ligand or adhesion molecule interactions between species. Third, these metastasis models generally require that tumor cells be injected directly into the bloodstream (cardiac or tail vein injection) to investigate organ-specific metastases to the bone or lung, which obviates the first steps of the metastatic cascade, namely local invasion from the primary site and intravasation into the circulation. Finally, the spectrum of metastatic sites that can be examined using these xenograft models are limited and metastasis to additional organs, such as liver and brain, is rare. From this perspective, the 4T1 mouse mammary carcinoma cell populations have proven to be an excellent model system to study breast cancer metastasis [110–112]. The 4T1 mouse mammary carcinoma cell population was derived as one of several sublines from a single spontaneously arising mammary tumor in a Balb/cfC3H mouse [110–112]. Sublines with distinct biological properties were established including 67NR cells which are tumorigenic but non-metastatic, 168FAR and 4T07 cells which are tumorigenic and disseminate to distant organs and tissues but fail to establish metastatic lesions, 66cl4 cells that form tumors and metastasize to the lungs and 4T1 cells that are the most aggressive of the series. Indeed, as in human cancer, 4T1 cells form tumors that invade locally to the lymph nodes and metastasize distally to the bone, lung, liver and brain [113]. These cell models have been widely used to decipher mechanisms through which breast cancer cells spread to distant organs. Thus, this series of cell lines has been used to identify candidate genes that are important for the ability of breast cancer cells to spontaneously metastasize from the primary site. This approach has implicated numerous candidate genes that are involved in pathways such as apoptosis, inflammation or Wnt signaling as important mediators of breast cancer metastasis.

Bnip3: Using the 67NR, 4T07 and 4T1 breast cancer cells, a role for the Bcl2/Adenovirus E1B 19 kDa Interacting Protein-3 (Bnip3) as a negative regulator of general breast cancer metastasis has been proposed [114]. Indeed, expression of Bnip3 inversely correlated with the intrinsic metastatic ability of the individual cell populations. Of the three cell populations tested, the 67NR cells expressed the highest level of Bnip3 while the 4T1 cells expressed the lowest levels. Interestingly, the 4T07 breast cancer cells that are known to form primary mammary tumors but fail to establish macroscopic distant metastases expressed intermediate levels of Bnip3 [114]. A siRNA-based approach to diminish Bnip3 expression in 4T07 or 67NR cells resulted in enhanced primary tumor growth and the formation of metastases in multiple organs including the sternum, lungs and liver by a mechanism involving the evasion of Bnip3-induced cell death under hypoxic conditions [114]. Thus, Bnip3 appears to function as a negative regulator of generalized breast cancer metastasis.

CCL5: CCL5 is a pleiotropic chemokine that is able to recruit T cells, NK cells, dendritic cells, mast cells, eosinophils and basophils to sites of inflammation [115]. Moreover, elevated CCL5 plasma levels correlate with disease progression in breast cancer patients [116, 117]. This observation is further validated by the fact that normal breast epithelial ductal cells express negligible CCL5 levels, but this cytokine is readily detectable in breast tumor cells derived from both DCIS and IDC lesions [118]. Recent evidence also suggests that CCL5 may act directly on tumor cells to increase their migratory and invasive properties [118]. Using antisense approaches, reduced CCL5 levels in 4T1 breast cancer cells was shown to be associated with a diminished ability to form spontaneous lung and liver metastasis and correlated with diminished expression of downstream targets such as cathepsin-L, MMP-2, MMP-3, MMP-10 and MMP-17 [119]. These results suggest that tumor-derived CCL5 expression may contribute to breast cancer cell invasion and metastasis, in part, through its ability to upregulate the expression of numerous proteases [119]. These data also suggest that CCL5 does not function as a liver-specific metastasis mediator but acts as a general regulator of breast cancer metastasis.

Wnt-5a: Wnt family signaling proteins are involved in various pathways including cell proliferation and differentiation, embryonic patterning, maintenance and differentiation of stem cells, cell polarity and axon guidance and have also been implicated in carcinogenesis, including the development of breast cancer [120–126]. Wnt-5a, a member of the Wnt protein family, activates non-canonical signaling pathways such as the Wnt/Ca^{2+} pathway which involves stimulation of intracellular Ca^{2+} release via activation of Phospholipase C and Protein Kinase C [127]. Elevated Ca^{2+} levels activate the calcium-regulated phosphatase, Calcineurin and this leads to activation and nuclear accumulation of the transcription factor NF-AT1 [128]. Furthermore, NF-AT1 activity has been shown to suppress the canonical Wnt signaling pathway during *Xenopus* development, whileWnt-5a has been suggested to antagonize canonical Wnt activity in limb development, in part, through promoting β-catenin degradation [123, 129]. Altered expression of Wnt-5a has been reported in both colon and breast cancers [130, 131]. More specifically, Wnt-5a expression has been reported as a prognostic factor for long-term disease free survival in breast cancer patients [131]. Loss of Wnt-5a protein expression is associated with an aggressive tumor phenotype in IDC, such as higher histology grade and absence of ER and PR. Interestingly, no correlation has been found with ILC [132]. Moreover, the same study reported that Wnt-5a expression was lost in 78% of patients with recurrent cancer while loss of expression was found in only 35% of recurrence-free patients [132]. Finally, Wnt-5a repression has been shown to correlate with increased adhesion to collagen and reduced migration of HB2 ductal breast epithelial cells [124]. Together, these data identify a tumor suppressive role for Wnt-5a and predict that loss of Wnt-5a expression could increase the risk of early relapse, possibly by influencing cell adhesion and migration [124, 132].

The Wnt-5a signaling pathway has recently been identified as a negative regulator of breast cancer metastasis to the lung and the liver [133]. Indeed, intraperitoneal administration of Foxy-5, which mimics Wnt-5a signaling in 4T1 breast cancer cells, resulted in decreased metastasis to the lung and the liver [133]. In vitro studies further suggested that Foxy-5 can also impair breast cancer cell migration and invasion without affecting cell proliferation or apoptosis in 4T1 cells [133]. These results are in accordance with previous data, described above, suggesting that loss of Wnt-5a expression in the primary breast tumors correlates with an increased risk of metastatic spread [132]. While the majority of these studies have identified factors that affect the ability of breast cancer cells to metastasize to the liver and the lung, few appear to describe molecules that specifically regulate liver metastasis.

10.4 A Role for Tight Junctional Proteins in Breast Cancer Liver Metastasis

Loss of cell-cell adhesion complexes appears to constitute a hallmark of a more aggressive phenotype in cancer. Based on their intercellular adhesion role, it has been hypothesized that reduced expression of adhesion molecules in metastatic cancers would enhance tumor cell motility and invasion. Tight junctions create a seal between adjacent epithelial cells to regulate the paracellular movement of water, solutes and macromolecules [134]. Claudins are key transmembrane proteins that promote cell-cell adhesion through homo- and heteromeric interactions between adjacent cells. Given this function, Claudin levels are predicted to be reduced in metastatic cancers. Indeed, many Claudins are down-regulated during cancer progression, including Claudin-1 and Claudin-7 in breast cancer [135–137]. The importance of modulating cell-cell adhesion complexes in general and a specific role for tight junctional proteins in the process of breast cancer liver metastasis has recently been highlighted (Fig. 10.3). A 4T1-derived cell subpopulation (4THM) that exhibits an elevated ability to metastasize to the liver when compared to the parental 4T1 cells was used to compare the gene expression profiles of liver metastases with those of 4THM-derived primary tumors [138]. This approach revealed that gene expression profiles of primary tumors arising from 4T1 and 4HTM cells

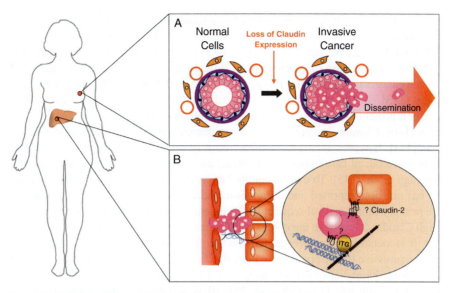

Fig. 10.3 Potential effects of differential Claudin expression on breast cancer liver metastasis. (**a**) Loss of tight junction components facilitates transition to invasive cancer and may enable breast cancer cells to spread to distant organs [139, 141]. (**b**) Claudin-2 may mediate breast cancer cell/hepatocyte adhesion or help breast cancer cell/ECM interactions that promote cancer cell survival and growth in the liver. ITG; integrin-containing complex

were very similar while the breast cancer liver metastasis profile was more divergent. Indeed a 16 gene signature was identified that was specifically reduced in 4THM primary tumors and their liver metastases compared to parental 4T1 tumors. Among these genes, several encode proteins that are normally involved in the formation of cell-cell junctions. Indeed, claudin-3, claudin-4 and ZO-1 participate in the formation of tight junctions while γ-catenin is involved in the formation of adherens junctions and desmosomes [139]. Although these data identify loss of intercellular interactions as an important factor during breast cancer liver metastasis, a causal role for the loss of these junctional proteins in this process has yet to be firmly established.

In a similar manner, we have utilized an in vivo selection approach to enrich for breast cancer cells that aggressively grow in the liver and identify novel breast tumor cell intrinsic genes that are important for the development of hepatic metastases. Following two rounds of splenic injection, we have isolated 4T1 breast cancer cells that display either a weak or aggressive growth phenotype in the liver. Gene expression profiling identified several tight junction proteins that are specifically lost in the liver-aggressive breast cancer cells (Fig. 10.3). Interestingly, in the context of diminished expression of several tight junction proteins, we also observed that Claudin-2 levels are specifically elevated in our liver-aggressive 4T1 sub-populations [140].

We observed a coordinated loss of Claudin-3, -4, -7 and Occludin in our liver aggressive breast cancer cells and this is in line with a recent study that has identified the presence of a "claudin-low" subtype in a small portion of human breast cancers that is characterized by low expression of numerous tight junctional genes including *ZO-2*, *OCLN*, *CLDN3* and *CLDN7* (Fig. 10.3) [141]. However, Claudin expression is highly variable and often elevated in different cancer types [142]. In fact, colorectal cancers that frequently metastasize to the liver display high Claudin-1 and -2 levels [143]. Significantly, we also observed that, within the context of reduced tight junction protein expression, Claudin-2 is elevated in liver-aggressive breast cancer cells [140]. *Claudin-2* expression has been demonstrated in 52% of breast carcinomas [144]; however, its expression has recently been shown to be down-regulated in invasive ductal carcinomas of the breast associated with lymph node metastasis and high grade [145]. To date, *Claudin-2* expression in breast cancer liver metastasis has not been reported and correlation studies between *Claudin-2* expression in the primary tumor and subsequent development of liver metastases are unavailable. High Claudin-2 levels, in the context of impaired tight junction formation, may permit its association with novel proteins in the plasma membrane and contribute to a more aggressive tumor phenotype. Indeed, Claudin-2 overexpression was sufficient to enhance the ability of breast cancer cells to establish and grow in the liver, suggesting a causal role in this process (Fig. 10.3). Moreover, stable diminishment of Claudin-2 expression in the liver-aggressive 4T1 populations resulted in impaired liver outgrowth following splenic injection [140]. These observations point to an important role for Claudin-2 in promoting the establishment and growth of breast cancer cells within the liver microenvironment (Fig. 10.3).

Recent evidence suggests that Claudins may have important functions outside of their prototypical roles within the tight junction complex. Indeed, the formation of tetraspanin-enriched membrane microdomains (TEMs) composed of *EpCAM*, *Claudin-7*, CD44 and tetraspanin CO-029 has been reported in metastatic pancreatic and colorectal adenocarcinomas [146] (for a more extensive discussion of TEM, see Chapter 4 of this volume). Interestingly, tetraspanins are Claudin-binding partners within TEMs that are essential for adhesion strengthening of integrin-containing complexes. Indeed, individual tetraspanins have been found in complexes with numerous integrin partners [147, 148]. In most cases, tetraspanins have been found to interact with integrin complexes containing the β1 chain, a major component for attachment to the extra-cellular matrix. Direct integrin-mediated cell adhesion to extracellular matrix components in the Space of Disse is required for the successful formation of liver metastases of colorectal cancer cells. Interestingly, Claudin-2 is not normally expressed in normal mammary epithelial cells but is abundantly expressed in hepatocytes [134]. In this regard, breast cancer cells that are metastatic to the liver can directly form tight junctions with hepatocytes [76].

Our research, focused on the identification of tumor intrinsic factors that control the ability of breast cancer cells to grow in the liver, has identified the coordinated loss of tight junctional proteins and the emergence of Claudin-2 expression in breast cancer cells selected in vivo [140]. The identification and functional validation of such candidate genes that are important for the ability of breast cancer cells to colonize the liver will provide insights into the pathways required for breast cancer cells to metastasize to this organ. These candidates and the knowledge of how they function will serve to identify targets for therapeutic intervention.

10.5 Emerging Areas of Interest

DNA microarray analysis has played an important role in identifying tumor intrinsic factors that regulate breast cancer metastasis [83–91]. However, recent studies have revealed that infiltrating cell types within the stroma of the primary tumor, as well as at the metastatic site, also play critical roles in the metastatic process. Therefore, it is important to consider not only the intrinsic properties of cancer cells, but also the stromal context within which they emerge [149, 150]. Increasing evidence suggests that cancer cells recruit stromal cells into the primary tumor that are essential in generating a permissive microenvironment to promote tumor growth [151, 152]. Solid tumor stroma consists of endothelial cells, fibroblasts, infiltrating haematopoietic cells and the ECM in which they are embedded. In addition to this complexity, recent work has highlighted an important role for diverse bone marrow derived cells, including endothelial progenitor cells, myeloid suppressor cells and haematopoietic stem cells that are required for a variety of different functions in both the primary tumor as well as distant metastases [153].

10.5.1 The Pre-metastatic Niche

Recently, Kaplan and colleagues have suggested that tumour metastasis may be facilitated by the formation of pre-metastatic niches in distant organs [154]. One key role of bone marrow derived cells (BMDCs) is to mark the location in sites, such as the lung, in which cancer cells will first establish themselves and promote the growth of these cells into macroscopic metastases. A variety of cell populations originating from the bone marrow have been implicated in promoting tumor formation and metastasis, including haematopoietic progenitor cells (HPCs) that express VEGFR1 [154]. Using mouse models, it was observed that VEGFR-1$^+$ positive cells formed clusters within the lung parenchyma that specified the future site of lung metastases. The establishment of VEGFR1$^+$ cells within the lungs preceded the arrival of tumor cells, creating privileged sites for the deposition, survival and growth of cancer cells. The emerging metastatic lesions were then populated with VEGFR2$^+$ endothelial progenitor cells that migrated into the cancer cell/VEGFR1$^+$ HPC clusters, resulting in an angiogenic switch to fuel the growth of these early lesions into macrometastases [154]. One of the earliest changes observed within distant sites of prospective metastases is a local accumulation of fibronectin [154]. VEGFR1$^+$ bone marrow derived cells express VLA-4, which can serve as a receptor for fibronectin and promote the adhesion of HPCs at sites of fibronectin deposition and the establishment of the pre-metastatic niche.

The recruitment of other BMDCs, such as CD11b+ myeloid cells, to form a pre-metastatic niche is also promoted by deposition and cross-linking of ECM components. It has recently been shown that Lysyl Oxidase (LOX), an amine oxidase known to crosslink collagen and elastin, is secreted by hypoxic tumor cells at the primary site and accumulates along with fibronectin at sites of future metastases, including the lungs. LOX functions to crosslink collagen IV and increases adhesion of CD11b$^+$ myeloid cells within the lung tissue and causes the myeloid cells to secrete matrix metalloproteinases, such as MMP-2. The MMP-2 produced by these cells degrades Collagen IV and further increases CD11b$^+$ and ultimately tumor cell invasion into the lung tissue [155].

10.5.2 Recruitment of Myeloid Cells

In addition to the recruitment of CD11b$^+$ cells into sites of metastasis [156], primary tumors have been shown to recruit CD11b$^+$Gr-1$^+$ myeloid cells [157]. CD11b$^+$ Gr-1$^+$ cells have been described as myeloid suppressor cells that are able to inhibit specific T-cell mediated anti-tumor immunity and are able to incorporate into tumor endothelium to enhance angiogenesis [158, 159]. It has recently been reported that 4T1 cells expressing the chemokine, CCL5, promoted the formation of a leukemoid reaction that was associated with splenomegaly, suggesting that myeloid cell infiltrates may be orchestrated by 4T1-derived chemokines or by chemokines secreted by tumor infiltrating HPCs. Histological analysis of both lung and liver metastases revealed the presence of granulocytic infiltrations at the tumor margins. Less than 15% of the liver area in control mice was composed of this granulocytic infiltrate (Gr1$^+$CD45$^+$ cells) while more than 50% of the liver area in 4T1 tumor-bearing mice consisted of accumulated granulocytes. Similar results were also reported in lung tissue [158]. Finally, CD11b$^+$Gr1$^+$ cell numbers were found to be increased in the livers of mice bearing 4T1-derived mammary tumors, where they interacted with resident Kupffer cells [160]. In response to these cellular interactions, Kupffer cells were found to enhance the expression of PD-L1, a co-inhibitory molecule that acts as a ligand of Programmed death-1. Engagement of PD-1 results in the downregulation of T-cell responses and immunosuppression, as reported in various cancers [160]. Thus, the contribution of BMDCs to the establishment and outgrowth of liver metastases has just recently gained appreciation as an important aspect of this process.

10.5.3 Factors that Mobilize Bone Marrow Cells

Studies aimed at identifying the factors responsible for establishing the pre-metastatic niche or inducing the migration of bone marrow derived cells to sites of metastasis are just now being reported. It was previously known that, in response to signals produced by the primary tumors, MMP-9 expression in lung tissue is upregulate prior to the formation of lung metastases [161]. Thus, identifying candidate molecules that are responsible for inducing these types of responses has become a research priority. Recently, Osteopontin has been characterized as a tumor-derived factor capable of inducing the mobilization of bone marrow cells to both the growing primary tumor and sites of metastasis in the lung [162]. These results were interesting given the long-standing association between Osteopontin expression and the metastatic ability of a wide variety of cancers [163–165].

Mesenchymal stem cells (MSCs) are pluripotent progenitor cells that contribute to the maintenance and regeneration of a variety of connective tissues. MSCs are involved in tissue remodeling after injury or inflammation. It has been reported that the conditioned media collected from MDA-MB-231 breast cancer cells may act as a chemoattractant for MSCs [151]. Breast cancer cells were shown to induce MSCs to secrete CCL5, which then acted in a paracrine fashion to increase motility of breast cancer cells expressing CCR5, a known CCL5 receptor. The result of this paracrine interaction between the breast cancer and mesenchymal stem cells resulted in enhanced breast cancer cell invasion and metastasis to the lung [151]. Similarly, MDA-MB-231 breast cancer cells have been shown to display an increase in their invasive abilities in the presence of MSCs derived from adipose tissue (ASCs), another stem cell population that may influence breast cancer progression and metastasis [166]. The observed enhancement of breast cancer cell invasion was again proposed to be mediated via CCL5 expression from the infiltrating MSCs. Moreover, co-culture of ASCs with MDA-MD-231 breast cancer cells has been shown to increase the activity of MMP-9, a molecule known to be enhanced in the presence of CCL5 [166, 167]. Given the close proximity of the ASCs with the emerging breast tumor, it is conceivable that these adipose-derived cells represent one of the earliest stromal influences on the breast cancer cells. It is thought that ASCs are responsible for producing CCL5, which in turn enhances breast cancer cell migration and invasion in a paracrine fashion [166]. Previous studies have proposed that the organotropism displayed during the metastatic spread of breast cancer cells could be explained, in part, by the pairing of chemokines in the metastatic site and chemokine receptors on the breast cancer cells. Indeed, breast cancer cells expressing high levels of CXCR4 preferentially target organs that produce SDF-1, its natural ligand; such as the bone marrow, the lungs and the liver [19, 77] (as discussed in greater detail above). It has been proposed that the SDF-1/CXCR4 axis could also play a role in facilitating communication between ASCs and 4T1 breast cancer cells. Co-injection of ASCs with 4T1 cells can lead to enhanced tumor growth of the breast cancer cells compared to injections of the tumor cells alone. It was determined that SDF-1 secreted from the ASCs could stimulate the CXCR4 receptor expressed on the breast cancer cells [168]. This suggests that, in addition to BMSCs, local stem cells situated in the breast microenvironment may be involved in tumor growth and metastasis.

In summary, migration of BMSCs, such as VEGFR1$^+$ HPCs is required to prime distant metastatic sites to receive cancer cells. In response to soluble stimuli produced by the primary tumor, including chemokines and other factors, bone marrow derived cells are mobilized and recruited to prospective sites of metastasis. These bone marrow cells establish a pre-metastatic niche that will allow tumors cells that encounter these niches to productively grow into macrometastases [154, 169]. It is clear that the molecular determinants and processes that control the ability of breast cancer cells to metastasize to the liver will not be fully understood unless both tumor intrinsic properties and the influence of the metastatic microenvironment are taken into consideration.

10.6 Conclusion

The liver is one of the most common sites of spread for various cancers including gastrointestinal and breast cancer. Indeed, the liver represents the third most frequent site for breast cancer metastasis. Systemic chemotherapy, loco-regional treatments and progress in surgical techniques has led to moderate increases in median survival time for patients with this disease. Despite these developments, the emergence of liver metastases in breast cancer patients remains associated with a poor prognosis.

Fortunately, experimentation using pre-clinical animal models for breast cancer liver metastasis has begun to elucidate molecular mechanisms and identify candidate molecules that function to regulate liver metastasis. In addition, microarray-based profiling has led to the identification of potential prognostic markers and/or therapeutic targets that may be common to different types of liver-metastatic cancers or specific to BCLivM. Indeed, we and others have highlighted both tumor intrinsic factors as well as aspects of the metastatic microenvironment that contribute to the establishment and growth of breast cancer liver metastases. Continued research into the identification of molecular mediators of breast cancer metastasis, using a combination of clinical samples and pre-clinical models, will be required to identify and validate potential therapeutic targets for the management of breast cancer patients that have developed liver metastases.

References

1. CCS (2009) Canadian Cancer Statistics 2009. Toronto, Canada, pp 1–124.
2. Edlich RF, Cross CL, Wack CA, Chase ME, Lin KY, Long WB 3rd (2008) Breast cancer and ovarian cancer genetics: an update. J Environ Pathol Toxicol Oncol 27:245–256
3. Singletary SE and Connolly JL (2006) Breast cancer staging: working with the sixth edition of the AJCC Cancer Staging Manual. CA Cancer J Clin 56:37–47; quiz 50–31
4. Ugnat AM, Xie L, Morriss J, Semenciw R, Mao Y (2004) Survival of women with breast cancer in Ottawa, Canada: variation with age, stage, histology, grade and treatment. Br J Cancer 90:1138–1143
5. Perou CM, Sorlie T, Eisen MB, van de Rijn M, Jeffrey SS, Rees CA, Pollack JR, Ross DT, Johnsen H, Akslen LA, Fluge O, Pergamenschikov A, Williams C, Zhu SX, Lonning PE, Borresen-Dale AL, Brown PO, Botstein D (2000) Molecular portraits of human breast tumours. Nature 406:747–752
6. Sorlie T, Perou CM, Tibshirani R, Aas T, Geisler S, Johnsen H, Hastie T, Eisen MB, van de Rijn M, Jeffrey SS, Thorsen T, Quist H, Matese JC, Brown PO, Botstein D, Eystein Lonning P, Borresen-Dale AL (2001) Gene expression patterns of breast carcinomas distinguish tumor subclasses with clinical implications. Proc Natl Acad Sci USA 98: 10869–10874

7. Sorlie T, Tibshirani R, Parker J, Hastie T, Marron JS, Nobel A, Deng S, Johnsen H, Pesich R, Geisler S, Demeter J, Perou CM, Lonning PE, Brown PO, Borresen-Dale AL, Botstein D (2003) Repeated observation of breast tumor subtypes in independent gene expression data sets. Proc Natl Acad Sci USA 100:8418–8423

8. Sotiriou C, Neo SY, McShane LM, Korn EL, Long PM, Jazaeri A, Martiat P, Fox SB, Harris AL, Liu ET (2003) Breast cancer classification and prognosis based on gene expression profiles from a population-based study. Proc Natl Acad Sci USA 100:10393–10398

9. Sims AH, Howell A, Howell SJ, Clarke RB (2007) Origins of breast cancer subtypes and therapeutic implications. Nat Clin Pract Oncol 4:516–525

10. Parker JS, Mullins M, Cheang MC, Leung S, Voduc D, Vickery T, Davies S, Fauron C, He X, Hu Z, Quackenbush JF, Stijleman IJ, Palazzo J, Marron JS, Nobel AB, Mardis E, Nielsen TO, Ellis MJ, Perou CM, Bernard PS (2009) Supervised risk predictor of breast cancer based on intrinsic subtypes. J Clin Oncol 27:1160–1167

11. Foulkes WD, Brunet JS, Stefansson IM, Straume O, Chappuis PO, Begin LR, Hamel N, Goffin JR, Wong N, Trudel M, Kapusta L, Porter P, Akslen LA (2004) The prognostic implication of the basal-like (cyclin E high/p27 low/p53+/glomeruloid-microvascular-proliferation+) phenotype of BRCA1-related breast cancer. Cancer Res 64:830–835

12. Haffty BG, Yang Q, Reiss M, Kearney T, Higgins SA, Weidhaas J, Harris L, Hait W, Toppmeyer D (2006) Locoregional relapse and distant metastasis in conservatively managed triple negative early-stage breast cancer. J Clin Oncol 24:5652–5657

13. Kurebayashi J (2009) Possible treatment strategies for triple-negative breast cancer on the basis of molecular characteristics. Breast Cancer 16:275–280

14. Rodriguez-Pinilla SM, Sarrio D, Honrado E, Hardisson D, Calero F, Benitez J, Palacios J (2006) Prognostic significance of basal-like phenotype and fascin expression in node-negative invasive breast carcinomas. Clin Cancer Res 12:1533–1539

15. Smid M, Wang Y, Zhang Y, Sieuwerts AM, Yu J, Klijn JG, Foekens JA, Martens JW (2008) Subtypes of breast cancer show preferential site of relapse. Cancer Res 68:3108–3114

16. Hu M, Polyak K (2008) Molecular characterisation of the tumour microenvironment in breast cancer. Eur J Cancer 44:2760–2765

17. Kleer CG, Bloushtain-Qimron N, Chen YH, Carrasco D, Hu M, Yao J, Kraeft SK, Collins LC, Sabel MS, Argani P, Gelman R, Schnitt SJ, Krop IE, Polyak K (2008) Epithelial and stromal cathepsin K and CXCL14 expression in breast tumor progression. Clin Cancer Res 14:5357–5367

18. Kim JB, Stein R, O'Hare MJ (2005) Tumour-stromal interactions in breast cancer: the role of stroma in tumourigenesis. Tumour Biol 26:173–185

19. Allinen M, Beroukhim R, Cai L, Brennan C, Lahti-Domenici J, Huang H, Porter D, Hu M, Chin L, Richardson A, Schnitt S, Sellers WR, Polyak K (2004) Molecular characterization of the tumor microenvironment in breast cancer. Cancer Cell 6:17–32

20. Finak G, Bertos N, Pepin F, Sadekova S, Souleimanova M, Zhao H, Chen H, Omeroglu G, Meterissian S, Omeroglu A, Hallett M, Park M (2008) Stromal gene expression predicts clinical outcome in breast cancer. Nat Med 14:518–527

21. van de Vijver MJ, He YD, van't Veer LJ, Dai H, Hart AA, Voskuil DW, Schreiber GJ, Peterse JL, Roberts C, Marton MJ, Parrish M, Atsma D, Witteveen A, Glas A, Delahaye L, van der Velde T, Bartelink H, Rodenhuis S, Rutgers ET, Friend SH, Bernards R (2002) A gene-expression signature as a predictor of survival in breast cancer. N Engl J Med 347:1999–2009

22. Cardoso F, Van't Veer L, Rutgers E, Loi S, Mook S, Piccart-Gebhart MJ (2008) Clinical application of the 70-gene profile: the MINDACT trial. J Clin Oncol 26:729–735

23. Paik S, Shak S, Tang G, Kim C, Baker J, Cronin M, Baehner FL, Walker MG, Watson D, Park T, Hiller W, Fisher ER, Wickerham DL, Bryant J, Wolmark N (2004) A multigene assay to predict recurrence of tamoxifen-treated, node-negative breast cancer. N Engl J Med 351:2817–2826

24. Sparano JA, Paik S (2008) Development of the 21-gene assay and its application in clinical practice and clinical trials. J Clin Oncol 26:721–728

25. Farmer P, Bonnefoi H, Anderle P, Cameron D, Wirapati P, Becette V, Andre S, Piccart M, Campone M, Brain E, Macgrogan G, Petit T, Jassem J, Bibeau F, Blot E, Bogaerts J, Aguet M, Bergh J, Iggo R, Delorenzi M (2009) A stroma-related gene signature predicts resistance to neoadjuvant chemotherapy in breast cancer. Nat Med 15:68–74

26. Desmedt C, Haibe-Kains B, Wirapati P, Buyse M, Larsimont D, Bontempi G, Delorenzi M, Piccart M, Sotiriou C (2008) Biological processes associated with breast cancer clinical outcome depend on the molecular subtypes. Clin Cancer Res 14:5158–5165

27. Er O, Frye DK, Kau SW, Broglio K, Valero V, Hortobagyi GN, Arun B (2008) Clinical course of breast cancer patients with metastases limited to the liver treated with chemotherapy. Cancer J 14:62–68

28. Chambers AF, Groom AC, MacDonald IC (2002) Dissemination and growth of cancer cells in metastatic sites. Nat Rev Cancer 2:563–572

29. Hess KR, Varadhachary GR, Taylor SH, Wei W, Raber MN, Lenzi R, Abbruzzese JL (2006) Metastatic patterns in adenocarcinoma. Cancer 106:1624–1633

30. Rabbani SA, Mazar AP (2007) Evaluating distant metastases in breast cancer: from biology to outcomes. Cancer Metastasis Rev 26:663–674

31. Paget S (1889) Distribution of secondary growths in cancer of the breast. Lancet 1: 571–573

32. Paterson AH, Powles TJ, Kanis JA, McCloskey E, Hanson J, Ashley S (1993) Double-blind controlled trial of oral clodronate in patients with bone metastases from breast cancer. J Clin Oncol 11:59–65

33. Plunkett TA, Smith P, Rubens RD (2000) Risk of complications from bone metastases in breast cancer. implications for management. Eur J Cancer 36:476–482

34. Nielsen OS, Munro AJ, Tannock IF (1991) Bone metastases: pathophysiology and management policy. J Clin Oncol 9:509–524

35. Elder EE, Kennedy CW, Gluch L, Carmalt HL, Janu NC, Joseph MG, Donellan MJ, Molland JG, Gillett DJ (2006) Patterns of breast cancer relapse. Eur J Surg Oncol 32:922–927

36. Lu X, Kang Y (2007) Organotropism of breast cancer metastasis. J Mammary Gland Biol Neoplasia 12:153–162

37. Clark GM, Sledge GW Jr, Osborne CK, McGuire WL (1987) Survival from first recurrence: relative importance of prognostic factors in 1,015 breast cancer patients. J Clin Oncol 5:55–61

38. Insa A, Lluch A, Prosper F, Marugan I, Martinez-Agullo A, Garcia-Conde J (1999) Prognostic factors predicting survival from first recurrence in patients with metastatic breast cancer: analysis of 439 patients. Breast Cancer Res Treat 56:67–78

39. Pentheroudakis G, Fountzilas G, Bafaloukos D, Koutsoukou V, Pectasides D, Skarlos D, Samantas E, Kalofonos HP, Gogas H, Pavlidis N (2005) Metastatic breast cancer with liver metastases: a registry analysis of clinicopathologic, management and outcome characteristics of 500 women. Breast Cancer Res Treat 97:237–244

40. Eichbaum MH, Kaltwasser M, Bruckner T, de Rossi TM, Schneeweiss A, Sohn C (2006) Prognostic factors for patients with liver metastases from breast cancer. Breast Cancer Res Treat 96:53–62

41. Selzner M, Morse MA, Vredenburgh JJ, Meyers WC, Clavien PA (2000) Liver metastases from breast cancer: long-term survival after curative resection. Surgery 127:383–389

42. Samaan NA, Buzdar AU, Aldinger KA, Schultz PN, Yang KP, Romsdahl MM, Martin R (1981) Estrogen receptor: a prognostic factor in breast cancer. Cancer 47:554–560

43. Arai Y, Sone Y, Inaba Y, Ariyoshi Y, Kido C (1994) Hepatic arterial infusion chemotherapy for liver metastases from breast cancer. Cancer Chemother Pharmacol 33:S142–144

44. Caralt M, Bilbao I, Cortes J, Escartin A, Lazaro JL, Dopazo C, Olsina JJ, Balsells J, Charco R (2008) Hepatic resection for liver metastases as part of the "oncosurgical" treatment of metastatic breast cancer. Ann Surg Oncol 15:2804–2810

45. Li XP, Meng ZQ, Guo WJ, Li J (2005) Treatment for liver metastases from breast cancer: results and prognostic factors. World J Gastroenterol 11:3782–3787

46. Lubrano J, Roman H, Tarrab S, Resch B, Marpeau L, Scotte M (2008) Liver resection for breast cancer metastasis: does it improve survival? Surg Today 38:293–299

47. Ercolani G, Grazi GL, Ravaioli M, Ramacciato G, Cescon M, Varotti G, Del Gaudio M, Vetrone G, Pinna AD (2005) The role of liver resections for noncolorectal, non-neuroendocrine metastases: experience with 142 observed cases. Ann Surg Oncol 12: 459–466

48. Adam R, Aloia T, Krissat J, Bralet MP, Paule B, Giacchetti S, Delvart V, Azoulay D, Bismuth H, Castaing D (2006) Is liver resection justified for patients with hepatic metastases from breast cancer? Ann Surg 244:897–907; discussion 907–898

49. Thelen A, Benckert C, Jonas S, Lopez-Hanninen E, Sehouli J, Neumann U, Rudolph B, Neuhaus P (2008) Liver resection for metastases from breast cancer. J Surg Oncol 97: 25–29

50. Sakamoto Y, Yamamoto J, Yoshimoto M, Kasumi F, Kosuge T, Kokudo N, Makuuchi M (2005) Hepatic resection for metastatic breast cancer: prognostic analysis of 34 patients. World J Surg 29:524–527

51. Diamond JR, Finlayson CA, Borges VF (2009) Hepatic complications of breast cancer. Lancet Oncol 10:615–621

52. Jakobs TF, Hoffmann RT, Schrader A, Stemmler HJ, Trumm C, Lubienski A, Murthy R, Helmberger TK, Reiser MF (2009) CT-guided radiofrequency ablation in patients with hepatic metastases from breast cancer. Cardiovasc Intervent Radiol 32:38–46

53. Umeda T, Abe H, Kurumi Y, Naka S, Shiomi H, Hanasawa K, Morikawa S, Tani T (2005) Magnetic resonance-guided percutaneous microwave coagulation therapy for liver metastases of breast cancer in a case. Breast Cancer 12:317–321

54. Milano MT, Philip A, Okunieff P (2009) Analysis of patients with oligometastases undergoing two or more curative-intent stereotactic radiotherapy courses. Int J Radiat Oncol Biol Phys 73:832–837

55. Lee MT, Kim JJ, Dinniwell R, Brierley J, Lockwood G, Wong R, Cummings B, Ringash J, Tse RV, Knox JJ, Dawson LA (2009) Phase I study of individualized stereotactic body radiotherapy of liver metastases. J Clin Oncol 27:1585–1591

56. Jemal A, Murray T, Ward E, Samuels A, Tiwari RC, Ghafoor A, Feuer EJ, Thun MJ (2005) Cancer statistics CA Cancer J Clin 55:10–30

57. Mayo SC, Pawlik TM (2009) Current management of colorectal hepatic metastasis. Expert Rev Gastroenterol Hepatol 3:131–144

58. Saif MW (2009) Secondary hepatic resection as a therapeutic goal in advanced colorectal cancer. World J Gastroenterol 15:3855–3864

59. Sharma S, Camci C, Jabbour N (2008) Management of hepatic metastasis from colorectal cancers: an update. J Hepatobiliary Pancreat Surg 15:570–580

60. Steele G, Jr, Ravikumar TS (1989) Resection of hepatic metastases from colorectal cancer. Biologic perspective. Ann Surg 210:127–138

61. Greenway CV, Stark RD (1971) Hepatic vascular bed. Physiol Rev 51:23–65

62. Auguste P, Fallavollita L, Wang N, Burnier J, Bikfalvi A, Brodt P (2007) The host inflammatory response promotes liver metastasis by increasing tumor cell arrest and extravasation. Am J Pathol 170:1781–1792

63. Gout S, Huot J (2008) Role of cancer microenvironment in metastasis: focus on colon cancer. Cancer Microenviron 1:69–83

64. Haier J, Nicolson GL (2001) The role of tumor cell adhesion as an important factor in formation of distant colorectal metastasis. Dis Colon Rectum 44:876–884

65. Phillips NC (1989) Kupffer cells and liver metastasis. Optimization and limitation of activation of tumoricidal activity. Cancer Metastasis Rev 8:231–252

66. Braet F, Wisse E (2002) Structural and functional aspects of liver sinusoidal endothelial cell fenestrae: a review. Comp Hepatol 1:1

67. Martinez-Hernandez A, Amenta PS (1993) The hepatic extracellular matrix. I. Components and distribution in normal liver. Virchows Arch A Pathol Anat Histopathol 423:1–11

68. Rosenow F, Ossig R, Thormeyer D, Gasmann P, Schluter K, Brunner G, Haier J, Eble JA (2008) Integrins as antimetastatic targets of RGD-independent snake venom components in liver metastasis [corrected]. Neoplasia 10:168–176

69. Enns A, Gassmann P, Schluter K, Korb T, Spiegel HU, Senninger N, Haier J (2004) Integrins can directly mediate metastatic tumor cell adhesion within the liver sinusoids. J Gastrointest Surg 8:1049–1059; discussion 1060

70. Kemperman H, Driessens MH, La Riviere G, Meijne AM, Roos E (1995) Adhesion mechanisms in liver metastasis formation. Cancer Surv 24:67–79

71. Schluter K, Gassmann P, Enns A, Korb T, Hemping-Bovenkerk A, Holzen J, Haier J (2006) Organ-specific metastatic tumor cell adhesion and extravasation of colon carcinoma cells with different metastatic potential. Am J Pathol 169:1064–1073

72. Yoshimura K, Meckel KF, Laird LS, Chia CY, Park JJ, Olino KL, Tsunedomi R, Harada T, Iizuka N, Hazama S, Kato Y, Keller JW, Thompson JM, Chang F, Romer LH, Jain A, Iacobuzio-Donahue C, Oka M, Pardoll DM, Schulick RD (2009) Integrin alpha2 mediates selective metastasis to the liver. Cancer Res 69:7320–7328

73. Vermeulen PB, Colpaert C, Salgado R, Royers R, Hellemans H, Van Den Heuvel E, Goovaerts G, Dirix LY, Van Marck E (2001) Liver metastases from colorectal adeno-carcinomas grow in three patterns with different angiogenesis and desmoplasia. J Pathol 195:336–342

74. Stessels F, Van den Eynden G, Van der Auwera I, Salgado R, Van den Heuvel E, Harris AL, Jackson DG, Colpaert CG, van Marck EA, Dirix LY, Vermeulen PB (2004) Breast ade-nocarcinoma liver metastases, in contrast to colorectal cancer liver metastases, display a non-angiogenic growth pattern that preserves the stroma and lacks hypoxia. Br J Cancer 90:1429–1436

75. Mook OR, Van Marle J, Vreeling-Sindelarova H, Jonges R, Frederiks WM, Van Noorden CJ (2003) Visualization of early events in tumor formation of eGFP-transfected rat colon cancer cells in liver. Hepatology 38:295–304

76. Roos E, Van de Pavert IV, Middelkoop OP (1981) Infiltration of tumour cells into cultures of isolated hepatocytes. J Cell Sci 47:385–397

77. Muller A, Homey B, Soto H, Ge N, Catron D, Buchanan ME, McClanahan T, Murphy E, Yuan W, Wagner SN, Barrera JL, Mohar A, Verastegui E, Zlotnik A (2001) Involvement of chemokine receptors in breast cancer metastasis. Nature 410:50–56

78. Zeelenberg IS, Ruuls-Van Stalle L, Roos E (2003) The chemokine receptor CXCR4 is required for outgrowth of colon carcinoma micrometastases. Cancer Res 63:3833–3839

79. Matsusue R, Kubo H, Hisamori S, Okoshi K, Takagi H, Hida K, Nakano K, Itami A, Kawada K, Nagayama S, Sakai Y (2009) Hepatic Stellate Cells Promote Liver Metastasis of Colon Cancer Cells by the Action of SDF-1/CXCR4 Axis. Ann Surg Oncol 16:2645–2653

80. Bessette DC, Qiu D, Pallen CJ (2008) PRL PTPs: mediators and markers of cancer progression. Cancer Metastasis Rev 27:231–252

81. Radke I, Gotte M, Kersting C, Mattsson B, Kiesel L, Wulfing P (2006) Expression and prog-nostic impact of the protein tyrosine phosphatases PRL-1, PRL-2, PRL-3 in breast cancer. Br J Cancer 95:347–354

82. Wang L, Peng L, Dong B, Kong L, Meng L, Yan L, Xie Y, Shou C (2006) Overexpression of phosphatase of regenerating liver-3 in breast cancer: association with a poor clinical outcome. Ann Oncol 17:1517–1522

83. Kang Y, Siegel PM, Shu W, Drobnjak M, Kakonen SM, Cordon-Cardo C, Guise TA, Massague J (2003) A multigenic program mediating breast cancer metastasis to bone. Cancer Cell 3:537–549

84. Lee H, Lin EC, Liu L, Smith JW (2003) Gene expression profiling of tumor xenografts: In vivo analysis of organ-specific metastasis. Int J Cancer 107:528–534

85. Minn AJ, Kang Y, Serganova I, Gupta GP, Giri DD, Doubrovin M, Ponomarev V, Gerald WL, Blasberg R, Massague J (2005) Distinct organ-specific metastatic potential of individual breast cancer cells and primary tumors. J Clin Invest 115:44–55

86. Minn AJ, Gupta GP, Siegel PM, Bos PD, Shu W, Giri DD, Viale A, Olshen AB, Gerald WL, Massague J (2005) Genes that mediate breast cancer metastasis to lung. Nature 436:518–524

87. Montel V, Huang TY, Mose E, Pestonjamasp K, Tarin D (2005) Expression profiling of primary tumors and matched lymphatic and lung metastases in a xenogeneic breast cancer model. Am J Pathol 166:1565–1579

88. Rose AA, Pepin F, Russo C, Abou Khalil JE, Hallett M, Siegel PM (2007) Osteoactivin promotes breast cancer metastasis to bone. Mol Cancer Res 5:1001–1014

89. Bos PD, Zhang XH, Nadal C, Shu W, Gomis RR, Nguyen DX, Minn AJ, van de Vijver MJ, Gerald WL, Foekens JA, Massague J (2009) Genes that mediate breast cancer metastasis to the brain. Nature 459:1005–1009

90. Hu Z, Fan C, Livasy C, He X, Oh DS, Ewend MG, Carey LA, Subramanian S, West R, Ikpatt F, Olopade OI, van de Rijn M, Perou CM (2009) A compact VEGF signature associated with distant metastases and poor outcomes. BMC Med 7:9

91. Cai D, Cao J, Li Z, Zheng X, Yao Y, Li W, Yuan Z (2009) Up-regulation of bone marrow stromal protein 2 (BST2) in breast cancer with bone metastasis. BMC Cancer 9:102

92. Bellet RE, Danna V, Mastrangelo MJ, Berd D (1979) Evaluation of a "nude" mouse-human tumor panel as a predictive secondary screen for cancer chemotherapeutic agents. J Natl Cancer Inst 63:1185–1188

93. Zhang Y, Pu X, Shi M, Chen L, Song Y, Qian L, Yuan G, Zhang H, Yu M, Hu M, Shen B, Guo N (2007) Critical role of c-Jun overexpression in liver metastasis of human breast cancer xenograft model. BMC Cancer 7:145

94. Zhang Y, Pu X, Shi M, Chen L, Qian L, Song Y, Yuan G, Zhang H, Yu M, Hu M, Shen B, Guo N (2007) c-Jun, a crucial molecule in metastasis of breast cancer and potential target for biotherapy. Oncol Rep 18:1207–1212

95. Honjo Y, Nangia-Makker P, Inohara H, Raz A (2001) Down-regulation of galectin-3 suppresses tumorigenicity of human breast carcinoma cells. Clin Cancer Res 7:661–668

96. Raz A, Zhu DG, Hogan V, Shah N, Raz T, Karkash R, Pazerini G, Carmi P (1990) Evidence for the role of 34-kDa galactoside-binding lectin in transformation and metastasis. Int J Cancer 46:871–877

97. Song YK, Billiar TR, Lee YJ (2002) Role of galectin-3 in breast cancer metastasis: involvement of nitric oxide. Am J Pathol 160:1069–1075

98. Moon BK, Lee YJ, Battle P, Jessup JM, Raz A, Kim HR (2001) Galectin-3 protects human breast carcinoma cells against nitric oxide-induced apoptosis: implication of galectin-3 function during metastasis. Am J Pathol 159:1055–1060

99. Wai PY, Kuo PC (2004) The role of Osteopontin in tumor metastasis. J Surg Res 121: 228–241

100. Lackner C, Moser R, Bauernhofer T, Wilders-Truschnig M, Samonigg H, Berghold A, Zatloukal K (1998) Soluble CD44 v5 and v6 in serum of patients with breast cancer. Correlation with expression of CD44 v5 and v6 variants in primary tumors and location of distant metastasis. Breast Cancer Res Treat 47:29–40

101. Ouhtit A, Abd Elmageed ZY, Abdraboh ME, Lioe TF, Raj MH (2007) In vivo evidence for the role of CD44s in promoting breast cancer metastasis to the liver. Am J Pathol 171:2033–2039

102. Buck MB, Knabbe C (2006) TGF-beta signaling in breast cancer. Ann N Y Acad Sci 1089:119–126

103. Derynck R, Akhurst RJ, Balmain A (2001) TGF-beta signaling in tumor suppression and cancer progression. Nat Genet 29:117–129

104. Siegel PM, Massague J (2003) Cytostatic and apoptotic actions of TGF-beta in homeostasis and cancer. Nat Rev Cancer 3:807–821

105. Shi Y, Massague J (2003) Mechanisms of TGF-beta signaling from cell membrane to the nucleus. Cell 113:685–700

106. Heldin CH, Miyazono K, ten Dijke P (1997) TGF-beta signalling from cell membrane to nucleus through SMAD proteins. Nature 390:465–471

107. Morimoto J, Imai S, Haga S, Iwai Y, Iwai M, Hiroishi S, Miyashita N, Moriwaki K, Hosick HL (1991) New murine mammary tumor cell lines. In Vitro Cell Dev Biol 27A:349–351

108. Azuma H, Ehata S, Miyazaki H, Watabe T, Maruyama O, Imamura T, Sakamoto T, Kiyama S, Kiyama Y, Ubai T, Inamoto T, Takahara S, Itoh Y, Otsuki Y, Katsuoka Y, Miyazono K, Horie S (2005) Effect of Smad7 expression on metastasis of mouse mammary carcinoma JygMC(A) cells. J Natl Cancer Inst 97:1734–1746

109. Ehata S, Hanyu A, Hayashi M, Aburatani H, Kato Y, Fujime M, Saitoh M, Miyazawa K, Imamura T, Miyazono K (2007) Transforming growth factor-beta promotes survival of mammary carcinoma cells through induction of antiapoptotic transcription factor DEC1. Cancer Res 67:9694–9703

110. Aslakson CJ, Miller FR (1992) Selective events in the metastatic process defined by analysis of the sequential dissemination of subpopulations of a mouse mammary tumor. Cancer Res 52:1399–1405

111. Dexter DL, Kowalski HM, Blazar BA, Fligiel Z, Vogel R, Heppner GH (1978) Heterogeneity of tumor cells from a single mouse mammary tumor. Cancer Res 38:3174–3181

112. Heppner GH, Dexter DL, DeNucci T, Miller FR, Calabresi P (1978) Heterogeneity in drug sensitivity among tumor cell subpopulations of a single mammary tumor. Cancer Res 38:3758–3763

113. Lelekakis M, Moseley JM, Martin TJ, Hards D, Williams E, Ho P, Lowen D, Javni J, Miller FR, Slavin J, Anderson RL (1999) A novel orthotopic model of breast cancer metastasis to bone. Clin Exp Metastasis 17:163–170

114. Manka D, Spicer Z, Millhorn DE (2005) Bcl-2/adenovirus E1B 19 kDa interacting protein-3 knockdown enables growth of breast cancer metastases in the lung, liver, and bone. Cancer Res 65:11689–11693

115. Soria G, Ben-Baruch A (2008) The inflammatory chemokines CCL2 and CCL5 in breast cancer. Cancer Lett 267:271–285

116. Niwa Y, Akamatsu H, Niwa H, Sumi H, Ozaki Y, Abe A (2001) Correlation of tissue and plasma RANTES levels with disease course in patients with breast or cervical cancer. Clin Cancer Res 7:285–289

117. Schall TJ, Jongstra J, Dyer BJ, Jorgensen J, Clayberger C, Davis MM, Krensky AM (1988) A human T cell-specific molecule is a member of a new gene family. J Immunol 141: 1018–1025

118. Soria G, Yaal-Hahoshen N, Azenshtein E, Shina S, Leider-Trejo L, Ryvo L, Cohen-Hillel E, Shtabsky A, Ehrlich M, Meshel T, Keydar I, Ben-Baruch A (2008) Concomitant expression of the chemokines RANTES and MCP-1 in human breast cancer: a basis for tumor-promoting interactions. Cytokine 44:191–200

119. Stormes KA, Lemken CA, Lepre JV, Marinucci MN, Kurt RA (2005) Inhibition of metastasis by inhibition of tumor-derived CCL5. Breast Cancer Res Treat 89:209–212

120. Fanto M, McNeill H (2004) Planar polarity from flies to vertebrates. J Cell Sci 117:527–533

121. Bienz M (2005) beta-Catenin: a pivot between cell adhesion and Wnt signalling. Curr Biol 15:R64–67

122. Keeble TR, Halford MM, Seaman C, Kee N, Macheda M, Anderson RB, Stacker SA, Cooper HM (2006) The Wnt receptor Ryk is required for Wnt5a-mediated axon guidance on the contralateral side of the corpus callosum. J Neurosci 26:5840–5848

123. Topol L, Jiang X, Choi H, Garrett-Beal L, Carolan PJ, Yang Y (2003) Wnt-5a inhibits the canonical Wnt pathway by promoting GSK-3-independent beta-catenin degradation. J Cell Biol 162:899–908

124. Jonsson M, Andersson T (2001) Repression of Wnt-5a impairs DDR1 phosphorylation and modifies adhesion and migration of mammary cells. J Cell Sci 114:2043–2053

125. Smalley MJ, Dale TC (2001) Wnt signaling and mammary tumorigenesis. J Mammary Gland Biol Neoplasia 6:37–52

126. Hatsell S, Rowlands T, Hiremath M, Cowin P (2003) Beta-catenin and Tcfs in mammary development and cancer. J Mammary Gland Biol Neoplasia 8:145–158

127. Huelsken J, Behrens J (2002) The Wnt signalling pathway. J Cell Sci 115:3977–3978
128. Dejmek J, Safholm A, Kamp Nielsen C, Andersson T, Leandersson K (2006) Wnt-5a/Ca2+-induced NFAT activity is counteracted by Wnt-5a/Yes-Cdc42-casein kinase 1alpha signaling in human mammary epithelial cells. Mol Cell Biol 26:6024–6036
129. Saneyoshi T, Kume S, Amasaki Y, Mikoshiba K (2002) The Wnt/calcium pathway activates NF-AT and promotes ventral cell fate in Xenopus embryos. Nature 417:295–299
130. Dejmek J, Dejmek A, Safholm A, Sjolander A, Andersson T (2005) Wnt-5a protein expression in primary dukes B colon cancers identifies a subgroup of patients with good prognosis. Cancer Res 65:9142–9146
131. Dejmek J, Leandersson K, Manjer J, Bjartell A, Emdin SO, Vogel WF, Landberg G, Andersson T (2005) Expression and signaling activity of Wnt-5a/discoidin domain receptor-1 and Syk plays distinct but decisive roles in breast cancer patient survival. Clin Cancer Res 11:520–528
132. Jonsson M, Dejmek J, Bendahl PO, Andersson T (2002) Loss of Wnt-5a protein is associated with early relapse in invasive ductal breast carcinomas. Cancer Res 62:409–416
133. Safholm A, Tuomela J, Rosenkvist J, Dejmek J, Harkonen P, Andersson T (2008) The Wnt-5a-derived hexapeptide Foxy-5 inhibits breast cancer metastasis in vivo by targeting cell motility. Clin Cancer Res 14:6556–6563
134. Turksen K, Troy TC (2004) Barriers built on claudins. J Cell Sci 117:2435–2447
135. Kramer F, White K, Kubbies M, Swisshelm K, Weber BH (2000) Genomic organization of claudin-1 and its assessment in hereditary and sporadic breast cancer. Hum Genet 107: 249–256
136. Kominsky SL, Argani P, Korz D, Evron E, Raman V, Garrett E, Rein A, Sauter G, Kallioniemi OP, Sukumar S (2003) Loss of the tight junction protein claudin-7 correlates with histological grade in both ductal carcinoma in situ and invasive ductal carcinoma of the breast. Oncogene 22:2021–2033
137. Sauer T, Pedersen MK, Ebeltoft K, Naess O (2005) Reduced expression of Claudin-7 in fine needle aspirates from breast carcinomas correlate with grading and metastatic disease. Cytopathology 16:193–198
138. Erin N, Zhao W, Bylander J, Chase G, Clawson G (2006) Capsaicin-induced inactivation of sensory neurons promotes a more aggressive gene expression phenotype in breast cancer cells. Breast Cancer Res Treat 99:351–364
139. Erin N, Wang N, Xin P, Bui V, Weisz J, Barkan GA, Zhao W, Shearer D, Clawson GA (2009) Altered gene expression in breast cancer liver metastases. Int J Cancer 124: 1503–1516
140. Tabariès S, Dong Z, Annis MG, Omeroglu A, Pepin F, Ouellet V, Russo C, Hassanain M, Metrakos P, Diaz Z, Basik M, Bertos N, Park M, Guettier C, Adam R, Hallett M, Siegel PM (2010) Claudin-2 is selectively enriched in and promotes the formation of breast cancer liver metastases through engagement of integrin complexes. Oncogene aop. doi:10.1038/onc.2010.518
141. Herschkowitz JI, Simin K, Weigman VJ, Mikaelian I, Usary J, Hu Z, Rasmussen KE, Jones LP, Assefnia S, Chandrasekharan S, Backlund MG, Yin Y, Khramtsov AI, Bastein R, Quackenbush J, Glazer RI, Brown PH, Green JE, Kopelovich L, Furth PA, Palazzo JP, Olopade OI, Bernard PS, Churchill GA, Van Dyke T, Perou CM (2007) Identification of conserved gene expression features between murine mammary carcinoma models and human breast tumors. Genome Biol 8:R76
142. Morin PJ (2005) Claudin proteins in human cancer: promising new targets for diagnosis and therapy. Cancer Res 65:9603–9606
143. Kinugasa T, Huo Q, Higashi D, Shibaguchi H, Kuroki M, Tanaka T, Futami K, Yamashita Y, Hachimine K, Maekawa S, Nabeshima K, Iwasaki H (2007) Selective up-regulation of claudin-1 and claudin-2 in colorectal cancer. Anticancer Res 27:3729–3734
144. Soini Y (2004) Claudins 2, 3, 4, 5 in Paget's disease and breast carcinoma. Hum Pathol 35:1531–1536

145. Kim TH, Huh JH, Lee S, Kang H, Kim GI, An HJ (2008) Down-regulation of claudin-2 in breast carcinomas is associated with advanced disease. Histopathology 53:48–55

146. Ladwein M, Pape UF, Schmidt DS, Schnolzer M, Fiedler S, Langbein L, Franke WW, Moldenhauer G, Zoller M (2005) The cell-cell adhesion molecule EpCAM interacts directly with the tight junction protein claudin-7. Exp Cell Res 309:345–357

147. Hemler ME (2005) Tetraspanin functions and associated microdomains. Nat Rev Mol Cell Biol 6:801–811

148. Lazo PA (2007) Functional implications of tetraspanin proteins in cancer biology. Cancer Sci 98:1666–1677

149. Bissell MJ, Kenny PA, Radisky DC (2005) Microenvironmental regulators of tissue structure and function also regulate tumor induction and progression: the role of extra-cellular matrix and its degrading enzymes. Cold Spring Harb Symp Quant Biol 70: 343–356

150. DiMeo TA, Kuperwasser C (2006) The evolving paradigm of tissue-specific metastasis. Breast Cancer Res 8:301

151. Bhowmick NA, Neilson EG, Moses HL (2004) Stromal fibroblasts in cancer initiation and progression. Nature 432:332–337

152. Karnoub AE, Dash AB, Vo AP, Sullivan A, Brooks MW, Bell GW, Richardson AL, Polyak K, Tubo R, Weinberg RA (2007) Mesenchymal stem cells within tumour stroma promote breast cancer metastasis. Nature 449:557–563

153. Psaila B, Kaplan RN, Port ER, Lyden D (2006) Priming the 'soil' for breast cancer metastasis: the pre-metastatic niche. Breast Dis 26:65–74

154. Kaplan RN, Psaila B, Lyden D (2006) Bone marrow cells in the 'pre-metastatic niche': within bone and beyond. Cancer Metastasis Rev 25:521–529

155. Erler JT, Bennewith KL, Cox TR, Lang G, Bird D, Koong A, Le QT, Giaccia AJ (2009) Hypoxia-induced lysyl oxidase is a critical mediator of bone marrow cell recruitment to form the premetastatic niche. Cancer Cell 15:35–44

156. Hiratsuka S, Watanabe A, Aburatani H, Maru Y (2006) Tumour-mediated upregulation of chemoattractants and recruitment of myeloid cells predetermines lung metastasis. Nat Cell Biol 8:1369–1375

157. Yang L, Huang J, Ren X, Gorska AE, Chytil A, Aakre M, Carbone DP, Matrisian LM, Richmond A, Lin PC, Moses HL (2008) Abrogation of TGF beta signaling in mam-mary carcinomas recruits Gr-1+CD11b+ myeloid cells that promote metastasis. Cancer Cell 13:23–35

158. DuPre SA, Redelman D, Hunter KW Jr (2007) The mouse mammary carcinoma 4T1: char-acterization of the cellular landscape of primary tumours and metastatic tumour foci. Int J Exp Pathol 88:351–360

159. Yang L, DeBusk LM, Fukuda K, Fingleton B, Green-Jarvis B, Shyr Y, Matrisian LM, Carbone DP, Lin PC (2004) Expansion of myeloid immune suppressor Gr+CD11b+ cells in tumor-bearing host directly promotes tumor angiogenesis. Cancer Cell 6: 409–421

160. Ilkovitch D, Lopez DM (2009) The liver is a site for tumor-induced myeloid-derived suppressor cell accumulation and immunosuppression. Cancer Res 69:5514–5521

161. Hiratsuka S, Nakamura K, Iwai S, Murakami M, Itoh T, Kijima H, Shipley JM, Senior RM, Shibuya M (2002) MMP9 induction by vascular endothelial growth factor receptor-1 is involved in lung-specific metastasis. Cancer Cell 2:289–300

162. McAllister SS, Gifford AM, Greiner AL, Kelleher SP, Saelzler MP, Ince TA, Reinhardt F, Harris LN, Hylander BL, Repasky EA, Weinberg RA (2008) Systemic endocrine instigation of indolent tumor growth requires osteopontin. Cell 133:994–1005

163. Jung T, Castellana D, Klingbeil P, Hernandez IC, Vitacolonna M, Orlicky DJ, Roffler SR, Brodt P, Zoller (2009) M CD44v6 dependence of premetastatic niche preparation by exosomes. Neoplasia 11:1093–1105

164. Rodrigues LR, Teixeira JA, Schmitt FL, Paulsson M, Lindmark-Mansson H (2007) The role of osteopontin in tumor progression and metastasis in breast cancer. Cancer Epidemiol Biomarkers Prev 16:1087–1097

165. Tuck AB, Chambers AF, Allan AL (2007) Osteopontin overexpression in breast cancer: knowledge gained and possible implications for clinical management. J Cell Biochem 102:859–868

166. Pinilla S, Alt E, Abdul Khalek FJ, Jotzu C, Muehlberg F, Beckmann C, Song YH (2009) Tissue resident stem cells produce CCL5 under the influence of cancer cells and thereby promote breast cancer cell invasion. Cancer Lett 284:80–85

167. Chabot V, Reverdiau P, Iochmann S, Rico A, Senecal D, Goupille C, Sizaret PY, Sensebe L (2006) CCL5-enhanced human immature dendritic cell migration through the basement membrane in vitro depends on matrix metalloproteinase-9. J Leukoc Biol 79:767–778

168. Muehlberg FL, Song YH, Krohn A, Pinilla SP, Droll LH, Leng X, Seidensticker M, Ricke J, Altman AM, Devarajan E, Liu W, Arlinghaus RB, Alt EU (2009) Tissue-resident stem cells promote breast cancer growth and metastasis. Carcinogenesis 30:589–597

169. Scadden DT (2006) The stem-cell niche as an entity of action. Nature 441:1075–1079

Part II
Clinical Management

Chapter 11
Imaging of Hepatic Metastases

Mohamed El Khodary, Laurent Milot, and Caroline Reinhold

Abstract Both benign and malignant focal liver lesions are common occurrences and imaging the liver for focal lesions especially in cancer patients is one of the most frequent tasks in everyday radiological practice. Metastasis from other organs is the most common liver malignancy, so familiarity with appearances of liver metastases and knowledge of the best imaging tool is a necessity. In this chapter we provide detailed information on the choice of imaging modalities available for imaging liver metastases, describe liver metastases as they appear using these modalities, and highlight the preferred imaging techniques in different clinical scenarios. Recent advances in imaging of liver metastases including new MRI contrast agents, contrast enhanced ultrasound and PET/CT are described and discussed in detail. Imaging is increasingly being used as a problem solving tool for the clinical team and a better understanding of the imaging capabilities presently available is essential for improving patient care and providing personalized medicine for the cancer patient.

Keywords Liver · Metastasis · Imaging · Contrast · MRI

Abbreviations

IVC	inferior vena cava
CT	computed tomography
MRI	magnetic resonance imaging
US	ultrasound
FLL's	focal liver lesions
THI	tissue harmonic imaging
IOUS	intraoperative ultrasound
PRF	pulse repetition frequency
CEUS	contrast-enhanced ultrasound
PIM	phase inversion mode

M. El Khodary (✉)
Department of Radiology, McGill University Health Center, 1650 Cedar Ave., Montreal, QC, Canada H3G 1A4
e-mail: mohamed.khodary@gmail.com

P. Brodt (ed.), *Liver Metastasis: Biology and Clinical Management*, Cancer Metastasis – Biology and Treatment 16, DOI 10.1007/978-94-007-0292-9_11, © Springer Science+Business Media B.V. 2011

PPI	power pulse inversion
CPS	contrast pulse sequences
CEIOUS	contrast enhanced intraoperative ultrasound
EFSUMB	European Federation of Societies for Ultrasound in Medicine and Biology
FNH	focal nodular hyperplasia
HCC	hepatocellular carcinoma
MDCT	multi-detector row CT
GIST	gastrointestinal stromal tumor
RF	radiofrequency
RECIST	Response Evaluation Criteria in solid tumors
NCCTG	North Central Cancer Treatment Group
NSABP	National Surgical Adjuvant Breast and Bowel Project
SSFP	steady-state free precision
FIESTA	fast imaging employing steady-state acquisition
bFFFE	balanced fast-field echo
True FISP	true fast imaging with steady precision
True SSFP	true steady-state free precision
Gd-BOPTA	gadobenate dimeglumine benzyloxypropionctetraacetate
SNR	signal to noise ratio
CNR	contrast to noise ratio
3D	three dimensional
THID	transient hepatic intensity difference
SAR	specific absorption rate
Gd-DTPA	gadopentetate dimeglumine
Gd-DOTA	gadolinium-tetraazacyclododecanetetraacetic acid
Gd-DTPA-BMA	gadolinium diethylenetriaminepentaacetic acid bis
Gd-HP-DO3A	gadolinium hydroxypropyl tetraazacyclododecane
RES	reticuloendothelial system
SPIO	superparamagnetic particles of iron oxide
DWI	diffusion-weighted MR imaging
PET	positron emission tomography
BGO	bismuth germinate
LSO	lutetium oxyorthosilicate
GSO	gadolinium silicate
SUV	standardized uptake value

Contents

11.1 Introduction

11.1.1 The Anatomy of the Liver

The anatomy of the liver can be described based on the external appearance of the organ (external or descriptive anatomy) or based on its vascular and biliary architecture (vascular or functional anatomy).

11.1.2 Descriptive Anatomy

The liver is the largest organ in the abdomen, occupying most of the right upper quadrant. Superiorly, laterally, and anteriorly, the liver is bordered by, and conforms to the undersurface of the diaphragm. Prominent diaphragmatic leaves may indent the surface of the liver as they insert on the ribs, producing hypoattenuating or low-signal-intensity defects that should not be misinterpreted as intrahepatic lesions [1]. The liver is covered by peritoneum, except for the surfaces apposed to the inferior vena cava (IVC), the gallbladder fossa, and the posterosuperior aspect of the diaphragm (bare area) [2].

The liver is divided into right and left lobes. Three hepatic fissures help define the margins of the hepatic lobes and the major hepatic segments. The interlobar fissure forms the inferior margin of the border between the right and left hepatic lobes. The fissure for the ligamentum teres divides the left lobe into medial and lateral segments. The fissure for the ligamentum venosum, is oriented in a coronal or oblique plane between the posterior aspect of the left lateral hepatic segment and the anterior aspect of the caudate lobe [3].

11.1.3 Functional and Radiological Anatomy

An understanding of the segmental anatomy of the liver is critical for localization and appropriate management of hepatic neoplasms. The system proposed by Goldsmith and Woodburne [4] and used by most North American radiologists does not provide a level of detail that is adequate for the surgical planning of subsegmental hepatic resections. The classification proposed by Couinaud [5] and

Table 11.1 Nomenclature of Liver Segments [148]

Anatomic subsegment	Nomenclature		
	Couinaud	Bismuth	Goldsmith and Woodburne
Caudate	I	I	Caudate lobe
Left lateral superior subsegment	II	II	Left lateral segment
Left lateral inferior subsegment	III	III	Left lateral segment
Left medial subsegment	IV	IVa-IVb	Left medial segment
Right anterior inferior subsegment	V	V	Right anterior segment
Right anterior superior subsegment	VIII	VIII	Right anterior segment
Right posterior inferior subsegment	VI	VI	Right posterior segment
Right posterior superior subsegment	VII	VII	Right posterior segment

later modified by Bismuth [6], provides the surgically relevant information and is easily applicable to cross-sectional imaging techniques such as computed tomography (CT), magnetic resonance imaging (MRI), and ultrasound (US). In Europe and Japan, this nomenclature is the most commonly used by surgeons and radiologists (Table 11.1).

In the Bismuth classification, the plane separating the right and the left liver runs from the middle hepatic vein, to the inferior vena cava, to the gallbladder. The segments in the right liver, those that are anterior and to the left of the right hepatic vein will be in the right anterior sector (segments 5 and 8) and those posterior and to the right will be in the right posterior sector (segments 6 and 7). The inferior segments (5 and 6) lie caudal to the portal bifurcation, and the superior segments (7 and 8) lie cranial to it. Therefore in the right anterior sector, segment 5 will be below and segment 8 above, and in the posterior sector, segment 6 below and segment 7 above.

In the left liver, the main landmark is the left portal vein and the second landmark is the left hepatic vein. The left portal vein demarcates a smooth arch from the main bifurcation to the umbilical ligament. All liver tissue circumscribed by the concavity of the arch and the middle hepatic vein are segment 4. On the convexity of the arch, the distal part of the left hepatic vein will separate segment 2 (posteriorly and superiorly) from segment 3 (more anteriorly and inferiorly) on the left side [7].

11.2 Imaging of Liver Metastases

11.2.1 Background

Both benign and malignant focal liver lesions are very common and imaging the liver for focal lesions, particularly in cancer patients is one of the most frequent tasks in everyday radiological practice. The most common malignant lesions in the liver are metastases from other organs: 25–50% patients with a known non-haematological malignancy have liver metastases at the time of diagnosis originating from (with decreasing frequency) colon, gastric, pancreatic, breast and lung

Table 11.2   Types of complex or solid liver lesions [11]

Types of focal liver lesions:	Metastases
	Hepatocellular carcinoma
	Cholangiocarcinoma
	Hepatoblastoma
	Fibrolamellar carcinoma
	Undifferentiated (embryonal) sarcoma
	Biliary cystadenoma/cystadenocarcinoma
Malignant	Cavernous hemangioma
	Focal nodular hyperplasia
Non malignant	Focal fatty infiltration
	Abscess
	Echinococcal cyst
	Hemangioendothelioma

cancer [8, 9] and there are multiple metastases in up to 98% of these patients. This is because the special features of the portal vein circulation favour haematogenous metastasis to the liver [10] (see Table 11.2).

Liver imaging of cancer patients requires an imaging modality that is not only highly sensitive in detection but also provides reliable characterization of the lesions and thus allows differentiation of malignant from benign tumors. Accurate and timely detection of hepatic metastases has far-reaching therapeutic and prognostic implications. Liver imaging has become increasingly demanding in view of recent improvements to liver resection and local ablation of metastases, particularly from colorectal carcinoma. Accurate assessment of the number, size and segmental location of metastases is required to identify patients suitable for surgical or interventional therapy, for treatment planning and for follow-up imaging during chemotherapy [12], (The reader is also referred to Chapters 12 for an extensive review of current approaches to the management of colorectal cancer liver metastasis).

The radiologic diagnosis of liver metastases involves detection, characterization and tumor staging. Knowledge of the histopathological changes that occur with metastases provides the best approach to the accurate interpretation of radiologic imaging, and in particular, radiologists need to choose appropriate imaging methods based on such knowledge. Liver metastases need to be screened for when an extrahepatic malignancy is confirmed. Moreover, liver metastases from an unknown origin need to be evaluated with the view to identifying the primary source, as well as for diagnosing the liver metastases. During the preoperative workup, it should be determined which liver segments are involved and how the tumors are anatomically associated with hepatic vessels, bile ducts, and extrahepatic structures [13].

11.2.2 Imaging modalities for Liver Metastases

The imaging techniques most commonly used today for liver metastasis are US, CT, MR and FDG PET. The sensitivity for detection of liver metastases is currently

55% for US, 72% for CT, 76% for MR imaging, and 90% for FDG PET, as per meta-analysis by Kinkel K, et al. [14, 15].

11.2.2.1 Sonography of Liver Metastasis

General Background

The ability of ultrasound to detect focal lesions depends on numerous factors including size, location, echogenicity, and mass effect. The size of the metastases can range from only microscopically detectable (cellular) infiltration to large masses measuring more than 20 cm. Detection depends on a combination of spatial and contrast resolutions. Typically, small echogenic lesions are easily detectable, while larger but isoechoic lesions are more difficult to image, with mass effect being more important for the diagnosis of the latter. The characterization of focal liver lesions and thus the specificity of the ultrasound rely on gray scale imaging, Doppler, and contrast agent appearance [16]. The echogenicity of liver metastases also varies widely. The majority of liver metastatic lesions have a target appearance with an echogenic or isoechoic center and a hypoechoic halo. A thin halo may represent peritumoral sinusoids or compressed liver parenchyma. Thick halos represent proliferating tumor. Other causes of target lesions are hepatocellular carcinoma and less likely are lymphoma, abscesses, adenoma and FNH [17, 16].

Examination Techniques

(i) *Grey Scale US*: Despite technical advances involving both spatial and contrast resolution, gray-scale ultrasound (US) is still considered a non-specific technique in the diagnosis of focal liver lesions (FLLs] [16]. The liver is best scanned using a curved array or sector probe with a center frequency ranging from 2 to 5 MHz. Higher frequency linear array transducers may be employed to image superficial parts of the liver surface on deep inspiration [16]. US appearances of metastases may vary within a given patient as well as over time and especially following chemotherapy. Most metastases are round with well-defined margins. Hypoechoic metastases are more common (approximately 65%) than hyper- or isoechoic. A hypoechoic halo surrounding the lesions is seen in 40%; it is usually associated with iso- or hyperechoic metastases (Fig. 11.1) [18]. For a summary of the common sonographic patterns of metastatic liver disease please see Table 11.3.

(ii) *Tissue Harmonic Imaging*: Tissue harmonic imaging (THI) is a grey-scale technique that uses information from harmonic signals (multiples of the insonating frequency) generated by non-linear propagation of a sound wave, as it passes through tissue. THI improves spatial and contrast resolution of B-mode US in the majority of cases, and the conspicuity of focal liver lesions is often improved. However, the detection rate of focal lesions is only slightly improved. THI should be part of every state-of-the-art sonogram of the liver and abdomen [19].

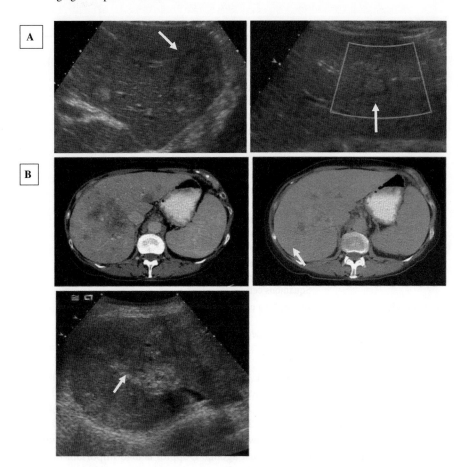

Fig. 11.1 Ultrasound and CT images of hepatic metastases of colorectal cancer. Shown in (**a**) are hepatic metastases of an 80 years old male with classical target appearance on US. Central increased echogenicity and peripheral hypoechoic rim are indicated by arrow (*left*). The lesion appears hypovascular on Doppler US as shown on the right (*arrow*). Shown in (**b**) are hepatic metastases of a 70 years-old female showing progressive central enhancement. Axial CT images in portovenous phase showing hypodense metastases with progressive central enhancement on the equilibrium phase are shown on the top and ultrasound images showing the metastasis as a heterogenous, hyperechoic focal lesion can be seen on the bottom

(iii) *Intraoperative Ultrasound*: Intraoperative US (IOUS) provides highly accurate information to the surgeon, influencing surgical management. IOUS detects 10–15% more metastases than CT arterial portography and 19–32% more than SPIO enhanced MR [20, 21]. One prospective study showed IOUS impact on the surgical management of primary or secondary liver malignancies in almost 50% of the cases [22].

(iv) *Doppler Ultrasound*: When using color Doppler, the setting should be optimized to achieve greatest sensitivity to detect low flow by increasing color

Table 11.3 Echogenic properties of different hepatic lesions [16]

1. Echogenic	Colon carcinoma
	Neuroendocrine tumours, i.e. carcinoid, pancreatic islet cell tumours
	Renal cell carcinoma
	Choriocarcinoma
	Multifocal hepatocellular carcinoma
2. Echopoor	Breast cancer
	Lung cancer
	Lymphoma
	Pancreas
3. Target pattern (halo)	Most common lung cancer
	May occur in many others
4. Calcified metastasis	Common; mucinous adenocarcinoma: colon, ovary, stomach, breast (treated)
	Rare; osteosarcoma, chondrosarcoma
5. Cystic	Ovary, pancreas, colon cancer
	Sarcomas-necrosis
	Squamous cell
6. Infiltrative	Breast, lung cancer
	Melanoma
	Multifocal hepatocellular carcinoma

gain to a level just below that which would create artifact. Also, the color box should be made as small as possible, and the wall filter and pulse repetition frequency (PRF) should be lowered [16, 23]. Conventional color and spectral Doppler are unable to image the vascularity of the majority of the metastases because it is too low (Fig. 11.2). This may be rectified with the use of power Doppler and contrast agents. Doppler is also important in detecting vascular invasion [16]. On color Doppler imaging, metastases are as a rule, poorly vascularised and their essential characteristic is a predominantly arterial blood supply (with little or no portal venous blood supply). Like echogenicity, the vascularisation depends on the size, the biological behavior and the nature of the primary tumour. Irregular vascularisation is often observed, with broken-off vessels and peripherally situated arterio-venous shunt formation. The metastases of neuroendocrine tumours (but also others such as metastases of renal cell carcinoma) may be more richly vascularised than other metastases. However, no conclusions are possible regarding the primary tumour on the basis of the observed vascularisation pattern [10].

(v) *Contrast-Enhanced Ultrasound*: Contrast-enhanced ultrasound (CEUS) represents a significant breakthrough in sonography and is being increasingly used for the evaluation of focal liver lesions (FLLs). The unique feature of CEUS for non-invasively assessing liver perfusion throughout the vascular phase has led to a dramatic improvement in the diagnostic accuracy of US for both detection and characterization of FLLs, as well as in the guidance and evaluation of response to therapeutic procedures. Currently, CEUS is included as a part of the

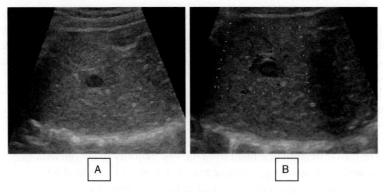

Fig. 11.2 Ultrasound images of hepatic metastases of esophageal cancer. Images are from a 53 years old male with metastatic esophageal carcinoma showing a hypoechoic focal lesion on grey scale US (**a**) which is hypovascular on Doppler scan (**b**)

suggested diagnostic work-up of FLLs, resulting in better patient management and more cost-effective therapy [24].

Ultrasound contrast agents consist of microbubbles of gas with a protein, lipid or polymer shell. The microbubbles are approximately 1–10 μm in diameter i.e. the size of red blood cells. Both the gas they contain (usually air or a perfluoro compound) and the stabilizing shell (denatured albumin, surfactants or phospholipids) are critical to their effectiveness as contrast agents and to rendering them sufficiently stable to "survive" for several minutes after injection. These agents flood the blood pool after intravenous injection and are confined to the vascular compartment (unless there is ongoing bleeding) [25]. They are too large to pass through the vascular endothelium and, as such, are considered pure blood pool agents [26]. After several minutes in the circulation, the microbubbles dissolve, the gas is exhaled and the shell is metabolized, mainly in the liver [27, 28, 29].

When subjected to an US wave, the microbubbles respond by changing their size: they expand during the rarefaction phase and contract during the pressure phase. These changes are much greater than the minor changes that occur in the soft tissues. The bubbles, like every oscillating system, have a natural frequency (the resonance frequency) at which their response is maximal. Fortunately, the bubbles resonate at frequencies used for diagnostic US imaging. This coincidence accounts for their high reflectivity, even when they are present in a small concentration. Furthermore, the expansion of these bubbles during the rarefaction phase exceeds their contraction during the pressure phase. This asymmetric oscillation produces a returning signal (echo) that contains harmonics, i.e. multiples of the driving frequency [30]. The echo is detected by different imaging techniques such as stimulated acoustic enhancement (SAE), phase inversion mode (PIM), power pulse inversion (PPI) and contrast pulse sequences (CPS) [31–34].

With up-to-date technology, CEUS sensitivity and specificity in staging liver metastases (80–95% and 84–98%, respectively) approach those of CT and MRI

[35, 36]. CEUS was shown to be particularly useful to improve the conspicuity and detection rate of metastases smaller than 1 cm or of those lesions that are isoechoic with respect to adjacent liver parenchyma and thus barely visible with conventional US [37, 38]. US contrast agents are safe, well-tolerated and have very few contraindications [39].

Metastases may show various contrast enhancement patterns in the arterial phase (absent, rim-like, dotted, or diffuse) and they invariably present as hypoechoic lesions in the late phase. Metastases consistently show rapid and complete contrast washout and appear as enhancement defects on late phase scans (Fig. 11.3) [40, 41], thus differentiating them from the vast majority of benign liver tumors that usually appear as iso- or hyperechoic masses because of sustained retention of contrast agent. This pattern is likely related to the abnormal blood supply (i.e., mainly arterial) of metastases, with rapid wash-out in the portal-venous phase [42, 43].

Metastases in all three phases show characteristic dynamic features after contrast injection. In the *arterial phase* the appearances is twofold: hypovascular metastases appear as hyporeflective lesions usually with a typical rim enhancement of varying size [44, 45] whereas *hypervascular_*metastatic deposits appear as brightly enhancing hyperreflective and homogeneous lesions, sometimes with non-enhancing necrotic areas. At the beginning of the *portal venous phase*, the (rim) enhancement fades and the entire lesion becomes increasingly hyporeflective. In the *delayed phase* both hypo- and hypervascular metastases invariably show as hyporeflective defects, while the enhancement persists in normal liver parenchyma. This imaging appearance during the delayed phase of acquisition is independent of the contrast agent and imaging technique used [18]. During the delayed phase, metastases are usually particularly well defined, often with sharp (punched out) borders. Both portal venous and delayed phase imaging markedly increase the contrast between the enhancing normal liver and the non-enhancing metastases and thus improve detection, especially of small lesions that are less than 1 cm in diameter and of lesions that are isoechoic at baseline imaging.

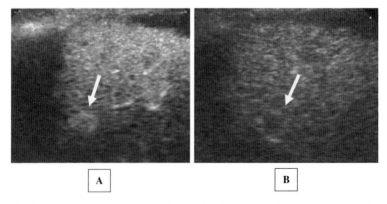

Fig. 11.3 Contrast enhanced US in a patient with colorectal carcinoma metastases. Shown are intense enhancement on the arterial phase (**a**) and washout in the delayed phase (**b**) (*arrows*). Courtesy of Mostafa Atri, University of Toronto, Toronto, CAN

It should be noted that the administration of contrast agents has also been shown to improve the accuracy of intraoperative ultrasound (CEIOUS) with important implications for surgical strategy [46, 47].

It has been proposed by the European Federation of Societies for Ultrasound in Medicine and Biology (EFSUMB) that any US staging study of the liver should be contrast enhanced. However the cost and feasibility of implementing this recommendation remain a challenge [48].

11.2.3 Imaging of Liver Metastasis by Computed Tomography

11.2.3.1 General Background

CT is the most commonly used imaging modality for both detection and characterization of hepatic metastases. Hepatic metastases generally present the histologic type of the primary neoplasm and are therefore histologically diverse and distinct from local hepatic cancers. In patients with suspected liver metastases four questions are important:

1. Does the liver contain focal lesions?
2. What is the number and location of the lesions
3. What are the characteristics of the lesions
4. If metastases are detected, are they treatable by resection or interventional therapy?

Patients with equivocal findings at sonography are often referred for definitive evaluation with computed CT or magnetic resonance imaging (MR). Indications for liver CT imaging include differentiation of benign liver lesions, i.e. simple cysts, hemangiomas, adenomas or focal nodular hyperplasia (FNH) from malignant lesions, such as metastases, hepatocellular carcinoma (HCC) or cholangiocarcinoma. CT is also used for early detection of liver metastases because of its better detection rates in comparison to conventional ultrasound that has more variable sensitivity and is more operator- dependent, particularly in the setting of a technically suboptimal exam.

11.2.3.2 Technical Aspects of CT

Multi-detector row CT (MDCT) has transformed CT from a transaxial cross-sectional technique into a 3D imaging modality. Whereas single-slice CT took at least 5 years to gain general acceptance, MDCT has been more rapidly accepted in the radiological community, with exponential growth in the use of these scanners in clinical practice. Major improvements (z-axis coverage, speed and longitudinal resolution) translated into rapid hepatic imaging and the use of new imaging protocols, not possible with single-slice spiral CT. Thin sections that can now be routinely used within a single breathhold, resulted in improved lesion detection and nearly isotropic image acquisition, providing high-resolution datasets for multiplanar reformations [49]. Whole liver scanning performed in 5–10 s offers in addition, high temporary resolution. Three dimensional display and multiplanar image reformatting are readily performed and facilitate image interpretation of liver segments with a tumor burden and the relation between tumors and hepatic vessels. This is critical information that allows the surgeons to preoperatively map out anatomical information associated with tumor resections [13].

Theoretically, a complete liver examination might include five phases of a contrast enhanced MDCT protocol. A pre-contrast scan, followed by a contrast-enhanced acquisition obtained during the arterial phase (sometimes split into early and late arterial phases), a portal venous phase and a delayed equilibrium phase. For several reasons, including radiation exposure and data explosion with complex image viewing and storing, not all five phases are acquired in each patient. Although there is no clear consensus over this issue, the selection and combination of acquisition phases generally depends on the clinical questions explored.

Contrast administration to acquire different liver phases can be achieved using fixed delay (35–40 s) for late arterial phase and 60 s for the portal venous phase. The other method is bolus tracking which enables calculation of the circulation time and planning of the optimal scanning delay.

To detect liver metastases, scanning in the portal venous phase is generally sufficient. The authors recommend scanning the whole liver at any time from 55 to 70 s after initiation, when liver parenchymal and portal venous enhancement are most intense. An arterial phase might be needed if hypervascular metastasis is suspected. For follow up patients, a single phase CT protocol can also be used in the portovenous phase. For evaluation of liver lesions, a triphasic liver protocol (arterial, portovenous and delayed phases) is recommended. A precontrast phase can also be added to this protocol.

It has been observed that slice thicknesses of 2 or 4 mm are the most effective for detection of focal liver lesions, with an identical detection rate of 96% for both. Thinner (1 mm) and thicker (6, 8 and 10 mm) slices showed significantly lower detection rates (85, 84, 75 and 70%, respectively). Moreover, 1 mm slice thickness generated the highest number of false positive findings [50, 51].

11.2.3.3 Appearance of Liver Metastasis in CT Imaging

It is important to stress that small benign hepatic masses are very common. In patients without a known malignancy, and without liver cirrhosis, the likelihood that a small mass (less than, or equal to 10 mm) is a metastasis is very low. These patients can be evaluated with serial follow-up imaging because nearly all of them will have benign lesions [52]. Even in a patient with known malignant disease, the chance that such a lesion is malignant is less than 20% [53, 54]. One study has demonstrated that in patients with colorectal and gastric cancer, the probability of one or more hypoattenuating liver lesions measuring 15 mm or less in diameter being malignant, in the absence of evidence of larger metastases, is less than 3% [55]. Another study demonstrated that among breast cancer patients with hepatic lesions considered too small to characterize and no definite liver metastases at initial CT, 93–96% had benign lesions [54].

A total of 3–10% of all colorectal cancer patients will develop liver metastases that are resectable [56, 57]. Unlike patients with other metastatic malignancies, the presence of distant metastases in colorectal cancer patients does not preclude curative treatment [58]. Twenty-five percent of patients who have colorectal carcinoma liver metastases have no other distant metastases. Of these, 10–25% are candidates for surgical resection. In fact, while patients with untreated liver metastases have a 5-year survival rate of 0–3% [59], in patients that undergo a resection with curative intent, the 5-year survival rate can be as high as 25–40% [13, 59]. Accurate detection and characterization of hepatic focal lesions in these patients is therefore critical.

The appearance of imaged metastases depends on a number of factors including lesion histology, vascularity and size, as well as the presence of necrosis, fibrosis, calcification, or hemorrhage within the mass.

In contrast to the liver parenchyma, hepatic metastases obtain their blood supply almost exclusively from the hepatic artery. Only small metastases with a diameter of less than 1.5 cm may be found to have a residual portal venous blood supply. In general, the vascularity of metastases is classified according to their contrast behavior in the arterial-dominant phase scan. Metastases which are hyperdense to normal liver parenchyma in this phase are called hypervascular. Hypervascular metastases are less frequently seen in the liver than hypovascular metastases and typically originate from renal cell carcinomas, carcinoids, pancreatic islet cell carcinomas, sarcomas, pheochromocytomas, melanomas, thyroid carcinomas, choriocarcinomas and occasionally breast cancer [60, 61]. The best phase for detection of hypervascular metastases is the arterial phase. While metastases receive strong contrast enhancement via the hepatic artery, the liver parenchyma enhances only minimally in the arterial phase. Small hypervascular metastases usually present with homogeneous enhancement, whereas larger lesions appear heterogeneous or show an enhancing peripheral rim surrounding a central area of necrosis. In the portal venous phase, most hypervascular metastases show isodense attenuation, because the tumor still receives some contrast from the hepatic artery and the liver parenchyma also receives contrast from the portal vein. Therefore, these hypervascular metastases become difficult to detect during the portal venous phase of enhancement [62, 63, 64, 65], (see Fig. 11.4).

Most hepatic metastases are hypovascular and they generally originate from adenocarcinomas of the gastrointestinal tract, lung and breast carcinomas. Metastases from squamous cell carcinomas (head and neck, esophagus, lung) are also typically hypovascular. Hypovascular metastases receive only minimal arterial and portal venous blood supply due to confluent dense cellularity, fibrosis or necrosis. They show low attenuation compared with normal liver parenchyma during both arterial and subsequent portal venous phases (see Fig. 11.5) [66, 13]. The detection of hypovascular metastases is therefore highest, during the portal venous phase at which time the lesion to liver contrast is optimal. In one study the overall sensitivity of portal venous phase helical CT for demonstrating hepatic neoplasms was

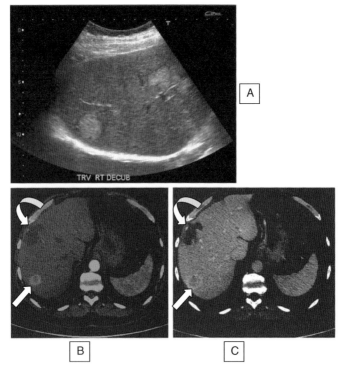

Fig. 11.4 Multi-modality imaging of a patient with hemangiomas and metastases from carcinoid tumors. (**a**) On ultrasound, hyperechoic lesions are seen, hemangiomas (*curved arrows*, (b)) and metastases (*straight arrows*, (b)) are difficult to differentiate. (**b**) CT on arterial phase demonstrates the carcinoid metastasis as hypervascular, whereas the hemangioma demonstrates a typical peripheral globular enhancement. (**c**) CT on the portal phase shows partial wash-out of the metastasis. (**d**) T2WI demonstrates mild heterogeneous hyperintensity of the metastasis whereas the hemangioma shows typical high signal intensity. (**e, f**) DWI MRI with ADC map show restriction of diffusion in the metastasis, no restriction in a small hemangioma and mild restriction in the large hemangioma. On the map, the metastasis demonstrates a decreased ADC. (**g, h**) MRI with contrast injection with strong enhancement of the metastasis and progressive filling of the hemangiomas

81% and for lesions larger than 1 cm, 91% [67]. The portal venous phase also has the advantage of demonstrating portal venous thrombosis, differentiating neoplasms from vessels, and identifying varices and shunts [63].

At times, hypovascular metastases show a target appearance with a hyperattenuating rim and a hypoattenuating center during the arterial and portal venous phases. The "complete ring" pattern is defined as circumferential ring enhancement surrounding a predominant central region with low attenuation seen in metastases, with a PPV of 98% and specificity of 93% (see Fig. 11.6), [64]. In the delayed phase, the outer rim may become isodense to surrounding liver parenchyma, so that the lesion appears smaller than it is in reality (Fig. 11.7). This finding can lead to problems in preoperative staging or follow-up examinations after chemotherapy [65].

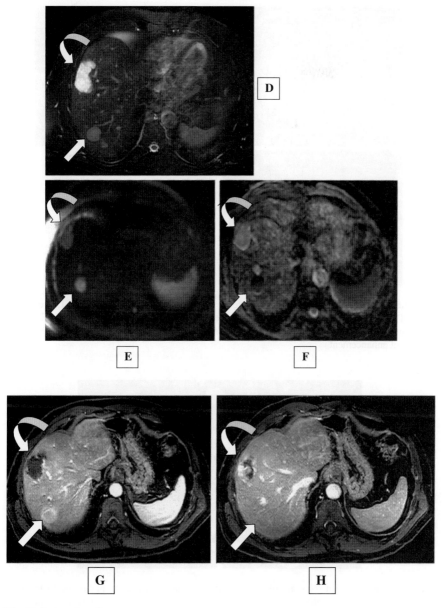

Fig. 11.4 (continued)

Precontrast images are useful to identify calcified and hemorrhagic metastases (Figs. 11.5 and 11.8). Calcification occurs most commonly in metastases from muci-nous colon carcinoma, but can be seen with other primary tumors including gastric, ovarian, breast, thyroid, lung, renal, carcinoid tumor and melanoma, in addition to a variety of less common neoplasms [60, 68, 69].

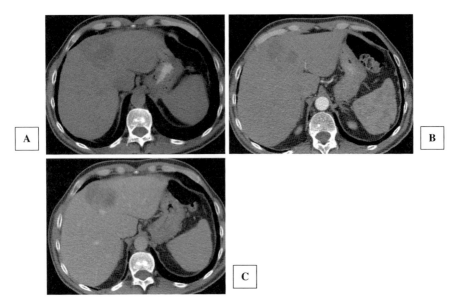

Fig. 11.5 Imaging of female patient with colon cancer and liver metastases by CT. Precontrast axial CT hypodense focal lesion with central hyperdenisty representing amorphous calcification is shown in (**a**). Lesion is persistently hypodense on arterial (**b**) and portovenous (**c**) phase with no significant enhancement

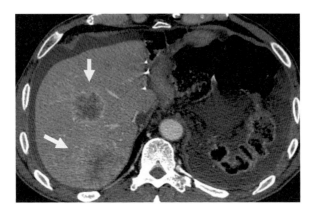

Fig. 11.6 Imaging of a 67 years old male with esophageal carcinoma metastatic to the liver. Axial CT in portovenous phase showing two metastatic focal lesions with classical peripheral rim enhancement (*arrows*)

Metastases of cystic malignant tumors, such as ovarian carcinoma or mucinous cystadenocarcinoma of the pancreas occasionally develop cystic liver metastases. Other primary malignancies that may present with cystic liver metastases include gastrointestinal stromal tumor (GIST), leiomyosarcoma, malignant melanoma,

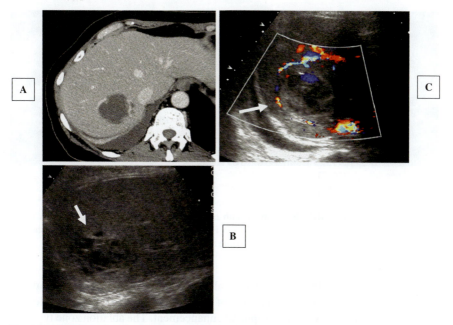

Fig. 11.9 Imaging of a 62 years old female with liposarcoma. Seen in (**a**) is a CT portovenous phase image showing a cystic metastases with rim enhancement. Seen in (**b**) is grey scale US of the liver and colored Doppler (C) showing a complex cystic lesion (*arrow*) and peripheral vascularity (*arrow*)

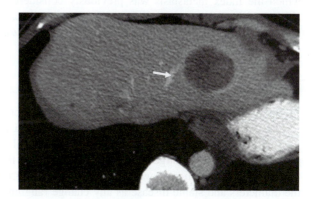

Fig. 11.10 Imaging of a 45 years old female with metastatic anal carcinoma. Shown is a hypodense necrotic liver metastasis with rim enhancement (*arrow*)

response to thermal injury, is usually transient and disappears over time, usually within one month [80]. On immediate follow-up CT images, the zone of ablation also often contains a central area of high attenuation along the electrode needle tract. This area of increased attenuation, which is believed to represent greater cellular disruption, usually disappears by the subsequent follow-up CT.

In addition to these characteristic findings, tiny air bubbles produced during ablation may be seen at immediate follow-up CT and should not be confused with a

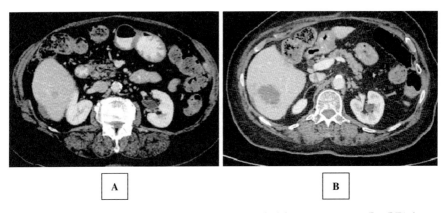

Fig. 11.11 Pre and post RFA in a patient with metastatic leiomyosarcoma. A Pre RFA image showing a hypodense hypovascular focal lesion is seen in (**a**) and a post RFA image showing successful ablation, with hypodense ablation zone and no evidence of tumor is seen in (**b**)

hepatic abscess [81]. These air bubbles also usually resolve within 1 month. At the one month follow-up CT, the zone of RF ablation appears as a well-defined area of low attenuation without peripheral enhancement. The ablation zone typically involutes gradually, but the rate of involution varies from case to case (Fig. 11.11).

Regular follow-up with CT is important for the detection of local tumor progression in order to facilitate timely treatment. At follow-up CT, local tumor progression appears as a newly developed focal enhancing lesion within an ablation zone in which the index metastasis was previously considered to have been completely ablated. If the index tumor was hypovascular, any distortion in the smooth interface of the ablation zone or any increase in the size of the zone is considered indicative of local tumor progression.

Evaluation of Response to Treatment in Patients with Liver Metastasis

In 2000, an international group agreed on standard criteria for measuring tumor response termed Response Evaluation Criteria in Solid Tumors (RECIST). A complete response was defined as the disappearance of all target tumors and a partial response as a 30% or larger decrease in the sum of the largest diameters of the tumors. Progressive disease was defined as a 20% or greater increase in the sum of the diameters and stable disease as any change ranging from a 30% decrease to a 20% increase in tumor size [82].

A more recently developed standard, termed the Choi criteria, appears to better predict survival than RECIST in a subgroup of patients. A good response by the Choi criteria is defined as a 10% decrease in tumour size or a 15% decrease in tumor density on contrast-enhanced CT scan. The Choi criteria also more accurately predicted disease-specific overall survival than the RECIST criteria. Although the Choi criteria were initially developed to evaluate Gastrointestinal Stromal Tumor "GIST" patients, a reanalysis of previously published clinical trial data for renal cell cancer patients has shown that they may potentially have value in other diseases. Recently, additional criteria have been developed for metastatic colorectal cancer based on progression-free survival or time to progression rather than the assessment of tumor response by groups such as the North Central Cancer Treatment Group (NCCTG) and the National Surgical Adjuvant Breast and Bowel Project (NSABP's).

The RECIST criteria have more recently been revised (RECIST 1.1) as follows: 1. The number of lesions required to assess tumour burden for response determination has been reduced from a maximum of 10 to a maximum of five total (and from a maximum of five to two per organ) 2. Assessment of pathological lymph nodes is now incorporated; nodes with a short axis of ≥15 mm are considered measurable and assessable as target lesions and the short axis measurements are included in the sum of lesions for calculation of tumour response. Nodes that shrink to <10 mm (short axis) are considered normal. 3. Confirmation of response is required for trials with response as primary endpoint but is no longer required in randomized studies because the control arm serves as an appropriate control for data interpretation. 4. The definition of "disease progression" has been clarified in several ways: (i) in addition to the previous definition of increase of 20% in target disease diameter, a 5 mm absolute increase is now required to prevent overcalling PD when the total sum is very small and (ii) the revised RECIST offers guidance as to what constitutes 'unequivocal progression' of non-measurable/non-target disease - a source of confusion in the original RECIST guidelines. Finally, the revised RECIST includes a section on detection of new lesions, including the interpretation of FDG-PET scan assessment and a new imaging appendix with updated recommendations on the optimal anatomical assessment of lesions.

A key question considered by the RECIST Working Group in developing RECIST 1.1 was whether it was appropriate to move from anatomic unidimensional assessment of tumour burden to either anatomical volumetric assessment or to functional assessment with PET or MRI. It was concluded that, at present, there is no sufficient standardization or evidence to abandon anatomical assessment of tumour burden. The only exception to this is in the use of FDG-PET imaging (see below) as an adjunct to the determination of progression [83].

Post Treatment Appearance

After the initiation of chemotherapy, some metastases can exhibit a less aggressive enhancement pattern that mimics hemangiomas, including early peripheral nodular enhancement and delayed retention of contrast material. This appearance has been postulated to be the result of chemotherapy-induced anti angiogenic effects, with the early peripheral nodular enhancement caused by altered vascularity and the retention of contrast material on the 10-minute delayed post-contrast images reflecting an enlarged extracellular space or decreased venous drainage. A key distinguishing feature of chemotherapeutically-treated metastases is an early, intact peripheral rim of enhancement unlike the discontinuous peripheral enhancement seen in hemangiomas [84].

11.2.4 Imaging Liver Metastases by MRI

11.2.4.1 General Background

As a result of major advances in field gradient technology and multi-channel surface coils, MR imaging is playing an increasingly greater role in the accurate,
noninvasive detection and characterization of hepatic lesions. MR imaging is frequently used as a problem solving modality and many patients are referred for MR
imaging for the evaluation of lesions considered indeterminate on other imaging
modalities [85].

However, because MR imaging displays the same lesion contrast enhancement
patterns as CT, but with superior lesion-to-liver contrast and without the use of
ionizing radiation [86], there has been increasing interest in, and experience with
MR imaging in this regards. In addition, the use of newer pulse sequences, such as
diffusion-weighted and steady-state free precession (SSFP) (fast imaging employing steady-state acquisition [FIESTA; GE Healthcare, Waukesha, Wis]), balanced
fast-field-echo (bFFE; Philips Medical Systems, Best, The Netherlands), true fast
imaging with steady precession (TrueFISP; Siemens Medical Solutions, Erlangen,
Germany), and true steady-state free precession (TrueSSFP; Toshiba America
Medical Systems, Tustin, Calif) sequences, along with hepatocyte-specific contrast
agents (e.g., gadobenate dimeglumine [Gd-BOPTA {benzyloxypropionictetraac-
etate}] [MultiHance; Bracco Diagnostics, Princeton, NJ]) may facilitate a more
specific diagnosis of the lesion in question [87, 88].

Technical advances in (MR) hardware and software have allowed the introduction of faster pulse sequences void of motion artifacts that previously posed
limitations to abdominal MR imaging. Plain imaging is useful for revealing the
morphology and the inherent structure of focal liver lesions and provides essential
information for the diagnosis. However, in most cases, these features are not enough
to correctly detect and characterize liver tumors [89]. MR imaging contrast agents
are currently used to accentuate the differences in signal intensity between the liver
lesion and the adjacent tissue and to highlight different enhancement patterns.

MR imaging is considered the most accurate modality for the detection and
characterization of focal and diffuse liver disease. The superiority of MR imaging to other imaging modalities for liver evaluation has become even more apparent
recently because of substantial improvements in 1.5T magnets, with faster image
acquisition and better image quality [90].

11.2.4.2 Technical Aspects of MRI Imaging

To obtain high quality liver MR examinations, the technical specifications of the MR
scanner, the choice of pulse sequence and the use of the most appropriate contrast
agent should all be taken into consideration. The use of high field strength MR
scanners (≥ 1.0 T) with fast gradients and phased-array surface coils is now standard
for liver MR imaging [91, 92]. Phased-array coils provide a great improvement in
the signal to noise ratio (SNR) and a better image quality. Rapidly switched gradient

systems are needed to obtain fast sequences. The selection of the MR sequence and the manipulation of parameters are fundamental to avoid motion artifacts and increase the SNR and contrast to noise (CNR) ratio.

Motion artifacts have been traditionally considered an important limitation in performing liver MR. Two strategies have been pursued to obtain high quality MR images: (1) suppression of the movement artifacts; (2) reduction of the acquisition time. To avoid motion artifacts, respiratory triggered imaging was introduced. Images are acquired in a fixed point of the expiratory breathing phase; the limitation of this kind of sequence is its inefficacy in patients with irregular breathing and its long acquisition time, which is also related to the respiratory frequency of the patient (Fig. 11.12) [93]. Fat suppression is another tool to reduce motion artifacts. On the other hand, strong gradients accelerate image encoding times and enable fast and ultrafast imaging, including fast dynamic, parallel and echo-planar imaging. Fast imaging with breath hold sequences can eliminate the respiratory artifacts and blurring, and greatly reduce the acquisition time [94]. More recently, parallel acquisition techniques have allowed a 2–4 fold faster acquisition of the entire liver when compared to other pulse sequences. Most importantly, the parallel MR approach may accelerate any imaging sequence [95].

At 1.5T, the current standard MR liver protocol includes a T2-weighted sequence, a T1-weighted sequence and serial postgadolinium GRE sequences. Imaging properties, demonstrated by their appearance on T1, T2, and early and late postgadolinium images, allow highly detailed evaluation of diffuse and focal liver abnormalities [90]. The predominant information provided by T2 weighted sequences is about fluid content, fibrotic tissue, and iron content (reflected by high, low, and very low signal intensity, respectively). Half-Fourier single-shot techniques should be used routinely because they are relatively insensitive to breathing artifacts. Fat suppression is generally applied for at least one set of images (e.g. to accentuate the high signal intensity of focal liver lesions on T2-weighted images). Fat suppression also improves visualization of regions bordered by fat, such as subcapsular parenchyma [90].

Pre-contrast T1-weighted sequences are extremely important in lesion characterization. Spoiled gradient-echo (SGE) sequences are important and versatile for studying liver disease, providing T1-weighted imaging in a short period of time and allowing chemical shift imaging in the same dual echo acquisition with spatially matched slices. Most lesions are mildly or moderately low in signal intensity, particularly lesions with high fluid or fibrous tissue content. Hemorrhagic lesions, those with high protein or fat content and well-differentiated melanoma metastases are high in signal intensity. The routine use of an additional fat attenuating technique facilitates reliable characterization of fatty lesions (90). Newer sequences allow combination of high spatial and temporal resolution, with use of a complex method of filling the k_{space} [96].

Gadolinium chelate enhancement is performed routinely with three-dimensional (3D) GRE breathhold sequences. 3D GRE imaging provides acquisition of thinner sections than typically used for 2D images, with contiguous slices allowing detection of smaller lesions. Furthermore, there is multiplanar capacity, allowing

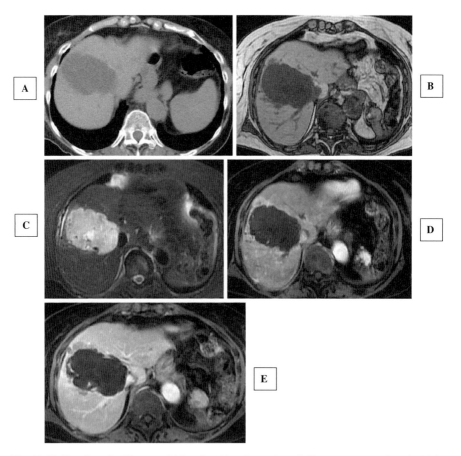

Fig. 11.12 Imaging of a 72 years old female with colorectal cystic liver metastases. Seen in (**a**) is an unenhanced CT showing hypodense cystic liver metastasis. Seen in (**b**) is an axial T1 FSPGR breathhold showing low T1 liver metastasis with high T2 signal (**c**) on the axial T2 Fast Recovery Fast Spin Echo with FATSAT. Seen in (**d**) is peripheral rim enhancement on the arterial and portal venous phase of the axial dynamic 3D FATSAT LAVA sequence

assessment of liver vascular anatomy [97]. Fat suppression usually is used to reduce motion artifacts and increase lesion conspicuity. Adequate delay between initiation of contrast injection and initiation of 3D GRE sequence is crucial (15–20 s for most patients). This allows visualization of the early enhancement pattern of lesions to aid in characterization and optimizes the detection of hypervascular lesions. The optimal time for early hepatic venous phase is less critical (45–75 s), showing enhancement of the entire vascular system. The early hepatic venous phase maximizes contrast between hypovascular lesions and the liver and can be used to evaluate the contrast washout pattern, which is a useful discriminating feature. Images acquired 1.5–10 min after contrast injection are in the interstitial phase of enhancement, which aids in evaluating persistent enhancement of hemangiomas, washout characteristics of liver lesions, or delayed enhancement of fibrotic tissue or tumors, such as cholangiocarcinoma. There is no demonstrated benefit to routinely waiting longer than 5 min [98].

11.2.4.3 Appearance of Liver Metastases in MR Imaging

Metastases may appear as solitary, multiple, or confluent masses and, on rare occasions, may appear infiltrative. Metastases that derive their predominant blood supply from hepatic arterial branches and enhance substantially on immediate postgadolinium images are termed "hypervascular" and are visualized best during the hepatic arterial – dominant phase of liver enhancement. Hypovascular tumors may be more conspicuous on images obtained one minute post contrast. Moreover, most hypovascular metastases can also be seen clearly on the hepatic arterial – dominant phase. Most diagnostic information can be derived from the hepatic arterial – dominant phase, with correct timing verified by observing contrast enhancement of the central portal veins, whereas hepatic veins remain un-enhanced [99].

Hypovascular metastases are the most common and colon adenocarcinoma is the most frequent source of these metastases. Imaging features of hypovascular liver metastases include variable T2 signal, low signal on T1-weighted images and mild to moderate enhancement on postgadolinium images. Typically, these lesions are most conspicuous on T1-weighted GRE pre- and post gadolinium sequences, and these latter data acquisition provide maximal sensitivity and specificity for detection and diagnosis. Post gadolinium images characteristically show mild early enhancement, most often with a ring pattern (see Fig. 11.12), with progressive venous-interstitial phase enhancement, predominantly filling in from the outer margins. Perilesional enhancement of adjacent liver is frequently seen with adenocarcinoma metastases on immediate post gadolinium images, most commonly with mucinous types from the colon, stomach or pancreas, usually fading over time. On T2-weighted images, the internal tumor anatomy of medium-large sized colorectal metastases has a target-like configuration: (1) highest (fluid-like) signal intensity is in the center of the lesion as a result of coagulative necrosis; (2) lower signal intensity is in a broad zone outside the center because of the presence of a desmoplastic reaction that facilitates the formation of the tumor matrix in which strands of tumor cells can grow; and (3) a slightly higher signal intensity is in the outermost zone as a result of more compact tumor cells with more vessels and less desmoplasia [100].

Hypervascular metastases show intense early enhancement (Fig. 11.4). Hypervascular metastases can result from neuroendocrine tumors, including carcinoid and islet cell tumors, renal cell carcinoma, melanoma or thyroid cancer. Breast cancer more commonly gives rise to liver metastases, but the metastases are not as consistently hypervascular. Imaging features may vary, but hypervascular metastases are typically markedly hyperintense on T2-weighted images, and may be cystic or necrotic [101]. Hypervascular metastases are usually of low T1 signal. On SSFP and diffusion-weighted images, these lesions are hyperintense [102]. Post gadolinium enhancement is most pronounced on arterial-phase images as a

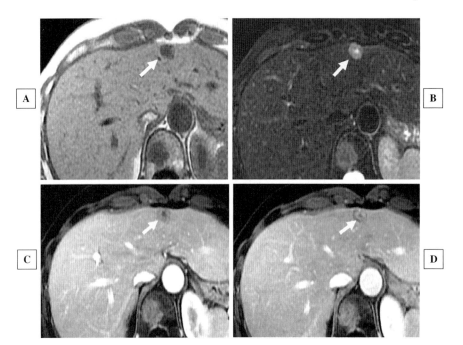

Fig. 11.13 Imaging of a 58 years old female breast cancer patient with liver metastases showing classic target and peripheral washout signs. Axial T1 FSPGR (**a**) shows a hypointense focal lesion with target sign on axial heavy T2 FRFSE (**b**), with low intensity rim and central necrotic high signal. Axial T1 3D dynamic LAVA portovenous phase (**c**) shows peripheral enhancement with non enhancing center. On the delayed phase, the lesion shows characteristic washout sign (**d**) (*arrow*)

peripheral ring or less likely, uniform or heterogeneous. On delayed postgadolinium images, contrast enhancement progresses in a centripetal fashion and fades peripherally [90, 102].

The "peripheral washout sign" is a specific but insensitive sign for both metastases and HCC (Figs. 11.13 and 11.14). This sign refers to contrast material preferentially washing out from the periphery of a hepatic mass on delayed scans, resulting in the periphery appearing hypointense relative to the center of the lesion. It is thought to be related to the degree of tumor vascularity, with increased vascularity peripherally (viable tumor) and decreased vascularity centrally (necrotic or fibrotic region). Metastases are hypointense relative to the liver or demonstrate a "target" appearance on delayed images obtained 1–3 h after the administration of Gd-BOPTA, a hepatobiliary contrast agent [103].

Hemorrhagic (e.g. lung, kidney, testicle; melanoma) or calcified metastases can demonstrate T1 hyperintensity (Fig. 11.15). In addition, perilesional fat deposition has been specifically described with hepatic metastases from a primary pancreatic insulinoma and is thought to be related to the effects of insulin, that is, the inhibition of fatty acid oxidation and the promotion of hepatocyte triglyceride accumulation [104].

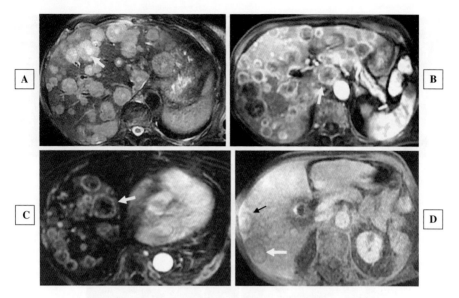

Fig. 11.14 Imaging of a 78 years old female patient with breast cancer and liver metastases. Axial T2 FRFSE with FATSAT (**a**) shows multiple metastatic hepatic lesions with peripheral hypointense signal and central high signal (necrosis) (*arrow*) with a classic target sign. Axial T1 dynamic FATSAT LAVA (**b**) and subtraction images (**c**) show classical peripheral ring enhancement (*arrow*). Delayed axial LAVA (**d**) shows central enhancement (*white arrow*) and peripheral washout (*black arrow*)

11.2.4.4 Pitfalls of MR Imaging

Transient Hepatic Intensity Difference areas of liver parenchyma enhancement (e.g., THID) from either non tumorous arterioportal shunts or obstruction of distal parenchymal portal venous flow, can cause homogeneous arterial phase enhancement that may mimic an underlying mass. Clues to the diagnosis include peripheral location, geographic or wedge shape, and non-displaced internal vasculature. Often, no abnormalities are seen on other sequences. Serial follow-up imaging can also be helpful because these lesions will invariably disappear [105].

11.2.4.5 Recent Developments in MR Imaging

3T MRI Imaging

Imaging at 3T is still in the early phases. The major expected advantage of 3T compared with 1.5T is the anticipated gain in signal strength and signal to noise ratio (SNR). Theoretically, this boost in SNR-an almost two-fold signal gain-could result in improved image quality or reduced examination time. However, several potential disadvantages, such as an increase in imaging artifacts, changes in relaxation kinetics [106, 107], and specific absorption rate (SAR) constraints, have to be considered [108, 109].

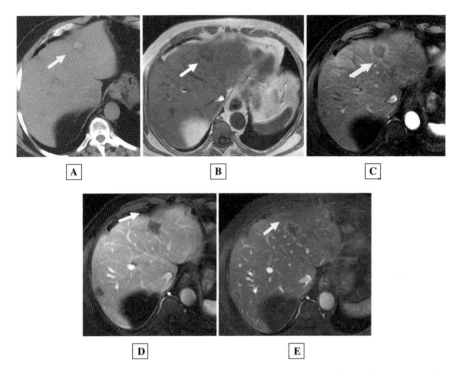

Fig. 11.15 CT imaging of calcified colorectal metastases. Images were from a 66 years old male. Shown in (**a**) is central hyperdense calcification on non enhanced CT. Shown in (**b**) is axial T1 FSPGR in phase with central high signal representing calcification. Axial dynamic 3D LAVA with peripheral enhancement on the arterial (**c**) and portovenous phases (**d**) are shown. Persistent rim enhancement on delayed phase is shown in (**e**)

The main advantage of liver imaging at 3T is the ability to acquire high-quality, relatively artifact free, thin-section post gadolinium T1-weighted, 3D GRE sequences (Fig. 11.16). This high spatial resolution is comparable to current-generation multidetector CT, but with the advantage of unmatched intrinsic soft tissue contrast resolution [90]. A drawback of 3T is an increased number and types of artifacts. Certain imaging artifacts are more prominent at 3T than at 1.5T, mainly because their physical parameters are dependent on the main magnetic field strength [90].

Imaging at 3T still requires optimization of the pulse sequence parameters normally used at 1.5T in order to compensate for different relaxation kinetics. In addition, modifications should be developed to overcome major disadvantages of higher field imaging, particularly SAR restriction [90].

New MRI Contrast Agents

The contrast agents available for liver imaging can be divided into three categories according to the biodistribution namely, (a) extracellular (b) hepatobiliary and (c) RES-targeted contrast agents [65, 110].

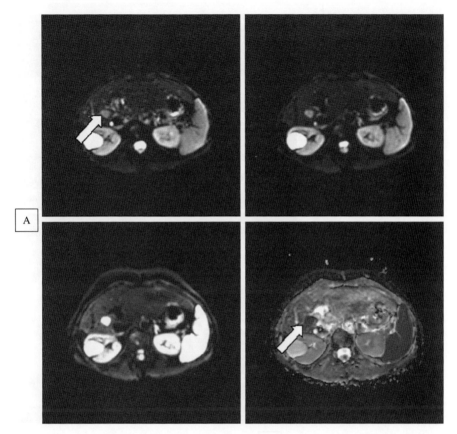

Fig. 11.16 Recurrence of metastases from neuroendocrine tumors after right hepatectomy. Illustrated in (**a**) is a typical increase in contrast of the metastasis (*straight arrows*) on background liver on DWI with increased strength of the diffusion gradient (b0, b50, b1000) and low ADC. Shown in (**b**) is arterial enhancement and discrete washout. The lesion would be difficult to see without the arterial phase

Extracellular contrast agents are hydrophilic, small molecular weight gadolinium chelates. After intravenous administration, these substances are rapidly cleared from the intravascular space to the interstitial space. They do not penetrate into intact cells and are eliminated via the urinary system. Several gadolinium complexes are currently available including gadopentetate dimeglumine (Gd-DTPA, Magnevist, Schering AG/Berlex Laboratories), gadoterate meglumine (Gd-DOTA, Dotarem, Laboratoires Guerbet), gadodiamide (Gd-DTPA-BMA, Omniscan, Amersham Health), and gadoteridol (Gd-HP-DO3A, ProHance, Bracco). The usual clinical dose of these gadolinium chelates is 0.1 mmol/kg. Extracellular contrast agents provide information on vascularization and perfusion similar to that of iodinated contrast media used for CT [111].

Liver-specific contrast agents may be classified as reticuloendothelial system (RES)- specific or hepatocyte-specific. RES-specific contrast agents are

Fig. 11.16 (continued)

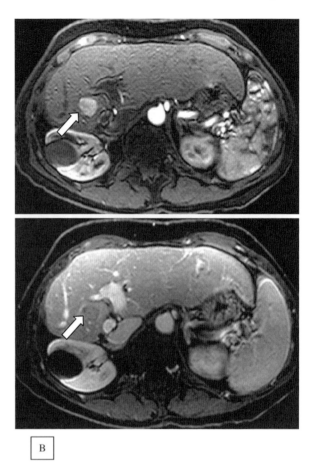

B

superparamagnetic particles of iron oxide (SPIO) that distort the local magnetic field, causing signal loss on T2-weighted images. These agents are removed from circulation mainly by functioning Kupffer cells that accumulate iron within the intracellular space. Metastases without Kupffer cells, and with mild to moderately increased signal on T2-weighted images, become more conspicuous relative to the very low signal intensity of liver parenchyma. These agents are not widely used in daily clinical practice [112] and the only agent in this class that is approved in the United States is SPIO ferumoxides. A number of articles have concluded that SPIO-enhanced MR imaging is the most appropriate preoperative imaging procedure for liver metastasis screening [113]. However, others have found difficulty in differentiating thin vessels, small cysts, hemangiomas and metastases on SPIO enhanced MR images [114].

Hepatobiliary or hepatocyte-selective contrast agents are paramagnetic compounds that are partially taken up by the hepatocytes and excreted in the biliary tract [115]. Contrast agents with combined perfusion and tissue selective properties

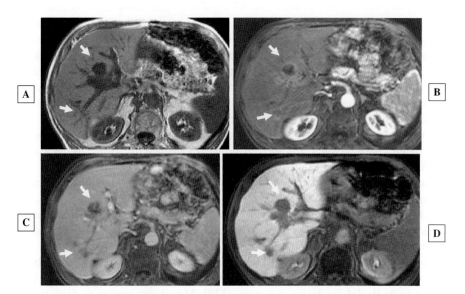

Fig. 11.17 Multiple metastases from colorectal cancer on liver specific (Gadoxetate/primovist) contrast. Axial T1 in phase (**a**) show hypointense focal lesions (arrows), arterial (**b**) and portovenous (**c**) phases show peripheral enhancement. Delayed 20 min images are shown in (**d**) (*arrows*). Courtsey of Christoph Zech, Klinikum der Universität Müchen-Grobhadern

are of great clinical interest. Two contrast agents that have achieved clinical use and that combine the properties of a non-specific gadolinium-based contrast agent with that of a hepatocyte-specific (specific) agent are Gd-BOPTA and Gd- EOB-DTPA (not approved by the US Food and Drug Administration). These chelates are administered as a bolus injection, allowing hemodynamic early perfusional data and late hepatobiliary contrast enhancement. The main difference between these agents is the degree of biliary excretion. Approximately 4% of the administered dose of Gd-BOPTA is excreted in the bile, whereas 50% of Gd-EOB-DTPA undergoes biliary excretion, providing sustained enhancement of liver parenchyma of approximately 1–2 h and 10–20 min after injection, respectively. Hepatospecific phase imaging can accordingly be performed at 20 min after the injection of Gd-EOB-DTPA and at 40 min after the injection of Gd-BOPTA (see Fig. 11.17) [116]. One major indication is the differentiation between FNH, which contains bile ducts, and HCA as well as other hepatic focal lesions, which do not [117]. In general, focal lesions that are not bile duct-containing hepatocellular lesions, such as metastases, show improved conspicuity by the increase in background signal of liver tissue, while the lesions remain unenhanced.

MRI Diffusion/Perfusion

Diffusion-weighted MR imaging (DWI) is a recently introduced technique to depict differences in molecular diffusion caused by the random motion of molecules that is known as Brownian motion. Intravoxel incoherent motion in the field gradients produces incoherent phase shifts that result in signal attenuation [118]. One of the attractive merits in DWI is that it provides excellent tissue contrast based on molecular diffusion, which is different from ordinary T1- and T2-weighted images. In addition, DWI is performed without the administration of a contrast agent. In recent years, owing to the development of fast imaging techniques such as echoplanar imaging and the parallel imaging technique, the image quality of DWI in body regions such as the abdomen has remarkably improved.

DWI yields qualitative and quantitative information that provides unique insight into tumor characteristics, and there is growing evidence for its use in the assessment of the patient with cancer. Tumors are frequently more cellular than the tissue from which they originate and thus appear to be of relatively high signal intensity (restricted diffusion) at DWI [119].

The technique can be applied widely for tumor detection and tumor characterization. In addition, DWI appears to have the ability to predict the response to chemotherapy and radiation treatment [119].

In the liver, low b-value images (e.g., b 50–150 s/mm^2) that suppress the high-signal flow from the hepatic vessels, resulting in black blood images, have been found to be useful for lesion detection [120]. Metastases appear as high signal-intensity foci at DWI (see Fig. 11.18). Nasu et al. found that DWI was more accurate than superparamagnetic iron oxide – enhanced MRI for the detection of liver metastases. In that study, the sensitivity and specificity of SPIO-enhanced MRI was 66 and 90%, respectively. By comparison, DWI was found to have a higher sensitivity of 82% and a specificity of 94% [121]. DWI was also shown to be helpful for liver lesion characterization [122]. To characterize lesions in the liver using DWI, b values ranging between 0 and 500 s/mm^2 are appropriate [123, Fig. 11.19]. Qualitative visual assessment can help to distinguish cystic from solid lesions. However, it is often difficult to distinguish different types of solid lesions in the liver by visual

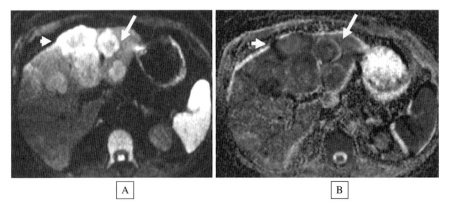

| A | B |

Fig. 11.18 Colorectal liver metastases diagnosed with breath hold single shot EPI diffusion. Shown are multiple liver metastases, some bright at 500 with decreased ADC (*arrows*) and some with a bright rim at b500 with decreased ADC, indicating a cellular rim (*short arrows*). Courtsey of Bachir Taouli, University of New York, New York, USA

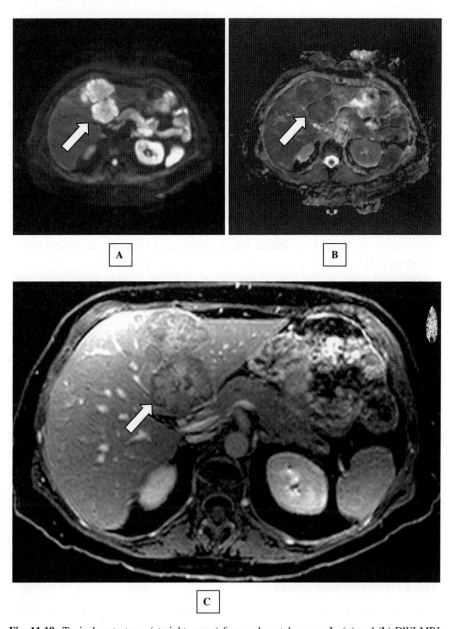

Fig. 11.19 Typical metastases (straight arrow) from colorectal cancer. In (**a**) and (**b**) DWI MRI with ADC map show restriction of diffusion in the metastases with decreased ADC. In (**c**) MRI with gadolinium on the delayed phase shows typical enhancement of the metastases with filling of the inner part of the lesion (contrast leakage), whereas the periphery washes-out

assessment alone. For example, a hemangioma will exhibit restricted diffusion and can mimic the appearance of a metastasis at DWI (Fig. 11.4). Using quantitative evaluation, investigators have found that benign liver lesions, such as cysts and hemangiomas, have higher mean ADC values (e.g., 2.45×10^{-3} mm^2/s) than malignant lesions, such as metastases and hepatocellular carcinoma (e.g., 1.08×10^{-3} mm^2/s) [124]. A team of investigators showed that for the diagnosis of malignant lesions, the use of a threshold ADC value less than 1.5×10^{-3} mm^2/s), with a diffusion factor (b) of 0 and 500 s/mm^2, would result in sensitivity, specificity, positive predictive value, and accuracy of 84, 89, 87 and 86%, respectively [124]. The ADC has also been used to distinguish abscesses which have low ADC values from cystic and necrotic metastases, which have higher ADC values [125].

The additional benefit of DWI is the ability to derive quantitative indices, which may be important in the assessment of disease response to novel therapeutics, including anti-vascular and anti-angiogenic therapy. Conventional assessment based on measuring lesion size is insensitive to early, treatment-related changes [123].

Perfusion study of the liver is possible with the single-shot echo-planar technique, by obtaining images at 1–2 s intervals after a bolus injection of paramagnetic contrast agent. On perfusion-weighted images (which are T2*-weighted images) gadolinium chelates serve as negative contrast agents decreasing the signal in the enhancing lesions [126]. In HCC and hemangiomas, a decrease in signal intensity was observed as the contrast agent reached the tumor. In contrast, the decrease in signal intensity in metastases was minimal [127]. Negative T2*-weighted enhancement may be advantageous in the evaluation of perfusion in tumors that are hyperintense on T1 images. MRI perfusion also helps in determining patient eligibility for various management procedures based on the intralesional perfusion. DCEMRI can also be performed with more conventional sequences, such as 3D ultrafast GRE sequences, with rapid acquisition of a targeted volume. DCEMRI allows the quantification of several perfusion indices, one of the most important being k$_{trans}$, as shown in numerous studies [128].

11.2.5 Technical Aspects of PET and PET CT Imaging of Liver Metastasis

11.2.5.1 General Background

Positron Emission Tomography (PET) is an imaging modality in which contrast is not based on intrinsic physical properties or on contrast media uptake and vascular behavior as is the case for in MRI or CT. Instead, PET provides unique information about the molecular and metabolic changes associated with any disease process, and more specifically, with tumoral metabolism. As such, it really allows "functional imaging" [129, 130].

The main molecular probe used in oncology is a glucose analog labeled with the positron emitter ^{18}F-FDG. This is based on the fact that cancer cells have an increased rate of glycolysis, and this alteration in glucose metabolism allows differentiation of tumor and normal tissue by the use of PET.

The precise role of PET in imaging of liver metastases remains unclear. Although its sensitivity for depiction of liver metastases on a per patient basis is very high, its sensitivity on a per lesion basis is low, especially for lesions smaller than a centimeter in diameter [131]. This technology is not suitable for liver resection planning. In the context of colorectal metastases, the role of PET is to avoid unnecessary surgery, based on its ability to detect extrahepatic foci of disease (nodal metastases, lung nodules) that are not depicted or characterized as malignant by other imaging methods [15].

11.2.5.2 Technical Aspects of PET CT Imaging

In PET, the images are generated by the detection of annihilation photons released when the positrons emitted by radionuclides, such as F-18, undergo annihilation with electrons [130, 131].

The annihilation photons are then detected by co-incidence. Detectors are made of crystals, such as bismuth germinate (BGO), cerium-doped lutetium oxyorthosilicate (LSO), or cerium-doped gadolinium silicate (GSO). Malignant cells demonstrate increased glucose utilization, secondary to increased activity of hexokinase(s). After uptake, glycolysis occurs with lactate formation under conditions of hypoxia. FDG is metabolized in the same manner, showing increased uptake in the tumor. It is important to stress that any hypermetabolic situation will result in increased uptake of glucose and therefore of FDG. Any inflammatory condition (e.g. infection, inflammatory diseases such as granulomatous disease, postoperative status) will result in FDG uptake and therefore in false positives [132].

Correlation with patient history and precise correlation with CT findings are mandatory in order to minimize the risk of false positive. This is especially critical when one considers the potential role of PET in denying surgery to patients that could be surgical candidates based on anatomic imaging.

PET in itself lacks anatomical landmarks. A PET and CT (PET CT) can be combined in order to provide fused images, allowing high spatial resolution and functional information in the same study [133]. There is however, some controversy regarding the acquisition of CT data. Some authors advocate its use only as an anatomic support to the PET data, whereas others advocate the combination of the PET with a multiphasic protocol involving contrast media injection. Since artifacts are generated by the injection of contrast material, the PET acquisition has to be performed after the CT without contrast and before the multiphasic acquisition [134–136].

One of the major advantages of PET, particularly useful in the oncology practice, is its ability to provide quantitative measurements of the metabolic activity in a tumor based on relatively simple measurements that are used to calculate the standardized uptake value (SUV) [129, 137]. The SUV is calculated based on the following equation: SUV= tracer activity in tissue/(injected radiotracer dose/patient weight).

Many studies have evaluated the SUV, and it appears that the simple measurements of the peak and decrease in SUV can be useful to define response to therapy [138].

It should be stressed, however that multiple factors can have an impact on the SUV. For example, partial volume, which depends on the spatial resolution can significantly alter the estimation of the true activity. Heterogeneous uptake, especially in large tumors that show a rim of uptake will also generate difficulty in the estimation. Other factors such as filtering, ROI selection, image noise, the time between the injection and acquisition (which should be the same in pre and post therapeutic evaluation) and changes in body weight can also affect SUV values [139, 140].

Plasma glucose levels will also alter the reproducibility of the SUV because glucose can compete with FDG for transport and phosphorylation. Diabetes and drugs that alter plasma glucose levels should therefore be taken into account when assessing the tumoral response.

In summary, while PET is still outside the scope of imaging for liver metastases, especially in the context of surgical planning, it is definitely a modality of choice in evaluation of early response to new therapeutic protocols.

11.2.5.3 Appearance of Liver Metastasis in PET and PET/CT Imaging

In PET and PET/CT imaging, the disease processes will be recognized based on uptake of FDG in foci of increased activity. As such, PET is highly sensitive, especially when anatomic criteria fail to positively identify a lesion as tumoral. As an example, this is especially true in nodal staging where PET overcomes the issue of size criteria that are important for both CT and MRI imaging. This explains the high success of this modality in staging of lung and head and neck cancer [141–143].

In PET imaging, most of the liver metastases will appear as discrete foci of increased activity in the liver. It is important to note, that the liver has a baseline level of FDG uptake due to its contribution to glucose metabolism [132]. Therefore large lesions, especially those with a necrotic center will appear with only a ring of increased activity. Lesions smaller than a centimeter in diameter will also rarely demonstrate uptake.

There are multiple studies that demonstrate the usefulness of PET and PET/CT in detecting liver metastases. Early studies were very optimistic with sensitivities and specificities of up to 88 and 92% respectively, in detection of liver metastases as compared to sensitivities ranging from 38 to 85% and specificity of 97% for CT [144, 145]. These results are controversial however, as more recent studies have documented significantly lower sensitivities. In a lesion-by-lesion analysis using the resected liver specimen for comparison, PET sensitivity was only 70%, with a documented inverse correlation between sensitivity and lesion size [146].

This issue has been well evaluated in the Meta analysis reported by Bipat and al. The authors of the study underlined that most of the studies on PET were based on a "per patient" analysis (only 22% of the PET studies were based on a "per lesion" analysis as compared to 73% for MRI studies). Their review demonstrated that in a "per patient" analysis, PET was the most sensitive technique, with a sensitivity of up to 95%. In a "per lesion" analysis, however, the results were different with PET showing a sensitivity of 76% comparable to helical CT (64% sensitivity) and 1.0-T and 1.5-T MRI (66 and 64%, respectively) [15, 131].

The inability of PET to depict small lesions of less than 1 cm is an important limitation. In this clinical scenario, every lesion is important. In other words, the major role of PET in the preoperative staging of patients with colorectal cancer will not likely be in the surgical planning of liver resection, but in depicting extrahepatic disease. In a review by Fletcher et al, it was estimated that the range of change in management of surgical planning for colorectal cancer related to PET was 7–68% (average, 20%). PET was influential in ruling out (unnecessary) surgery in 12% and influenced initiating surgery in 8% of patients [147]. *Note that this review was not specifically regarding management of metastases, but management of colorectal cancer, metastatic or not.*

In summary, it is clear that PET and PET/CT are useful techniques in the management of colorectal cancer, their role being different than that of the other modalities discussed. They are particularly useful for selecting patients suitable for surgery by excluding distant or unexpected metastases. The use of state of the art PET together with multi-slice detector CT and contrast media could improve detection by combining the advantages of these techniques. This however will need to be evaluated in large prospective trials that will demonstrate the added value of these combined modalities.

11.3 Summary: Challenges and Future Directions

Imaging metastases is a frequent task in current radiological practice. In this chapter we tried to provide a comprehensive overview of the imaging technology for, and imaging characteristics of liver metastases. Imaging techniques have evolved dramatically during the past decade. The combination of state of the art ultrasound, CT, MRI and PET allows earlier and more accurate diagnosis. But the goal of imaging has also changed with this increased capability, and this is well illustrated by the current management of metastases from colorectal cancer. While in the past, staging was the main focus of imaging, addressing the question "Does the patient present metastases"? The focus of imaging at present is to guide the treatment plan, with a curative intent and provide answers to the following new fundamental questions:

1. How many metastases does the patient have?
2. In which segments are they located and how much liver resection do they imply? and
3. How many of the depicted lesions are, in fact, benign and therefore should not cause unnecessary resection of the liver?

The current challenge of all the imaging modalities is to answer these questions with maximal accuracy and specificity. These challenges can be partially met with the use of newer contrast agents and new kinds of MR sequences or ultrasound modes, as outlined above.

Another challenge for imaging is to become an accurate surrogate biomarker, and aid in assessing the efficacy of new drugs, such as antiangiogenic therapy. In this setting, each modality provides its own benefits, and the future direction is likely to be the combination of these strengths for modeling and predicting the response to treatment.

In the future, imaging of liver metastases will likely be based on a multimodality/multiparametric approach, with a better understanding of the biology of the tumors and their characteristics translated into improved imaging. Co-analysis of perfusion data, diffusion maps and molecular probes should allow great progress in the ability of imaging to diagnose and possibly predict the appearance of liver metastases. It is important to stress, however, that only large prospective trials will determine whether indeed these new and appealing technologies can impact the prognosis of the disease at an acceptable cost.

Acknowledgements The authors thank Ms. Ruth Ramadeen, executive research secretary, Department of Radiology, McGill University Health Center for her help in the preparation of the manuscript. Dr. El-Khodary wishes to thank his lovely wife Marwa, daughter Zeina and son Aly.

References

1. Auh YH, Rubenstein WA, Zirinsky K et al (1984) Accessory fissures of the liver: CT and sonographic appearance. AJR Am J Roentgenol 143:565–572
2. Lazarchick J, De Souza e Silva NA, Nichols DR et al (1973) Pyogenic liver abscess. Mayo Clin Proc 48:349–355
3. Dawson J, Tan K (1992) Anatomy of the liver. In: Millward-Sadler GH, Wright R, Arthur MJP (eds) Wright's liver and biliary disease, vol 2, 3rd ed. WB Saunders, Philadelphia, PA, pp 3–11
4. Goldsmith M, Woodburne R (1957) Surgical anatomy pertaining to liver resection. Surg Gynecol Obstet 141:429–437
5. Couinaud C (1957) Le foie: etudes anatomiques et chirurgicales. Masson, Paris
6. Bismuth H (1982) Surgical anatomy and anatomical surgery of the liver. World J Surg 6:3–9
7. Fasel JH, Selle D, Evertsz CJ et al (1998) Segmental anatomy of the liver: poor correlation with CT. Radiology 206:151–156
8. Edmunson H, Craig J (1987) Neoplasms of the liver. In: Schiff l (ed) Diseases of the liver, 8th ed. Lippincott, Philadelphia, PA, p 1109
9. Cosgrove DO (2001) Malignant liver disease. In: Meire HB, Cosgrove DO, Dewbury KC, Farrant P (eds) Clinical ultrasound a comprehensive text, vol 1, 2nd edn. Abdominal and general ultrasound. Churchill livingstone, London, p 211–231
10. Dietrich CF (2004) Characterization of focal liver lesions with contrast enhanced ultrasonography. Eur J Radiol 51S:S9–S17
11. Eisenberg RL (2009) Clinical imaging: an atlas of differential diagnosis, 4th edn. Lippincott Williams & Wilkins, Philadelphia, PA, pp 626–632
12. Lencioni R, Cioni D, Bartolozzi C (2005) Focal liver lesions detection, characterization, ablation. Springer, New York, NY, pp 261–273
13. Kanematsu M, Kondo H, Goshima S et al (2006) Imaging liver metastases: review and update. Eur J Radiol 58:217–228
14. Kinkel K, Lu Y, Both M et al (2002) Detection of hepatic metastases from cancers of the gastrointestinal tract by using noninvasive imaging methods (US, CT, MR Imaging, PET): a meta-analysis. Radiology 224:748

15. Bipat S, van Leeuwen MS, Comans EF et al (2005) Colorectal liver metastases: CT, MR imaging, and PET for diagnosis—meta-analysis. Radiology 237:123–131
16. Harvey CJ, Albrecht T (2001) Ultrasound of focal liver lesions. Eur Radiol 11: 1578–1593
17. Middleton WD, Kurtz AB, Hertzberg BS (2004) Ultrasound: the requisites, 2nd edn. Mosby, St. Louis, MO, pp 35–38
18. Hohmann J, Skrok J, Puls R et al (2003) Characterization of focal liver lesions with contrast-enhanced low MI real time ultrasound and SonoVue. Rofo Fortschr Geb Rontgenstr Neuen Bildgeb Verfahr 175:835–843
19. Choudhry S, Gorman B, Charboneau JW et al (2000) Comparison of tissue harmonic imaging with conventional US in abdominal disease.1 RadioGraphics 20:1127–1135
20. Bluemke DA, Paulson EK, Choti MA et al (2000) Detection of hepatic lesions in candidates for surgery: comparison of ferumoxides-enhanced MR imaging and dual-phase helical CT. AJR 175:1653–1658
21. Schmidt J, Strotzer M, Fraunhofer S et al (2000) Intraoperative ultrasonography versus helical computed tomography and computed tomography with arterioportography in diagnosing colorectal liver metastases: lesion by lesion analysis. World J Surg 24:43–48
22. Clarke MP, Kane RA, Steele DG et al (1998) Prospective comparison of preoperative imaging and intraoperative ultrasonography in the detection of liver tumors. Surgery 106:849–855
23. Jeffrey RB Jr, Ralls PW (1995) The liver. In: JeffreyRB Jr, Ralls PW (eds) Sonography of the abdomen. Raven, New York, NY, p 71–177
24. Bartolotta TV, Taibbi A, Midiri M et al (2009) Focal liver lesions: contrast-enhanced ultrasound. Abdom Imag 34:193–209
25. Cosgrove D (2006) Ultrasound contrast agents: An overview. Eur J Radiol 60:324–330
26. Brannigan M, Burns PN, Wilson SR (2004) Blood flow patterns in focal liver lesions at microbubble-enhanced US. Radiographics 24:921–935
27. Cosgrove D, Blomley M (2004) Liver tumors: evaluation with contrast-enhanced ultrasound. Abdom Imag 29:446–454
28. Krishna PD, Newhouse VL (1997) Second harmonic characteristics of the ultrasound contrast agents albunex and FSO69. Ultrasound Med Biol 23:453
29. Schutt E, Klein D, Mattrey R, Riess J (2003) Injectable microbubbles as contrast agents for diagnostic ultrasound imaging: the key role of perfluorochemicals. Angew Chem Int Ed Eng 42:3218
30. Uhlendorf V, Scholle FD, Reinhardt M (2000) Acoustic behaviour of current ultrasound contrast agents. Ultrasonics 38:81–86
31. Burns PN, Wilson SR, Simpson DH (2000) Pulse inversion imaging of liver blood flow: improved method for characterizing focal masses with microbubble contrast. Invest Radiol 35:58
32. Burns PN, Hope-Simpson D, Averkiou MA (2000) Nonlinear imaging. Ultrasound Med Biol 26:S19–22
33. Burns P, Powers J, Hope-Simpson D et al (1994) Harmonic power mode Doppler using microbubble contrast agents: and improved method for small vessel flow imaging. Ultrasonic symposium 1994. In: Proceedings of the IEEE UFFC, p 1547 (online library)
34. Phillips P (2001) Contrast pulse sequences (CPS): Imaging nonlinear microbubbles. In: 2001 IEEE Ultrasonics Symposium: IEEE (online library)
35. Quaia E, D_Onofrio M, Palumbo A et al (2006) Comparison of contrast-enhanced ultrasonography versus baseline ultrasound and contrast-enhanced computed tomography in metastatic disease of the liver: diagnostic performance and confidence. Eur Radiol 16: 1599–1609
36. Piscaglia F, Corradi F, Mancini M et al (2007) Real time contrast enhanced ultrasonography in detection of liver metastases from gastrointestinal cancer. BMC Cancer 7:171
37. Konopke R, Bunk A, Kersting S (2007) The role of contrastenhanced ultrasound for focal liver lesion detection: an overview. Ultrasound Med Biol 33:1515–1526

38. Quaia E, Bertolotto M, Forga čs B et al (2003) Detection of liver metastases by pulse inversion harmonic imaging during Levovist late phase: comparison with conventional ultrasound and helical CT in 160 patients. Eur Radiol 13:475–483

39. Morin SHX, Lim AKP, Cobbold JFL et al (2007) Use of second generation contrast-enhanced ultrasound in the assessment of focal liver lesions. World J Gastroenterol 13:5963–5970

40. Leen E, Ceccotti P, Kalogeropoulou C et al (2006) Prospective multicenter trial evaluating a novel method of characterizing focal liver lesions using contrast enhanced sonography. AJR 186:1551–1559

41. Ding H, Wang WP, Huang BJ et al (2005) Imaging of focal liver lesions: low-mechanical-index real-time ultrasonography with SonoVue. J Ultrasound Med 24:285–297

42. Quaia E, Calliada F, Bertolotto M et al (2004) Characterization of focal liver lesions with contrast-specific US modes and sulphur hexafluoride-filled microbubble contrast agent: diagnostic performance and confidence. Radiology 232:420–430

43. Bartolotta TV, Taibbi A, Galia M et al (2007) Characterization of hypoechoic focal hepatic lesions in patients with fatty liver: diagnostic performance and confidence of contrast-enhanced ultrasound. Eur Radiol 17:650–661

44. Von Herbay A, Vogt C, Willers R et al (2004) Real-time imaging with the sonographic contrast agent SonoVue: differentiation between benign and malignant hepatic lesions. J Ultrasound Med 23:1557–1568

45. Jang HJ, Kim TK, Wilson SR (2006) Imaging of malignant liver masses: characterization and detection. Ultrasound Q 22:19–29

46. Fioole B, de Haas RJ, Wicherts DA et al (2008) Additional value of contrast enhanced intraoperative ultrasound for colorectal liver metastases. Eur J Radiol 67:169–176

47. Torzilli G, Del Fabbro D, Palmisano A et al (2005) Contrast-enhanced intraoperative ultrasonography during hepatectomies for colorectal cancer liver metastases. J Gastrointest Surg 9:1148–1153

48. Albrecht T, Blomley M, Bolondi L et al (2004) Guidelines for the use of contrast agents in ultrasound. Ultraschall Med 25:249–256

49. Kamel IR, Georgiades C, Fishman EK (2003) Incremental value of advanced image processing of multislice computed tomography data in the evaluation of hypervascular liverlesions. J Comput Assist Tomogr 27:652–656

50. Kopka L, Rodenwaldt J, Hamm B (2001) Biphasic multi-slice helical CT of the liver: intraindividual comparison of different slice thicknesses for the detection and characterization of focal liver lesions. Radiology 217:367

51. Haider MA, Amitai MM, Rappaport DC et al (2002) Multi-detector row helical CT in preoperative assessment of small (< or = 1.5 cm) liver metastases: is thinner collimation better? Radiology 225:137–142

52. Jones EC, Chezmar JL, Nelson RC et al (1992) The frequency and significance of small (less than or equal to 15 mm) hepatic lesions detected by CT. AJR 158:535–539

53. LH Swartz, Gandras EJ, Colangelo SM et al (1999) Prevalence and importance of small hepatic lesions found at CT in patients with cancer. Radiology 210:71–74

54. Khalil HI, Patterson SA, Panicek DM (2005) Hepatic lesions deemed too small to characterize at CT: prevalence and importance in women with breast cancer. Radiology 235:872–878

55. Jang HJ, Lim HK, Lee WJ et al (2002) Small hypoattenuating lesions in the liver on single-phase helical CT in preoperative patients with gastric and colorectal cancer: prevalence, significance, and differentiating features. J Comput Assist Tomogr 26:718–724

56. Fong Y, Sun RL, Jarnagin W et al (1999) An analysis of 412 cases of hepatocellular carcinoma at a western center. Ann Surg 229:790–799

57. Rose AT, Rose DM, Pinson CW et al (1998) Hepatocellular carcinoma outcomes based on indicate treatment strategy. Am J Surg 64:1128–1134

58. Yoon SS, Tanabe TK (1999) Surgical treatment and other regional treatments for colorectal cancer liver metastases. Oncologist 4:197–208
59. Wood CB, Gillis CR, Blumgart LH (1976) A retrospective study of the natural history of patients with liver metastases from colorectal cancer. Clin Oncol 2:285–288
60. Miller FH, Butler RS, Hoff FL et al (1998) Using triphasic helical CT to detect focal hepatic lesions in patients with neoplasms. AJR 171:643–649
61. Semelka RC, Hussain SM, Marcos HB et al (2000) Perilesional enhancement of hepatic metastases: correlation between MR imaging and histopathologic findings-initial observations. Radiology 215:89–94
62. DuBrow RA, David CL, Libshitz HI et al (1990) Detection of hepatic metastases in breast cancer: the role of nonenhanced and enhanced CT scanning. J Comput Assist Tomogr 14:366–369
63. Laghi A, Iannaccone R, Rossi P et al (2003) Hepatocellular carcinoma: detection with triplephase multi-detector row CT in patients with chronic hepatitis. Radiology 226:543–549
64. Nino-Murcia M, Olcott EW, Jeffrey RB Jr et al (2000) Focal liver lesions: Pattern-based classification Scheme for enhancement at arterial phase CT1. Radiology 215:746–751
65. Semelka RC, Helmberger TK (2001) Contrast agents for MR imaging of the liver. Radiology 218:327–332
66. Ferrucci JT (1991) Liver tumor imaging: current concepts. Keio J Med 40:194–205
67. Kuszyk BS, Bluemke DA, Urban BA et al (1996) Portal-phase contrast-enhanced helical CT for the detection of malignant hepatic tumors: sensitivity based on comparison with intraoperative and pathologic findings. AJR 166:91–95
68. Stoupis C, Taylor HM, Paley MR et al (1998) The Rocky liver: radiologic-pathologic correlation of calcified hepatic masses. Radiographics 18:675–685; quiz 726
69. Hale HL, Husband JE, Gossios K et al (1998) CT of calcified liver metastases in colorectal carcinoma. Clin Radiol 53:735–741
70. Michael C, Robert B, Paul S (2002) Cystic changes in hepatic metastases from gastrointestinal stromal tumors (GISTs) treated with Gleevec (imatinib mesylate). AJR 179:1059–1062
71. Muramatsu Y, Takayasu K, Moriyama N et al (1986) Peripheral low density area of hepatic tumors: CT-pathologic correlation. Radiology 1601:49–52
72. Gabata T, Matsui O, Kadoya M et al (1998) Delayed MR imaging of the liver: correlation of delayed enhancement of hepatic tumors and pathologic appearance. Abdom Imaging 23:309–313
73. Goldberg SN, Dupuy DE (2001) Image-guided radiofrequency tumor ablation: challenges and opportunities part I. J Vasc Interv Radiol 12:1020–1032
74. Dupuy DE, Goldberg SN (2001) Image-guided radiofrequency tumor ablation: challenges and opportunities part II. J Vasc Interv Radiol 12:1135–1148
75. Goldberg SN, Grassi CJ, Cardella JF et al (2005) Imageguided tumor ablation: standardization of terminology and reporting criteria. Radiology 235:728–739
76. Choi H, Loyer EM, DuBrow RA et al (2001) Radiofrequency ablation of liver tumors: assessment of therapeutic response and complications. RadioGraphics 21:S41–S54
77. Veit P, Antoch G, Stergar H et al (2006) Detection of residual tumor after radiofrequency ablation of liver metastasis with dual-modality PET/CT: initial results. Eur Radiol 16: 80–87
78. Anderson GS, Brinkmann F, Soulen MC (2003) FDG positron emission tomography in the surveillance of hepatic tumors treated with radiofrequency ablation. Clin Nucl Med 28: 192–197
79. Lim HK, Choi D, Lee WJ et al (2001) Hepatocellular carcinoma treated with percutaneous radio-frequency ablation: evaluation with follow-up multiphase helical CT. Radiology 221:447–454
80. Goldberg SN, Gazelle GS, Compton CC et al (2000) Treatment of intrahepatic malignancy with radiofrequency ablation: radiologicpathologic correlation. Cancer 88:2452–2463

81. Dromain C, de Baere T, Elias D et al (2002) Hepatic tumors treated with percutaneous radio-frequency ablation: CT and MR imaging follow-up. Radiology 223:255–262
82. Tuma RS (2006) sometimes size doesn't matter: reevaluating RECIST and tumor response rate endpoints. J Natl Cancer Inst 98:1272–1274
83. Eisenhauera EA, Therasseb P, Bogaertsc J (2009) New response evaluation criteria in solid tumours: Revised RECIST guideline (version 1.1), Eur J Cancer 45:228–247
84. Semelka RC, Worawattanakul S, Noone TC et al (1999) Chemotherapy-treated liver metastases mimicking hemangiomas on MR images. Abdom Imaging 24:378–382
85. Mueller GC, Hussain HK, Carlos RC et al (2003) Effectiveness of MR imaging in characterizing small hepatic lesions: routine versus expert interpretation. AJR 180:673–680
86. Semelka RC, Armao DM, Elias J Jr et al (2007) Imaging strategies to reduce the risk of radiation in CT studies, including selective substitution with MRI. J Magn Reson Imaging 25:900–909
87. Parikh T, Drew SJ, Lee VS et al (2008) Focal liver lesion detection and characterization with diffusionweighted MR imaging: comparison with standard breath-hold T2-weighted imaging. Radiology 246:812–822
88. Morana G, Salviato E, Guarise A (2007) Contrast agents for hepatic MRI. Cancer Imaging 7:S24–S27
89. Bartolozzi C, Cioni D, Donati F et al (2001) Focal liver lesions: MR imaging-pathologic correlation. Eur Radiol 11:1374–1388
90. Ramalho M, Altun E, Heredia V (2007) Liver MR Imaging: 1.5T versus 3T. Magn Reson Imaging Clin N Am 15:321–347
91. Keogan MT, Edelman RR (2001) Technologic advances in abdominal MR imaging. Radiology 220:310–320
92. Morrin MM, Rofsky NM (2001) Techniques for liver MR imaging. Magn Reson Imaging Clin N Am 9:675–696
93. Low RN, Alzate GD, Schimakawa A (1997) Motion suppression in MR imaging of the liver: comparison of respiratory-triggered and nontriggered fast spin-echo sequences. AJR 168:225–231
94. Kanematsu M, Hoshi H, Itoh K et al (1999) Focal hepatic lesion detection: comparison of four fat-suppressed T2-weighted MR imaging pulse sequences. Radiology 211:363–371
95. Heidemann RM, Ozsarlak O, Parizel PM et al (2003) A brief review of parallel magnetic resonance imaging. Eur Radiol 13:2323–2337
96. Coenegrachts K, Ghekiere J, Denolin V et al (2010) Perfusion maps of the whole liver based on high temporal and spatial resolution contrast-enhanced MRI (4D THRIVE): Feasibility and initial results in focal liver lesions. Eur J Radiol 74:529–535
97. Rofsky NM, Lee VS, Laub G et al (1999) Abdominal MR imaging with a volumetric interpolated breath-hold examination. Radiology 212:876–884
98. Martin DR, Semelka RC (2005) Magnetic resonance imaging of the liver: review of techniques and approach to common diseases. Semin Ultrasound CT MR 26:116–131
99. Kanematsu M, Semelka R, Matsuo M et al (2002) Gadolinium-enhanced MR imaging of the liver: optimizing imaging delay for hepatic arterial and portal venous phases—a prospective randomized study in patients with chronic liver damage. Radiology 225:407–415
100. Outwater E, Tomaszewski JE, Daly JM et al (1991) Hepatic colorectal metastases: correlation of MR imaging and pathologic appearance. Radiology 180:327–332
101. Danet IM, Semelka RC, Leonardou P et al (2003) Spectrum of MRI appearances of untreated metastases of the liver. AJR 181:809–17
102. Namasivayam S, Martin DR, Saini S (2007) Imaging of liver metastases: MRI Cancer Imag 7:2–9
103. Silva AC, Evans JM, McCullough AE (2009) MR Imaging of hypervascular liver masses: a review of current techniques. RadioGraphics 29:385–402
104. Sohn J, Siegelman E, Osiason A (2001) Unusual patterns of hepatic steatosis caused by the local effect of insulin revealed on chemical shift MR imaging. AJR 176:471–474

105. Colagrande S, Centi N, Galdiero R et al (2007) Transient hepatic intensity differences. II. Those not associated with focal lesions. AJR 188:160–166
106. Stanisz GJ, Odrobina EE, Pun J et al (2005) T1, T2 relaxation and magnetization transfer in tissue at 3.0T. Magn Reson Med 54:507–512
107. Bazelaire CM, Duhamel GD, Rofsky NM et al (2004) MR imaging relaxation times of abdominal and pelvic tissues measured in vivo at 3.0 T: preliminary results. Radiology 230:652–659
108. Merkle EM, Dale BM (2006) Abdominal MRI at 3.0 T: the basics revisited. AJR 186: 1524–1532
109. Morakkabati-Spitz N, Gieseke J, Kuhl C et al (2005) 3.0-T high-field magnetic resonance imaging of the female pelvis: preliminary experiences. Eur J Radiol 15:639–644
110. Lencioni R, Cioni D, Crocetti L et al (2004) Magnetic resonance imaging of liver tumors. J Hepatol 40:162–171
111. Bellin MF, Vasile M, Morel-Precetti S (2003) Currently usednon-specific extracellular MR contrast media. Eur Radiol 13:2688–2698
112. Balci NC, Semelka RC (2005) Contrast agents for MR imaging of the liver. Radiol Clin North Am;43:887–898
113. Vogl TJ, Schwarz W, Blume S et al (2003) Preoperative evaluation of malignant liver tumors: comparison of unenhanced and SPIO (Resovist)-enhanced MR imaging with biphasic CTAP and intraoperative US. Eur Radiol 13:262–272
114. Ward J, Feng C, Guthrie JA et al (2000) Hepatic lesion detection after superparamagnetic iron oxide enhancement: comparison of five T2-weighted sequences at 1.0 T by using alternative free response receiver operating characteristic analysis. Radiology 214:159–166
115. Reimer P, Schneider G, Schima W (2004) Hepatobiliary contrast agents for contrast-enhanced MRI of the liver: properties, clinical development and applications. Eur Radiol 14:559–578
116. Huppertz A, Balzer T, Blakeborough A et al (2004) Improved detection of focal liver lesions at MR imaging: multicenter comparison of gadoxetic acid-enhanced MR images with intraoperative findings. Radiology 230:266–275
117. Grazioli L, Morana G, Kirchin MA et al (2005) Accurate differentiation of focal nodular hyperplasia from hepatic adenoma at gadobenate dimeglumineenhanced MR imaging: prospective study. Radiology 236:166–177
118. Koyama T, Tamai K, Togashi K (2006) Current status of body MR imaging: fast MR imaging and diffusion-weighted imaging. Int J Clin Oncol 11:278–285
119. Koh DM, Collins DJ (2007) Diffusion-weighted MRI in the body: applications and challenges in oncology. AJR 188:1622–1635
120. Moteki T, Sekine T (2004) Echo planar MR imaging of the liver: comparison of images with and without motion probing gradients. J Magn Reson Imaging 19:82–90
121. Nasu K, Kuroki Y, Nawano S et al (2006) Hepatic metastases: diffusion-weighted sensitivity-encoding versus SPIO-enhanced MR imaging. Radiology 239:122–130
122. Ichikawa T, Haradome H, Hachiya J et al (1998) Diffusion-weighted MR imaging with a single-shot echoplanar sequence: detection and characterization of focal hepatic lesions. AJR 170:397–402
123. Koh DM, Scurr E, Collins DJ et al (2006) Colorectal hepatic metastases: quantitative measurements using single-shot echo-planar diffusion-weighted MR imaging. Eur Radiol 16:1898–1905
124. Taouli B, Vilgrain V, Dumont E et al (2003) Evaluation of liver diffusion isotropy and characterization of focal hepatic lesions with two single-shot echo-planar MR imaging sequences: prospective study in 66 patients. Radiology 226:71–78
125. Chan JH, Tsui EY, Luk SH et al (2001) Diffusion weighted MR imaging of the liver: distinguishing hepatic abscess from cystic or necrotic tumor. Abdom Imaging 26:161–165
126. Padhani AR, Husband JE (2001) Dynamic contrast-enhanced MRI studies in oncology with an emphasis on quantification, validation and human studies. Clin Radiol 56:607–620

127. Ichikawa T, Haradome H, Hachiya J et al (1998) Characterization of hepatic lesions by perfusion-weighted MR imaging with an echoplanar sequence. AJR 170:1029–1034

128. Tofts PS, Brix G, Buckley DL et al (1999) Estimating kinetic parameters from dynamic contrast-enhanced T(1)-weighted MRI of a diffusable tracer: standardized quantities and symbols. J Magn Reson Imaging 10:223–232

129. Strauss LG, Conti PS (1991) The applications of PET in clinical oncology. J Nucl Med 32:623–648

130. Rohren EM, Turkington TG, Coleman RE (2004) Clinical applications of PET in oncology. Radiology 231:305–332

131. Selzner M, Hany TF, Wildbrett P et al (2004) Does the novel PET/CT imaging modality impact on the treatment of patients with metastatic colorectal cancer of the liver? Ann Surg 240:1027–1034

132. Shreve PD, Anzai Y, Wahl RL (1999) Pitfalls in oncologic diagnosis with FDG PET imaging: physiologic and benign variants. Radiographics 19:61–77

133. Reinartz P, Wieres FJ, Schneider W et al (2004) Side-by-side reading of PET and CT scans in oncology: which patients might profit from integrated PET/CT? Eur J Nucl Med Mol Imaging 31:1456–1461

134. Burger C, Goerres G, Schoenes S et al (2002) PET attenuation coefficients from CT images: experimental evaluation of the transformation of CT into PET 511-keV attenuation coefficients. Eur J Nucl Med Mol Imaging 29:922–927

135. Yau YY, Chan WS, Tam YM et al (2005) Application of intravenous contrast in PET/CT: does it really introduce significant attenuation correction error? J Nucl Med 46:283–291

136. Brechtel K, Klein M, Vogel M et al (2006) Optimized contrast-enhanced CT protocols for diagnostic whole-body ^{18}F-FDG PET/CT: technical aspects of single-phase versus multiphase CT imaging. J Nucl Med 47:470–476

137. Mankoff DA, Muzi M, Krohn KA (2003) Quantitative positron emission tomography imaging to measure tumor response to therapy: what is the best method? Mol Imaging Biol 5:281–285

138. Weber WA, Ziegler SI, Thodtmann R et al (1999) Reproducibility of metabolic measurements in malignant tumors using FDG PET. J Nucl Med 40:1771–1777

139. Keyes JW (1995) SUV: standard uptake or silly useless value? J Nucl Med 36:1836–1839

140. Sugawara Y, Zasadny KR, Neuhoff AW et al (1999) Reevaluation of the standardized uptake value for FDG: variations with body weight and methods for correction. Radiology 213: 521–525

141. Gambhir SS, Czernin J, Schwimmer J et al (2001) A tabulated summary of the FDG PET literature. J Nucl Med 42:1S–93S

142. Kitagawa Y, Nishizawa S, Sano K et al (2003) Prospective comparison of 18F-FDG PET with conventional imaging modalities (MRI, CT, and 67 Ga scintigraphy) in assessment of combined intraarterial chemotherapy and radiotherapy for head and neck carcinoma. J Nucl Med 44:198–206

143. Gould MK, Maclean CC, Kuschner WG et al (2001) Accuracy of positron emission tomography for diagnosis of pulmonary nodules and mass lesions: a meta-analysis. JAMA 285:914–924

144. Abdel-Nabi H, Doerr RJ, Lamonica DM et al (1998) Staging of primary colorectal carcinomas with fluorine-18 fluorodeoxyglucose whole-body PET: correlation with histopathologic and CT findings. Radiology 206:755–760

145. Hustinx R, Paulus P, Jacquet N et al (1998) Clinical evaluation of whole-body ^{18}F-fluorodeoxyglucose positron emission tomography in the detection of liver metastases. Ann Oncol 9:397–401

146. Fong Y, Saldinger PF, Akhurst T et al (1999) Utility of ^{18}F-FDG positron emission tomography scanning in selection of patients for resection of hepatic colorectal metastases. Am J Surg 178:282–287

147. Fletcher JW, Djulbegovic B, Soares HP et al (2008) Recommendations on the use of 18F-FDG PET in oncology. J Nucl Med 49:480–508
148. Soyer P (1993) Segmental Anatomy of the liver: utility of a nomenclature accepted worldwide. AJR Am J Roentgenol 161:572–573

Chapter 12
Colorectal Carcinoma Liver Metastasis: Surgical Clinical Perspective

Adrian M. Fox, Steven Gallinger, and Carol-Anne Moulton

Abstract Few malignancies have their prognosis changed by resection of their metastatic deposits. Why this should be possible with colorectal cancer is being investigated by researchers worldwide. This observation, however, has seen surgical therapy of colorectal liver metastases witness revolutionary changes over the past years. Historically, liver resection was seen as a formidable operation fraught with complications. Perioperative safety has improved and specialist centers performing liver resection for colorectal liver metastases are reporting operative mortality rates of less than 1%. A challenge for the future is to make more patients eligible for curative intent surgery by downstaging the tumours with chemotherapy to make them resectable. Specialist centers are expanding the operations applied to this disease with vein resection, interposition vascular grafting, in-vivo liver isolation even ex vivo resections with re-implantation of the liver. Surgery is becoming safer for the patient and chemotherapy is slowing the progress of metastatic colorectal cancer to allow surgery to add more effectively to increase patient survival. Five year survival rates continue to improve. Chemotherapy does have effects on the liver which at times limit the possibilities for resection; however, newer therapies, combinations of therapies, timing and shorter courses of therapy see similar tumour responses without the deleterious effects. The amount of liver remaining after resection also limits which tumours are technically resectable. The volume of residual liver required has been further defined. Portal vein embolization can preoperatively selectively hypertrophy the future liver which the patient will be dependant upon. Better imaging and volumetric analysis has seen an extension of the criteria of what is thought resectable. Tumour margins of the resected specimen have been shown to be important only if less than 1 mm, therefore expanding the indications for resection. The evolving field of chemotherapeutics will continue to push the limits of tumour response. These improvements will see dynamic changes in the roles of the members of the multidisciplinary cancer care team.

A.M. Fox (✉)
University Health Network, University of Toronto, Toronto, ON, Canada
e-mail: adrian.fox@uhn.on.ca

P. Brodt (ed.), *Liver Metastasis: Biology and Clinical Management*, Cancer Metastasis – Biology and Treatment 16, DOI 10.1007/978-94-007-0292-9_12, © Springer Science+Business Media B.V. 2011

Keywords Colorectal carcinoma · Liver metastasis · Surgical resection · Chemotherapy

Abbreviations

CLMs   colorectal liver metastases
CEA   carcinoembryonic antigen
CT   computerized tomography
MRI   magnetic resonance imaging
FAP   familial adenomatous polyposis
FLR   future liver remnant
NAFLD   non-alcoholic fatty liver disease
PET   positron emission tomographic scan
MCC   Multidisciplinary Cancer Conference
IVC   inferior vena cava
PVE   portal vein embolization
RFA   radiofrequency ablation

Contents

12.1 Introduction

Recent developments in the treatment of metastases from colorectal cancer are changing the approach to a disease that has traditionally been viewed with pessimism. Advances in surgery, chemotherapeutics and targeted biologic therapies have altered metastatic colorectal cancer to a state of slowly progressive "chronic disease" in many patients [1]. The role of surgery in this context is becoming increasingly important and the indications for surgical intervention in advanced stage disease are expanding. Although prospective, randomized clinical trials are lacking, retrospective and comparative studies clearly support hepatic resection as first-line treatment providing long-term survival for many patients with colorectal carcinoma that has metastasized to the liver [2].

Recent reports have shown an almost doubling of disease free and overall survival rates for patients undergoing liver resection for metastatic colorectal cancer. Prior to 1992, overall survival was 30–40% increasing to almost 60% more recently [3]. For patients with solitary colorectal liver metastases (CLMs) who have a resection, up to 70% 5-year survival may be expected. Long term survival with chemotherapy alone is rare [4].

It is not well understood why resection of metastatic deposits improves survival in metastatic colorectal cancer. The concept that liver-only metastases is the result of a "regionally confined" process while extrahepatic disease is systemic, has justified a regional approach to treatment such as surgery [5].

12.1.1 Justification for Liver Resection as a Therapeutic Option

Historically liver resection was seen as a formidable operation fraught with complications. Perioperative safety has improved and specialist centers performing liver

Table 12.1 Used by permission from Springer [8]

Investigator	Year	Years included in study	5-year survival (%)
Huges	1988	1948–1985	24
Sheele	1991	1960–1988	31
Sheele	1995	1960–1992	39
Fong	1999	1985–1998	37
Minagawa	2000	1980–1997	38
Choti	2002	1993–1999	58
Okano	2002	1992–1996	67.88
Abdalla	2004	1992–2002	58
Fernandez	2004	1992–2002	58
Pawlik	2005	1990–2004	58
Tanaka	2008	1990–2006	45.7

resection for CLMs are reporting operative mortality rates of less than 1% [6]. The relative safety of surgery combined with improved 5 year survival data for resection has encouraged the use of this procedure. Advances in chemotherapeutics have extended survival of many patients with metastatic disease from colorectal cancer [7]. However, the effect of surgery is even greater for patients eligible for liver resection of hepatic metastases (see Table 12.1).

12.1.2 The Patient Referral

Metastatic liver disease from colorectal cancer can present at any time in the treatment pathway. It is more common to find a metastasis on surveillance early after resection of the primary, usually within the first 2 years [9]. Slightly less frequently, the patient presents with synchronous liver disease and a colorectal primary. Surveillance post colonic resection consisting of clinical review, serial Carcinoembryonic Antigen (CEA) measurements and imaging by computerized tomography (CT), ultrasound or magnetic resonance imaging (MRI) regularly identify metastatic deposits before they become clinically apparent, reinforcing the importance of post colorectal cancer surgery surveillance. Of note, a survival benefit of surveillance has been shown in three separate meta-analyses [10–12]. Other modes of presentation are changing due to developing technologies. CT or ultrasound scanning performed for other reasons are discovering liver lesions sometimes before the primary disease becomes symptomatic. These scenarios pose new and increasingly complex issues for the surgeon (for a more detailed discussion of imaging modalities for liver metastases, see Chapter 11 in this volume).

12.1.3 Unexpected Presentation on the Operating Table

Although population-based colorectal cancer screening is becoming commonplace, compliance and public education remain challenging [13], therefore, primary colorectal cancer continues to present as acute abdominal emergencies [14]. Colonic perforation or obstruction may warrant urgent surgical intervention prior to adequate radiological work-up. Therefore, liver lesions are sometimes identified unexpectedly at the time of emergency surgery. If colonic perforation is the presenting problem, the patient's clinical condition may preclude prolonged intraoperative assessment. Brief liver palpation and the judicious use of liver biopsy might be considered. Biopsy of suspicious lesions should be performed only if the results will alter the treatment algorithm. Increasing use of CT in the workup of acute abdominal conditions has seen an increase in the immediate preoperative recognition of synchronous liver lesions. Less common is the radiologically misinterpreted or overlooked liver lesion that becomes evident at surgery for the primary. These situations are less of an emergency and allow the surgeon to make a more thorough assessment of the liver (including intra-operative ultrasound) and the abdominal cavity. Occasionally, the presence of widespread and incurable metastatic disease is identified and the patient is considered for palliative treatment only. Decisions of incurability on the operating room table that affect the surgical plan have to be made with caution, because chemotherapeutic agents offer the chance for significant response and possibly cure, even in some cases of widespread disease.

12.2 Preoperative Evaluation

12.2.1 Multidisciplinary Cancer Conference (MCC)

The decision to resect CLMs is individualized based on the specific clinical situation, with adherence to oncologic principles and based on the highest level of available evidence. A multidisciplinary team is ideally composed of all of the health care providers that deliver care to the cancer patient, including representation from medical oncology, surgery, radiation oncology, pathology, diagnostic radiology, palliative care, nursing staff and social work.

The MCC constitutes a multidisciplinary clinical discussion to ensure the evaluation, management and follow-up of all cancer patients and to arrive at patient care recommendations through consensus decision making and institutional protocols or trials [15].

12.2.2 Fitness for Major Surgery

The general and lifestyle risk factors that predispose to colorectal cancer are also present in patients with colorectal cancer liver metastases. The epidemiologic links between diet, weight, exercise and colorectal cancer risk are some of the strongest for any type of cancer [16]. Therefore these patients represent a cohort of the population with a higher rate of obesity-related co-morbidities.

The liver resection patient is relatively young compared to the average patient undergoing surgery for primary colorectal cancer. For the years 2002 through to 2006, median age at diagnosis for cancer of the colon and rectum was 71 years according to SEER data [17]. The mean age of patients having liver surgery for CLMs is 10 years younger at 61 years [18]. Even with co-morbidities, the patient with advanced colorectal cancer may still be fit to withstand a major oper-ation. If deemed medically unfit for surgery, patients are considered for alternative treatments, e.g., ablative therapy [19].

12.3 Required Investigations

12.3.1 Imaging

Most hepatic surgical oncologists perform a CT scan of the chest, abdomen and pelvis utilizing a liver-specific protocol for the purposes of identifying and charac-terizing the number and location of hepatic metastases prior to planning surgery. Some centers also advocate the use of Magnetic Resonance Imaging (MRI) [20]. MRI can be helpful in patients with fatty liver or in patients who have had extensive chemotherapy because the demonstration of CLMs in these situations is some-times confounded by the background changes in the surrounding liver parenchyma. Ultrasound is particularly useful for the characterization of cystic lesions in the liver (see Chapter 11 for more on this subject).

12.3.2 Tumour Markers/Other Biochemistry

Baseline measurement of CEA [19] and liver function tests should be performed as well as blood typing for possible blood transfusions perioperatively.

12.3.2.1 Endoscopy

Complete examination of the colon should have been performed within the preced-ing 18 months leading up to a liver resection [19]. This is especially important if the primary tumour presented as an acute emergency and a colonoscopy was either not performed or was incomplete. The rate of synchronous colonic lesions is not insignificant with adenocarcinoma occurring in at least 2% of patients and benign polyps even more frequently [21]. Less than 5% of patients will have a highly pen-etrant genetic predilection for colorectal cancer [22] and these patients may, in some circumstances, benefit from an update of their other surveillance regimens. As an example, Familial Adenomatous Polyposis (FAP) patients will require upper endoscopy to screen for duodenal lesions and this could be performed at the time of colonic assessment.

12.4 Special Investigations

12.4.1 Liver Functional Reserve Assessment

A major liver resection puts the patient at risk of liver failure, often leading to death, if functional reserve is inadequate. The following variables have been shown to influence how the remnant liver will perform after hepatic resection:

- Volume of liver remaining after a proposed resection,
- Underlying liver disease
- Duration and type of chemotherapy already delivered.

The best method for determining liver volume utilizes computer modeling to measure the future liver remnant (FLR) directly on a three-dimensional CT reconstruction of the liver [3]. Standard liver volume is estimated based on a formula that relates liver volume to patient size (body surface area). CT volumetric analysis is often required when planning complex liver resections. Realization that the FLR determines surgical outcome (including duration of hospital stay, complications and risk for liver failure and death) has been one of the major advances allowing extensive resection, particularly for CLMs [3].

Minimum requisite FLR volume for safe recovery after resection will be affected by chronic liver disease, steatosis or steatohepatitis and the effects of chemotherapy (discussed in detail below). As a guide, with normal liver size and function, most patients can safely have 80% of the liver volume resected [23]. After extensive chemotherapy or with other causes of moderate liver damage, more remnant volume is required [23].

Standard liver biochemical tests do not have a predictive value in determining which patients will suffer liver failure after resection [24]. Other methods for testing liver function include measurement of uptake of organic anions [such as bromsulphthalein, rose Bengal, and indocyanine green (ICG)], the arterial ketone body ratio, redox tolerance test, the aminopyrine breath test and the amino acid clearance test [2].

The ICG clearance test seems to be the best discriminating investigation and most often used. Hepatectomy involving resection of up to 60% of the parenchyma can be tolerated in patients who have retention of less than 20% of ICG at 15 min. Minor hepatectomies can be accomplished if ICG retention at 15 min is less than 25% [2]. Histopathology in the form of a core biopsy of liver tissue will sometimes help decision making, especially if a case is borderline. Intraoperative factors such as inflow clamp times combine with post-operative factors such as sepsis and hypotension to have an impact on hepatic function.

12.4.1.1 Hepatic Steatosis

Steatosis is a subtype of Non-Alcoholic Fatty Liver disease (NAFLD) and is a common pathological change in the liver characterized by lipid deposition within the hepatocytes. These histopathological findings meet the criteria for steatohepatitis when associated with lobular inflammation and cellular changes of hepatocyte ballooning. The "Kleiner score" is used to histologically evaluate liver specimens for NAFLD. The score is based on three objective factors using routine hematoxylin and eosin-stains:

- percentage parenchymal involvement by steatosis,
- degree of lobular inflammation, and
- degree of ballooning of hepatocytes.

Up to 34% of the Western population has hepatic steatosis [25]. The prevalence increases to up to 74% in the obese and to over 90% in the morbidly obese populations [26]. Diabetes mellitus is also strongly associated. Certain chemotherapy regimens have been reported to increase the incidence of steatosis and steatohepatitis [27] (see Section 12.12 below).

The adverse impact of hepatic steatosis on perioperative outcomes after liver resection is quite well recognized [28]. Uncomplicated steatosis is associated with more bleeding during parenchymal transection and more postoperative complications, including sepsis. Steatosis alone has not been associated with a significant increase in mortality. In contrast, patients with steatohepatitis are at higher risk for liver failure and death after major hepatectomy [27].

12.4.2 Laparoscopic Staging

The role of pre-resection laparoscopic staging is evolving since peritoneal carcinomatosis is a common type of extrahepatic disease in patients with CLMs, representing about one third of the cases of extrahepatic disease [29] (see Fig. 12.1). When peritoneal disease is found at laparotomy, this would usually contraindicate hepatic resection. Therefore, the aim of laparoscopy is to spare the occasional patient a futile laparotomy and start systemic therapy earlier.

The probability of laparoscopy altering the treatment algorithm increases in patients with more advanced disease. Prognostic markers used to decide which patients undergo laparoscopy are discussed below. Laparoscopy can be used in the patient with a fatty liver to assess the liver macroscopically and to obtain core biopsies under vision which may decrease the risk of bleeding associated with blind transcutaneous biopsies.

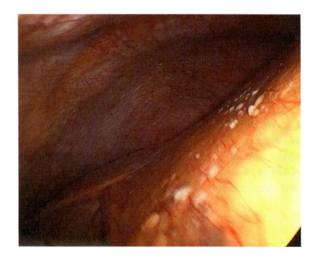

Fig. 12.1 Laparoscopic imgae of small peritoneal tumour nodules on the faliciform ligament

Pilkington et al. reported criteria for laparoscopic staging are as follows:

- Unfavorable primary tumour where there are concerns regarding the risk of locoregional recurrence, i.e. pT4 stage or circumferential resection margin involvement on histopathology, and/or perforation and/or acute obstruction at the index operation.
- Multiple bilobar metastases where there is concern regarding the feasibility or safety of liver resection and where radiological imaging is indeterminate.
- Hepatic parenchymal assessment where there is concern regarding the magnitude of the planned liver resection and, specifically, the quantity and/or quality of the liver remnant.
- In addition to the above, where there are concerns regarding medical co-morbidity and the fitness of the patient for major resectional surgery under prolonged general anesthesia, laparoscopic staging serves as a "test of anesthesia" [30].

However, in the report by Pilkington et al., two inadvertent enterotomies and one port site metastasis were documented in a series of 77 patients, highlighting the potential hazards of laparoscopy after colorectal cancer surgery [30].

Fong and colleagues, by applying multivariate analysis to their data on 1001 patients, determined that the following factors were predictive of poor, long term outcome after liver resection for CLMs:

- positive nodal status of the primary disease,
- short disease-free interval,
- increased number of hepatic metastases (more than one metastasis),
- large metastases,
- high carcinoembryonic antigen level [18].

When these five criteria were used as a preoperative scoring system, assigning one point for each criterion, the total score was highly predictive of outcome ($p < 0.0001$). No patient with a score of 5 was a long-term survivor [18]. As well as being predictive of outcome, this scoring system has been used by others to guide in the work up of patients with CLMs, with laparoscopy reserved for patients with "higher Fong scores" as described by Mann et al. [31].

12.4.3 PET Scanning

The Positron Emission Tomographic (PET) scan has potential utility in the preoperative investigation of a structural abnormality seen on CT that if metabolically active changes the treatment algorithm. Often combined with CT, the PET/CT scan may detect unsuspected disease, both within the liver and in extra-hepatic sites. There is limited evidence that PET scanning has contributed to improved 5-year survival following liver resection by preventing patients with occult extrahepatic disease from receiving a non-therapeutic liver resection [32]. The reliability of PET/CT to screen for occult disease, to meaningfully add to the routine workup and to do so economically, are questions currently being addressed in an ongoing multi-center randomized controlled trial in Ontario, Canada referred to as PETCAM [33].

12.4.4 Portal Vein Embolization (PVE)

Described as "liver enhancement", PVE is a procedure that allows most of the portal blood flow to be diverted to the FLR, consequently promoting liver hypertrophy of the high flow areas; although the physiological mechanisms are not fully understood. When the predicted FLR volume is inadequate, PVE is considered [3]. PVE also acts as a dynamic preoperative test of the capacity of the liver to recover after insult. When the degree of hypertrophy is greater than 5%, the risk of post resection liver failure is low [34]. Standard chemotherapy does not seem to affect PVE-induced liver hypertrophy [3]. Bevacizumab (Avastin®) has been reported in small studies to possibly impair PVE liver hypertrophy [3, 35], however, more studies are needed to address this question. Analysis of hepatic regeneration after PVE in patients without cirrhosis reveals an early phase of regeneration during the first 3 weeks followed by a plateau during which the FLR volume increases only slightly [34].

12.5 Defining Resectability

Patients with metastatic colorectal cancer suitable for resection still represent the minority of all colorectal cancer patients with Stage IV disease, although criteria are expanding. Patients with solitary, multiple, or bilobar disease who have had curative intent treatment of their primary tumors are candidates for liver resection [19]. The current approach to resectability focuses on achieving an R0[1] resection, including resection of limited extrahepatic disease [32]. If necessary, this is achieved in combination with ablative methods, portal vein embolization PVE (see below), preoperative downstaging chemotherapy or as a two-stage procedure.

Traditional criteria for resection are giving way to a new approach to this disease. No longer are surgeons counting lesions or measuring their size; rather, the question

---

[1] The tumor status following treatment is described by the residual tumor (R) classification: R0, no residual tumor; R1, microscopic residual tumor; R2, macroscopic residual tumor. Residual tumor may be found in the area of primary tumor and its regional lymph nodes and/or at distant sites. The R classification reflects the effects of treatment and influences further treatment planning. Furthermore, the R classification is a strong predictor of prognosis. An acceptable long-term prognosis can be expected only in R0 patients. Although there exist clear correlations between stage and R classification, the differences in prognosis of R0 versus R1, 2 cannot be explained by differences in stage alone. The prognostic significance of R classification is demonstrated by respective data for non-small cell lung carcinoma, squamous cell carcinoma of oesophagus, gastric carcinoma, ductal adenocarcinoma of the pancreas, colorectal carcinoma, lung and liver metastases [80].

is, "Can all disease be resected while leaving a functional liver remnant?" – i.e. the current "what is left" paradigm [36]. This new approach has been fueled by recent reports of good results even in patients with multiple bilateral CLMs. With a combination of careful selection, systemic chemotherapy, PVE, and two-stage surgery, 3-year survival has been reported to be as high as 85% [37]. Factors that are considered important include: sufficient functional hepatic reserve with adequate portal inflow, adequate hepatic venous outflow and adequate biliary drainage.

Pawlik et al. have expanded on the "what is left" paradigm by defining resectability based on four criteria:

1. The disease needs to be completely resected. An R0 resection of both the intra- and extrahepatic disease sites must be feasible.
2. At least two adjacent liver segments need to be spared.
3. Vascular inflow and outflow, as well as biliary drainage to the remaining segments, must be preserved.
4. The volume of the liver remaining after resection (i.e., the future liver remnant) must be adequate:

    a. at least 20% of the total estimated liver volume if normal parenchyma,
    b. at least 30–60% if the liver is injured by chemotherapy, steatosis, or hepatitis, or
    c. at least 40–70% in the presence of cirrhosis, depending on the degree of underlying hepatic dysfunction [29].

Liver metastases are generally considered non-resectable if there is invasion of the two main portal pedicles, if there is invasion of one portal pedicle and the contra-lateral hepatic vein, if the three major hepatic veins are invaded (except in rare circumstances where reimplantation of an hepatic vein is possible) or if total removal of liver deposits will leave less than 20% of functional liver [38].

12.5.1 Extra-Hepatic Disease

CLM patients with even limited hepatic disease and any extrahepatic disease (except perhaps lung metastases) were traditionally considered ineligible for radical surgery. However, recent evidence suggests that with careful patient selection, surgical resection of CLMs with limited extrahepatic disease may result in survival rates of 78% at 3 years and 56% at 5 years [39]. However, the sites and amount of extrahepatic disease considered resectable, with curative intent, is controversial, with no Level 1 evidence to support a dogmatic approach.

With the criteria expanding, current recommendations for patients with extrahepatic disease that should be considered for liver resection include:

- resectable or ablatable pulmonary metastases
- resectable, isolated extrahepatic sites for example:

o portal lymph nodes

o resectable local recurrence

• local direct extension of liver metastases to, for example, diaphragm/adrenal that can be resected [19].

12.5.1.1 Pulmonary Metastases

Patients may be considered for pulmonary resection, as long as it is technically feasible and there is no evidence of hilar or pericardial lymphadenopathy [39]. Patients with liver and lung metastases can be treated with sequential resection of both disease sites. The liver metastases are usually resected first to ensure there is no unsuspected extrahepatic disease in the abdomen. Five year overall survival rates of 30% have been reported for patients with liver and lung metastases [40]. These complicated cases benefit from the involvement of thoracic surgical specialists in the MCC session.

12.5.1.2 Hepatic Pedicle Nodal Metastases

Hepatectomy combined with resection of metastatic regional portal lymph node metastases results in cures in well selected patients [40]. However, as the involved nodes extend to the celiac axis – the distal field – survival rates approach 0% [2] (see Fig. 12.2).

12.5.1.3 Peritoneal Metastases

The role of resection of peritoneal carcinomatosis, including limited disease, is not yet clear. Several small studies reported encouraging results, however, the benefit of this approach is still unproven [41]. As such, it cannot be considered standard therapy and should be offered only in the form of a clinical trial [39].

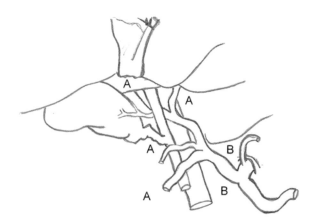

Fig. 12.2 Portal lymph node fields. (**A**) Proximal field and (**B**) distal field (celiac nodes)

12.6 When to Operate; When to Use Neoadjuvant Chemotherapy

Patients with a low clinical risk (Fong) score for recurrence are often offered immediate surgery. Those with unfavorable primary pathology such as perforated primary tumour or extensive nodal involvement may be considered for neoadjuvant chemotherapy prior to liver resection and then re-staged at three months [19]. However, the decision to give chemotherapy before or after liver surgery should be individualized and based on local policy [8].

The recently completed EORTC 40983 trial did not demonstrate a clearly significant advantage of pre-operative chemotherapy for initially resectable liver metastases [8]. The use of a no-chemotherapy control arm also compromises the significance of EORTC 40983, because the trial could not really answer the question of whether neoadjuvant (preoperative) chemotherapy is superior (or equal) to postoperative chemotherapy, or to both preoperative and postoperative "sandwich" chemotherapy. Opponents of the neoadjuvant approach claim that pre-operative chemotherapy only delays definitive curative treatment (surgical resection). Proponents place emphasis on the possible information that can be inferred from the in vivo tumor response to chemotherapy regarding the drug that may be most beneficial postoperatively. Responders to neo-adjuvant chemotherapy have been shown to represent a group that has particularly good survival after subsequent resection [43]. Non-responders to chemotherapy are a worse prognostic group that does not benefit as much from surgery. However, the decision not to operate on this cohort of patients, based on their response to preoperative chemotherapy would not be supported by current evidence.

Novel protein or genetic biomarkers may, in the future, better define cohorts of patients suitable for one treatment pathway or another. This could avoid the over treatment of patients with aggressive biology and enable a more tailored approach for individual patients [8]. (The reader is referred to Chapter 14 in this volume for a review on the use of proteomics as an approach for individualization of treatment).

Preoperative (or neoadjuvant) chemotherapy in the resectable patient may cause concern to the hepatic surgeon. Operating on the chemotherapy-affected liver can be difficult. The fatty mottled liver is often rigid, difficult to handle, friable and may bleed excessively. A report published in 2008 helps to quantify the risks and benefits of these regimens [42]. This Intergroup trial may dispel concerns regarding preoperative chemotherapy in a resectable patient since:

1. Resectable patients did not progress to unresectable on treatment; an identical proportion of patients proceeded to resection in each group
2. Hepatotoxicity was minimized with short duration of therapy
3. Complications were similar between groups and operative mortality identical
4. There was improved survival in the chemotherapy arm [42].

These and other results have prompted a recent expert panel to conclude:

"In a major change to clinical practice, the panel's recommendation was that the majority of patients with colorectal cancer liver metastases should be treated up front with chemotherapy, irrespective of the initial resectability status of their metastases" [44]. Nevertheless, prospective randomized trials are necessary to definitively answer the question whether preoperative (neoadjuvant) chemotherapy is equivalent or superior to post-operative chemotherapy for patients with resectable colorectal cancer hepatic metastases. These trials must include well-defined criteria for resectability and clear reporting of the extent of resection [45].

12.7 Downstaging

Chemotherapy for downstaging liver-only metastatic disease that is otherwise judged to be non-resectable technically has recently shown promise, with up to 44% of initially unresectable patients coming to surgery for successful, potentially curative, resection [46]. These patients have acceptable outcomes of up to 17%, 10 year survivorship [47]. This is important in view of the fact that close to 80% of patients presenting with CLMs do not have technically resectable disease. Usual reasons for non-resectability include ill located lesions, proximity to, or invasion of major portal structures and/or hepatic veins, or when resection of all disease will leave the patient with an insufficient liver remnant for survival. The hope for these patients is that their disease will respond to chemotherapy to a degree that allows surgical excision. Over the last ten years, combination chemotherapeutic regimens have been shown to downsize tumour burden to an extent that sometimes allows initially unresectable metastases to be resected (see Fig. 12.3). Giachetti et al. reported a 5-year survival rate of 50% in 77 downstaged cases [48], which compared favorably with the 5-year survival rate for non-operated patients that ranged between 0 and 5% [49].

12.8 The "Ghost" Lesion

Some liver metastases may no longer be visible on imaging after neoadjuvant or downstaging chemotherapy. Whether these metastases are completely eradicated or remain viable at a microscopic/histologic level is a matter of current debate (see Fig. 12.4). To address this question, 38 patients with 66 liver metastases that had disappeared on CT scan were reviewed [50]. This study showed that viable cancer cells persisted at the initial site of liver metastases in over 80% of cases that had disappeared on imaging, suggesting that complete radiologic response does not mean cure of the disease [50]. This also provides some insight into why current chemotherapy does not cure CLM's. The current approach to "ghost lesions" at

Initial Appearance   After downstaging chemotherapy

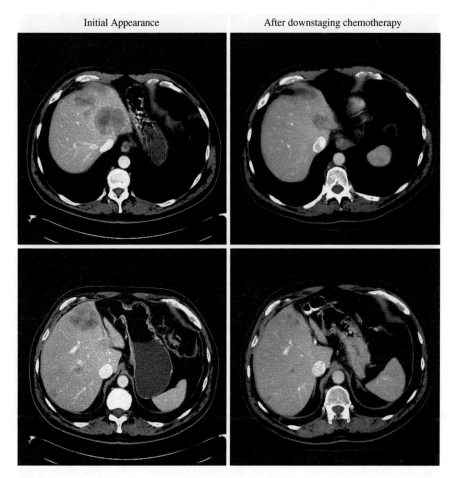

Fig. 12.3 Successful downstaging with chemotherapy of initially unresectable disease. *Left* computerized tomography images show the initial appearance. *Right* – after seven cycles of FOLFIRI and Bevacizumab

surgery is to remove as many as possible. This is sometimes difficult because the lesion is often not palpable, nor can it be seen with intra-operative ultrasound to guide the plane of transection [4].

This CT image of the same patient as above, shows three lesions. One large lesion in segment 4B and two smaller lesions in segment 6. The centrally located lesion is placed just behind the right hepatic vein, the other more peripherally located.

After downstaging chemotherapy and left trisegmentectomy the anterior lesion near the right hepatic vein is barely visible. The more peripheral segment 6 lesion has disappeared.

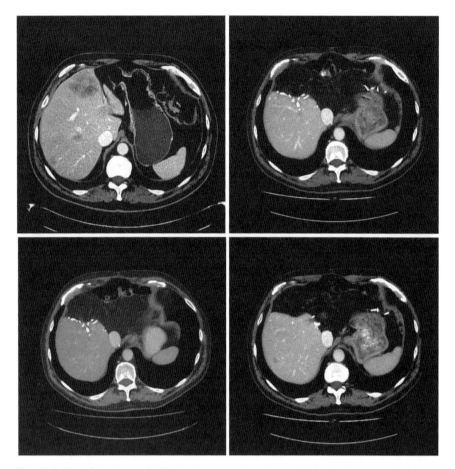

Fig. 12.4 The "Ghost Lesion". This is the same patient shown in Fig. 12.3. Note the first image shows two lesions in segment 6 that initially responded to chemotherapy and then 3 months later have reappeared

Now seen on two separate slices of the CT – the anterior lesion near the right hepatic vein is more visible 3 months later.

On another slice of the CT, the recurrence of the peripheral lesion is also evident.

12.9 Intraoperative Techniques

A better understanding of internal hepatic anatomy and improved techniques for liver transection and hemostasis have resulted in improved safety of liver resections [51–52]. Low central venous pressure anesthesia is accepted widely as a safe method to minimize blood loss during liver resection [3]. Operative mortality rates of less than 5 per cent are consistently being reported from high-volume centers [27].

The authors of this chapter have developed a liver anatomy learning resource for trainees to understand hepatic anatomy; a 3 dimensional graphic web-based teaching tool known as the *Virtual Liver Project*. This site can be found at: http://pie.med.utoronto.ca/VLiver/index.htm

12.9.1 Resection Margins

Achieving margins of 1 cm or more may be less important than previously appreciated [29]. While adequate surgical margins around the tumour are important, the actual width may not be as critical. This is because liver metastases are usually histopathologically well circumscribed [53], only 16% have satellitosis [54], Glisson sheath extension is uncommon (14.5%) and limited (5 mm or less) [55], and micrometastases are rare (2%) [55]. Therefore, currently available data support the concept of limited complete resection that encompasses all tumor-bearing liver parenchyma [29]. As a result, there are two principles that are currently important regarding margins around a resected colorectal cancer liver metastasis.

- a clear margin is important
- a margin width of greater than 1 mm is not as important

Local recurrence, disease free and overall survival are the same when the margin is greater than 1 mm versus greater than 1 cm [3]. For practical and safety reasons, a margin of 1 cm around a CLM should be the surgical goal. A non-anatomic or wedge resection generates the same results as a more formal anatomical resection and a wedge resection may actually be preferable in some cases where future resectable hepatic recurrences may necessitate a contralateral lobectomy or major wedge resection [56].

12.9.2 Hanging Maneuver

Surgeons who use this technique aim to place a sling behind the liver sliding it in front of the inferior vena cava (IVC) to gain vascular control to allow splitting the liver before wide mobilization of either lobe. The method was initially described in 2001 by Belghiti et al. [57]. The liver hanging maneuver is commonly applied to right hepatectomy as a possible improvement to the anterior approach described in 1996 by Lai et al. [58].

The method involves blunt and blind insinuation of a clamp along the front of the IVC from the caudal aspect of the liver, exiting cranially between the right hepatic vein and the middle hepatic vein. An elastic tape is then passed allowing the liver to be lifted which compresses vascular structures and allows a guide for transection. There is the theoretical potential that oncologic outcomes may be improved because of the initial control of hepatic venous outflow before mobilization and perhaps reduced shedding of tumor cells into the circulation during the resection.

12.9.3 Hepatic Inflow Control

The use of the "Pringle maneuver" (hepatic pedicle clamping) is variable. It can be helpful to reduce intraoperative blood loss [3] but decreases the perfusion of the remnant liver.

12.9.4 Intraoperative Ultrasound

Intraoperative ultrasound is used to control margins, locate lesions, and confirm vascular anatomy [3].

12.10 Two-Stage Hepatectomy

This approach has gained acceptance because it avoids two common problems associated with trying to clear extensive metastases from both lobes of the liver at once.

1. Post operative liver failure – addressed by utilizing the capacity of the liver to regenerate between two operations, often assisted by PVE.
2. Unwanted tumour progression in the FLR- managed by removing or ablating tumour deposits in the FLR first.

A two stage hepatectomy may be useful in a patient with multiple bilobar metastases that would otherwise not be curable by single stage surgery because of an insufficient liver remnant. This operation can be applied to different combinations of bilobar disease patterns.

The steps usually include:

1. First stage resection: the lobe with least disease is cleared (resection and/or ablation)
2. Intervening PVE of opposite lobe
3. Often intervening chemotherapy
4. CT assessment to confirm that the cleared lobe has now hypertrophied
5. Second stage resection: definitive hepatectomy of the embolized lobe

The prototype of this operation was a two stage procedure that did not utilize an intervening PVE [59]. The results were encouraging but morbidity was high due mostly to insufficient functional liver remnant [60]. PVE after the first procedure has been proposed to induce compensatory hypertrophy of the FLR and encouraging results have resulted in increasing popularity of this approach.

It has been feared (and debated) that when an area of liver is induced to hypertrophy, the tumour within that segment may also be induced to grow, perhaps at a greater rate than the surrounding liver [61]. Therefore, metastases located in the FLR should be ideally resected or ablated before PVE.

12.10.1 First-Stage

The first-stage consists of complete clearance of metastases located in one hemiliver. Depending on the distribution of the metastases, this could be either lobe; however, the first procedure is most commonly applied to the left hemiliver. If there are three or fewer metastases in this lobe they may be resected non-anatomically, if there are more than three metastases, radiofrequency ablation (RFA) may be added to ablate the lesions as an adjunct, complementing or replacing surgery.

Two to five weeks after the first-stage hepatectomy is probably the optimal time to perform percutaneous PVE [62]. To control tumor growth between the two hepatectomies, chemotherapy may be administered, generally starting 3 weeks after the first hepatectomy. FLR hypertrophy needs to be evaluated with three-dimensional CT scan, 5–8 weeks after PVE [59]. If the estimated volume of the FLR is considered insufficient (less than 0.5% of body weight), a second evaluation, 3–4 weeks later can be performed before excluding the patient from the second-stage hepatectomy.

12.10.2 Second-Stage Hepatectomy

A right or an extended right hepatectomy is the operation most commonly performed in these cases; resection of caudate lobe can be performed when it is involved. The dissection of liver parenchyma is again preferably performed without clamping or under selective right pedicle clamping. In case of development of further metastases in the left FLR, further non anatomic resection or RFA can be performed during the second-stage hepatectomy.

12.11 Follow Up After Liver Resection

Follow up after liver resection should continue for at least five years at regular intervals and consist of clinical review, chest and abdomen CT and serial CEA measurements. The risk of liver recurrence decreases with time. About 70% of recurrences will be observed within the first 12 months after resection and 92% will be apparent within 24 months [63].

12.11.1 Re-resection for Recurrence

If tumour recurs in the liver, well selected patients will benefit from repeat resection. Yan et al. [64] have shown that after a third resection for isolated hepatic recurrence, 5-year overall survival rates of 16–68% may be achieved, and postoperative morbidity and mortality are no greater than after the first hepatectomy. Patients who have repeat resections do not have a significantly different overall survival compared with those who only had a single resection. In comparison, salvage surgery after RFA

Reference	Treatment Status	Median Survival

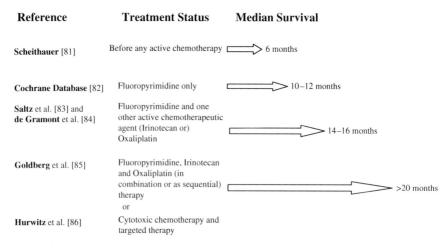

Fig. 12.5 Trends in the median survival of patients with advanced colorectal cancer. With permission from Meyerhardt and Mayer [66]

failure does not appear to provide survival rates similar to those of salvage surgery of recurrence following resection [3].

12.12 Chemotherapy

Chemotherapy for the patient with non resectable CLMs is effective in prolonging life, but is not curative. Figure 12.5 provides an historical overview of progress in chemotherapy for metastatic colorectal cancer and related survival. The data show survival approaching 2 years with current regimens in patients who never qualify for surgery [7].

12.12.1 5-Fluorouracil (5-FU)

Over 50 years have elapsed since the discovery of 5-FU in 1957 [71]. The drug 5-FU is converted by the enzyme thymidine phosphorylase into fluorodeoxyuridine monophosphate, which, in the presence of reduced folate, forms a complex with thymidylate synthase, thus interfering with DNA synthesis and causing apoptosis in rapidly dividing tumor cells. Leucovorin (folinic acid), an agent that enhances the binding of fluorodeoxyuridine monophosphate to thymidylate synthase, is frequently added to 5-FU to enhance its efficacy [72]. When first introduced, bolus administration of these two agents was widely adopted as first-line treatment in the United States. Infusional 5-FU has since been shown to be safer than bolus administration and to lead to higher response rates and it is now the preferred delivery method [73]. Administration of 5-fluorouracil may also be associated with increased risk of steatosis in this patient population [74].

12.12.2 Irinotecan

In the history of colorectal cancer chemotherapeutics, one of the important developments was the introduction in 1996 of the topoisomerase inhibitor – irinotecan. Irinotecan is activated by hydrolysis to SN-38, an inhibitor of topoisomerase I. The inhibition of topoisomerase I eventually leads to inhibition of both DNA replication and transcription. The common colorectal cancer regimen, FOLFIRI, consists of infusional 5-FU, leucovorin, and irinotecan.

12.12.3 Oxaliplatin

Oxaliplatin is a platinum-based chemotherapeutic drug that is commonly combined with 5-FU in a regimen known as FOLFOX. Oxaliplatin was introduced in 2004 and both irinotecan and oxaliplatin have emerged as critical partners with 5-FU in improving the treatment outcome for patients with Stage IV colorectal cancer. An analysis of several large, phase III trials demonstrated that use of all three agents namely, irinotecan, oxaliplatin, and 5-FU plus Leucovorin at some point during treatment, significantly improves the overall survival time, reaching an average of 20 months [73].

12.12.4 Bevacizumab

Bevacizumab was the first clinically available angiogenesis inhibitor. It is a monoclonal antibody that targets vascular endothelial growth factor. Potential unwanted side-effects such as increased operative and postoperative bleeding, impaired wound healing and liver regeneration, prohibits its use 5–6 weeks prior to liver resectional surgery. Interestingly, this compound in addition to improving pathologic tumour response may also protect against Oxaliplatin-induced sinusoidal injury [75].

12.12.5 Cetuximab

Also a monoclonal antibody, Cetuximab targets the epidermal growth factor-mediated cell growth regulatory pathway [73]. Cetuximab first received approval for use, either in combination with irinotecan for the treatment of EGFR-expressing, irinotecan-refractory metastatic colorectal cancer or as a single agent in patients who cannot tolerate irinotecan. In 2007, it was also approved as mono-therapy for EGFR-expressing metastatic colorectal cancer after failure of irinotecan and oxaliplatin-based regimens [73]. The EGFR ligand-receptor complex on the cell surface transmits its growth-promoting signal via the K-ras G protein pathway. Not surprisingly therefore, Cetuximab and other EGFR inhibitors are only effective against tumors that do not express a mutated K-ras (which maintains a constitutively activated pathologic growth pathway in these cancer cells) [76].

12.12.6 Chemotherapy Induced Hepatic Injury

Chemotherapy can damage the liver in a dose and duration-related manner with effects that may be regimen, and likely patient-specific [67]. Vauthey et al. [67] showed that oxaliplatin was associated with sinusoidal dilation at a rate of 18.9% versus 1.9% for patients with no chemotherapy. Irinotecan was associated with steatohepatitis: 20.2% versus 4.4% in those with no chemotherapy.

Sinusoidal injury has not been shown to cause death from liver failure in patients having liver resection, although prolonged oxaliplatin therapy (six to nine cycles) leads to severe sinusoidal injury, fibrosis, and splenomegaly that may classify some patients as non-resectable [3]. When oxaliplatin is used as a short course, there is no increase in morbidity [67].

There is an ongoing debate regarding the relationship between chemotherapy and steatosis – it appears that steatosis may be linked to demographic patient factors rather than to treatment [37]. Co-morbid conditions that can, of themselves, increase the risk of complications, such as obesity and diabetes are common in patients with steatosis. In a study of patients who had major liver resections, patients with steatosis had increased postoperative complications such as blood loss and longer intensive-care-unit stays compared with matched control patients with healthy livers. Also, 26% of patients with steatosis were obese (BMI ≥ 30 kg/m^2) as compared to only 2% of control individuals, which might have contributed to the worse outcome for those with steatosis [68].

Hepatic steatosis without inflammation (simple steatosis) may be present in patients having chemotherapy. Irrespective of the possible links with chemotherapy, hepatic resection can be performed safely even in patients with severe (>30%) steatosis [69].

Steatohepatitis is a more significant liver injury, characterized by fatty change and portal inflammation. It has been associated with perioperative morbidity and mortality, likely secondary to insufficient hepatic regeneration that is due to the inflammatory component of the disease [67]. Steatohepatitis linked to irinotecan is associated with increased 90-day mortality due to liver failure after surgery [67]. The duration of irinotecan therapy is important. When used for less than 3 months (six cycles), there was no increase in morbidity [70].

12.13 Ablative Therapy

Radiofrequency ablation (RFA) is the best studied and most widely used method for in situ tumor destruction in the liver [3]. Its early use was greeted with great enthusiasm as initial results were encouraging; however, more recent reports revealed that this method has several limitations. First and most significant is a local recurrence rate of 37% [39]. By comparison, the rate after resection (with a negative margin) is 3–5% [77]. Another limitation is the treatment area. Although newer technologies have seen the treatable lesion size increase to close to 5 cm, the standard has been 3 cm which excludes many larger sized metastases. RFA cannot be used near certain structures (e.g. major bile ducts) for fear of causing thermal injury. Blood flow in nearby major vessels may dissipate the thermal energy of RFA, thus reducing effectiveness when used close to these structures. There are problems with surveillance after RFA. The resultant scar is often radiologically apparent for many years. PET scanning is sometimes required to discriminate scar from recurring tumour at an ablation site edge.

In situ destructive techniques such as RFA are useful in selected cases. This method, when combined with resection, can be of importance to clear the liver of metastatic disease when the surgeon is trying to preserve hepatic volume. Percutaneous RFA also has a role in the occasional non-resectable case or in patients with restricted operability due to co-morbidities. Consistent reports of local failure in nearly one third of CLMs cases suggest that this procedure is of limited utility as a "curative" treatment modality for this disease, even for small lesions [3].

12.14 Questions, Controversies and Future Developments

There are many important fundamental questions that remain unanswered concerning the management of colorectal cancer liver metastases. One major question pertains to the source and significance of circulating tumor cells. Circulating tumour cells offer a unique glimpse into the metastatic process and their presence is an opportunity to study the dynamics of tumour dissemination and the host immune responses and the factors required for metastases to occur. Important to their use as a research tool, circulating tumour cells are accessible in the peripheral blood [78]. Their presence raises several intriguing questions including: (1) Do these circulating cells originate from the liver metastases themselves and does their presence imply a worse outcome? (2) Do liver metastases metastasize? and (3) Why do CRC tumours preferentially spread to the liver if tumour cells can be found circulating freely in the bloodstream? There are other remaining enigmas for example; why does surgical excision of metastatic deposits improve survival for colon carcinoma when this is not apparent with most other gastrointestinal malignancies?

12.15 Conclusion

Major advances in chemotherapeutics and surgical techniques have revolutionized the current approach to colorectal cancer liver metastases. As a result, many more patients are now eligible for curative-intent surgery. Current challenges include identifying appropriate prognostic indicators for the selection of patients who will benefit from an aggressive surgical approach, as well as identifying biomarkers that will help tailor available chemotherapeutic options based on the patients' profile.

Acknowledgement Adrian M. Fox was supported by an educational grant from Sanofi-Aventis pharmaceuticals.

References

1. Goldberg RM, Rothenberg ML, Van Cutsem E, Benson AB 3rd, Blanke CD, Diasio RB et al (2007) The continuum of care: a paradigm for the management of metastatic colorectal cancer. Oncologist 12:38–50
2. Jaeck D, Pessaux P (2008) Bilobar colorectal liver metastases: treatment options. Surg Oncol Clin N Am 17:553–568, ix
3. Berri RN, Abdalla EK (2009) Curable metastatic colorectal cancer: recommended paradigms. Curr Oncol Rep 11:200–208
4. Benoist S, Nordlinger B (2009) The role of preoperative chemotherapy in patients with resectable colorectal liver metastases. Ann Surg Oncol 16:2385–2390
5. Carpizo DR, Are C, Jarnagin W, Dematteo R, Fong Y, Gonen M et al (2009) Liver resection for metastatic colorectal cancer in patients with concurrent extrahepatic disease: results in 127 patients treated at a single center. Ann Surg Oncol 16:2138–2146
6. Lochan R, White SA, Manas DM (2007) Liver resection for colorectal liver metastasis. Surg Oncol 16:33–45
7. Tournigand C, Andre T, Achille E, Lledo G, Flesh M, Mery-Mignard D et al (2004) FOLFIRI followed by FOLFOX6 or the reverse sequence in advanced colorectal cancer: a randomized GERCOR study. J Clin Oncol 22:229–237
8. Shimada H, Tanaka K, Endou I, Ichikawa Y (2009) Treatment for colorectal liver metastases: a review. Langenbeck's Arch Surg/Deutsche Gesellschaft fur Chirurgie. Langenbecks Arch Surg 394:973–983. http://www.ncbi.nlm.nih.gov/pubmed/19582473. Epub 7 Jul 2009
9. Kimura T, Akazai Y, Iwagaki H, Nonaka Y, Ariki N, Fuchimoto S et al (1995) Metachronous liver metastasis of colorectal cancer: timing of occurrence and efficacy of adjuvant portal chemotherapy. Anticancer Res 15:1585–1588
10. Jeffery M, Hickey BE, Hider PN (2007) Follow-up strategies for patients treated for non-metastatic colorectal cancer. Cochrane Database Syst Rev, CD002200
11. Renehan AG, Egger M, Saunders MP, O'Dwyer ST (2002) Impact on survival of intensive follow up after curative resection for colorectal cancer: systematic review and meta-analysis of randomised trials. BMJ 324:813
12. Figueredo A, Rumble RB, Maroun J, Earle CC, Cummings B, McLeod R et al (2003) Follow-up of patients with curatively resected colorectal cancer: a practice guideline. BMC Cancer 3:26
13. Mauri D, Pentheroudakis G, Milousis A, Xilomenos A, Panagoulopoulou E, Bristianou M et al (2006) Colorectal cancer screening awareness in European primary care. Cancer Detect Prev 30:75–82
14. Smothers L, Hynan L, Fleming J, Turnage R, Simmang C, Anthony T (2003) Emergency surgery for colon carcinoma. Dis Colon Rectum 46:24–30
15. Wright F (2006) Multidisciplinary Cancer Conference Standards: The Evidentiary Review [Developed by the Expert Panel on Multidisciplinary Cancer Conference Standards, Cancer Care Ontario, Report Date: June 1, 2006]; Available from: http://www.cancercare.on.ca/common/pages/UserFile.aspx?fileId=36872. Accessed Oct 2009
16. http://www.cancer.org/docroot/CRI/content/CRI_2_4_2X_What_are_the_risk_factors_for_colon_and_rectum_cancer.asp. http://www.cancer.org/docroot/CRI/content/CRI_2_4_2X_What_are_the_risk_factors_for_colon_and_rectum_cancer.asp. Available from: http://www.cancer.org/docroot/CRI/content/CRI_2_4_2X_What_are_the_risk_factors_for_colon_and_rectum_cancer.asp. Accessed Oct 2009
17. http://seer.cancer.gov/statfacts/html/colorect.html. http://seer.cancer.gov/statfacts/html/colorect.html. http://seer.cancer.gov/statfacts/html/colorect.html; Available from: http://seer.cancer.gov/statfacts/html/colorect.html. Accessed Oct 2009
18. Fong Y, Fortner J, Sun RL, Brennan MF, Blumgart LH (1999) Clinical score for predicting recurrence after hepatic resection for metastatic colorectal cancer: analysis of 1001 consecutive cases. Ann Surg 230:309–318; discussion 18–21

19. Garden OJ, Rees M, Poston GJ, Mirza D, Saunders M, Ledermann J et al (2006) Guidelines for resection of colorectal cancer liver metastases. Gut 55:iii1–8
20. Blyth S, Blakeborough A, Peterson M, Cameron IC, Majeed AW (2008) Sensitivity of magnetic resonance imaging in the detection of colorectal liver metastases. Ann R Coll Surg Engl 90:25–28
21. Nikoloudis N, Saliangas K, Economou A, Andreadis E, Siminou S, Manna I et al (2004) Synchronous colorectal cancer. Tech Coloproctol 8:S177–S179
22. Gatalica Z, Torlakovic E (2008) Pathology of the hereditary colorectal carcinoma. Fam Cancer 7:15–26
23. Abdalla EK, Barnett CC, Doherty D, Curley SA, Vauthey JN (2002) Extended hepatectomy in patients with hepatobiliary malignancies with and without preoperative portal vein embolization. Arch Surg 137:675–680; discussion 80–81
24. Hemming AW, Scudamore CH, Shackleton CR, Pudek M, Erb SR (1992) Indocyanine green clearance as a predictor of successful hepatic resection in cirrhotic patients. Am J Surg 163:515–518
25. Browning JD, Szczepaniak LS, Dobbins R, Nuremberg P, Horton JD, Cohen JC et al (2004) Prevalence of hepatic steatosis in an urban population in the United States: impact of ethnicity. Hepatology 40:1387–1395
26. Nomura H, Kashiwagi S, Hayashi J, Kajiyama W, Tani S, Goto M (1988) Prevalence of fatty liver in a general population of Okinawa, Japan. Jpn J Med 27:142–149
27. Gomez D, Malik HZ, Bonney GK, Wong V, Toogood GJ, Lodge JP et al (2000) Steatosis predicts postoperative morbidity following hepatic resection for colorectal metastasis. Br J Surg 94:1395–1402
28. Cho CS, Curran S, Schwartz LH, Kooby DA, Klimstra DS, Shia J et al (2008) Preoperative radiographic assessment of hepatic steatosis with histologic correlation. J Am Coll Surg 206:480–488
29. Pawlik TM, Schulick RD, Choti MA (2008) Expanding criteria for resectability of colorectal liver metastases. Oncologist 13:51–64
30. Pilkington SA, Rees M, Peppercorn D, John TG (2007) Laparoscopic staging in selected patients with colorectal liver metastases as a prelude to liver resection. HPB (Oxford) 9: 58–63
31. Mann CD, Neal CP, Metcalfe MS, Pattenden CJ, Dennison AR, Berry DP (2007) Clinical risk score predicts yield of staging laparoscopy in patients with colorectal liver metastases. Br J Surg 94:855–859
32. Grundmann RT, Hermanek P, Merkel S, Germer CT, Grundmann RT, Hauss J et al (2008) Diagnosis and treatment of colorectal liver metastases – workflow. Zentralbl Chir 133: 267–284
33. Gallinger S (2010) The impact of positron emission tomography (PET) imaging prior to liver resection for colorectal adenocarcinoma metastases: a prospective, multicentre randomized clinical trial. Available from: http://clinicaltrials.gov/ct2/show/study/NCT00265356 (ahead of print)
34. Ribero D, Abdalla EK, Madoff DC, Donadon M, Loyer EM, Vauthey JN (2007) Portal vein embolization before major hepatectomy and its effects on regeneration, resectability and outcome. Br J Surg 94:1386–1394
35. Aussilhou B, Dokmak S, Faivre S, Paradis V, Vilgrain V, Belghiti J (2009) Preoperative liver hypertrophy induced by portal flow occlusion before major hepatic resection for colorectal metastases can be impaired by bevacizumab. Ann Surg Oncol 16:1553–1559
36. Charnsangavej C, Clary B, Fong Y, Grothey A, Pawlik TM, Choti MA (2006) Selection of patients for resection of hepatic colorectal metastases: expert consensus statement. Ann Surg Oncol 13:1261–1268
37. Chun YS, Vauthey JN, Ribero D, Donadon M, Mullen JT, Eng C et al (2007) Systemic chemotherapy and two-stage hepatectomy for extensive bilateral colorectal liver metastases: perioperative safety and survival. J Gastrointest Surg 11:1498–1504; discussion 504–505

38. Lupinacci R, Penna C, Nordlinger B (2007) Hepatectomy for resectable colorectal cancer metastases – indicators of prognosis, definition of resectability, techniques and outcomes. Surg Oncol Clin N Am 16:493–506, vii–viii

39. Adams RB, Haller DG, Roh MS (2006) Improving resectability of hepatic colorectal metastases: expert consensus statement by Abdalla et al. Ann Surg Oncol 13:1281–1283

40. de Haas RJ, Wicherts DA, Adam R (2008) Resection of colorectal liver metastases with extrahepatic disease. Dig Surg 25:461–466

41. Elias D, Liberale G, Vernerey D, Pocard M, Ducreux M, Boige V et al (2005) Hepatic and extrahepatic colorectal metastases: when resectable, their localization does not matter, but their total number has a prognostic effect. Ann Surg Oncol 12:900–909

42. Nordlinger B, Sorbye H, Glimelius B, Poston GJ, Schlag PM, Rougier P et al (2008) Perioperative chemotherapy with FOLFOX4 and surgery versus surgery alone for resectable liver metastases from colorectal cancer (EORTC Intergroup trial 40983): a randomised controlled trial. Lancet 371:1007–1016

43. Tamandl D, Gruenberger B, Herberger B, Kaczirek K, Gruenberger T (2009) Surgery after neoadjuvant chemotherapy for colorectal liver metastases is safe and feasible in elderly patients. J Surg Oncol 100:364–371

44. Nordlinger B, Van Cutsem E, Gruenberger T, Glimelius B, Poston G, Rougier P et al (2009) Combination of surgery and chemotherapy and the role of targeted agents in the treatment of patients with colorectal liver metastases: recommendations from an expert panel. Ann Oncol 20:985–992

45. Pozzo C, Barone C, Kemeny NE (2008) Advances in neoadjuvant therapy for colorectal cancer with liver metastases. Cancer Treat Rev 34:293–301

46. Pozzo C, Basso M, Cassano A, Quirino M, Schinzari G, Trigila N et al (2004) Neoadjuvant treatment of unresectable liver disease with irinotecan and 5-fluorouracil plus folinic acid in colorectal cancer patients. Ann Oncol 15:933–939

47. Adam R, Delvart V, Pascal G, Valeanu A, Castaing D, Azoulay D et al (2004) Rescue surgery for unresectable colorectal liver metastases downstaged by chemotherapy: a model to predict long-term survival. Ann Surg 240:644–657; discussion 57–58

48. Giacchetti S, Itzhaki M, Gruia G, Adam R, Zidani R, Kunstlinger F et al (1999) Long-term survival of patients with unresectable colorectal cancer liver metastases following infusional chemotherapy with 5-fluorouracil, leucovorin, oxaliplatin and surgery. Ann Oncol 10: 663–669

49. Van den Eynde M, Hendlisz A (2009) Treatment of colorectal liver metastases: a review. Rev Recent Clin Trials 4:56–62

50. Benoist S, Brouquet A, Penna C, Julie C, El Hajjam M, Chagnon S et al (2006) Complete response of colorectal liver metastases after chemotherapy: does it mean cure? J Clin Oncol 24:3939–3945

51. Imamura H, Seyama Y, Kokudo N, Maema A, Sugawara Y, Sano K et al (2003) One thousand fifty-six hepatectomies without mortality in 8 years. Arch Surg 138:1198–1206; discussion 206

52. Heriot AG, Karanjia ND (2002) A review of techniques for liver resection. Ann R Coll Surg Engl 84:371–380

53. Yamamoto J, Sugihara K, Kosuge T, Takayama T, Shimada K, Yamasaki S et al (1995) Pathologic support for limited hepatectomy in the treatment of liver metastases from colorectal cancer. Ann Surg 221:74–78

54. Scheele J, Stang R, Altendorf-Hofmann A, Paul M (1995) Resection of colorectal liver metastases. World J Surg 19:59–71

55. Kokudo N, Miki Y, Sugai S, Yanagisawa A, Kato Y, Sakamoto Y et al (2002) Genetic and histological assessment of surgical margins in resected liver metastases from colorectal carcinoma: minimum surgical margins for successful resection. Arch Surg 137: 833–840

56. Zorzi D, Mullen JT, Abdalla EK, Pawlik TM, Andres A, Muratore A et al (2006) Comparison between hepatic wedge resection and anatomic resection for colorectal liver metastases. J Gastrointest Surg 10:86–94

57. Belghiti J, Guevara OA, Noun R, Saldinger PF, Kianmanesh R (2001) Liver hanging maneuver: a safe approach to right hepatectomy without liver mobilization. J Am Coll Surg 193:109–111

58. Lai EC, Fan ST, Lo CM, Chu KM, Liu CL (1996) Anterior approach for difficult major right hepatectomy. World J Surg 20:314–317; discussion 8

59. Adam R, Laurent A, Azoulay D, Castaing D, Bismuth H (2000) Two-stage hepatectomy: a planned strategy to treat irresectable liver tumors. Ann Surg 232:777–785

60. Jaeck D, Oussoultzoglou E, Rosso E, Greget M, Weber JC, Bachellier P (2004) A two-stage hepatectomy procedure combined with portal vein embolization to achieve curative resection for initially unresectable multiple and bilobar colorectal liver metastases. Ann Surg 240: 1037–1049; discussion 49–51

61. Elias D, De Baere T, Roche A, Mducreux, Leclere J, Lasser P (1999) During liver regeneration following right portal embolization the growth rate of liver metastases is more rapid than that of the liver parenchyma. Br J Surg 86:784–788

62. Jaeck D, Abdalla EK (2009) Curable metastatic colorectal liver metastases. Ann Surg 11: 200–208

63. Langenhoff BS, Krabbe PF, Ruers TJ (2009) Efficacy of follow-up after surgical treatment of colorectal liver metastases. Eur J Surg Oncol 35:180–186

64. Yan TD, Sim J, Black D, Niu R, Morris DL (2007) Systematic review on safety and efficacy of repeat hepatectomy for recurrent liver metastases from colorectal carcinoma. Ann Surg Oncol 14:2069–2077

65. Karanjia ND, Lordan JT, Fawcett WJ, Quiney N, Worthington TR (2009) Survival and recurrence after neo-adjuvant chemotherapy and liver resection for colorectal metastases: a ten year study. Eur J Surg Oncol 35:838–843

66. Meyerhardt JA, Mayer RJ (2005) Systemic therapy for colorectal cancer. N Engl J Med 352:476–487

67. Vauthey JN, Pawlik TM, Ribero D, Wu TT, Zorzi D, Hoff PM et al (2006) Chemotherapy regimen predicts steatohepatitis and an increase in 90-day mortality after surgery for hepatic colorectal metastases. J Clin Oncol 24:2065–2072

68. Chun YS, Laurent A, Maru D, Vauthey JN (2009) Management of chemotherapy-associated hepatotoxicity in colorectal liver metastases. Lancet Oncol 10:278–286

69. Abdalla EK, Vauthey JN (2008) Chemotherapy prior to hepatic resection for colorectal liver metastases: helpful until harmful? Dig Surg 25:421–429

70. Parikh AA, Gentner B, Wu TT, Curley SA, Ellis LM, Vauthey JN (2003) Perioperative complications in patients undergoing major liver resection with or without neoadjuvant chemotherapy. J Gastrointest Surg 7:1082–1088

71. Shirasaka T, Taguchi T (2006) Timeline from discovery of 5-FU to development of an oral anticancer agent S-1 and its drug concept. Gan To Kagaku Ryoho 33:4–18

72. Piedbois P, Buyse M, Rustum Y, Machover D, Erlichman C, Carlson RW, Valone F, Labianca R, Doroshow JH, Petrelli N (1992, June) Modulation of fluorouracil by leucovorin in patients with advanced colorectal cancer: evidence in terms of response rate. Advanced Colorectal Cancer Meta-Analysis Project. J Clin Oncol 10:896–903

73. Kohne CH, Lenz HJ (2009) Chemotherapy with targeted agents for the treatment of metastatic colorectal cancer. Oncologist 14:478–488

74. Peppercorn PD, Reznek RH, Wilson P, Slevin ML, Gupta RK (1998) Demonstration of hepatic steatosis by computerized tomography in patients receiving 5-fluorouracil-based therapy for advanced colorectal cancer. Br J Cancer 77:2008–2011

75. Ribero D, Wang H, Donadon M, Zorzi D, Thomas MB, Eng C et al (2007) Bevacizumab improves pathologic response and protects against hepatic injury in patients treated with oxaliplatin-based chemotherapy for colorectal liver metastases. Cancer 110:2761–2767

76. Van Cutsem E, Kohne CH, Hitre E, Zaluski J, Chang Chien CR, Makhson A et al (2009) Cetuximab and chemotherapy as initial treatment for metastatic colorectal cancer. N Engl J Med 360:1408–1417

77. Pawlik TM, Scoggins CR, Zorzi D, Abdalla EK, Andres A, Eng C et al (2005) Effect of surgical margin status on survival and site of recurrence after hepatic resection for colorectal metastases. Ann Surg 241:715–722; discussion 22–24

78. Cohen SJ, Punt CJ, Iannotti N, Saidman BH, Sabbath KD, Gabrail NY et al (2009) Prognostic significance of circulating tumor cells in patients with metastatic colorectal cancer. Ann Oncol 20:1223–1229

79. Nagasue N, Yukaya H, Ogawa Y, Higashi T (1983) Portal pressure following partial to extensive hepatic resection in patients with and without cirrhosis of the liver. Ann Chir Gynaecol 72:18–22

80. Hermanek P, Wittekind C (1994) Residual tumor (R) classification and prognosis. Semin Surg Oncol 10:12–20

81. Scheithauer W, Rosen H, Kornek GV, Sebesta C, Depisch D (1993) Randomised comparison of combination chemotherapy plus supportive care with supportive care alone in patients with metastatic colorectal cancer. BMJ 306:752–755

82. Best L, Simmonds P, Baughan C, Buchanan R, Davis C, Fentiman I, George S, Gosney M, Northover J, Williams C, Collaboration Colorectal Meta-analysis (2000) Palliative chemotherapy for advanced or metastatic colorectal cancer. Cochrane Database Syst Rev, CD001545

83. Saltz LB, Cox JV, Blanke C, Rosen LS, Fehrenbacher L, Moore MJ et al (2000) Irinotecan plus fluorouracil and leucovorin for metastatic colorectal cancer. Irinotecan Study Group. N Engl J Med 343:905–914

84. de Gramont A, Figer A, Seymour M, Homerin M, Hmissi A, Cassidy J et al (2000) Leucovorin and fluorouracil with or without oxaliplatin as first-line treatment in advanced colorectal cancer. J Clin Oncol 18:2938–2947

85. Goldberg RM, Sargent DJ, Morton RF, Fuchs CS, Ramanathan RK, Williamson SK et al (2004) A randomized controlled trial of fluorouracil plus leucovorin, irinotecan, and oxaliplatin combinations in patients with previously untreated metastatic colorectal cancer. J Clin Oncol 22:23–30

86. Hurwitz H, Fehrenbacher L, Novotny W, Cartwright T, Hainsworth J, Heim W et al (2004) Bevacizumab plus irinotecan, fluorouracil, and leucovorin for metastatic colorectal cancer. N Engl J Med 350:2335–2342

Chapter 13
Evaluation and Management of Liver Metastases from Non-gastrointestinal Cancer

Khaled Elgadi, Trevor Reichman, and Sean P. Cleary

Abstract Tumor metastasis is considered a late stage of cancer progression and has traditionally been associated with a poor overall prognosis. The liver is one of the most common sites for the development of distant metastases from many different solid malignancies. The management of liver metastases has evolved significantly over the last several decades. Early experience with aggressive resection of hepatic metastases was associated with high morbidity and poor overall survival. These initial, poor outcomes with aggressive therapy led to some resistance in many centers to consider a surgical approach to hepatic metastases of non-gastrointestinal (non-GI) origin, and as a result treatment strategies tended to focus on palliative chemotherapy to slow disease progression and improve overall survival. However, recent advances in the field of hepatobiliary surgery have led to a renewed, albeit cautious, interest in the use of surgical resection for hepatic metastases of non-gastrointestinal malignancies. This chapter will review the available literature for each of several malignancies in the hope of providing guidance for clinical decision-making and will also highlight some of the areas in which data is clearly lacking.

Keywords Liver metastases · Liver resection · Non-gastrointestinal tumors · Selection criteria

Abbreviations

CRC	colorectal cancer
CSC	cancer stem cells
FRL	future remnant liver
HSC	hematopoietic stem cells
Non-GI	non-gastrointestinal

S.P. Cleary (✉)
Hepatobiliary and Pancreatic Surgical Oncology and Transplantation, Division of General Surgery, University Health Network-10EN212 Toronto General Hospital, 200 Elizabeth Street, Toronto, ON, Canada M5G 2C4
e-mail: sean.cleary@uhn.on.ca

P. Brodt (ed.), *Liver Metastasis: Biology and Clinical Management*, Cancer Metastasis – Biology and Treatment 16, DOI 10.1007/978-94-007-0292-9_13, © Springer Science+Business Media B.V. 2011

MELD	model for endstage liver disease
ICG	isocyanine green
RCC	renal cell carcinoma
TIL	tumor-infiltrating lymphocytes

Contents

13.1 Introduction

In the past 15 years, there have been significant improvements in the prognosis of patients with metastatic colorectal cancer (CRC) or neuroendocrine cancer confined to the liver. This is due to a combination of early detection, improved chemotherapy and surgical resection. The 5 year survival rate for patients with metastatic CRC to the liver improved from 9.1% in the early 1990s to 19.2% between 1998 and 2003 and coincided with increases in the use of liver resection to treat CRC liver metastases [1]. Similarly, patients with metastatic neuroendocrine tumors (NET) to the liver showed improved survival following hepatic resection. The 5-year survival for patients with NET liver metastases ranged from 61–73% following hepatic resection, which compared favorably to 25–29% in the non-surgical group [2–4]. The progress seen in metastatic colorectal and GI-NET cancer has encouraged many to reconsider their reluctance to apply a surgical approach to metastatic disease of non-GI cancers.

Despite significant improvement in the survival of patients with colorectal and neuroendocrine cancer liver metastases, resection of non-gastrointestinal tumors still remains controversial. Several factors may play a role in shifting the pendulum towards a more aggressive surgical approach to the management of non-colorectal and non-neuroendocrine liver metastases. First, the natural history of tumor metastasis is heterogeneous in nature and a percentage of patients may have metastatic disease confined to the liver that may benefit from surgical resection. For example, 7–9% of breast cancer metastases are confined to the liver [5]. Secondly, improvements in chemotherapy have led to increased tumor response rates in many diseases and successful control or reduction of tumor burden in certain cases. This enhanced effectiveness of chemotherapy has increased the percentage of patients with responsive or controllable oligometastatic disease. Thirdly, the increased safety of liver resection has improved the risk-benefit balance in these cases, rendering resection justifiable in selected instances.

Isolated reports of improved survival for patients undergoing liver resection for diseases such as metastatic breast cancer have led to cautious optimism in several centers regarding hepatic resection for non-GI cancers. However, all currently published studies are retrospective reviews, small case series or isolated case reports. These retrospective series report outcomes in a highly selected population and lack meaningful control groups or well defined eligibility criteria. This raises the possibility that the observed improvements in survival may not be directly attributed to the benefit of resection and are potentially due to multiple other factors including improved chemotherapy, improved imaging modalities leading to earlier detection (lead time bias) or improved patient selection. Unfortunately, scenarios in which patients present with optimal characteristics that warrant resection are rare. Therefore, the likelihood that an adequate prospective study can be performed remains low, unless a coordinated, well controlled multi-centered study is undertaken.

Surgical intervention for non-GI cancer liver metastases is still an evolving treatment option with a potential for improving overall and disease-free survival, in a select group of patients. As chemotherapeutic options for systemic disease continue to advance and progress, patients will continue to have improved control of the disease and improved survival. This improved response could increase the proportion of patients with controllable oligometastatic disease that might benefit from surgical resection. Therefore, the indications for liver resection will likely continue to evolve as discoveries are made in systemic treatment. In the future, better studies should help define tumor-related factors and patient characteristics which could identify patients likely to benefit from hepatic resection. Until more evidence is available, surgical decision-making will rely heavily on careful multidisciplinary review of each case on an individual basis. Below, we review the available literature for several malignancies in the hope of providing guidance for clinical decision-making and also highlight some of the areas in which data is clearly lacking.

13.2 Pathophysiology of Liver Metastasis

The process of tumor metastasis is complex and its underlying molecular mechanisms are not fully understood. Recent advances in molecular biology and stem cell research have shed new light on this complex process. The conventional model of tumor metastasis postulated that continued accumulation of genetic mutations in cancer cells resulted in the development of more aggressive cancer cells with metastatic capability. However, this model failed to account for some key features of the metastatic process such as tumor cell dormancy and the appearance of more differentiated cells in the metastatic lesions. Pioneering work in the field of leukemia led to the discovery of a subpopulation of leukemic cells with metastatic potential that share features with hematopoietic stem cells (HSC) [6]. These cells were therefore termed cancer stem cells (CSC). Since the publication of this work in the mid 1990s, cells with similar stem cell characteristics have been identified in several solid tumors including breast [7], pancreatic [8], and colon cancers [9].

Similar to HSCs, CSCs are capable of self-renewal and self-proliferation and can give rise to more differentiated cancer cells. Normal stem cells are generally found in a specialized microenvironment termed the stem cell "niche". Trumpp and Wiestler hypothesized that similarly to normal stem cells, the CSC also interact with their microenvironment to regulate their fate [10]. They further postulated that CSC may convert a normal stem-cell niche into tumor stroma to support self-renewal and survival. This may explain why disseminating tumor cells often migrate and seed areas characteristically occupied by somatic stem cells. Sites for preferential seeding of metastatic CSCs include stem-cell niches in the bone marrow, liver or brain.

This changing paradigm of the metastatic process has a major impact on the surgical approach to metastatic lesions of the liver. For example, the pathophysiology of CRC and gastrointestinal neuroendocrine liver metastases is traditionally viewed differently than that of non-GI cancers. In an anatomic model of CRC liver metastases, the spread of colorectal cancer proceeds predominantly along the regional lymph node (LN) basin and to the liver via lymphatic and portal venous drainage. Consequently, up to 50% of CRC patients will develop liver metastases and in up to half of these cases, the disease may be confined to the liver. This anatomic model attributes liver metastases to entrapment of free CRC cells in the portal venous system of the liver and as a result, they are viewed as an extension of locoregional disease justifying the aggressive approach for potential cure. Non-GI cancer cells, on the other hand, would implant in the liver from the general circulation via the hepatic arterial and portal/venous systems and are considered a systemic disease, discouraging many from adopting a similar aggressive approach. However, CRC cells have been detected in the systemic circulation during the very early stages of the disease [11, 12], challenging the conventional anatomic view of metastasis in this disease. Furthermore, emerging data suggest that selective and complex interactions take place between cancer cells and the liver microenvironment, leading to the recruitment of hematopoietic and resident stromal cells, initiation of an inflammatory response and activation of matrix metalloproteinases that together support preferential tumour seeding to the liver, regardless of the route (The reader is referred to several chapters in this book including Chapters 3, 5, 6 and 7 for additional information on the role of the microenvironment in liver metastasis). This pathophysiologic model implies that liver metastasis from different solid malignancies may be regulated by common mechanisms and may be more similar than originally appreciated. Therefore, similar treatment strategies, including an aggressive surgical approach may also be justified for non-GI liver metastases.

13.3 A Surgical Approach to Liver Metastases

Most patients are evaluated by a multidisciplinary team consisting of hepato-biliary surgical oncologists, radiologists, medical and radiation oncologists. The patient's complete history, tumor pathology, treatment and response are considered along with careful review of all current and previous imaging studies. Patients must first and foremost be medically fit for hepatic resection with no obvious contraindications to surgery.

A thorough radiologic assessment of each patient is essential for staging their disease and determining resectability. All patients should have recent and complete staging investigations done at the time of their assessment for hepatic resection. Imaging techniques with high sensitivity should be used to assess each patient for common sites of metastatic disease according to the primary tumor type (e.g. breast, renal cell) in order to identify extrahepatic sites of disease. This may include a thorough evaluation of the thoracic and abdominal cavities with CT of the chest/abdomen/pelvis, CT or MRI of the skull and brain, as well as a bone scan. The use of a [14]FDG-PET scan is particularly useful in the search for extrahepatic disease in [14]FDG-avid tumors but the sensitivity of this modality is limited in the detection of small (<1 cm) or intrahepatic metastatic deposits. The development of combined [14]FDG-PET/CT imaging has increased the sensitivity, as well as the anatomic precision of this imaging modality. The assessment of peritoneal carcinomatosis is particularly challenging in tumour types prone to this mode of spread such as lobular breast and ovarian cancer. Traditional imaging techniques may fail to detect small volume peritoneal disease and diagnostic laparoscopy, with or without laparoscopic ultrasound should be considered in cases or disease types where peritoneal spread is suspected. At present, the presence of extrahepatic disease is likely to render patients ineligible for resection in many centers and for several tumor types. However, in selected circumstances and for specific tumor types including neuroendocrine, colorectal and breast cancers, hepatic resection may still be considered if extrahepatic disease is controlled and/or resectable.

For assessment of hepatic disease, contrast enhanced CT scan with arterial, portal venous and delayed venous phase imaging provide detailed images of the lesions, as well as arterial and portal inflow, along with views of the hepatic outflow that are critical for proper operative planning and assessment of resectability. Abdominal MRI is a complementary imaging modality that can provide additional information on the characteristics of the lesions and may be particularly useful in differentiating benign and malignant lesions in cases where CT is equivocal. Ultrasound is an additional complementary imaging modality used in the assessment of hepatic lesions. It is frequently used for screening of metastatic disease in several cancers due to its relatively high sensitivity and low cost. Ultrasound performed by centers with extensive experience in hepatic ultrasonography can provide useful diagnostic information on suspected hepatic lesions. The use of contrast-enhanced ultrasound and Doppler vascular imaging can supplement ultrasound data providing further characterization of the lesions and determining their spatial relationship to intrahepatic vascular structures (for an extensive discussion of imaging modalities for liver metastasis see Chapter 11 in this volume).

Once the presence of additional disease has been ruled out and the patient has been deemed medically fit, careful planning is undertaken and the type of liver resection is determined. The degree of liver resection is based primarily on the location of the tumor, with the size of the lesion representing a secondary consideration. Peripheral lesions that are located far from major vascular structures are typically amenable to a wedge resection that removes only the metastatic lesion leaving sufficient surrounding parenchyma to obtain a negative microscopic margin (R0 resection). Lesions that are centrally located and/or close to major vascular structures typically require a formal anatomic hepatic resection (e.g., right hepatectomy) to adequately and safely remove the tumor and obtain negative margins (R0 resection). The size of the margin between the resection plane and the gross tumor required to obtain an R0 resection is the subject of some debate and may depend on a tumor's propensity for infiltrative growth or vascular invasion. There is no evidence that obtaining larger negative margins is of significant benefit [13]. In addition, for certain cancers such as ovarian cancer, the aim of the surgery is a debulking to decrease tumor load before chemotherapy. Technical planning of hepatic resection must include an assessment of hepatic function, as well as the anticipated future remnant liver (FRL) volume after resection to minimize the risk of post-operative hepatic dysfunction. The assessment of hepatic function is difficult as many techniques and scores are available including Childs-Pugh score, MELD score, ICG clearance but none have been conclusively validated or universally used. The evaluation of FRL volume may predict post-operative hepatic dysfunction and can be assessed by liver volumetry [14]. Ensuring the preservation of at least two contiguous Couinaud segments with FRL volumes >20% in patients with normal hepatic function and >30% in patients with chronic liver disease or extensive chemotherapy may reduce the risk of post-operative liver failure. Sparing as much liver as possible minimizes the risk of potential post-operative liver dysfunction, and also preserves liver for the eventuality that additional resections are entertained at a later time. The technical planning of a liver resection requires detailed knowledge of the intrahepatic vascular and biliary anatomy. Selection of an anatomic resection and/or a non-anatomic resection must be made in each patient by balancing factors such as the potential achievement of an adequate resection margin, the propensity for intraoperative blood loss and the preservation of adequate future remnant liver. Anatomic resections may be associated with better oncologic margins, lower blood loss and removal of larger liver volumes as compared to parenchyma–preserving, non-anatomic resections.

Exposure of the liver is typically via a right subcostal incision with a midline extension to the level of the xiphoid. Intraoperative ultrasound is routinely performed just prior to resection to determine the presence of additional metastatic lesions and define the proximity of the known lesion to major vascular structures. Wedge resections do not require isolation and ligation of any major vascular structures. However, in our institute, we routinely establish access to the porta hepatis, should control of vascular inflow be required via a pringle maneuver to control bleeding. For formal liver resections (e.g. sectionectomies, segmentectomies), complete vascular isolation of the resected segment(s) is performed to minimize blood loss during parenchymal transection. Arterial and portal inflow to the resected segments are isolated and ligated in the porta hepatis followed by control and/or division of the hepatic venous outflow, whenever possible. Low central venous pressure is maintained during parenchymal division to minimize blood loss and is standard for almost all liver resections. Parenchymal transection can then be carried out in several ways ranging from simple techniques (e.g. clamp-crush, finger fracture) to techniques requiring specific devices (e.g. CUSA). Our center's preference is to use hydrodissection routinely for liver parenchyma transection. This technique allows swift selective division of the liver parenchyma with preservation of important structures (such as branches of the portal vein or tributaries of the biliary system), which are carefully defined, identified and preserved when necessary. Once the liver resection is complete, the patient's central venous pressure is restored to normal levels and the cut surface of the liver is inspected again for hemostasis and the presence of a bile leak. The abdomen is then closed using the standard technique. Drains are not routinely left in place. Patients typically are in the hospital for 4–7 days, depending on the degree of resection. In experienced centers, perioperative morbidity and mortality from major liver resections are very low [15, 16].

The unique challenges, practices and outcomes associated with the management of hepatic metastasis of specific tumor types are discussed below.

13.3.1 Breast Cancer

Twenty five percent of women with breast cancer develop liver metastases during the course of their disease [17]. Liver metastases usually develop in the context of widespread systemic disease with multi-organ involvement. Zinser et al. [18] retrospectively reviewed 233 cases of breast cancer with liver metastases treated at MD Anderson in the 1970s. Synchronous liver metastases were present at the time of initial diagnosis of breast cancer in 15% of these cases. For patients who developed metachronous metastases, liver metastases were restricted to the liver in 12% of the cases, found in liver and bone in 15%, part of a diffuse multi-organ involvement (more than three organs) in 38% and, associated with different metastatic combinations including bone and bone marrow, lung and pleura or bone and central nervous system in the remaining 35%. A more recent report by Atalay et al. [5] retrospectively analyzed the outcome of two chemotherapeutic trials for metastatic breast cancer conducted in the 1990s. Liver metastases were found in 160 out of 331 (48%) and in 115 out of 275 (42%) of the patients, in the first and second trials and metastases were confined to the liver in 9 and 7% of cases, respectively. The observed small but significant number of isolated liver metastases encouraged many surgeons to consider liver resection in these highly selected cases of liver-only or oligometastatic disease.

Table 13.1 Liver resection for the management of metastatic breast cancer – retrospective studies

	Period	Number of patients	Median survival (months)	3-year survival (%)	5-year survival (%)
Raab et al. [47]	1983–1996	34	27	50	18.4
Siefert et al. [48]	1985–1997	15	57	53.6	–
Selzner et al. [49]	1987–1999	17	24	35	22
Yoshimoto et al. [50]	1985–1998	25	34.3	–	27
Pocard et al. [23]	1988–1999	65	41	71	46 (4 years)
Elias et al. [20]	1986–2000	54	34	50	34
Carlini et al. [51]	1990–1999	17	53	–	46
Vlastos et al. [52]	1991–2002	31	63	–	61
Sakamoto et al. [24]	1985–2003	34	36	52	21
d'Annibale et al. [53]	1984–1999	18	36	–	30
Adam et al. [54]	1984–2004	85	32	–	37
Adam et al. [16]	1984–2003	454	45	–	41
Caralt et al. [21]	1988–2006	12	35.9	79	33
Lubrano et al. [55]	1989–2004	16	14	61	33
Thelen et al. [25]	1988–2006	39		50 (68 for R0)	42 (61 for R0)

Current studies reporting on the use of liver resection for management of metastatic breast cancer are retrospective and without appropriate control groups. Table 13.1 summarizes the results of some of these studies. The indications for surgery in these series were highly variable and often poorly described. Adam et al. [19] adopted an aggressive approach, offering liver resection to patients who previously received chemotherapy, had resectable liver disease with no extrahepatic disease or had extrahepatic disease that was resectable and/or well-controlled. In a second study [20], liver resection was offered to patients with breast cancer metastases confined to the liver or liver and bone who had demonstrated stable disease or had a partial response during prehepatectomy chemotherapy. A third group [21] offered liver resection only to those patients with good performance status and no extrahepatic disease. The 3 and 5 year overall survival reported in these series ranged from 35 to 79% and from 18 to 61% respectively. Not surprisingly, the outcomes reported in these studies were highly variable and this is likely attributable to variations in selection criteria and differences in the chemotherapeutic regimens utilized in these series. Nevertheless, these outcomes compared favorably to the 0% 5-year survival rates for patients with hepatic metastases from breast cancer who did not undergo surgical resection [22].

Due to the small numbers of patients in most of these studies, it is difficult to arrive at a clear consensus regarding which prognostic criteria would improve patient selection. Positive prognostic criteria include >48 month disease free period between diagnosis of breast cancer and appearance liver metastases [23], response to prehepatectomy chemotherapy [19], R0 or R1 hepatic resection [19], absence of

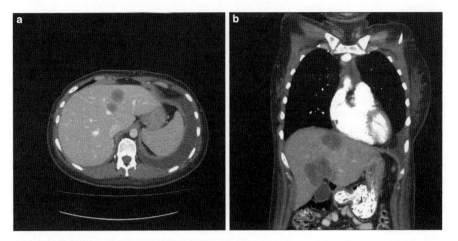

Fig. 13.1 (**a**, **b**) Resectable liver metastases from breast cancer

extrahepatic disease [24, 25] and positive hormone receptor status (estrogen, progesterone or both) [20] although it is not clear whether the hormone receptor status of the primary or metastatic tumor) or both are of importance. The largest study by Adam et al. [16] included 454 breast cancer patients as part of a larger study of non-colorectal, non-neuroendocrine liver metastases. This study did not provide sufficient detail on the subgroup of breast cancer patients and it is therefore difficult to deduce prognostic criteria from the findings.

In conclusion, while the limited results from liver resections for hepatic metastases of breast cancer are encouraging, the heterogeneity in the patient populations studied and the lack of controls makes extracting meaningful operative indications, prognostic factors and outcomes difficult. Existing literature appears to support a role for hepatic resection for patients with liver-only disease with a long disease-free interval (see Fig. 13.1). Patients with limited extrahepatic disease and with disease that is stable or responsive to chemotherapy should be selected carefully because the long-term results are variable.

13.3.2 Renal Cell Cancer

Renal cell carcinoma (RCC) metastasis is usually a delayed process after treatment of the primary tumor. About 50% of patients with RCC develop metastases with the lung being the most common site of spread followed by liver, which is involved in 20% of cases. Liver metastases are usually associated with widespread disease and poor prognosis with 1-year survival rates approaching 10%. Several groups have recognized a small subset of patients with liver metastases (up to 5% of cases) who have liver-only limited disease and who may be amenable to liver resection. The reported studies on the outcome of these resections are limited, retrospective and based on small numbers patients, making it very difficult to draw any conclusions about prognostic criteria. Table 13.2 summarizes some of these studies. Adam et al. [16] reported on the largest group of patients (85) who underwent resection between 1983 and 2004. Unfortunately, these cases were reported as part of a larger study examining non-neuroendocrine, non-colorectal liver metastases and the prognostic criteria were analyzed for the entire group. Nevertheless the study did show that patients with metastatic RCC to the liver had a median overall survival of 36 months and an overall 5-year survival of 38%. Aloia et al. [26] reported the results of 19 liver resections for metastatic RCC during the time period of 1982–2005. The mean disease-free period between nephrectomy and diagnosis of liver metastases in this series was 53 months (9–137 months). Seven patients were treated previously or presented concurrently with resectable extra-hepatic metastases. The median and 5-year disease-free survival were 13 months and 25%, respectively. The median and 5 year overall survival were 36 months and 26%, respectively. Positive prognostic criteria included male gender, age group of 30–36 years old, tumor size ≤ 5 cm in diameter, disease-free period between nephrectomy and liver metastases > 24 months and repeat hepatectomy for liver recurrence.

In contrast to distant liver metastases, a smaller group of patients present with direct liver invasion during initial presentation. A recent report from the Memorial Sloan Kettering Cancer Center on aggressive surgical treatment for advanced renal cell carcinoma during the time period of 1998–2006 included 10 patients (out of 38) who underwent concurrent liver resections [27]. The median survival for the whole group was 11.9 months with only one patient alive and disease free at 60 months (the time of the analysis). Achievement of a R0 resection was the only identifiable positive prognostic factor. The authors concluded that the outcome of aggressive surgical management of this select group of patients was very poor and suggested considering entry of these patients into neoadjuvant or adjuvant clinical trials with new targeted systemic agents. However, Margulis et al. [28] cautioned about overstaging as they identified only 40% (12 out of 30 patients) in their series who had true invasion in the final pathological assessment.

Recent results in the treatment of advanced RCC with tyrosine kinase inhibitor therapy (sunitinib) have demonstrated improvements in the prognosis of patients with metastatic disease. A phase III trial randomized 670 patients with metastatic RCC to receive either sunitinib or interferon-α [29]. Thirty one percent of patients

Table 13.2 Liver resection for the management of metastatic renal cancer – retrospective studies

	Time period	Number of patients	Median time before liver metastases (months)	Median disease free period after hepatectomy (months)	Median overall survival (months)	5-year overall survival (%)
Aloia et al. [26]	1982–2005	19	53	13	36	26
Adam et al. [16]	1984–2003	85			36	38
Alves et al. [56]	1982–2001	14			26	26[a]

[a]3-year survival

Fig. 13.2 Liver metastases
from renal cell carcinoma

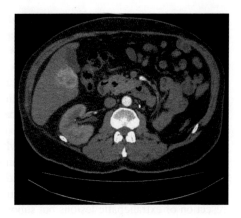

who received sunitinib had objective response rates as compared to only 6% who received interferon-α and the progression-free survival was 11 months in the sunitinib-treated group vs 5 months in the interferon-α group. Based on these results, sunitinib is emerging as first line treatment for advanced RCC. Results of resection of hepatic RCC metastases following, or in combination with, tyrosine kinase inhibitor therapy have not yet been reported.

In conclusion, liver resection for metastatic RCC may be associated with increased survival in those patients with liver-only or limited extrahepatic disease (see Fig. 13.2). While the current available data are limited to case reports and small retrospective series, long-term outcomes of patients undergoing resection of RCC liver metastases compare favorably to those of patients with unresectable metastatic disease. The treatment of locally advanced RCC requiring liver resection to achieve adequate tumour clearance has been associated with poor long-term results. Finally, the impact of treatment with tyrosine kinase inhibitor therapy (sunitinib) on patient selection and outcomes of liver resection needs to be assessed.

13.3.3 Gynecological Cancer

Among gynecological cancers, epithelial ovarian cancer is the most likely tumour to present with liver metastases. Ovarian cancer typically spreads via the peritoneal cavity and lymphatic routes. Parenchymal liver involvement from either direct extension of the peritoneal disease or via hematogenous spread occurs during the advanced stages of the disease (stage IV). Ovarian cancer is a chemosensitive disease with high response rates to platinum-based regimens. While many with metastatic disease develop chemoresistance, the median survival of these patients can approach 40 months or more. The current goals of surgical treatment for advanced ovarian cancer (stage III and IV) are to achieve optimal cytoreduction of intra-abdominal and extra-abdominal disease with residual lesions less than 1 cm prior to chemotherapy. Though randomized, prospective evidence is lacking, an aggressive attempt at primary cytoreductive surgery followed by combination chemotherapy has evolved as the cornerstone of initial treatment for advanced epithelial ovarian cancer. Several studies suggested that disease-free interval and overall survival are inversely related to the amount of residual disease present prior to chemotherapy [30, 31]. Historically, liver involvement precluded aggressive surgery given the associated morbidity with hepatic resection. However, with recent improved survival following hepatic resection for colon cancer, several groups included liver resections as part of cytoreductive surgery. Bristow et al. [32] reported the results of 37 patients who underwent liver resection as part of a primary cytoreductive surgery for ovarian cancer. Six patients underwent optimal hepatic and extrahepatic resection (residual disease <1 cm in maximal diameter) and had a median survival of 50.1 months. Patients who underwent optimal resection of extrahepatic lesions but suboptimal hepatic resection (11 patients) had a median survival of 27.0 months while those who underwent suboptimal hepatic and extrahepatic resections (20 patients) had a median survival of only 7.6 months.

Secondary cytoreductive surgery for recurrent ovarian cancer is controversial. Two prospective, randomized trials showed contradictory results. In the study by Rose et al. [33], patients with residual ovarian cancer greater than 1 cm in maximal diameter were randomized to either having surgery (201 patients) with pre and post operative chemotherapy or receiving chemotherapy alone (208 patients). There were no significant differences in the overall survival and progression-free survival in these groups. On the other hand, van der Burg et al. [34] showed that patients who underwent surgery (140) when compared to patients who underwent chemotherapy alone (138) had significantly longer overall and progression free survival (median overall survival and median progression free survival were 26 vs. 20 months and 18 vs. 13 months, respectively).

There are retrospective studies addressing the value of liver resection as a part of secondary cytoreduction surgery. Table 13.3 summarizes the results of some of these studies. The median period between diagnosis of primary disease and liver resection is 29–68 months. Many of these patients underwent several surgical procedures for cytoreduction before their liver resection. Merideth et al. [35] reported the results of a study of 26 patients who underwent hepatic resection as part of a secondary cytoreductive procedure. Six patients had the disease confined to the liver and 20 had extrahepatic disease. Twenty-one patients had optimal resection of the hepatic and extrahepatic disease and five had suboptimal resection. Patients who underwent optimal resection had a median survival of 27.3 vs. 8.6 months for patients who underwent suboptimal resection. The authors also found that those patients whose primary operation was performed at least 12 months before hepatic resection had significantly better median survival than those whose primary operation was performed less than 12 months before resection (27.3 vs. 5.7 months). In a more updated report by the same group [36], 35 patients underwent hepatic resection as part of a secondary cytoreductive procedure and the median disease specific survival for those who underwent optimal versus suboptimal surgery was 41.3 vs. 5.7 months, respectively. These studies suggest that in selected cases, liver

Table 13.3 Liver resection in the management of ovarian cancer

	Time period	Number of patients	Median interval from primary diagnosis to liver resection (months)	Median overall survival (months)	5-year overall survival (%)
Yoon et al. [57]	1988–2001	24 (21 ovarian, 3 fallopian tube) (metachronous)	68.5	62	40
Merideth et al. [35]	1976–1999	26 patients (metachronous)	29.4	26.3	
Bosquet [36][a]	1976–2003	35 (metachronous)		27.4 (41.3 months for patients without any macroscopic residual disease)	

[a]Updated report of a previous study by Merideth et al. [35]

resection as part of a secondary cytoreductive treatment is associated with prolonged survival.

In conclusion, survival in advanced ovarian cancer correlates with the response to chemotherapy, as well as the success and degree of disease debulking. Liver resection is indicated as part of primary cytoreduction surgery to prolong both overall and progression-free survival. On the other hand, the indication for liver resection for recurrent ovarian cancer remains controversial. There is some evidence that achieving optimal cytoreduction is associated with prolonged overall survival. However, conflicting results of the randomized controlled trials cast some doubt on the value of secondary cytoreductive surgery. Given the current evidence, decisions regarding resection of metachronous or residual disease involving the liver are best managed on an individual basis, through multidisciplinary tumour boards.

13.3.4 Melanoma

Both primary cutaneous and uveal melanomas have significant metastatic potential, with the risk of developing metastases persisting for several years after diagnosis and treatment of the primary lesion. Cutaneous melanomas metastasize either via lymphatics to lymph nodes or hematogenously to distant organs [37]. The liver is the third most common site of metastases preceded only by lymph nodes and the lungs. Isolated liver metastases occur rarely and are usually associated with widespread organ involvement. In contrast, metastasis from uveal melanoma is purely hematogenous because the uveal tract is devoid of lymphatics. These tumors commonly metastasize to the liver. Liver is involved in 80% of metastatic uveal

melanoma followed by the lungs, lymph nodes, skin, and bones [38]. Palliative systemic chemotherapy is the mainstay of treatment for both advanced cutaneous and
uveal melanoma and it is associated with 5-year survival rates of approximately
9% [39]. Several retrospective studies have been published on hepatic resection
for metastatic melanoma and the results are summarized in Table 13.4. Patients
reported in these series were considered for resection based on the resectability
of the liver lesions and good performance status. The disease-free interval from
resection of the primary tumor and diagnosis of metastases was documented in
some studies and ranged from 58 to 63 months. Following resection of hepatic
metastases, the median overall survival and disease-free survival ranged from 21 to
28 months and 4.7 to 12 months, respectively, with 5-year overall survival ranging
from 0 to 29%. Uveal melanoma was more frequently associated with liver recurrence while cutaneous melanoma was associated with more systemic recurrence [15,
16]. Prognostic criteria for overall survival included disease confined to liver, prolonged disease-free period between diagnosis of melanoma and detection of liver
metastases, tumor size <5 cm, and R0 resection. Taken together, liver resection for
metastatic melanoma may be associated with increased survival. However in the
absence of control groups, the observed survival rates could all be attributed to a
selection bias of a subgroup with favorable tumor biology.

More recently, Ripley et al. [40] reported on the use of liver resection to obtain
metastatic tissue to isolate tumor-infiltrating lymphocytes (TIL) for post-operative
TIL therapy. In this study, nine patients underwent R0 resection without TIL therapy
with 3 years overall and disease free survival of 80 and 56%, respectively. Fifteen
patients had resections with residual disease and TIL therapy. Of these patients 40%
had a partial response and their overall 3 years survival was 65%. Seven patients had
resections with residual disease and no TIL therapy because their isolated lymphocytes did not grow in culture. This group had a median survival of only 4.6 months.

Table 13.4 Liver resection for melanoma – results of retrospective studies

	Time Period	Number of patients	Median time to systemic disease (months)	Median time for recurrence after liver resection (months)	Median overall survival (months)	5-year overall survival (%)
Pawlik et al. [15]	1988–2004	16 ocular	62.9	8.8	29.4	20.5
Pawlik et al. [15]	1988–2004	24 cutaneous	63.1	4.7	23.6	0
Frenkel et al. [58]	1988–2008	35 ocular			23	
Rose et al. [59]	1971–1999	24	58	12	28	29
Adam et al. [16]	1983–2004	44 cutaneous			22	27
Adam et al. [16]	1983–2004	104 ocular			21	19

The authors cautioned that due to lack of randomization, observed differences could be due to tumor biology and not to the intervention.

In conclusion, liver resection should be considered for isolated melanoma liver metastases. There is no strong evidence for justifying liver resection in the context of widespread metastases. Further research is warranted to verify the outcome of liver resection combined with TIL therapy. Prolonged disease free period from the primary tumor and R0 resection are associated with better survival and less recurrence rate.

13.3.5 Bronchopulmonary Neuroendocrine Tumors

Bronchopulmonary neuroendocrine tumours represent a spectrum of disease ranging from indolent bronchopulmonary carcinoid (both low grade typical carcinoid and intermediate grade atypical carcinoid tumors) to aggressive high-grade malignancies (large cell carcinoma and small cell carcinoma). These cancers originate from pulmonary neuroendocrine cells that exist as solitary cells or are clustered into neuroepithelial bodies. The normal function of these cells remains somewhat unclear but the neuroendocrine bundles are thought to function as airway chemoreceptors, nociceptors, and mechanosensory cells. Small cell lung cancer is a rapidly advancing disease that is most often metastatic at the time of presentation. As a result, surgical resection is rarely an option and systemic chemotherapy is standard of care. In contrast, carcinoids are slow growing cancers with a fairly good prognosis. They are not known to be very chemosensitive and surgical excision is the only known curative treatment for primary tumors.

Approximately 3% of typical carcinoids and 20% of atypical carcinoids present as stage IV disease. Distant metastases are known to occur in the liver, bone, central nervous system, mammary glands, and skin [41]. Approximately 2% of patients will develop hepatic metastases. The approach to treatment of carcinoid tumors of all origins (gastrointestinal and bronchopulmonary) has undergone significant change over the past century. Recently, debulking surgery (removing >90% of metastatic disease) has been shown to improve not only the quality of life but also survival [3]. However, recurrence is the norm in this group of malignancies, with most patients recurring with hepatic metastases.

There are no isolated studies examining the role of surgical resection for bronchopulmonary carcinoid tumors. These tumors are often examined as part of larger studies of neuroendocrine hepatic metastases. In these series, both curative (R0) and palliative (R2) resections were performed. The sample size of bronchopulmonary tumors within these series is usually very small, representing only 5–25% of all patients [3, 42, 43]. In the series by Hibi et al. [42], patients with metastatic liver disease from bronchopulmonary carcinoid had lower survival rates than patients with primaries from other sites and no patients survived 5 years. In contrast, Nave et al. [43] compared survival of patients who underwent hepatic resection of liver metastases for primary tumors of the midgut, lung, and pancreas. Patients with pulmonary metastases were found to have a similar mean survival (53 months) to patients with midgut primaries, and had a longer median survival than patients with pancreatic cancer. In the largest study by Sarmiento et al., 170 patients were examined and of these 5% (nine patients) had primary tumors in the lung. While the patients with primary lung tumors were not studied independently, the overall 5 year survival for the group was 61% with a recurrence rate of 84% [3]

Although the evidence is sparse, management of bronchopulmonary hepatic metastases can be extrapolated from the management of neuroendocrine tumors in general. Therefore, hepatic metastases should be resected if greater then 90% of the disease can be successfully removed. Patients can achieve improvement in both survival and symptomatic control.

13.3.6 Testicular Cancer

Testicular cancers are classified into seminomas, non-seminomas, and teratomas and are associated with a favorable overall prognosis, even for metastatic disease. Among these subtypes, seminomas carry the most favorable prognosis. The excellent overall survival is largely due to the chemoresponsiveness of the tumors. However, a proportion of these patients will have either an incomplete response to chemotherapy or will develop a recurrence. Testicular cancer is known to metastasize to several organ systems including the lungs, liver, brain, and bone. The presence of hepatic metastases is a known predictor of poor outcome. However, the surgical resection of residual deposits of metastatic disease after chemotherapy is considered beneficial based on several published series. Hahn et al. reviewed 57 patients who underwent hepatic resection, and noted a 69% 2-year survival rate with no evidence of active disease in 63% of patients. The authors went on to recommend the use of hepatic resection post chemotherapy for residual disease in patients whose tumor markers returned to normal levels [44]. Another group examined a cohort of 37 patients who underwent hepatic resection for germ cell tumors, of whom 35 had complete (R0) resections. Resections were performed as an adjunct to primary surgery ($n = 18$) or as a salvage procedure ($n = 19$) for residual disease after chemotherapy. Following a median follow up period of 66 months, 23/37 patients were alive with no evidence of disease with a 5-year overall survival of 62%. Factors predictive of poor survival were the presence of pure embryonal carcinoma in the primary tumor, liver metastases $\geq$ 30 mm and the presence of viable active residual disease. Patients with tumors of $\leq$ 10 mm were recommended for close follow up because of a high probability of tumor necrosis [45]. More recently, You et al. reported on 15 patients who underwent hepatic resection for testicular germ cell metastases. The overall 10-year survival for this cohort was 62%. No predictors of survival were identified but the study size was small [46].

In conclusion, hepatic metastases from testicular cancer should be resected if technically feasible, because patients outcome and survival are excellent for a stage IV cancer.

13.4 Conclusions

The indication for surgical resection of non-gastrointestinal liver metastases is still evolving. As chemotherapeutic options for systemic disease continue to improve, patients will continue to have better control of systemic disease and improved overall survival. However, these same patients will potentially be at risk for development of liver metastases, as they survive longer. To date, malignancies in which good systemic chemotherapy is available appear to derive some benefit from surgical excision of residual or recurrent disease. These patients should be carefully selected and have isolated disease present only in their liver. In addition, those patients with long disease-free intervals appear to derive the most benefit from hepatic metastasectomy. As newer chemotherapeutic options continue to emerge (e.g. sorafanib), the indications for surgical excision may continue to expand. However for now, only a very select group of patients should undergo surgical excision of non-gastrointestinal liver metastases.

References

1. Kopetz S et al (2009) Improved survival in metastatic colorectal cancer is associated with adoption of hepatic resection and improved chemotherapy. J Clin Oncol 27:3677–3683
2. Touzios JG et al (2005) Neuroendocrine hepatic metastases: does aggressive management improve survival? Ann Surg 241:776–783; discussion 783–785
3. Sarmiento JM et al (2003) Surgical treatment of neuroendocrine metastases to the liver: a plea for resection to increase survival. J Am Coll Surg 197:29–37
4. Chen H et al (1998) Isolated liver metastases from neuroendocrine tumors: does resection prolong survival? J Am Coll Surg 187:88–92; discussion 92–93
5. Atalay G et al (2003) Clinical outcome of breast cancer patients with liver metastases alone in the anthracycline-taxane era: a retrospective analysis of two prospective, randomised metastatic breast cancer trials. Eur J Cancer 39:2439–2449
6. Bonnet D, Dick JE (1997) Human acute myeloid leukemia is organized as a hierarchy that originates from a primitive hematopoietic cell. Nat Med 3:730–737
7. Al-Hajj M et al (2003) Prospective identification of tumorigenic breast cancer cells. Proc Natl Acad Sci USA 100:3983–3988
8. Li C et al (2007) Identification of pancreatic cancer stem cells. Cancer Res 67:1030–1037
9. O'Brien CA et al (2007) A human colon cancer cell capable of initiating tumour growth in immunodeficient mice. Nature 445:106–110
10. Trumpp A, Wiestler OD (2008) Mechanisms of disease: cancer stem cells – targeting the evil twin. Nat Clin Pract Oncol 5:337–347
11. Engell HC (1959) Cancer cells in the blood; a five to nine year follow up study. Ann Surg 149:457–461
12. Sadahiro S et al (2001) Detection of tumor cells in the portal and peripheral blood of patients with colorectal carcinoma using competitive reverse transcriptase-polymerase chain reaction. Cancer 92:1251–1258
13. de Haas RJ et al (2008) R1 resection by necessity for colorectal liver metastases: is it still a contraindication to surgery? Ann Surg 248:626–637
14. Vauthey JN et al (2000) Standardized measurement of the future liver remnant prior to extended liver resection: methodology and clinical associations. Surgery 127:512–519
15. Pawlik TM et al (2006) Hepatic resection for metastatic melanoma: distinct patterns of recurrence and prognosis for ocular versus cutaneous disease. Ann Surg Oncol 13:712–720

16. Adam R et al (2006) Hepatic resection for noncolorectal nonendocrine liver metastases: analysis of 1,452 patients and development of a prognostic model. Ann Surg 244:524–535
17. Tampellini M et al (1997) Relationship between CA 15-3 serum levels and disease extent in predicting overall survival of breast cancer patients with newly diagnosed metastatic disease. Br J Cancer 75:698–702
18. Zinser JW et al (1987) Clinical course of breast cancer patients with liver metastases. J Clin Oncol 5:773–782
19. Adam R et al (2006) Is liver resection justified for patients with hepatic metastases from breast cancer? Ann Surg 244:897–907; discussion 907–908
20. Elias D et al (2003) An attempt to clarify indications for hepatectomy for liver metastases from breast cancer. Am J Surg 185:158–164
21. Caralt M et al (2008) Hepatic resection for liver metastases as part of the "oncosurgical" treatment of metastatic breast cancer. Ann Surg Oncol 15:2804–2810
22. Wyld L et al (2003) Prognostic factors for patients with hepatic metastases from breast cancer. Br J Cancer 89:284–290
23. Pocard M et al (2001) Hepatic resection for breast cancer metastases: results and prognosis (65 cases). Ann Chir 126:413–420
24. Sakamoto Y et al (2005) Hepatic resection for metastatic breast cancer: prognostic analysis of 34 patients. World J Surg 29:524–527
25. Thelen A et al (2008) Liver resection for metastases from breast cancer. J Surg Oncol 97:25–29
26. Aloia TA et al (2006) Outcome following hepatic resection of metastatic renal tumors: the Paul Brousse Hospital experience. HPB (Oxford) 8:100–105
27. Karellas ME et al (2009) Advanced-stage renal cell carcinoma treated by radical nephrectomy and adjacent organ or structure resection. BJU Int 103:160–164
28. Margulis V et al (2007) Renal cell carcinoma clinically involving adjacent organs: experience with aggressive surgical management. Cancer 109:2025–2030
29. Motzer RJ et al (2007) Sunitinib versus interferon alfa in metastatic renal-cell carcinoma. N Engl J Med 356:115–124
30. Griffiths CT et al (2002) The effect of residual mass size on response to chemotherapy after surgical cytoreduction for advanced ovarian cancer: long-term results. Int J Gynecol Cancer 12:323–331
31. Griffiths CT (1975) Surgical resection of tumor bulk in the primary treatment of ovarian carcinoma. Natl Cancer Inst Monogr 42:101–104
32. Bristow RE et al (1999) Survival impact of surgical cytoreduction in stage IV epithelial ovarian cancer. Gynecol Oncol 72:278–287
33. Rose PG et al (2004) Secondary surgical cytoreduction for advanced ovarian carcinoma. N Engl J Med 351:2489–2497
34. van der Burg ME et al (1995) The effect of debulking surgery after induction chemotherapy on the prognosis in advanced epithelial ovarian cancer. Gynecological Cancer Cooperative Group of the European Organization for Research and Treatment of Cancer. N Engl J Med 332:629–634
35. Merideth MA et al (2003) Hepatic resection for metachronous metastases from ovarian carcinoma. Gynecol Oncol 89:16–21
36. Bosquet JG et al (2006) Hepatic resection for metachronous metastases from ovarian carcinoma. HPB (Oxford) 8:93–96
37. Patel JK et al (1978) Metastatic pattern of malignant melanoma. A study of 216 autopsy cases. Am J Surg 135:807–810
38. Einhorn LH, Burgess MA, Gottlieb JA (1974) Metastatic patterns of choroidal melanoma. Cancer 34:1001–1004
39. Balch CM et al (2001) Final version of the American Joint Committee on Cancer staging system for cutaneous melanoma. J Clin Oncol 19:3635–3648

40. Ripley RT et al (2010) Liver resection for metastatic melanoma with post-operative tumor-infiltrating lymphocyte therapy. Ann Surg Oncol 17:163–170
41. Gustafsson BI et al (2008) Bronchopulmonary neuroendocrine tumors. Cancer 113:5–21
42. Hibi T et al (2007) Surgery for hepatic neuroendocrine tumors: a single institutional experience in Japan. Jpn J Clin Oncol 37:102–107
43. Nave H et al (2001) Surgery as primary treatment in patients with liver metastases from carcinoid tumors: a retrospective, unicentric study over 13 years. Surgery 129:170–175
44. Hahn TL et al (1999) Hepatic resection of metastatic testicular carcinoma: a further update. Ann Surg Oncol 6:640–644
45. Rivoire M et al (2001) Multimodality treatment of patients with liver metastases from germ cell tumors: the role of surgery. Cancer 92:578–587
46. You YN, Leibovitch BC, Que FG (2009) Hepatic metastasectomy for testicular germ cell tumors: is it worth it? J Gastrointest Surg 13:595–601
47. Raab R et al (1998) Liver metastases of breast cancer: results of liver resection. Anticancer Res 18:2231–2233
48. Seifert JK et al (1999) Liver resection for breast cancer metastases. Hepato-Gastroenterology 46:2935–2940
49. Selzner M et al (2000) Liver metastases from breast cancer: long-term survival after curative resection. Surgery 127:383–389
50. Yoshimoto M et al (2000) Surgical treatment of hepatic metastases from breast cancer. Breast Cancer Res Treat 59:177–184
51. Carlini M et al (2002) Liver metastases from breast cancer. Results of surgical resection. Hepato-Gastroenterology 49:1597–1601
52. Vlastos G et al (2004) Long-term survival after an aggressive surgical approach in patients with breast cancer hepatic metastases. Ann Surg Oncol 11:869–874
53. d'Annibale M et al (2005) Liver metastases from breast cancer: the role of surgical treatment. Hepato-Gastroenterology 52:1858–1862
54. Adam R et al (2006) Is liver resection justified for patients with hepatic metastases from breast cancer?[see comment]. Ann Surg 244:897–907; discussion 907–908
55. Lubrano J et al (2008) Liver resection for breast cancer metastasis: does it improve survival? Surg Today 38:293–299
56. Alves A et al (2003) Hepatic resection for metastatic renal tumors: is it worthwhile? Ann Surg Oncol 10:705–710
57. Yoon SS et al (2003) Resection of recurrent ovarian or fallopian tube carcinoma involving the liver. Gynecol Oncol 91:383–388
58. Frenkel S et al (2009) Long-term survival of uveal melanoma patients after surgery for liver metastases. Br J Ophthalmol 93:1042–1046
59. Rose DM et al (2001) Surgical resection for metastatic melanoma to the liver: the John Wayne Cancer Institute and Sydney Melanoma Unit experience. Arch Surg 136:950–955

Chapter 14
Proteomic Profiling of Hepatic Metastases: Paving the Way to Individualized Therapy

Alessandra Silvestri, Emanuel F. Petricoin, Lance A. Liotta, and Mariaelena Pierobon

Abstract Cancer development, like most other human diseases, is the consequence of functional cellular alterations that drive to deregulation of tissue homeostasis. These modifications translate into stronger survival abilities and profound re-adjustments of the subtle balance between proliferative rates and regulated cell death programs. Moreover, further alterations in selected cell sub-clones allow specific cells not only to invade into the local surrounding tissue, but also to enter the systemic circulation – via lymphatic or blood vessels – and to establish new cancer colonies in a host organ. Because of the central role that the protein network plays in cellular function and in maintenance of normal cellular homeostasis, proteomics has become an intense focus of study in oncology today. In this context, technological approaches such as Reverse Phase Protein Microarray that utilize small input samples such as fine needle aspirants or tiny core biopsy samples, routinely used for analysis of metastatic lesions, could have a dramatic impact at the bedside as the gatekeeper for therapeutic selection for each patient. Several studies revealed discrepancies between pathway activation in the primary tumor and in the hepatic metastases, indicating an influence not only of the primary tumor but also of the host microenvironment in the development of metastases. These findings highlight the importance of metastatic lesion profile analysis and suggest its potential in selecting patients for therapy. The use of data derived not only from the primary tumor but also from tumors in secondary sites that ultimately drive the course of the disease is fundamental for clinical decision to increase therapeutic efficacy as well as in the development of new, more specific, compounds for the treatment of metastatic cancer.

Keywords Hepatic metastases · Individualized therapy · Host organ influence · Cell signaling · Phosphoproteomic profile · Reverse phase protein microarray

M. Pierobon (✉)
Center for Applied Proteomics and Molecular Medicine, George Mason University,
10900 University Blvd, MS 1A9, Bull Run Hall, Room 325, Manassas VA 20110, USA
e-mail: mpierobo@gmu.edu

P. Brodt (ed.), *Liver Metastasis: Biology and Clinical Management*, Cancer
Metastasis – Biology and Treatment 16, DOI 10.1007/978-94-007-0292-9_14,
© Springer Science+Business Media B.V. 2011

Abbreviations

FDA	Food and Drug Administration
IHC	immunohistochemistry
FPM	forward phase microarrays
RPPA	reverse phase protein microarrays
EDT	post-excision delay time
PDT	processing delay time
LCM	laser capture microdissection
EGF	epidermal growth factor
EGFR	epidermal growth factor receptor
COX-2	cyclooxygenase 2

Contents

14.1 Introduction

Neoplastic progression has been widely described as a gradual, long-term and multistep process, during which normal epithelium acquires novel geno/phenotypical characteristics responsible for the transformation of the mucosa's structures to atypical lesions and further to malignant neoplasms [1].

These newly acquired genetic and molecular properties translate into stronger survival abilities and profound re-adjustments of the subtle balance between proliferative rates and regulated cell death programs. In addition, within a cancer cell population, only selected sub-clones acquire further molecular modifications that bestow them with abilities not only to invade into the local surrounding tissue, but also to enter the systemic circulation – via lymphatic or blood vessels – and to establish new cancer colonies in a host organ [2–4]. Less than 1% of the cancer cells that enter the systemic and lymphatic circulations present with the ability to successfully survive through anoikis, extravasion and adaption to the host microenvironment indicating that profound and very selective molecular derangements are required to establish distant colonies. A series of molecular adaptations, characterized by specific temporal and biological shifting, is the condition "sine qua non" needed to achieve successful metastatic advancement [5, 6]. The new molecular setting needs to provide the cancer cells with the ability not only to survive in the local microenvironment, but also to adapt to the unique host organ microenvironment [7].

As the malignant cells become embedded in the new microenvironment -through favorable interactions between transformed cells and host setting- a gradual replacement of the endogenous tissue occurs causing progressive loss of organ architecture and physiological functions [8]. Steady decline of tissue functions and consequent organ failure rather than the primary tumor itself are the causes of death in more than 90% of patients affected by advanced disease [9]. Indeed, the development of distant metastasis is still considered the most important prognostic factor for long term survival of cancer patients [10, 11].

American Cancer Society epidemiologists estimated that in 2008 there were 565,650 cancer related deaths in the USA – 294,120 of them male and 271,530 female. The impact this illness has on modern societies and the intricacy of the metastatic progression have been considered two essential reasons for promoting incessant development of new and more elaborate technologies to investigate cell function, gene suppression, gene modification and more recently, protein expression and activation. A greater understanding of the phenomena driving neoplastic evolution has been an urgent priority in order to better comprehend the different stages of cancer invasion and dissemination, to identify specific cellular markers able to inform on the presence of the tumor at early stages of development and to discover new prognostic and therapeutic targets.

A very fine and constant input from genetic abnormalities to consequent protein encoding alterations and vice versa are one of the pivotal causes of cancer development and progression. The study of genetic duplications, amplifications and deletions allowed the identification of underlying phenomena that drive cell deregulation such as cell proliferation and survival, migration and apoptosis [12, 13]. Although DNA and RNA expression analyses provide information regarding potential genetic alterations, it is the proteins that "do the work" of the cell and are the molecular machines that provide functional output: i.e. transmit signals for death, growth, motility, etc. Moreover, alterations occurring in specific posttranslational modifications during tumor development, such as phosphorylation, glycosylation and ubiquitination, protein cleavage or conformational alterations are currently the main focus of interest in translational research aiming to design new theranostic modalities for diagnosis and treatment [14–16]. Indeed, proteins do not operate as single molecules, but constant molecular interactions and consequential changes in protein activation status lead to innumerable cellular functions. Intra- and extra-cellular communications are both participating and influencing this complex protein network. Posttranslational modifications, particularly phosphorylation and de-phosphorylation events, are the consequences of the continuous cross talk within cells and the surrounding microenvironment and are accountable for signal pathway activation and molecular derangement.

Because of the central role that the protein network plays in cellular function and in maintenance of normal cellular homeostasis, proteomics has become an intense focus of study in oncology today. Undeniably, the analysis of protein derangement not only provides specific explanations for the dynamic phenomena driving cancer progression, but it also allows the identification of novel diagnostic and prognostic factors and the discovery of groundbreaking therapeutic targets. In fact, in recent decades several new molecularly-targeted therapeutics, such as monoclonal antibodies and small molecule protein kinase inhibitors, have already been approved as standard of care for the treatment of different types and stages of cancer [17–21].

The capability of producing synthetic molecules targeting specific proteins and protein activities expressed exclusively by the neoplastic lesion or the surrounding microenvironment has progressively persuaded the scientific and medical community about the necessity to sub-classify patients based on the distinctive pathways activated in each malignant lesion. In the last decade the concept of *Individualized therapy* has represented the goal of most investigations in the cancer field. The advantage of treating patients based on their exclusive molecular profile could have a tremendous impact on cancer treatment. These novel therapeutic strategies have

Table 14.1 FDA-approved kinase inhibitors for the treatment of neoplastic disease

Chemotherapeutic agent	Target	Application
Bevacizumab	VEGFR-1/VEGFR-2	Metastatic colorectal cancer Non-small cell lung cancer Metastatic breast cancer
Sorafenib	VEGFR-1/VEGFR-2/VEGFR-3 PDGFR-β Raf-1	Metastatic renal carcinoma Unresectable hepatocarcinoma
Sunitinib	VEGFR-1/VEGFR-2/VEGFR-3 PDGFR-β RET	Metastatic renal carcinoma Gastrointestinal stromal tumor – imatinib resistant
Cetuximab	EGFR (extracellular domain)	Metastatic colorectal cancer Metastatic head and neck cancer
Panitumumab	EGFR	Resistant metastatic colorectal cancer
Trastuzumab	HER-2	Breast cancer over-expressing the HER-2
Imatinib	c-Kit c-Abl PDGFR	Chronic myelogenous leukemia Gastro-intestinal stromal tumor
Temsirolimus	mTOR	Metastatic renal carcinoma
Bortezomib	Proteosome	Multiple myeloma Mantle cell lymphoma

Listed in the table are some of the FDA approved kinase inhibitors and their clinical applications. Compounds targeting different pathways and substrates are currently considered standard of care for the treatment of neoplastic disease.

the advantage to specifically target proteins that are over-expressed or hyperacti-vated in each patient's tumor specimen. By treating neoplastic lesions according to the patients' unique molecular profiles, these innovative pharmaceutical compounds act selectively only on the malignant elements and could spare the normal cells lacking in target molecule activity. This selectivity could lead to profound reduc-tions in chemotherapeutic side effects and may ameliorate cancer patients' quality of life [22]. Moreover, through accurate and aimed selection of patients that will benefit from a specific treatment, the cost-welfare management of cancer patients' care could greatly improve (Table 14.1).

14.2 Proteomic Analysis in Clinical Practice: The Present and the Future

Currently, in clinical practice patient diagnosis and therapeutic decision are largely based on morphological and histological analyses of the neoplastic specimens. Pathological classification of tumors, regardless the site of origin is principally based on tumor size, grade of cellular differentiation, presence of lymph node or dis-tant metastases and in some selected subtypes of cancer, on the presence of specific membrane receptors known to be targets of FDA approved molecularly-targeted inhibitors. Molecular diagnosis of protein expression in the clinical setting utilizes mostly immunohistochemistry (IHC)-based procedures able to identify the presence of selective targets within the tissue framework [23–25].

Although IHC is considered a standard procedure in cancer diagnosis, this tech-nique presents several limitations. Firstly, IHC is a non-quantitative, relatively subjective analysis and differences in pathologist-to-pathologist staining interpreta-tions can introduce inaccuracies into the diagnostic process [26]. The pathologist's experience in the field and medical practice can profoundly influence the results of the test, and although different and more sophisticated scoring systems have been developed over time [27], quantitative or semi-quantitative measurement of the analyte of interest still represents an unattained goal. Moreover, fixation of surgical specimens at the time of tumor removal, commonly performed with for-malin, still represents an important hurdle to IHC analysis of cytosolic and nuclear proteins and to the capability of correctly measuring post-translational modifications that can themselves change as a result of post-excision delay time [28]. Furthermore, although tissue antigen retrieval protocols can uncover masked antigens by reversing protein cross-linking due to the formalin fixation, complete exposure of all antigenic sites is very difficult to achieve, and the reproducible measurement of analytes is still problematic.

Furthermore, when IHC is applied for clinical investigations of post-translational modifications such as phosphorylation, it is important to recognize that the phospho-proteome is subjected to continuous variation due to the presence of phosphatases and kinases in the cellular microenvironment. Formalin penetration of surgical spec-imens proceeds at roughly one to three hours per centimeter of tissue, and it is now known that during the fixation process, protein phosphorylation levels can change dramatically [28]. Such time-dependent rather than disease-dependent alterations may lead to profound misinterpretation of the molecular profiles of tumor cells and can impact therapeutic decisions. Due to the central role that proteins play in cancer progression and their potential use as novel targets for pharmaceutical compounds, a number of techniques for the investigation of protein expression and post-translational rearrangements have been developed and applied for tissue protein profile examination.

14.3 Novel Tools for Proteomics Investigation

Proteomics generally uses two overarching upfront techniques: those that require labeling for detection and those that are label-free. Indeed, 2D gel electrophoresis [29] and mass spectrometry are examples of label-free techniques. Both technologies are utilized for broad screening of protein content in a given sample; investigations based on these methodologies do not focus on quantification or identification of single or multiple known analytes, but generate extensive protein profiles from the input sample [30–33].

Conversely, labeled probe methods, such as protein microarray technology, are fundamental for the investigation and/or quantification of specific and previously identified analytes within the context of cell or tissue lysates. This type of technique usually requires the availability of one or more validated antibodies to target the protein of interest and a fluorescent or chromogen-based detection system. In selected cases, an amplification system for signal detection can be applied for successful outcome of the procedure.

Below, two protein microarray methods will be briefly described: the Forward Phase Microarrays and the Reverse Phase Protein Microarrays.

The Forward Phase Microarray (FPM) is also defined as a "Fix detector/Free analyte system" assay. It is based on immobilization onto a solid matrix (e.g. nitrocellulose) of multiple bait molecules -such as antibodies, nucleic acids or lipids- that allows simultaneous comparison of different analytes in a given sample. The analytes of interest, usually denatured cell or serum proteins, can be detected through prior fluorescent labeling of the analyte or by incubating the sample with two distinct antibodies. In the latter case, the first antibody binds the analyte to the solid substrate and the second identifies a second epitope of the same protein and is used for detection purposes in a so-called "sandwich assay". The necessity to obtain multiple antibodies that target different epitopes within the same protein is the major limitation of the sandwich assay technique [34–35] (Fig. 14.1).

The Reverse Phase Protein Microarrays (RPPA) is also defined as a "Free detector/Immobilized analyte" technique. This multiplex platform has the exceptional capacity to concurrently evaluate the proteomic profile of hundreds of samples, allowing direct comparison of cellular signaling between multiple individuals. Numerous samples are directly spotted onto an inert substratum -usually nitrocellulose coated glass- and protein detection is based on single, specific antibody-epitope interactions. A few microliters of a denatured cell lysate – collected from whole

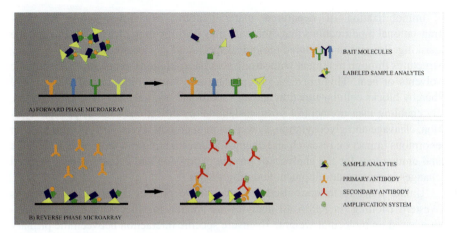

Fig. 14.1 Comparison between Forward Phase Microarray (*panel A*) and Reverse Phase Protein Microarray (*panel B*). While forward phase microarray is based on immobilization of antibodies onto a solid support i.e. "Fix detector/Free analyte system", reverse phase protein microarray is characterized by immobilization of analytes into the substrate i.e. "Free detector/Immobilized analyte" – allowing direct comparison of hundreds of samples

tissue or microdissected material – or body fluids such as serum, cerobrospinal fluid, synovial fluid, vitreous or sweat all represent adequate sources for protein analysis through RPPA [35–38]. This technology has the advantage of detecting picograms of analytes in a biological mixture thanks to the development of a highly sensitive tyramide-based avidin/biotin amplification system (Fig. 14.2).

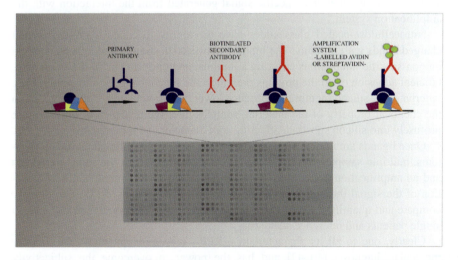

Fig. 14.2 An example of RPPA. Cellular lysate is spotted directly onto a nitrocellulose-coated slide and multiple samples are simultaneously probed with the same antibody. In the top part of the figure the staining procedure is illustrated. The bottom of the figure shows an actual image of an example RPPA slide. Incubation with primary and secondary antibodies is followed by an amplification reaction

Immobilization of denatured material allows the investigation of post-translational modifications that otherwise may be difficult to measure due to epitope masking. Proteins in denatured biological specimens can lose secondary and tertiary structures through treatment with strong acid/base solutions, inorganic salts, organic solvents or heat. This prevents phosphatase and kinase binding and activity and thereby blocks cellular function and any additional posttranslational modifications. By enabling measurement of posttranslational modifications such as phosphorylation, cleavage and glycosylation, as well as total protein levels, RPPA could have an enormous impact on research and diagnostic investigation and represents a valuable and unique tool for the analysis of protein expression and cell signaling -induced changes in disease development and progression.

Unlike other techniques used for quantitative protein investigations, such as Western Blotting, in RPPA all analytes are spotted together without any separation based on molecular weight. To ensure specific interaction between the primary antibody and the protein of interest, it is therefore mandatory to determine if binding between the antibodies and non-specific proteins can occur. To this end, each antibody needs to be thoroughly validated through Western Blotting to verify its specificity. A single band on the blot, at the specified molecular weight, provides indication of specific and unique affinity between the antibody and the protein of interest.

Ideal inert substrata, provided with chemical properties that facilitate the immobilization of cell lysates or other biological material, are nitrocellulose coated glass slides, although nylon or silanized silica represents suitable alternatives. A careful evaluation of the substratum is crucial in the RPPA since it determines the quality of the spots and it dramatically impacts the signal to noise ratio. The composition of the inert support should allow high affinity bonds formation with the analytes and minimize non-specific signal generated from the interaction with the amplification system.

Nitrocellulose-coated glass slides have the ability to create hydrophobic and charged bonds with proteins. The binding between substratum and ligands is based on non-specific interactions ensuring a minimal and uniform but, at the same time, efficient adhesion of all the proteins present in the specimen to the substratum [39]. Alternatively, silicon membranes produce lower background noise, although due to the chemical property of the material, samples have the tendency to diffuse more profusely into silicon substrata affecting spot diameter and reproducibility.

Once ligands are immobilized on the substratum, using different automated systems, multiple samples can be analyzed simultaneously with the same antibodies and an amplification system based on a streptavidin-biotin complex allows detection of the signal through fluorescent or colorimetric systems. RPPA can directly compare and quantify the analyte of interest either within a population or between single patients and reference standards.

Clearly, due to all its characteristics, RPPA represents an innovative tool for molecular diagnosis [40–42] and has the power to overcome the subjectivity associated with the IHC procedure, circumvent the main obstacle of the FPM i.e. the necessity for multiple antibodies, and provide quantification of the analyte measured.

14.4 Sample Preparation and Proteome Stability

Sample preparation and collection still represent an immense obstacle and ongoing problem in clinical practice. Molecular investigation and histological-morphological analysis of surgical specimens require different procedures for sample collection and conservation. In order to introduce molecular analyses as standard diagnostic procedures in clinical practice, sample collection and preservation procedures that can stabilize unstable molecules such as proteins and RNA need to be put into practice. Indeed, when fresh samples are collected in the operating room and left on a bench or fixed in formalin, the specimen is still alive: effectively a wound, now reacting to the ex-vivo environment. Cells within the tissue react to the environmental stresses and activate several pathways in response to the absence of vascular perfusion, hypoxia, temperature changes, etc. Enzymes involved in cellular activity remain activated and induce modifications of proteins and nucleic acids. The new cellular setting is a dynamic environment that is constantly changing as time passes and temperature fluctuates.

Sample collection is characterized by different key moments; the time between surgical excision and tissue stabilization (through freezing or chemical fixation) represents the post-excision delay time (EDT), while the time between tissue fixation and processing is considered the processing delay time (PDT). Depending on the length of EDT and PDT, different molecular derangements can be triggered by the recruitment of different pathways that readjust constantly as time passes.

For all of these reasons, prompt and adequate tissue fixation is critical to obtain proper and accurate results from analysis of clinical specimens. The most common tissue fixation procedures are snap freezing in liquid nitrogen and the formalin fixation discussed above. Both of these techniques have limitations such as the difficulty and availability of liquid nitrogen management in the hospital and physician's office for the former and slow penetration of the formalin, causing a delay in intracellular inactivation in the latter.

There is an urgent need therefore to develop new fixative solutions able not only to preserve and instantly "freeze" cellular activity, but also to preserve cell morphology and tissue histology for standard diagnostic procedures. A fixative based on a combination of alcohol, kinase/phosphatase inhibitors and cell culture media has recently been developed by Espina and colleagues [28]. This innovative fixative meets all the requirements for high quality sample collection for molecular diagnosis, while also preserving tissue morphology.

An additional problem encountered in surgical specimen analysis is due to tissue heterogeneity. Tissue composition can markedly influence the results of specimen analysis and generate misleading conclusions. Tissues are complex structures composed of different cell types with different characteristics, function and therefore, cellular signaling. Tissue composition can profoundly influence the molecular profile of a cancer specimen and hinder correct understanding of cellular modifications occurring in transformed cells.

For example in protein profiling studies performed for drug target identification, the signal of the subpopulation of interest within the whole tissue may be obscured by signals derived from other types of cells present within the tissue.

In the late 1990s the introduction of laser capture microdissection (LCM) technology overcame this problem. Indeed, through this technology, it is now possible to selectively isolate specific cell types from the whole tissue and obtain homogeneous cell populations for tissue analysis [43].

Most of the criticism against the applicability of LCM in clinical practice is related to the fact that it is a time consuming technique and that only a small amount of material can be obtained. RPPA represents the perfect downstream and linked tool for LCM material analysis because hundreds of proteins and protein activities can be measured at once from only a few thousand LCM-derived cells.

14.5 Proteomics in Neoplastic Progression, What Are We Learning from Clinical Experience and Where Are We Going?

In the past decades, the development of more sophisticated biomolecular technologies has led to more accurate and incisive investigations and, as a consequence, more precise and specific understanding of the molecular alterations that characterize cancer development and progression. New discoveries concerning genetic modifications and, more recently, alteration of the cellular proteome have provided biological explanations for therapeutic failures and successes, as well as insight into drug resistance.

A recent illustration of this is the valuable lesson the scientific community recently learned from studies evaluating the correlation between response rate to Cetuximab – a FDA approved monoclonal antibody that targets the epidermal growth factor (EGF) receptor – and K-Ras mutations in patients affected by hepatic dissemination of colorectal cancer. To establish the benefit of Cetuximab when added to standard of care, patients' overall and disease-free survival were compared within subgroups of patients with mutant or wild type K-Ras expression in their tumors. Whereas in patients with K-Ras mutations, the overall survival was 4.5 months in the group that received Cetuximab as compared to 4.6 months in the group that received standard of care only (i.e. no clinical benefit), patients whose tumors expressed wild type K-Ras had a median overall survival of 9.5 months when treated with the monoclonal antibody as compared to 4.8 months for patients that received best supportive care only (i.e. a clear clinical benefit) [44]. These studies highlighted the necessity for appropriately selecting patients based on their molecular profiles.

In more recent studies, different immunoassays were used to establish the relationship between protein derangement and response to Cetuximab in order to identify a subgroup of patients with metastatic colorectal cancer whose tumors express activated proteins in the EGF pathway that is targeted by this pharmaceutical compound. In the framework of developing efficient individualized therapy,

Loupakis and colleagues analyzed the expression and activation status (i.e. phosphorylation) of several key cellular proteins in colorectal cancer patients with hepatic metastases in order to identify possible correlations between response to Cetuximab and protein status. In this cutting edge study, signaling pathways were analyzed not only in the primary tumors (as is generally the case in clinical practice) but also in liver metastases [45]. The study revealed discrepancies between pathways activated in the primary lesion and in the hepatic metastases, highlighting the importance of selecting patients based on data derived not only from the primary tumor but also from tumors in secondary sites that ultimately drive the progressive, and too often irreversible and lethal course of the disease. Indeed, as hypothesized by Paget in his *seed and soil* theory published at the end of the nineteen century, metastatic tumor cells have a unique ability to grow in a foreign and unfamiliar microenvironment and this is likely the consequence of molecular rearrangements within the tumor cells that are compatible with the new site of growth [46]. Target organ colonization, driven by unique cellular inter-communication and cytokines/chemokine production, promotes activation (or selection) of particular cellular circuits that can sustain cell survival and proliferation in the new microenvironments. Numerous studies support Paget's hypothesis and show that metastatic lesions are the consequence of molecular adjustments acquired first in the primary site of growth and then in the new setting [47].

Wulfkuhle and colleagues recently published an innovative study comparing the proteomic profiles of hepatic metastases generated by tumors from different primary organ sites. The comparison between protein signaling in liver metastases of breast cancer and other primary carcinomas provides an ideal study design to investigate the roles of the microenvironments in the original sites of growth and the liver in the augmentation and progression of aggressive lesions. In Wulfkuhle's analysis, liver metastases from malignant breast epithelium and other primary organs were subjected to RPPA following isolation of pure cancer cell populations through LCM. Various proteins involved in assorted pathways were analyzed. The results revealed that only a small number of endpoints were differentially expressed in the two groups, strongly suggesting that the microenvironment of the host organ plays a pivotal role in the activation of specific survival pathways and that protein activation in the metastatic lesion, although influenced by the origin of the primary tumor, is mainly driven by the target organ microenvironment [48]. These results were in line with the results of an earlier study of patient-matched primary and metastatic colorectal cancer tissue sets where large differences in molecular signaling were found between the primary tumors and matched hepatic metastases [49].

The ability to identify molecular targets that are specific for the metastatic lesions or that are present only in a subgroup of cancer patients represents a unique opportunity not only to identify patients that may benefit from specific therapeutic strategies, directed at known molecules, but also for the discovery of novel therapeutic targets and diagnostic or prognostic markers. Pierobon and colleagues reported that colorectal cancers presenting with synchronous liver metastases (i.e. at the time of diagnosis) are characterized by hyper-activation of pro-survival and anti-apoptotic pathways that promote local invasion and dissemination through the vascular bed [50].

These observations suggest that primary tumors with metastatic abilities have distinctive molecular programs that can initiate and sustain local invasion and progression at distant sites. In fact, colorectal tumors presenting with synchronous liver metastases displayed higher activation of the EGFR and COX-2 pro-survival pathways, when compared to large intestinal lesions that never metastasized. Both of these pathways are already targets of several agents that have either been approved or are under investigation for the treatment of cancer patients. The identification of colorectal cancer patients with high activation of EGFR signaling and COX-2, or their downstream substrates, represents an attractive prospective for novel preventive therapeutic strategies aimed at inactivating signaling and interfering with the establishment and growth of secondary lesions.

The capability to identify molecular derangements driving metastatic progression, as well as the possibility to utilize, in medical settings, novel molecular technologies that allow the identification of patients with aggressive lesions before metastases are clinically detectable represent the future direction of cancer treatment.

RPPA, associated with LCM, is a groundbreaking technology with extraordinary potential for clinical application because it allows the measurement of numerous analytes in surgical specimens, even when the biological material is limited. This capability provides physicians with comprehensive sets of data on specific molecular pathways activated in each individual tumor (patient). Currently RPPA is already utilized as an investigative tool in several clinical trials aimed either at the identification of patients that can benefit from innovative therapies or at examining cellular response to standard treatments in order to identify alternative pathways that allow cancer cell to escape from drug-induced cell death. This pioneering technology is an excellent tool for more efficient stratification and successful treatment of patients affected by liver metastases. Several crucial points have been highlighted by the results of RPPA application for the profiling of hepatic lesions. Because liver metastasis is the lethal aspect of the disease and current studies point to profound molecular differences between the primary and metastatic lesions [51], it becomes essential to perform molecular analysis on the metastatic lesions in order to select the most appropriate and tailored therapy for each patient. The isolation of pure cancer cell populations through LCM is critical to identify molecular derangements that are exclusive to the malignant cells and can minimize any misleading contribution by elements of the surrounding microenvironment. Ultimately, once specific subgroups of cellular derangements are identified within a cancer population, each patient, or subgroup can be treated specifically for the set of proteins that are aberrantly activated/expressed in their malignant lesions (Fig. 14.3). This individualized approach can be further empowered through monitoring the response to a given treatment clinically, as well as biologically (at the cell level). In this way the chemotherapeutic/targeted treatments can be improved according to additional molecular rearrangement(s), possibly acquired through exposure to chemical compounds that cause resistance to the therapy.

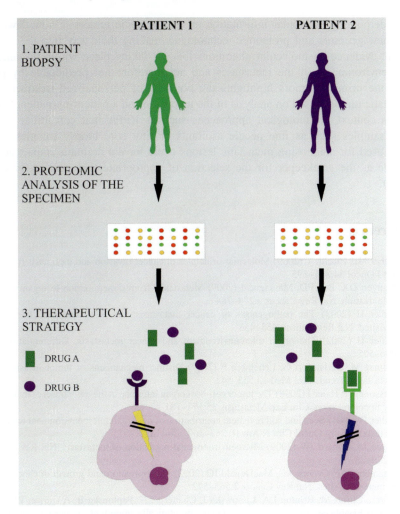

Fig. 14.3 New frontier for individualized therapy. Patients affected by histologically similar types of cancer can present distinct protein activation profiles and are treated according to their specific molecular profiles. Patient stratification based on the investigation of the metastatic lesion and identification of specific targets allows profound reduction of chemotherapeutic side effects and ameliorates cancer patients' quality of life

14.6 Conclusions and Future Directions

For decades, the misleading assumption that all patients with tumors originating from the same primary organ had to be considered and treated as homogeneous populations has profoundly affected the development of unique therapeutic strategies that can dramatically improve outcome and overall survival. A new era of personalized molecular medicine, whereby patients are selected and stratified based on underpinning molecular information on their specific tumors is now dawning with new genomic and proteomic technologies making their way into the clinic. Recent evidence on molecular alterations that are taking place within the unique microenvironments of the metastases and are therefore not predictable by profiling the primary tumors highlights the potential of personalized treatment for metastatic tumors based on analysis of the metastases on a patient-by-patient basis. In this context, technological approaches such as RPPA that can utilize small input samples such as fine needle aspirants or tiny core biopsy samples, routinely used for diagnosing metastatic lesions could have a dramatic impact at the bedside as the gatekeeper for the selection of appropriate therapeutics for each patient.

References

1. Leber MF, Efferth T (2009) Molecular principles of cancer invasion and metastasis (review). Int J Oncol 34:881–895
2. Nguyen DX, Bos PD, Massague J (2009) Metastasis: from dissemination to organ-specific colonization. Nat Rev Cancer 9:274–284
3. Fidler IJ (2003) The pathogenesis of cancer metastasis: the 'seed and soil' hypothesis revisited. Nat Rev Cancer, 453–458
4. Fidler IJ (2002) The organ microenvironment and cancer metastasis. Differentiation 70: 498–505
5. Yilmaz M, Christofori G, Lehembre F (2007) Distinct mechanisms of tumor invasion and metastasis. Trends Mol Med 13:535–541
6. Gassmann P, Haier J (2008) The tumor cell-host organ interface in the early onset of metastatic organ colonisation. Clin Exp Metastasis 25:171–181
7. Fidler IJ (2001) Seed and soil revisited: contribution of the organ microenvironment to cancer metastasis. Surg Oncol Clin N Am 10:257–269, vii–viiii
8. Joyce JA, Pollard JW (2009) Microenvironmental regulation of metastasis. Nat Rev Cancer 9:239–252
9. Chambers AF, Groom AC, MacDonald IC (2002) Dissemination and growth of cancer cells in metastatic sites. Nat Rev Cancer 2:563–572
10. Garcia-Closas M, Brinton LA, Lissowska J, Chatterjee N, Peplonska B, Anderson WF et al (2006) Established breast cancer risk factors by clinically important tumour characteristics. Br J Cancer 95:123–129
11. Morris M, Iacopetta B, Platell C (2007) Comparing survival outcomes for patients with colorectal cancer treated in public and private hospitals. Med J Aust 186: 296–300
12. Radinsky R (1995) Modulation of tumor cell gene expression and phenotype by the organ-specific metastatic environment. Cancer Metastasis Rev 14:323–338
13. Radinsky R, Ellis LM (1996) Molecular determinants in the biology of liver metastasis. Surg Oncol Clin N Am 5:215–229
14. Ideker T, Thorsson V, Ranish JA, Christmas R, Buhler J, Eng JK et al (2001) Integrated genomic and proteomic analyses of a systematically perturbed metabolic network. Science 292:929–934
15. Wulfkuhle J, Espina V, Liotta L, Petricoin E (2004) Genomic and proteomic technologies for individualisation and improvement of cancer treatment. Eur J Cancer 40:2623–2632
16. Nielsen UB, Cardone MH, Sinskey AJ, MacBeath G, Sorger PK (2003) Profiling receptor tyrosine kinase activation by using Ab microarrays. Proc Natl Acad Sci USA 100: 9330–9335

17. Dangle PP, Zaharieva B, Jia H, Pohar KS (2009) Ras-MAPK pathway as a therapeutic target in cancer – emphasis on bladder cancer. Recent Pat Anticancer Drug Discov 4: 125–136
18. Rini BI (2009) Vascular endothelial growth factor-targeted therapy in metastatic renal cell carcinoma. Cancer 115:2306–2312
19. Schenone S, Bruno O, Radi M, Botta M (2009) New insights into small-molecule inhibitors of Bcr-Abl. Med Res Rev. Published online Wiley InterScience. www.interscience.wiley.com. doi:10.1002/med.20175
20. Aguilera DG, Tsimberidou AM (2009) Dasatinib in chronic myeloid leukemia: a review. Ther Clin Risk Manag 5:281–289
21. Browne BC, O'Brien N, Duffy MJ, Crown J, O'Donovan N (2009) HER-2 signaling and inhibition in breast cancer. Curr Cancer Drug Targets 9:419–438
22. Arteaga CL (2003) EGF receptor as a therapeutic target: patient selection and mechanisms of resistance to receptor-targeted drugs. J Clin Oncol 21:289s–291s
23. Gown AM, Goldstein LC, Barry TS, Kussick SJ, Kandalaft PL, Kim PM et al (2008) High concordance between immunohistochemistry and fluorescence in situ hybridization testing for HER2 status in breast cancer requires a normalized IHC scoring system. Mod Pathol 21: 1271–1277
24. Umemura S, Osamura RY (2004) Utility of immunohistochemistry in breast cancer practice. Breast Cancer 11:334–338
25. Hanna W (2001) Testing for HER2 status. Oncology 61:22–30
26. Choudhury KR, Yagle KJ, Swanson PE, Krohn KA, Rajendran JG (2009) A robust automated measure of average antibody staining in immunohistochemistry images. J Histochem Cytochem. 58:95–107
27. Allred DC, Harvey JM, Berardo M, Clark GM (1998) Prognostic and predictive factors in breast cancer by immunohistochemical analysis. Mod Pathol 11:155–168
28. Espina V, Edmiston KH, Heiby M, Pierobon M, Sciro M, Merritt B et al (2008) A portrait of tissue phosphoprotein stability in the clinical tissue procurement process. Mol Cell Proteomics 7:1998–2018
29. Unlu M, Morgan ME, Minden JS (1997) Difference gel electrophoresis: a single gel method for detecting changes in protein extracts. Electrophoresis 18:2071–2077
30. Celis JE, Gromov P (2003) Proteomics in translational cancer research: toward an integrated approach. Cancer Cell 3:9–15
31. Aebersold R, Mann M (2003) Mass spectrometry-based proteomics. Nature 422:198–207
32. Lin D, Tabb DL, Yates JR 3rd (2003) Large-scale protein identification using mass spectrometry. Biochim Biophys Acta 1646:1–10
33. Chen CH (2008) Review of a current role of mass spectrometry for proteome research. Anal Chim Acta 624:16–36
34. Haab BB (2005) Antibody arrays in cancer research. Mol Cell Proteomics 4:377–383
35. Espina V, Woodhouse EC, Wulfkuhle J, Asmussen HD, Petricoin EF 3rd, Liotta LA (2004) Protein microarray detection strategies: focus on direct detection technologies. J Immunol Methods 290:121–133
36. Espina V, Mehta AI, Winters ME, Calvert V, Wulfkuhle J, Petricoin EF 3rd et al (2003) Protein microarrays: molecular profiling technologies for clinical specimens. Proteomics 3: 2091–2100
37. Charboneau L, Tory H, Chen T, Winters M, Petricoin EF 3rd, Liotta LA et al (2002) Utility of reverse phase protein arrays: applications to signalling pathways and human body arrays. Brief Funct Genomic Proteomic 1:305–315
38. Sheehan KM, Calvert VS, Kay EW, Lu Y, Fishman D, Espina V et al (2005) Use of reverse phase protein microarrays and reference standard development for molecular network analysis of metastatic ovarian carcinoma. Mol Cell Proteomics 4:346–355
39. Steinitz M, Tamir S (1995) An improved method to create nitrocellulose particles suitable for the immobilization of antigen and antibody. J Immunol Methods 187:171–177

40. Grubb RL, Calvert VS, Wulkuhle JD, Paweletz CP, Linehan WM, Phillips JL et al (2003) Signal pathway profiling of prostate cancer using reverse phase protein arrays. Proteomics 3:2142–2146

41. Wulfkuhle JD, Aquino JA, Calvert VS, Fishman DA, Coukos G, Liotta LA et al (2003) Signal pathway profiling of ovarian cancer from human tissue specimens using reverse-phase protein microarrays. Proteomics 3:2085–2090

42. Paweletz CP, Charboneau L, Bichsel VE, Simone NL, Chen T, Gillespie JW et al (2001) Reverse phase protein microarrays which capture disease progression show activation of pro-survival pathways at the cancer invasion front. Oncogene 20:1981–1989

43. Emmert-Buck MR, Bonner RF, Smith PD, Chuaqui RF, Zhuang Z, Goldstein SR et al (1996) Laser capture microdissection. Science 274:998–1001

44. Karapetis CS, Khambata-Ford S, Jonker DJ, O'Callaghan CJ, Tu D, Tebbutt NC et al (2008) K-ras mutations and benefit from cetuximab in advanced colorectal cancer. N Engl J Med 359:1757–1765

45. Loupakis F, Pollina L, Stasi I, Ruzzo A, Scartozzi M, Santini D et al (2009) PTEN expression and KRAS mutations on primary tumors and metastases in the prediction of benefit from cetuximab plus irinotecan for patients with metastatic colorectal cancer. J Clin Oncol 27:2622–2629

46. Paget S (1989) The distribution of secondary growths in cancer of the breast. 1889. Cancer Metastasis Rev 8:98–101

47. Ramaswamy S, Ross KN, Lander ES, Golub TR (2003) A molecular signature of metastasis in primary solid tumors. Nat Genet 33:49–54

48. Wulfkuhle JD, Speer R, Pierobon M, Laird J, Espina V, Deng J et al (2008) Multiplexed cell signaling analysis of human breast cancer applications for personalized therapy. J Proteome Res 7:1508–1517

49. Petricoin EF, 3rd, Bichsel VE, Calvert VS, Espina V, Winters M, Young L et al (2005) Mapping molecular networks using proteomics: a vision for patient-tailored combination therapy. J Clin Oncol 23:3614–3621

50. Pierobon M, Calvert V, Belluco C, Garaci E, Deng J, Lise M et al (2009) Multiplexed cell signaling analysis of metastatic and nonmetastatic colorectal cancer reveals COX2-EGFR signaling activation as a potential prognostic pathway biomarker. Clin Colorectal Cancer 8:110–117

51. Belluco C, Mammano E, Petricoin E, Prevedello L, Calvert V, Liotta L et al (2005 July) Kinase substrate protein microarray analysis of human colon cancer and hepatic metastasis. Clin Chim Acta 357:180–183

Chapter 15
Targeting Angiogenesis in the Treatment of Hepatic Metastasis

Christina M. Edwards, J. Joshua Smith, Nipun B. Merchant, and Alexander A. Parikh

Abstract The liver is the most common site for the development of metastases from gastrointestinal malignancies. Although the only potentially curative option for patients with liver metastases is resection, only a minority are candidates. In order to increase the number of patients who may be candidates for resection, preoperative systemic chemotherapy and targeted therapy approaches have been utilized. Angiogenesis has been shown to be integral for the growth and metastasis of many tumor types including the development of liver metastases. The development of anti-angiogenic approaches, particularly anti vascular endothelial growth factor (VEGF) therapy with bevacizumab, has shown great promise in the treatment of patients with liver metastases, particularly from colorectal cancer and to a lesser degree, neuroendocrine carcinoma. These approaches have allowed physicians to increase the number of patients that may be amenable for curative resection. As angiogenesis and VEGF have been shown to be important in liver hypertrophy and regeneration, however, the possible effects of anti-VEGF therapy on liver recovery may carry significant risks along with the potential benefits.

Keywords Angiogenesis · Liver · VEGF · Bevacizumab · Neoadjuvant

Abbreviations

Ang	angiopoietin
BEAT	Bevacizumab Expanded Access Trial
BV	bevacizumab
CRC	colorectal cancer
FDA	Food and Drug Administration
FGF	fibroblast growth factor
FLR	future liver remnant
5-FU	5-fluorouracil

A.A. Parikh (✉)
Division of Surgical Oncology, Department of Surgery, Vanderbilt University Medical Center, 597 Preston Building, 2220 Pierce Avenue, Nashville, TN 37232-2730, USA
e-mail: alexander.parikh@vanderbilt.edu

P. Brodt (ed.), *Liver Metastasis: Biology and Clinical Management*, Cancer
Metastasis – Biology and Treatment 16, DOI 10.1007/978-94-007-0292-9_15,
© Springer Science+Business Media B.V. 2011

GI   gastrointestinal
GIST   gastrointestinal stromal tumors
HCC   hepatocelluar carcinoma
HGF   hepatocyte growth factor
HIF   hypoxia-inducible factor
IGF   insulin growth factor
LV   leucovorin
mCRC   metastatic colorectal cancer
OS   overall survival
PD   progressive disease
PFS   progression-free survival
PlGF   placental growth factor
PR   partial response
PVE   portal vein embolization
PVO   portal vein occlusion
RCC   renal cell carcinoma
SD   stable disease
SWOG   Southwestern Oncology Group
TKI   tyrosine kinase inhibitor
VEGF   vascular endothelial growth factor

Contents

15.1 Introduction

The liver is the most common site of metastases from gastrointestinal (GI) malignancies including colorectal carcinoma (CRC), neuroendocrine carcinomas, pancreatic carcinomas as well as others. For example, it is estimated that for patients with CRC, between 20 and 70% will either have liver metastases at the time of diagnosis of the primary tumor or develop liver metastases after resection of the primary CRC [1]. Although complete surgical resection can be potentially curable in some patients and lead to very good long-term survival rates, up to 80% of patients with liver metastases are not candidates for resection due to extrahepatic disease or insufficient residual healthy liver tissue [1, 2]. Although the median survival for these (unresectable) patients has greatly improved over the past several years, long term survival remains rare.

Advances in multi-agent systemic chemotherapy regimens and targeted therapies have led to significant increases in the median survival of patients with metastatic disease to the liver – particularly in the case of colorectal cancer. Of the many pathways involved in the development of metastatic disease, angiogenesis has been shown to play an important role in the development of metastases from several cancers including colorectal cancer [3–6], neuroendocrine carcinomas as well as others [7, 8]. To that end, the development of biological agents that inhibit angiogenesis and their use in combination with multi-agent chemotherapy regimens has offered new possibilities, not only for improved response and survival rates, but also for rendering select patients with unresectable disease potential candidates for resectable metastases.

This chapter will focus on the biological and clinical aspects of angiogenesis and anti-angiogenic therapy in the treatment of liver metastases. As most of the clinical data and experience comes from metastatic colorectal cancer, and to a lesser degree, metastatic neuroendocrine cancer, we will focus our discussion on these disease subtypes.

15.2 Angiogenesis and Tumor Metastasis

Angiogenesis is the establishment of a neovascular blood supply from pre-existing blood vessels [9]. Once a tumor grows beyond a certain size, oxygen and other nutrients cannot reach areas beyond 1–2 mm from the nearest blood vessel. For continued growth, therefore, the development and expansion of the blood supply (i.e., angiogenesis) are necessary [7, 9–11]. Tumor angiogenesis is the result of a shift in the homeostatic balance of proangiogenic and antiangiogenic molecules (summarized in Table 15.1). When the activity of proangiogenic molecules exceeds the activity of antiangiogenic molecules, new blood vessels can form. Proangiogenic molecules may be constitutively expressed, or their expression may be increased by factors such as hypoxia, low pH, cytokines, growth factors, and tumor size [9].

Not only is angiogenesis essential for primary tumor growth, it also plays an important role in the development of metastases [7, 12]. Metastasis is a sequential, highly selective, non-random process which favors the survival of a small population of metastatic cells pre-existing within the primary tumor mass. In order for a primary tumor cell to become metastatic, it must first invade into the surrounding normal stroma. Once the invading cells penetrate the vascular or lymphatic circulation, the cells can then detach and are transported within the circulatory system, arrest in the capillary bed of a target organ, extravasate into the organ parenchyma, proliferate, and establish micrometastasis [12]. It is thought that angiogenesis facilitates tumor metastasis by providing a route for tumor cells to leave the primary site and enter the blood stream [13].

Table 15.1 Proangiogenic and antiangiogenic factors

Proangiogenic factors	Antiangiogenic factors
Vascular endothelial growth factor (VEGF)	Angiopoietin-2 (in the absence of VEGF)
Angiogenin	Angiostatin
Epidermal growth factor receptor (EGFR)	Endostatin
Hepatocyte growth factor	Interferon inducible protein-10
Hypoxia inducible factor alpha (HIF-alpha)	Interferon-α, Interferon-β
Fibroblast growth factor 1, 2	Platelet factor 4
Insulin-like growth factor 1	Prolactin fragment
Integrin $\alpha_5\beta_1$, Integrin $\alpha_v\beta_3$	Thrombospondin 1, 2
Interleukin-8	Tissue inhibitor of metalloproteinase
Mammalian target of rapamycin (mTOR)	Tumstatin
Neuropilin-2	Vasculostatin
Placenta growth factor	
Platelet-derived endothelial cell growth factor	
Transforming growth factor-α	
Tumor necrosis factor-α	

15.2.1 Angiogenic Factors

15.2.1.1 VEGF

Numerous proangiogenic growth factors have been discovered and among them the vascular endothelial growth factor (VEGF) family of proteins and receptors is the best characterized [7, 12, 14]. VEGF regulates both physiological and pathological growth of blood vessels. Expression of VEGF leads to increased vascular permeability and induction of endothelial cell migration, proliferation, invasion and survival [15, 16]. Overexpression of VEGF has been associated with tumor progression and poor prognosis in a variety of human carcinomas, including colon and neuroendocrine tumors [3, 17, 18].

The VEGF family consists of six secreted glycoproteins, VEGF-A, VEGF-B, VEGF-C, VEGF-D, VEGF-E, and placental growth factor (PIGF) [7, 15, 16]. VEGF-A (commonly referred to as VEGF) is the best characterized of the VEGF family members. The angiogenic effects of VEGF are mediated by the tyrosine kinase receptors, VEGF-R1 (Flt-1), VEGF-R2 (KDR/Flk-1) and VEGF-R3 (Flt-4) that are present on endothelial cells as well as on tumor cells themselves [15].

Role of VEGF in Tumor Metastasis

The role of VEGF in the growth and development of several different tumor types and metastases has been shown in numerous pre-clinical and clinical studies. For example, VEGF, as well as its receptor (KDR) are upregulated in colorectal carcinoma, and their expression correlates with increased proliferation, metastasis and neovascularisation, as well as an increased likelihood of metastatic spread and decreased long-term survival [3, 4, 7]. Neuroendocrine tumors are highly vascular lesions that also express VEGF [18]. In these tumors, VEGF expression has been shown to correlate with metastases and a decreased duration of progression-free survival [19]. Similar results have been found with several other tumor types including breast, pancreas and lung cancers [7].

15.2.1.2 Other Angiogenesis Factors

In addition to VEGF, there are several other angiogenic factors that appear to be involved in the pathogenesis of both primary and metastatic tumors. These include angiopoietins (Ang), platelet-derived growth factors (PDGFs), fibroblast growth factor-2 (FGF-2), hepatocyte growth factor (HGF), insulin-like growth factors (IGF) and adhesion receptors such as integrins [7, 20–23]. Clinical evidence supporting the role of these factors in the development of liver metastases, is however, still limited.

15.3 Angiogenesis Inhibitors

Several angiogenesis inhibitors that target different proangiogenic molecules including VEGF, PDGF, integrins and angiopoietins have been developed. These inhibitors are in various stages of pre-clinical and clinical development. By far the most extensive experience has been gained with the VEGF inhibitor bevacizumab (BV) (Avastin, Genentech/Roche) that was approved for the treatment of metastatic CRC, breast cancer and non-small cell lung cancer in combination with chemotherapy.

BV is a recombinant humanized monoclonal antibody that is 93% homologous to the human protein sequence and 7% to the murine ortholog and was approved by the United States Food and Drug Administration (FDA) in 2004 for the treatment of metastatic colorectal cancer in conjunction with 5-Fluorouracil (5-FU)-based chemotherapy [15, 16]. It binds and inactivates all 5 isoforms of VEGF to inhibit angiogenesis, tumor growth and proliferation. As indicated above, VEGF is often over-expressed in human tumors. In xenograft models of human carcinoid and colon carcinoma respectively, treatment with BV was shown to block tumor growth and reduce the size and number of liver metastases [24–26]. In both preclinical and clinical studies, the anti-tumor effect of BV was shown to be enhanced when combined with cytotoxic chemotherapy, radiation and other angiogenesis inhibitors [1, 5, 27–29].

In addition to VEGF neutralizing antibodies, other therapeutic strategies for VEGF targeting have included the development of soluble VEGF receptors, anti-VEGF receptor antibodies, tyrosine-kinase inhibitors (TKI) and anti-cellular signalling approaches [15, 16, 21, 30], and they are all in various stages of clinical development. In addition to BV, the VEGF receptor TKIs sorafenib (Nexavar, Bayer/Onyx) and sunitinib (Sutent, Pfizer) have been approved for clinical use [31–33]. Sorafenib has been approved for the treatment of renal cell carcinoma (RCC) and hepatocellular carcinoma (HCC), while sunitinib has been approved for the treatment of RCC and gastrointestinal stromal tumors (GISTs).

Several other agents that target other angiogenic factors are currently being studied in the pre-clinical and clinical settings. For example, angiopoietin-1 (Ang-1) regulates embryonic and postnatal neovascularization. Ang-1 interacts directly with endothelial cells and other angiogenic molecules to maintain and stabilize blood vessels [34]. Stoeltzing et al. [35] demonstrated that overexpression of Ang-1 in the human colon cancer cell line HT29 decreased vascular permeability, inhibited tumor-induced angiogenesis and reduced the growth of tumor cells implanted into the livers of mice , suggesting that vessel stabilization may act to limit angiogenesis and metastasis.

Integrins are dimeric cell surface receptors that mediate cell-matrix and cell-cell adhesion and are expressed in a cell type-specific manner on various cells including tumor and endothelial cells [36]. Integrin $\alpha_5\beta_1$ is expressed on endothelial cells and plays an important role in tumor angiogenesis. When CT26 colon cancer cells were injected into mice, it was noted that treatment with a novel integrin $\alpha_5\beta_1$ inhibitor, ATN-161, led to decreased liver metastases formation. The combination of ATN-161 with 5-FU resulted in a statistically significant increase in tumor cell apoptosis, decreased tumor cell proliferation, and improved overall survival [37]. Similar results were obtained with S247, an inhibitor of integrin $\alpha_v\beta_3$ that is expressed on proliferating endothelial cells. Mice treated with S247 developed significantly fewer liver metastases and had prolonged survival as compared to controls [38].

Similar studies have been reported with other angiogenesis inhibitors [7, 21, 23, 30, 39, 40]. Nevertheless, clinical experience remains limited and none have yet been approved for clinical use.

15.4 Clinical Studies

15.4.1 *Bevacizumab for Liver Metastatic Colorectal Cancer*

A phase III randomized control trial conducted by Hurwitz et al. led to the clinical approval of BV for the treatment of metastatic colorectal cancer (mCRC) in 2004. This study consisted of 813 patients with previously untreated metastatic colorectal cancer who were randomly assigned to receive irinotecan, 5-FU, and LV (IFL) plus BV or IFL plus placebo. The median overall survival (OS) was 20.3 months in the IFL plus BV group and 15.6 months in the IFL plus placebo group (HR = 0.66, $p < 0.001$) and the median progression-free survival (PFS) was 10.6 months vs. 6.2 months (HR = 0.54, $p < 0.001$). The RRs were 44.8 and 34.8% respectively ($p = 0.004$), and the median durations of response were 10.4 and 7.1 months ($p = 0.001$). Although this study did not specifically analyze patients with liver metastases, the results did suggest that the addition of BV to multi-agent systemic chemotherapy improved the efficacy of this treatment regimen for mCRC [31].

Emmanouilides et al. [41] investigated the efficacy and toxicity of 5-FU, LV, and oxaliplatin (FOLFOX4) combined with BV as front line treatment in patients with *inoperable* mCRC. Fifty-three patients were enrolled in the single arm study and complete responses were achieved in eight patients (15.1%), while partial responses were observed in 28 (52.8%) patients. Time to tumor progression was 11 months and the probability of 1-, 2-, and 3-year survival was 79.8, 63.8, and 58.3%, respectively. Six patients (11%) with initially unresectable metastatic lesions in the liver underwent margin-negative (R0) metastasectomy. All patients who underwent metastasectomy were alive at the time of the analysis (median follow up was 10 months) [41]. Although this was a small single arm trial, the results suggested that BV in combination with FOLFOX may change the status of matastases in a small percentage of patients from unresectable to resectable.

In a large phase III randomized trial, BV was added to FOLFOX or capecitabine/oxaliplatin (XELOX) in patients with unresectable mCRC [42]. A total of 1401 patients were randomly assigned to the 2×2 factorial design. Unlike other reported studies, in this study, the median overall survival was similar in the BV-containing and non containing arms (21.3 vs. 19.9 months, $p = 0.077$). Nevertheless, hepatic metastases were resectable in a larger percentage of all patients treated with BV (8.4% vs. 6.1%), as well as in a subgroup of patients with initially unresectable liver metastases (19.2% vs. 12.9%) [42]. Although margin and survival data are not available, this study suggested that a greater proportion of patients with unresectable hepatic metastases can convert to a "resectable" status with the addition of BV to systemic chemotherapy.

The Bevacizumab Expanded Access Trail (BEAT) was a large, multicenter registry evaluating the safety and efficacy of BV [29]. All patients had surgically inoperable mCRC and all received BV plus chemotherapy (physician's choice). Chemotherapy included 5-FU/LV plus oxaliplatin (29%), 5-FU/LV plus irinotecan (26%), capecitabine plus oxaliplatin (18%), and monotherapy (16%). The study enrolled 1965 patients from 41 countries worldwide (excluding the United States). A total of 704 patients (37%) had liver-only metastatic disease. The overall survival for all patients was 22.7 months – consistent with that of other studies. Curative hepatic resection was carried out in 107 patients with liver only disease (15.2%) and was margin-negative (R0) in 85 patients (12.1%). The resection rate was 20.3% in patients who received BV plus oxaliplatin with a R0 resection rate of 15.4%. For patients receiving BV plus irinotecan, the resection rate and R0 rates were 14.3 and 11.7%, respectively. Two-year OS was 89% in patients with curative-intent hepatic resection and 94% in those patients who received an R0 resection [29]. Although this study was non-comparative and observational, a very large number of patients were followed and the results further suggested that anti-VEGF therapy with BV when combined with systemic chemotherapy can convert the status of the disease for a significant number of patients from unresectable liver metastases to resectable and potentially curable disease and lead to excellent overall survival rates.

These studies also suggested that BV could be a useful adjunct to systemic chemotherapy in patients with *resectable* metastases in the neoadjuvant setting. Gruenberger et al. investigated the role of BV, capecitabine and oxaliplatin as neoadjuvant therapy for patients with *potentially curable* metastatic colorectal cancer. The study was a phase II, nonrandomized trial consisting of 56 patients [43]. Patients included in the study were at high-risk for metastatic disease (e.g., synchronous liver metastases, metastatic disease that developed within 1 year after primary resection, lymph node positive primary tumor, more than one liver metastasis, a liver metastasis larger than 5 cm or a positive carcinoembryonic antigen level). Patients received BV plus XELOX for six cycles and there was a 5-week interval between the last BV dose and surgery. BV and XELOX were restarted 5 weeks after surgery. The overall RR was 73%. Fifty-two (93%) patients underwent liver resection (41 underwent liver resection alone and 11 underwent primary tumor and liver resection). There was no increase in intraoperative bleeding events or wound-healing complications. Postoperative liver function and regeneration were normal in all but one patient and no postoperative mortality occurred [43]. Survival data for this trial are currently pending. Although this study was small and non-randomized, this report suggested that the use of BV in combination with systemic chemotherapy for patients with potentially resectable mCRC is safe and feasible and leads to excellent response and resectability rates. Additional studies, especially in comparison to resection alone are needed to further define the role of BV-containing regimens in the neoadjuvant setting for mCRC.

15.4.2 Bevacizumab for Neuroendocrine Tumors

Gastrointestinal neuroendocrine tumors including carcinoid tumors, account for only 2% of all GI malignancies [44–46]. Nevertheless, due to their often indolent nature, resection of hepatic metastases, when possible is usually recommended. As is the case with metastatic CRC, only a minority of patients have resectable disease and for the others, systemic treatment is necessary [44–46]. As mentioned previously, neuroendocrine carcinomas are vasculature-rich tumors and express VEGF. In 2008, Yao et al. [47] performed a randomized trial comparing BV and interferon α-2b as treatments for metastatic or unresectable GI carcinoid tumors. Forty-four patients receiving octreotide were randomly assigned to 18 weeks of treatment with BV or PEGylated interferon α-2b. After 18 weeks or at disease progression (whichever occurred first), patients received both BV and PEG-interferon. In the BV group, four patients (18%) achieved partial response (PR), 17 patients (77%) had stable disease (SD) and one patient (5%) had disease progression (PD). In the PEG-interferon group, 15 patients (68%) had SD and 6 patients (27%) had PD. PFS after 18 weeks of therapy were 95% in the BV group and 68% in the PEG interferon α-2b group. On functional CT, decreases of 49 and 28% in tumor blood flow, respectively were observed on day 2 and week 18 post treatment initiation among patients treated with BV as compared to baseline measurements, while no significant changes in tumor blood flow were observed in the PEG-interferon group [47]. This study demonstrated that the addition of BV to octreotide resulted in a higher response rate, a longer PFS and a reduction in tumor blood flow in patients with advanced carcinoid tumors. Although promising, this study was small and definitive conclusions cannot yet be reached. Currently, a larger study (S0518) sponsored by the Southwest Oncology Group (SWOG) is underway. This study will compare the PFS of patients treated with octreotide plus either BV or conventional dosing of interferon for patients with unresectable neuroendocrine carcinoma [47].

15.5 Hepatic Toxicity

Due to the unique mechanisms by which angiogenesis inhibitors work as compared to chemotherapeutic agents, their toxicity profiles are also unique. Angiogenesis and VEGF have been shown to play an important role in liver hypertrophy and healing after hepatic resection or chemical injury in several preclinical models [48–51]. This effect appears to be mediated through the increase in blood supply as well as through the regulation of other important growth factors. Furthermore, in several clinical studies, it has been shown that cytotoxic chemotherapy itself can lead to hepatic injury – including steatosis and sinusoidal congestion with a consequent increase in biliary complications following resection [52–54]. The addition of BV to systemic chemotherapy regimens may therefore lead to additional hepatic toxicity. Another unique and relevant property of BV is its very long half life. In contrast to standard chemotherapeutic agents (that have a relatively short half life, measured in minutes) the mean half-life of BV is approximately 20 days, ranging from 11 to 50 days. In addition, although BV doses of 5–10 mg/kg every 2 weeks are usually used, a dose as low as 0.3 mg/kg could reduce circulating VEGF to below detectable levels. Therefore, even after a period twice as long as the half-life (i.e. 25% activity) at a dose of 5–10 mg/kg, a significant amount of biologically active BV may still be present, reducing circulating VEGF to below detectable levels [55].

Remarkably however, there is no clinical evidence for a detrimental effect of BV on hepatic growth after resection. In general, BV was well tolerated when combined with chemotherapeutic agents, such as 5-FU, irinotecan and oxaliplatin [31, 42] in several large randomized trials, as well as observational studies. In the study by Gruenberger discussed above, patients who received neoadjuvant BV plus XELOX for up to 5 weeks prior to hepatic resection, had no apparent increase in biliary complications or impairment of liver regrowth as compared to historical data [43]. Similarly, in a study by D'Angelica, there was no increase in overall postoperative morbidity including biliary complications in patients having received preoperative BV, as compared to matched historical controls. In addition, estimated blood loss at the time of resection was actually decreased in patients who had received BV [56]. Reddy reported on 96 patients who received irinotecan or oxaliplatin-based neoadjuvant therapy (39 with BV) [57]. There was no difference in overall, severe, thromboembolic/bleeding or hepatic complications in those having received BV versus those who did not. Similar to the study by D'Angelica, preoperative BV treatment was also associated with less blood loss and lower transfusion rates after hepatic resection [57]. A study by Kesmodel et al. [58], reported on 81 patients who received chemotherapy plus BV versus 44 patients who received chemotherapy alone. In this retrospective study, there were no differences in the overall complication rate between the groups. In fact, there was a suggestion that biliary complications may actually be decreased in patients receiving BV as compared to those receiving chemotherapy alone (5% vs. 11%), although this did not reach statistical significance ($p = 0.28$) [58].

In combination with oxaliplatin regimens, BV may actually protect against sinusoidal obstruction syndrome (a known complication of oxaliplatin). In a study from Gruenbergers group, 50 patients who received oxaliplatin-based therapy were compared with the 56 patients (discussed above) who received BV-containing oxaliplatin regimens [59]. In this non-randomized study, the addition of BV led to a decrease in sinusoidal obstruction syndrome, as compared to oxaliplatin alone. Similarly, in another study by the group at M.D. Anderson, the addition of BV to 5-FU/oxaliplatin-based therapy also decreased the incidence and severity of hepatic sinusoidal injury while improving the overall pathologic response [60]. Although these results are intriguing, additional studies are needed to fully investigate the potential protective effect of BV on the liver. Nevertheless, with the data available, it does not appear that the addition of BV to systemic chemotherapy regimens leads to an increase in biliary complications or an impairment of hepatic regeneration, provided that BV is discontinued 5–8 weeks prior to hepatic resection.

The other potential complication of BV in association with hepatic resection is the potential effect on liver growth after portal vein embolization or occlusion (PVE/PVO), prior to resection. PVE is a technique that involves embolization of the portal vein supplying the lobe that is to be removed. The goal of this strategy is to divert portal flow away from the affected lobe while increasing the flow to the remaining lobe. This is performed when the future liver remnant (FLR) volume is too low to tolerate a major resection [61, 62]. Since VEGF and angiogenesis are important in liver hypertrophy and proliferation, the use of BV prior to PVE could potentially impair the growth of the FLR. The clinical evidence in support of this effect is however less clear. A study from M.D. Anderson reported on 65 patients who underwent PVE prior to resection [62]. Forty-three had received chemotherapy (26 with concurrent BV) and 22 had not. After a median of 4 weeks post PVE, there was no difference in the degree of FLR volume increase and liver growth among patients treated with or without chemotherapy or with or without BV. Furthermore, in agreement with other studies, there were no differences in morbidity or mortality amongst those patients who received chemotherapy or BV [62]. In contrast, however, a study from France suggested that hypertrophy after PVE may indeed be impaired by BV. In this prospective but non randomized study, 13 patients who received BV and chemotherapy prior to PVE were compared to 27 who received chemotherapy only [61]. In this study, the addition of BV to chemotherapy prior to PVE led to a significantly reduced increase in FLR volume as compared to the group having received chemotherapy alone [61]. At the time of resection, however, there were no differences in complications between the two groups. The different conclusions by these two studies may be due to a variety of reasons including the number of cycles of chemotherapy and BV received (which was higher in the French study), the mean age of the patients, as well as different volumetric techniques to calculate FLR volumes. Additional studies and experience using BV prior to PVE are needed before definitive conclusions can be reached. It is important to note, however, that the morbidity and mortality rates did not differ with the use of BV in either of these studies.

15.6 Conclusion

The liver remains the most common site of metastases from gastrointestinal malignancies. Angiogenesis has been shown to be an integral component in the development and progression of liver metastasis, as well as in liver growth and hypertrophy. VEGF is the best characterized proangiogenic factor and targeted therapy against VEGF with bevacizumab in combination with systemic chemotherapy has been shown to prolong survival in patients with metastatic colorectal cancer. In select patients, the use of bevacizumab with systemic chemotherapy may convert some unresectable hepatic metastases to potentially resectable tumors. Although the potential complications with the use of anti-VEGF therapy are significant and unique, clinical studies in general have suggested that the use of bevacizumab is safe and not associated with significant increases in complications. Many other anti-angiogenic agents remain in development and as data from ongoing clinical trials evolve, it is hoped that more targeted therapy options will exist for the treatment of hepatic metastases.

References

1. Alberts SR, Wagman LD (2008) Chemotherapy for colorectal cancer liver metastases. Oncologist 13:1063–1073
2. Scoggins CR, Campbell ML, Landry CS et al (2009) Preoperative chemotherapy does not increase morbidity or mortality of hepatic resection for colorectal cancer metastases. Ann Surg Oncol 16:35–41
3. Takahashi Y, Kitadai Y, Bucana CD, Cleary KR, Ellis LM (1995) Expression of vascular endothelial growth factor and its receptor, KDR, correlates with vascularity, metastasis, and proliferation of human colon cancer. Cancer Res 55:3964–3698
4. Warren RS, Yuan H, Matli MR, Gillett NA, Ferrara N (1995) Regulation by vascular endothelial growth factor of human colon cancer tumorigenesis in a mouse model of experimental liver metastasis. J Clin Invest 95:1789–97
5. Zuckerman DS, Clark JW (2008) Systemic therapy for metastatic colorectal cancer: current questions. Cancer 112:1879–1891
6. Duff SE, Jeziorska M, Rosa DD et al (2006) Vascular endothelial growth factors and receptors in colorectal cancer: implications for anti-angiogenic therapy. Eur J Cancer 42:112–117
7. Garcea G, Lloyd TD, Gescher A, Dennison AR, Steward WP, Berry DP (2004) Angiogenesis of gastrointestinal tumours and their metastases–a target for intervention? Eur J Cancer 40:1302–1313
8. Pourreyron C, Poncet G, Roche C et al (2008) The role of angiogenesis in endocrine liver metastases: an experimental study. J Surg Res 144:64–73
9. Reinmuth N, Parikh AA, Ahmad SA et al (2003) Biology of angiogenesis in tumors of the gastrointestinal tract. Microsc Res Tech 60:199–207
10. Folkman J (1990) What is the evidence that tumors are angiogenesis dependent? J Natl Cancer Inst 82:4–6
11. Folkman J (1995) Angiogenesis in cancer, vascular, rheumatoid and other disease. Nat Med 1:27–31
12. Takeda A, Stoeltzing O, Ahmad SA et al (2002) Role of angiogenesis in the development and growth of liver metastasis. Ann Surg Oncol 9:610–616

13. Zetter BR (1998) Angiogenesis and tumor metastasis. Annu Rev Med 49:407–24
14. Stoeltzing O, Liu W, Reinmuth N et al (2003) Angiogenesis and antiangiogenic therapy of colon cancer liver metastasis. Ann Surg Oncol 10:722–733
15. Ellis LM, Hicklin DJ (2008) VEGF-targeted therapy: mechanisms of anti-tumour activity. Nat Rev Cancer 8:579–591
16. Gaur P, Bose D, Samuel S, Ellis LM (2009) Targeting tumor angiogenesis. Semin Oncol 36:S12–S19
17. Lee JC, Chow NH, Wang ST, Huang SM (2000) Prognostic value of vascular endothelial growth factor expression in colorectal cancer patients. Eur J Cancer 36:748–753
18. Terris B, Scoazec JY, Rubbia L et al (1998) Expression of vascular endothelial growth factor in digestive neuroendocrine tumours. Histopathology 32:133–138
19. Zhang J, Jia Z, Li Q et al (2007) Elevated expression of vascular endothelial growth factor correlates with increased angiogenesis and decreased progression-free survival among patients with low-grade neuroendocrine tumors. Cancer 109:1478–1486
20. Bauer TW, Fan F, Liu W et al (2007) Targeting of insulin-like growth factor-I receptor with a monoclonal antibody inhibits growth of hepatic metastases from human colon carcinoma in mice. Ann Surg Oncol 14:2838–2846
21. Cao Y (2009) Tumor angiogenesis and molecular targets for therapy. Front Biosci 14: 3962–3973
22. Meyers MO, Watson JC (2003) Angiogenesis and hepatic colorectal metastases. Surg Oncol Clin N Am 12:151–63
23. Mi J, Sarraf-Yazdi S, Zhang X et al (2006) A comparison of antiangiogenic therapies for the prevention of liver metastases. J Surg Res 131:97–104
24. Kanai T, Konno H, Tanaka T et al (1998) Anti-tumor and anti-metastatic effects of human-vascular-endothelial-growth-factor-neutralizing antibody on human colon and gastric carcinoma xenotransplanted orthotopically into nude mice. Int J Cancer 77:933–936
25. Gerber HP, Ferrara N (2005) Pharmacology and pharmacodynamics of bevacizumab as monotherapy or in combination with cytotoxic therapy in preclinical studies. Cancer Res 65:671–680
26. Konno H, Arai T, Tanaka T et al (1998) Antitumor effect of a neutralizing antibody to vascular endothelial growth factor on liver metastasis of endocrine neoplasm. Jpn J Cancer Res 89: 933–939
27. Grothey A, Sugrue MM, Purdie DM et al (2008) Bevacizumab beyond first progression is associated with prolonged overall survival in metastatic colorectal cancer: results from a large observational cohort study (BRiTE). J Clin Oncol 26:5326–5334
28. Kinuya S, Yokoyama K, Koshida K et al (2004) Improved survival of mice bearing liver metastases of colon cancer cells treated with a combination of radioimmunotherapy and antiangiogenic therapy. Eur J Nucl Med Mol Imaging 31:981–985
29. Van Cutsem E, Rivera F, Berry S et al (2009) Safety and efficacy of first-line bevacizumab with FOLFOX, XELOX, FOLFIRI and fluoropyrimidines in metastatic colorectal cancer: the BEAT study. Ann Oncol 20:1842–1847
30. Mross K, Drevs J, Muller M et al (2005) Phase I clinical and pharmacokinetic study of PTK/ZK, a multiple VEGF receptor inhibitor, in patients with liver metastases from solid tumours. Eur J Cancer 41:1291–1299
31. Hurwitz H, Fehrenbacher L, Novotny W et al (2004) Bevacizumab plus irinotecan, fluorouracil, and leucovorin for metastatic colorectal cancer. N Engl J Med 350: 2335–2342
32. Miller K, Wang M, Gralow J et al (2007) Paclitaxel plus bevacizumab versus paclitaxel alone for metastatic breast cancer. N Engl J Med 357:2666–2676
33. Sandler A, Gray R, Perry MC et al (2006) Paclitaxel-carboplatin alone or with bevacizumab for non-small-cell lung cancer. N Engl J Med 355:2542–2550
34. Papapetropoulos A, Garcia-Cardena G, Dengler TJ, Maisonpierre PC, Yancopoulos GD, Sessa WC (1999) Direct actions of angiopoietin-1 on human endothelium: evidence for network

stabilization, cell survival, and interaction with other angiogenic growth factors. Lab Invest 79:213–223

35. Stoeltzing O, Ahmad SA, Liu W et al (2003) Angiopoietin-1 inhibits vascular permeability, angiogenesis, and growth of hepatic colon cancer tumors. Cancer Res 63:3370–3377

36. Giancotti FG, Ruoslahti E (1999) Integrin signaling. Science 285:1028–1032

37. Stoeltzing O, Liu W, Reinmuth N et al (2003) Inhibition of integrin alpha5beta1 function with a small peptide (ATN-161) plus continuous 5-FU infusion reduces colorectal liver metastases and improves survival in mice. Int J Cancer 104:496–503

38. Reinmuth N, Liu W, Ahmad SA et al (2003) Alphavbeta3 integrin antagonist S247 decreases colon cancer metastasis and angiogenesis and improves survival in mice. Cancer Res 63: 2079–2087

39. Daruwalla J, Nikfarjam M, Malcontenti-Wilson C, Muralidharan V, Christophi C (2005) Effect of thalidomide on colorectal cancer liver metastases in CBA mice. J Surg Oncol 91:134–140

40. te Velde EA, Reijerkerk A, Brandsma D et al (2005) Early endostatin treatment inhibits metastatic seeding of murine colorectal cancer cells in the liver and their adhesion to endothelial cells. Br J Cancer 92:729–735

41. Emmanouilides C, Sfakiotaki G, Androulakis N et al (2007) Front-line bevacizumab in combination with oxaliplatin, leucovorin and 5-fluorouracil (FOLFOX) in patients with metastatic colorectal cancer: a multicenter phase II study. BMC Cancer 7:91

42. Saltz LB, Clarke S, Diaz-Rubio E et al (2008) Bevacizumab in combination with oxaliplatin-based chemotherapy as first-line therapy in metastatic colorectal cancer: a randomized phase III study. J Clin Oncol 26:2013–2019

43. Gruenberger B, Tamandl D, Schueller J et al (2008) Bevacizumab, capecitabine, and oxaliplatin as neoadjuvant therapy for patients with potentially curable metastatic colorectal cancer. J Clin Oncol 26:1830–1835

44. Abood GJ, Go A, Malhotra D, Shoup M (2009) The surgical and systemic management of neuroendocrine tumors of the pancreas. Surg Clin North Am 89:249–266, x

45. Metz DC, Jensen RT (2008) Gastrointestinal neuroendocrine tumors: pancreatic endocrine tumors. Gastroenterology 135:1469–1492

46. Pasieka JL (2009) Carcinoid tumors. Surg Clin North Am 89:1123–1137

47. Yao JC, Phan A, Hoff PM et al (2008) Targeting vascular endothelial growth factor in advanced carcinoid tumor: a random assignment phase II study of depot octreotide with bevacizumab and pegylated interferon alpha-2b. J Clin Oncol 26:1316–1323

48. Assy N, Spira G, Paizi M et al (1999) Effect of vascular endothelial growth factor on hepatic regenerative activity following partial hepatectomy in rats. J Hepatol 30:911–915

49. Ellis LM, Curley SA, Grothey A (2005) Surgical resection after downsizing of colorectal liver metastasis in the era of bevacizumab. J Clin Oncol 23:4853–4855

50. Furnus CC, Inda AM, Andrini LB et al (2003) Chronobiology of the proliferative events related to angiogenesis in mice liver regeneration after partial hepatectomy. Cell Biol Int 27:383–386

51. Kraizer Y, Mawasi N, Seagal J, Paizi M, Assy N, Spira G (2001) Vascular endothelial growth factor and angiopoietin in liver regeneration. Biochem Biophys Res Commun 287: 209–215

52. Aloia T, Sebagh M, Plasse M et al (2006) Liver histology and surgical outcomes after preoperative chemotherapy with fluorouracil plus oxaliplatin in colorectal cancer liver metastases. J Clin Oncol 24:4983–4990

53. Parikh AA, Gentner B, Wu TT, Curley SA, Ellis LM, Vauthey JN (2003) Perioperative complications in patients undergoing major liver resection with or without neoadjuvant chemotherapy. J Gastrointest Surg 7:1082–1088

54. Vauthey JN, Pawlik TM, Ribero D et al (2006) Chemotherapy regimen predicts steatohepatitis and an increase in 90-day mortality after surgery for hepatic colorectal metastases. J Clin Oncol 24:2065–2072

55. Parikh AA, Ellis LM (2008) Targeted therapies and surgical issues in gastrointestinal cancers. Target Oncol 3:119–125
56. D'Angelica M, Kornprat P, Gonen M et al (2007) Lack of evidence for increased operative morbidity after hepatectomy with perioperative use of bevacizumab: a matched case-control study. Ann Surg Oncol 14:759–765
57. Reddy SK, Morse MA, Hurwitz HI et al (2008) Addition of bevacizumab to irinotecan- and oxaliplatin-based preoperative chemotherapy regimens does not increase morbidity after resection of colorectal liver metastases. J Am Coll Surg 206:96–106
58. Kesmodel SB, Ellis LM, Lin E et al (2008) Preoperative bevacizumab does not significantly increase postoperative complication rates in patients undergoing hepatic surgery for colorectal cancer liver metastases. J Clin Oncol 26:5254–5260
59. Klinger M, Eipeldauer S, Hacker S et al (2009) Bevacizumab protects against sinusoidal obstruction syndrome and does not increase response rate in neoadjuvant XELOX/FOLFOX therapy of colorectal cancer liver metastases. Eur J Surg Oncol 35:515–520
60. Ribero D, Wang H, Donadon M et al (2007) Bevacizumab improves pathologic response and protects against hepatic injury in patients treated with oxaliplatin-based chemotherapy for colorectal liver metastases. Cancer 110:2761–2767
61. Aussilhou B, Dokmak S, Faivre S, Paradis V, Vilgrain V, Belghiti J (2009) Preoperative liver hypertrophy induced by portal flow occlusion before major hepatic resection for colorectal metastases can be impaired by bevacizumab. Ann Surg Oncol 16:1553–1559
62. Zorzi D, Chun YS, Madoff DC, Abdalla EK, Vauthey JN (2008) Chemotherapy with bevacizumab does not affect liver regeneration after portal vein embolization in the treatment of colorectal liver metastases. Ann Surg Oncol 15:2765–2772

Chapter 16
Uveal Melanoma – A Paradigm of Site-Specific Liver Metastasis

Bruno F. Fernandes and Miguel N. Burnier Jr.

Abstract Uveal melanoma is the most frequent intra-ocular malignant tumor encountered in adults. Despite the advances in the initial diagnosis and treatment of the primary tumor, the mortality rates remain unchanged for the last several decades. This may be explained by the past and present treatment modalities, which target only the primary tumor. A systemic approach is required in uveal melanoma, a malignancy in which the cellular events leading to malignant transformation and progression are not well characterized. Metastatic melanoma has a clear predilection for the liver, which is involved in almost all patients and is often the first and only affected site. By exploring molecular pathways involved in the metastatic cascade, it may be possible to develop new strategies in the search for new therapeutic targets to treat metastatic uveal melanoma.

Keywords Uveal melanoma · Liver metastasis · Molecular targets · Circulating malignant cells · Metastasis suppressor genes

Abbreviations

UM	uveal melanoma
CMCs	circulating malignant cells
MRNA	messenger ribonucleic acid
RT-PCR	reverse transcriptase – polymerase chain reaction
HGF	hepatocyte growth factor
IGF-1	INSULIN-like growth factor
Grb2	growth factor receptor-bound protein 2
PI3-K	phosphatidylinositol 3-kinase
IRS	insulin-receptor substrate
ECM	extracellular matrix
PPP	picropodophyllin

B.F. Fernandes (✉)
Department of Ophthalmology, McGill University Health Center, McGill University,
3775 University Street, Room 216, Montreal, QC, Canada
e-mail: bruno.mtl@gmail.com

P. Brodt (ed.), *Liver Metastasis: Biology and Clinical Management*, Cancer
Metastasis – Biology and Treatment 16, DOI 10.1007/978-94-007-0292-9_16,
© Springer Science+Business Media B.V. 2011

SDF-1   stromal cell-derived factor-1
GAB-1   GRB2-associated-binding protein 1
APS   adapter protein with a pleckstrin homology (PH) and Src homology 2
         (SH2) domain
MAP   mitogen-activated protein
B RAF   V-raf murine sarcoma viral oncogene homolog B1
MSG   metastasis suppressor gene

Contents

16.1 Introduction

Uveal melanoma (UM) is the most common primary intraocular malignant tumor in adults, with an incidence of seven to nine cases per million in the western world [1]. Tumors arise in the uveal tract, which is comprised of the iris, ciliary body, and the choroid (Fig. 16.1). In contrast to skin melanoma, epidemiological studies have failed to show an association between exposure to sunlight and an increased incidence of UM [2–5]. Despite this lack of correlation, recent studies have implicated blue light exposure as a possible risk factor for uveal melanoma, but further studies are necessary to draw definitive conclusions [6–8].

Histopathologically, UMs are composed of spindle, epithelioid cells or a combination of both. The Callender's classification, modified at the Armed Forces Institute of Pathology (AFIP), is one of the most reliable prognosticators; tumors composed exclusively of spindle cells carry a better prognosis than those that contain epithelioid cells in any proportion [9, 10]. Tumor size, lymphocytic infiltration, vascular loops and cytomorphometry are some of the other histopathological features with prognostic relevance.

There are currently several modalities of treatment for primary UM. Historically, UM has been treated by enucleation of the affected globe, which in addition to loss of vision also requires the implantation of prosthesis. This has been supplanted by the use of globe-sparing treatments such as plaque radiotherapy, where a shield containing seeds of a radioactive isotope such as ruthenium or iodine is sutured to the sclera at the base of the tumor. No significant differences in patient mortality have

Fig. 16.1 A macroscopic image of an enucleated eye harboring a uveal melanoma. The tumor is seen as a pigmented *dome-shaped* mass with associated retinal detachment

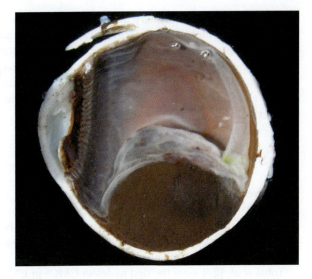

been documented when using either treatment options [11]. The majority of patients are treated by plaque radiotherapy, although a percentage of patients still undergo enucleation due to failure of the primary treatment or large tumor dimensions at the time of diagnosis. While treatment of the primary tumor is well established and usually results in high rates of local control and globe preservation, treating metastatic disease is a much more daunting task.

16.2 Liver Metastasis

At the time of diagnosis, very few patients present with clinically detectable metastatic lesions [12]. The outlook for patients becomes increasingly poor as follow-up time increases. Despite advances in the diagnosis and treatment of the primary tumor, the five-year mortality rate for UM patients has not changed significantly [13]. The survival rates at 5, 10 and 15 years are 65, 52 and 46%, respectively [14, 15]. The principal target organ for metastasis is the liver, involved in 71.4–87% of patients with metastatic disease [16–18]. The liver is the exclusive site of systemic metastasis in approximately 40% of the patients and is often the first metastatic site [19]. Unfortunately, when liver metastases are diagnosed, treatment options are limited and life expectancy is poor. Reports have differed on the median survival time, ranging between 2.2 and 12.5 months which probably reflects technological advances in finding metastases earlier [12, 18]. Minor improvements have been seen in some patients treated by surgical resection of liver metastases or by intra-hepatic arterial chemotherapy. Clinical trials assessing potential therapeutic agents, such as dacarbazine, treosulfan, in combination with gemcitabine, thalidomide with interferon alpha 2β, temoxolomide and 9-nitrocamtothecin, have also been disappointing with only minor improvements in survival of some patients [20–24].

Cells that escape the primary tumor do so by haematogenous dissemination, due to the lack of lymphatics in the eye [25]. The predominance of liver metastases cannot be explained solely by mechanical factors related to the circulation, as the lungs are the first set of capillary beds that these cells would encounter. Therefore, uveal melanoma offers a unique setting to study the haematogenous dissemination of cells and the subsequent homing of these cells, or their preferential survival, in the liver of patients.

16.3 Systemic Disease

The presence of circulating malignant cells (CMCs) in the peripheral blood is revealed by the detection of mRNA specific to neoplastic cells using quantitative real-time RT-PCR. Tyrosinase alone or with melan-A is the preferred markers for UM. Their expression in the primary tumor is high, with no correlation to prognostic factors or previous radiotherapy [26].

Tobal et al. [27] were the first to detect CMCs in UM patients. Subsequent studies found a correlation of CMCs with worst prognosis and eventual development of metastases [28–30]. Schuster et al. analyzed 110 patients with high-risk primary UM with a median follow-up of 22 months. Five of 11 PCR-positive patients (45%) relapsed and three died during the first year, in comparison with five relapses (5%) and no deaths in 99 PCR-negative patients. The detection of tyrosinase and melan-A transcripts in the peripheral blood of patients with UM was shown to be an independent prognostic factor for the development of metastases and survival [30]. Boldin et al. [28] studied a smaller cohort but with a minimal follow-up of 5 years. A prognostic value for these markers was also suggested by their studies.

In contrast, Callejo et al. [31] published a prospective study where 30 UM patients, without metastatic disease were tested every 3 months. Twenty-nine out of 30 patients had at least one positive test. CMCs could be identified in patients independently of tumor size; type of treatment (local radiation or enucleation) or period of time after the tumor was diagnosed. In other words, almost all patients had CMCs present in their blood, at some point in time during the study period. The discrepancy between these results and other studies may be explained by the different methodology applied. In this particular clinical study, Callejo et al. [31] performed multiple samplings, had a larger volume of blood per sample, and used two markers, melan-A and tyrosinase. The presence of CMCs in patients with small UM supports the idea that the dissemination occurs early, even before the primary lesion is diagnosed [32]. Knowing that neoplastic cells cannot survive more than a few hours in the circulation [33], it was of interest that CMCs were found even in patients that had been enucleated several years earlier. It may well be possible that CMCs are able to colonize distant organs, remain dormant for several years and sporadically seed new tumor cells into the circulation [34]. It is also of note that serial blood sampling showed negative results between two positive tests in the same patient, suggesting that the presence of neoplastic cells in the peripheral blood is not constant.

Although the method currently used is highly sensitive and can detect a single cell per ml of blood, it is conceivable that individual samplings may not contain UM cells even if those are present in the circulation. As the likelihood of detecting CMCs increases with tumor load, even a single positive test could have a prognostic significance, as shown in some studies [28–30]. Alternatively, a negative result may be due to loss of expression of the particular markers analyzed by RT-PCR. Studies using genetic profiling showed that while some genes are overexpressed during metastatic progression, others are downregulated. The latter group included markers of melanocytic differentiation such as Melan-A [35].

It is interesting to note that not all patients with positive CMCs developed metastasis during the study period. The intravasation of malignant cells is just one of the steps of the metastatic cascade. Reaching distant organs, extravasation, favorable interaction with the target organ microenvironment and establishment of a micrometastatic focus are subsequent necessary events for development of metastases [36]. During malignant progression, subpopulations of tumor cells within the developing tumor mass may have different gene expression profiles that could affect their metastatic potentials [37]. Molecular studies were able to identify patterns of gene expression in primary UM cells that could predict the development of metastases [38]. It is also important to understand the genetic variability within CMCs. Marshall et al. [39] studied changes in gene expression profiles of UM during malignant progression in an animal model. Recultured CMCs showed a gene expression profile distinct from the primary tumor and the metastases, suggesting that these cells represent an intermediate subpopulation in the metastatic cascade [40]. Therefore, it is likely that even after the malignant cells reach the systemic circulation, only a small proportion will have the appropriate "molecular machinery" to successfully form a metastasis [37]. For UM, the liver is the preferred site of metastasis even in the face of CMCs and this suggests that it is the most permissive organ for UM colonization and survival. This may be due to specific cross-talk signals between CMCs and the liver that create a microenvironment favorable for metastatic colonization and growth [41]. The isolation of CMCs from patients and the study of genetic changes involved in disease progression will provide insight into molecular mechanisms involved in this process and answer some of these questions.

16.4 Molecular Mediators of UM Progression and Metastasis

Several molecular mediators and downstream signaling pathways have been implicated in liver metastasis of UM. An understanding of these molecular pathways could lead to new opportunities to halt disease progression through molecular targeting in uveal melanoma and potentially other malignancies that disseminate haematogenously to the liver. It seems unlikely, given the evidence, that targeting only one of these molecular mediators would not be sufficient to improve patient survival [42] and a combined approach may therefore be required to achieve this goal.

16.4.1 HGF/SF and C-Met

One of the molecules that have long been implicated in specific growth of cells in the liver is the hepatocyte growth factor (HGF), also known as scatter factor, and its corresponding receptor, C-Met. Expression of C-Met by UM cells was shown to correlate with their expression of epithelial specific cytokeratin, previously described as the interconverted phenotype [43, 44].

Studies have shown that increased levels of C-Met expression in primary tumors significantly increased patients' risk of developing liver metastases [45]. UM cells have also been shown to be highly motile and invasive when HGF was used as a motility factor [46, 47]. The exposure of UM cells to tumor associated macrophages, the presence of which is an indicator of worse prognosis in UM, was also shown to increase the expression of HGF [48].

Upon activation of C-Met by HGF, C-Met is autophosphorylated on two tyrosine residues: Tyr 1234 and Tyr 1235. This results in the formation of a docking site for intracellular adapter proteins such as growth factor receptor bound protein 2 (Grb2), recruitment/activation of phosphatidylinositol 3-kinase (PI3-K), Shc, and Src [49] and activation of multiple downstream signaling pathways, including the Ras/Raf/ERK pathway. This leads to transcriptional activation, increased cellular proliferation, cell cycle progression, protection from apoptosis, cell motility and invasion [49].

However, the expression of HGF alone does not explain the predominance of liver-specific metastasis. A study by Economou et al. described the inter-relationship of insulin like growth factor 1 receptor (IGF1R) and C-Met expression in UM samples [50]. Interestingly, while the co-expression of these two molecules was highly predictive of liver metastasis by univariate analysis, only IGF-1R expression had a significant prognostic value when analyzed by multivariate analysis [50].

16.4.2 IGF-1 and IGF-1R

Other molecules of interest in UM are the insulin like growth factor 1 (IGF-1) and its receptor, expression of which has been shown to correlate with large tumor size [51] and worse prognosis [52]. Similar to HGF, IGF-1 is mainly produced by the liver and this may help explain the preferential growth of UM cells in this organ. IGF-1 binds to IGF-1R, a heterotetrameric plasma membrane glycoprotein, which is composed of two alpha and two beta subunits [53]. When stimulated by ligand binding, the intrinsic tyrosine kinase of the beta subunit is activated and phosphorylation of several intracellular proteins takes place [54] (The reader is referred to Chapter 9 for a more detailed discussion on the role of the IGF axis in liver metastasis).

At least nine substrates of the insulin/IGF-1 receptors have been described. It is believed that the phosphorylation of these diverse substrates may have different cellular effects depending on the substrate that is activated [55]. Activation of IGF-1R has been shown to play a role in cellular proliferation, protection from apoptosis, migration, integrin mediated adhesion to the ECM and invasion of basement membranes [56]. These are all essential steps in the formation of metastases. Among the downstream pathways that can be stimulated by IGF-1R is the phosphorylation of Akt via phosphatidylinositol 3-kinase (PI3-K). Phosphorylated Akt has also been shown to be a prognostic indicator of increased metastasis in patients with uveal melanoma. It is possible that this increased mortality rate may reflect the activation of Akt through the IGF-1 receptor pathway. Other downstream pathway which have been shown to be activated by IGF-1R is the Ras/mitogen-activated protein kinase (MAP kinase) pathway [55].

In vitro studies demonstrated a significant association between IGF-1R activity and cell proliferation and cell survival of uveal melanoma cells [52]. Moreover, it was shown that inhibition of N-linked glycosylation induced by treatment with tunicamycin and lovastatin caused decreased IGF-1R expression and consequently decreased tyrosine phosphorylation, inducing growth arrest and cell death in the three investigated uveal melanoma cell lines [52]. The use of IGF-1R as a potential therapeutic target has been confirmed by targeting this pathway with cyclolignan picropodophyllin (PPP) – a specific inhibitor of IGF-1R tyrosine phosphorylation. This was shown to cause tumor regression in a xenograft mouse model of UM [57].

16.4.3 CXCR4 and CXCL12

An emerging field of study has been the role of chemokines in tumor cell homing to sites of metastasis; of these the CXCL12 or stromal derived factor-1 (SDF1) may be the most relevant for UM. The major receptor for CXCL12 is CXCR4, a cell surface G protein-coupled seven span transmembrane receptor [58]. Expression of this receptor has been documented in different cancer types, including breast, prostate and colon carcinomas [59–61]. Currently, CXCL12 is the only ligand that has been described for CXCR4, which makes it unique among chemokines and chemokine receptors that typically can have several potential receptors and ligands, respectively [62] (see Chapter 5 in this volume for a review on the role of chemokines in liver metastasis).

Binding of CXCL12 by CXCR4 can lead to activation of several intracellular signal transduction pathways and the regulation of cellular survival, proliferation, migration and adhesion [63]. Among the pathways activated is the PI3-K pathway leading to Akt phosphorylation. As mentioned above, activated Akt is associated with worse prognosis in uveal melanoma and plays a role in cell proliferation and migration [64]. Other pathways of interest that have been shown to be activated by CXCL12/CXCR4 are the MAP kinase and JAK/STAT signaling pathways. Activation of the MAP kinase pathway is common in uveal melanoma, although a report by Zuidervaart et al. [65] showed that in contrast to cutaneous melanoma, this pathway is seldom activated by B-Raf or Ras. Future experiments will have to be carried out to establish whether the frequently observed MAP kinase activation in UM is due to CXCL12 signaling, IGF-1R [51], c-Met or involves other ligands.

Potential candidates would include the proangiogenic vascular endothelial growth factor (VEGF) [66] or a crosstalk with the PI3K/PTEN/AKT pathway [67].

Recently, it has been shown that cancer cells that express CXCR4 can migrate and intravasate in response to CXCL12 [68]. For example in an animal model of breast cancer, inhibition of the CXCR4/CXCL12 axis by a synthetic CXCR4 antagonist inhibited metastasis of the human breast carcinoma MDA-MB-231 cells [68]. It has been proposed that the CXCR4/CXCL12 mono-axis also plays a critical role in the migration of (CXCR4 positive) CMCs to organ sites where CXCL12 production is high such as the bone, brain, lungs and most importantly, the liver [59]. Recent work has shown that, while CXCL12 is not typically expressed in UM cells lines, expression of CXCR4 was detectable in clinical UM specimens and its expression correlated with markers of poor prognosis [46, 69], suggesting the UM cells could respond to organ-site derived CXCL12. Additional work will be required to identify chemokine/chemokine receptor pathways involved in UM metastasis and establish whether CXCL12 plays a role in liver-specific metastasis of this malignancy.

16.4.4 KISS1

When disseminated tumor cells reach the target organ, they can undergo apoptosis, proliferate and form metastases or remain dormant for years (Fig. 16.2). Tumor dormancy, namely, the prolonged survival of single cells or small micrometastases without apparent progression for extended periods of time has long been recognized clinically, particularly in breast and prostate cancers and melanoma [70, 71] (the reader is referred to Chapter 8 in this volume for an extensive discussion of the mechanisms of tumor dormancy) . Metastasis suppressor genes (MSGs) that have been identified can selectively suppress the formation of spontaneous, macroscopic metastases without affecting the growth rate of the primary tumors [72]. One of these MSGs, KISS1, is thought to be involved in tumor growth suppression during the dormancy phase. KISS1 encodes a 145-amino acid residue peptide that is further processed. One of the products, the 54-amino acid peptide named Metastin or Kisspeptin-54 is a natural ligand of a G-coupled receptor known as HOT7T175/AXOR12/GPR54 [73]. Although its mechanisms of action remain elusive, experimental evidence shows that KISS1 secretion is required for multiple organ metastasis suppression and for maintenance of disseminated cells in a dormant state [74].

The KISS1 gene was identified as a metastasis suppressor gene in human melanoma and breast cancer cells [72]. Nash et al. were the first to show that the introduction of *KISS1* into highly metastatic human melanoma cell lines C8161 and MelJuSo suppressed lung metastasis by more than 95% [75, 76]. Furthermore, introduction of *KISS1* into the metastatic breast cancer cell line MDA-MB-435 also resulted in a >95% suppression of metastases to the lung [77]. On the other hand, loss of KISS1 mRNA expression was shown to correlate with progression from the benign to the malignant phenotype in human melanoma [78].

Fig. 16.2 Evidence for uveal melanoma dormancy in a nude mouse model of hematogenous dissemination. Intravital microscopy of the liver reveals the presence of solitary, *green fluorescent protein*-tagged uveal melanoma cells 6 weeks after intravenous tumor cell injection, suggesting that these cells may have entered a state of dormancy

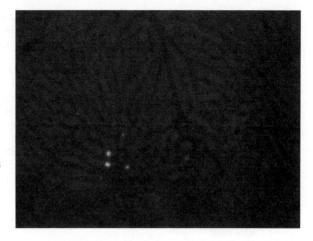

We have recently shown that KISS1 is also expressed in human UM. Eighty-four percent of the paraffin embedded specimens examined were positive for KISS1. Moreover, there was a statistically significant association between KISS1 expression levels and patient's survival. Namely, no cases of metastasis were found in a total of 12 patients whose tumors were highly KISS1 positive while in a group of 25 patients with low KISS1 staining, 13 (52%) had liver metastases [79].

16.5 Future Directions

The focus of uveal melanoma research has shifted to early detection and treatment of metastatic disease. Eventhough advances in the diagnosis and treatment of the primary tumor are essential, no impact on the prognosis is likely to be based on improved management of the primary tumor alone. The study of CMCs in UM provides evidence that the systemic dissemination of the tumor occurs before diagnosis and treatment of the primary tumors. By exploring the mechanisms involved in the metastatic cascade, it may be possible to develop new strategies and identify new therapeutic targets for the treatment of metastatic uveal melanoma.

References

1. Egan KM et al (1988) Epidemiologic aspects of uveal melanoma. Surv Ophthalmol 32: 239–251
2. Ivry GB, Ogle CA, Shim EK (2006) Role of sun exposure in melanoma. Dermatol Surg 32:481–492
3. Shah CP et al (2005) Intermittent and chronic ultraviolet light exposure and uveal melanoma: a meta-analysis. Ophthalmology 112:1599–1607
4. Holly EA et al (1990) Uveal melanoma in relation to ultraviolet light exposure and host factors. Cancer Res 50:5773–5777

5. Seddon JM et al (1983) A prognostic factor study of disease-free interval and survival following enucleation for uveal melanoma. Arch Ophthalmol 101:1894–1899

6. Manning WS Jr, Greenlee PG, Norton JN (2004) Ocular melanoma in a Long Evans rat. Contemp Top Lab Anim Sci 43:44–46

7. Fernandes BF, Marshall JC, Burnier MN Jr (2006) Blue light exposure and uveal melanoma. Ophthalmology 113:1062 e1; author reply 1062

8. Marshall JC et al (2006) The effect of blue light exposure and use of intraocular lenses on human uveal melanoma cell lines. Melanoma Res 16:537–541

9. Callender GR (1931) Malignant melanotic tumors of the eye: a study of histologic types of 111 cases. Trans Am Acad Ophthalmol Otolaryngol 36:131–142

10. McLean IW et al (1983) Modifications of Callender's classification of uveal melanoma at the Armed Forces Institute of Pathology. Am J Ophthalmol 96:502–509

11. Diener-West M et al (2001) The COMS randomized trial of iodine 125 brachytherapy for choroidal melanoma, III: initial mortality findings. COMS Report No. 18. Arch Ophthalmol 119:969–982

12. Rietschel P et al (2005) Variates of survival in metastatic uveal melanoma. J Clin Oncol 23:8076–8080

13. Singh AD, Topham A (2003) Survival rates with uveal melanoma in the United States: 1973–1997. Ophthalmology 110:962–965

14. Jensen OA (1982) Malignant melanomas of the human uvea: 25-year follow-up of cases in Denmark, 1943–1952. Acta Ophthalmol (Copenh) 60:161–182

15. Raivio I (1977) Uveal melanoma in Finland. An epidemiological, clinical, histological and prognostic study. Acta Ophthalmol Suppl 133:1–64

16. Kath R et al (1993) Prognosis and treatment of disseminated uveal melanoma. Cancer 72:2219–2223

17. Lorigan JG, Wallace S, Mavligit GM (1991) The prevalence and location of metastases from ocular melanoma: imaging study in 110 patients. AJR Am J Roentgenol 157:1279–1281

18. Rajpal S, Moore R, Karakousis CP (1983) Survival in metastatic ocular melanoma. Cancer 52:334–336

19. Bedikian AY (2006) Metastatic uveal melanoma therapy: current options. Int Ophthalmol Clin 46:151–166

20. O'Neill PA et al (2006) A prospective single arm phase II study of dacarbazine and treosulfan as first-line therapy in metastatic uveal melanoma. Melanoma Res 16:245–248

21. Schmittel A et al (2005) A two-cohort phase II clinical trial of gemcitabine plus treosulfan in patients with metastatic uveal melanoma. Melanoma Res 15:447–451

22. Solti M et al (2007) A pilot study of low-dose thalidomide and interferon alpha-2b in patients with metastatic melanoma who failed prior treatment. Melanoma Res 17:225–231

23. Bedikian AY et al (2003) Phase II evaluation of temozolomide in metastatic choroidal melanoma. Melanoma Res 13:303–306

24. Ellerhorst JA et al (2002) Phase II trial of 9-nitrocamptothecin (RFS 2000) for patients with metastatic cutaneous or uveal melanoma. Anticancer Drugs 13:169–172

25. Woll E, Bedikian A, Legha SS (1999) Uveal melanoma: natural history and treatment options for metastatic disease. Melanoma Res 9:575–581

26. Fernandes BF et al (2007) Immunohistochemical expression of melan-A and tyrosinase in uveal melanoma. J Carcinog 6:6

27. Tobal K et al (1993) Detection of melanocytes from uveal melanoma in peripheral blood using the polymerase chain reaction. Invest Ophthalmol Vis Sci 34:2622–2625

28. Boldin I et al (2005) Five-year results of prognostic value of tyrosinase in peripheral blood of uveal melanoma patients. Melanoma Res 15:503–507

29. Keilholz U et al (2004) Quantitative detection of circulating tumor cells in cutaneous and ocular melanoma and quality assessment by real-time reverse transcriptase-polymerase chain reaction. Clin Cancer Res 10:1605–1612

30. Schuster R et al (2007) Circulating tumor cells as prognostic factor for distant metastases and survival in patients with primary uveal melanoma. Clin Cancer Res 13:1171–1178

31. Callejo SA et al (2006) Identification of circulating malignant cells and its correlation with prognostic factors and treatment in uveal melanoma. A prospective longitudinal study. Eye (Lond) Jun 21:752–759. Epub 31 Mar 2006

32. Eskelin S et al (2000) Tumor doubling times in metastatic malignant melanoma of the Uvea: tumor progression before and after treatment. Ophthalmology 107:1443–1449

33. Fidler IJ (1970) Metastasis: quantitative analysis of distribution and fate of tumor embolilabeled with 125 I-5-iodo-2'-deoxyuridine. J Natl Cancer Inst 45:773–782

34. Demicheli R et al (1994) Local recurrences following mastectomy: support for the concept of tumor dormancy. J Natl Cancer Inst 86:45–48

35. Marshall J-CA et al (2005) Transcriptional profiling of the evolution of uveal melanoma from cell lines to intraocular tumors to metastasis. Invest Ophthalmol Vis Sci 46:E-Abstract 3390

36. Fidler IJ (2003) The pathogenesis of cancer metastasis: the 'seed and soil' hypothesis revisited. Nat Rev Cancer 3:453–458

37. Fidler IJ, Kripke ML (1977) Metastasis results from preexisting variant cells within a malignant tumor. Science 197:893–895

38. Onken MD et al (2004) Gene expression profiling in uveal melanoma reveals two molecular classes and predicts metastatic death. Cancer Res 64:7205–7209

39. Blanco PL et al (2005) Characterization of ocular and metastatic uveal melanoma in an animal model. Invest Ophthalmol Vis Sci 46:4376–4382

40. Marshall JC et al (2007) Transcriptional profiling of human uveal melanoma from cell lines to intraocular tumors to metastasis. Clin Exp Metastasis 24:353–362

41. Dittmar T et al (2007) Adhesion molecules and chemokines: the navigation system for circulating tumor (stem) cells to metastasize in an organ-specific manner. Clin Exp Metastasis 25:11–32. Epub 8 Sep 2007

42. Augsburger JJ, Correa ZM, Shaikh AH (2009) Effectiveness of treatments for metastatic uveal melanoma. Am J Ophthalmol 148:119–127

43. Hendrix MJ et al (1998) Regulation of uveal melanoma interconverted phenotype by hepatocyte growth factor/scatter factor (HGF/SF). Am J Pathol 152:855–863

44. Hendrix MJ et al (1998) Biologic determinants of uveal melanoma metastatic phenotype: role of intermediate filaments as predictive markers. Lab Invest 78:153–163

45. Mallikarjuna K et al (2007) Expression of epidermal growth factor receptor, ezrin, hepatocyte growth factor, and c-Met in uveal melanoma: an immunohistochemical study. Curr Eye Res 32:281–290

46. Di Cesare S et al (2007) Expression and migratory analysis of 5 human uveal melanoma cell lines for CXCL12, CXCL8, CXCL1, and HGF. J Carcinog 6:2

47. Woodward JK et al (2002) Stimulation and inhibition of uveal melanoma invasion by HGF, GRO, IL-1alpha and TGF-beta. Invest Ophthalmol Vis Sci 43:3144–3152

48. Cools-Lartigue J et al (2005) Secretion of hepatocyte growth factor and vascular endothelial growth factor during uveal melanoma-monocyte in vitro interactions. Melanoma Res 15: 141–145

49. Peruzzi B, Bottaro DP (2006) Targeting the c-Met signaling pathway in cancer. Clin Cancer Res 12:3657–3660

50. Economou MA et al (2005) Receptors for the liver synthesized growth factors IGF-1 and HGF/SF in uveal melanoma: intercorrelation and prognostic implications. Invest Ophthalmol Vis Sci 46:4372–4375

51. Mallikarjuna K et al (2006) Expression of insulin-like growth factor receptor (IGF-1R), c-Fos, and c-Jun in uveal melanoma: an immunohistochemical study. Curr Eye Res 31: 875–883

52. All-Ericsson C et al (2002) Insulin-like growth factor-1 receptor in uveal melanoma: a predictor for metastatic disease and a potential therapeutic target. Invest Ophthalmol Vis Sci 43:1–8

53. Pollak MN (2004) Insulin-like growth factors and neoplasia. Novartis Found Symp 262: 84–98; discussion 98–107, 265–268
54. Adhami VM, Afaq F, Mukhtar H (2006) Insulin-like growth factor-I axis as a pathway for cancer chemoprevention. Clin Cancer Res 12:5611–5614
55. Saltiel AR, Kahn CR (2001) Insulin signalling and the regulation of glucose and lipid metabolism. Nature 414:799–806
56. Riedemann J, Macaulay VM (2006) IGF1R signalling and its inhibition. Endocr Relat Cancer 13:S33–43
57. Girnita A et al (2006) The insulin-like growth factor-I receptor inhibitor picropodophyllin causes tumor regression and attenuates mechanisms involved in invasion of uveal melanoma cells. Clin Cancer Res 12:1383–1391
58. Burger JA, Kipps TJ (2006) CXCR4: a key receptor in the crosstalk between tumor cells and their microenvironment. Blood 107:1761–1767
59. Muller A et al (2001) Involvement of chemokine receptors in breast cancer metastasis. Nature 410:50–56
60. Wang J et al (2005) Diverse signaling pathways through the SDF-1/CXCR4 chemokine axis in prostate cancer cell lines leads to altered patterns of cytokine secretion and angiogenesis. Cell Signal 17:1578–1592
61. Zeelenberg IS, Ruuls-Van Stalle L, Roos E (2003) The chemokine receptor CXCR4 is required for outgrowth of colon carcinoma micrometastases. Cancer Res 63:3833–3839
62. Bertolini F et al (2002) CXCR4 neutralization, a novel therapeutic approach for non-Hodgkin's lymphoma. Cancer Res 62:3106–3112
63. Yasumoto K et al (2006) Role of the CXCL12/CXCR4 axis in peritoneal carcinomatosis of gastric cancer. Cancer Res 66:2181–2187
64. Saraiva VS et al (2005) Immunohistochemical expression of phospho-Akt in uveal melanoma. Melanoma Res 15:245–250
65. Zuidervaart W et al (2005) Activation of the MAPK pathway is a common event in uveal melanomas although it rarely occurs through mutation of BRAF or RAS. Br J Cancer 92:2032–2038
66. Graells J et al (2004) Overproduction of VEGF concomitantly expressed with its receptors promotes growth and survival of melanoma cells through MAPK and PI3K signaling. J Invest Dermatol 123:1151–1161
67. Tsao H et al (2004) Genetic interaction between NRAS and BRAF mutations and PTEN/MMAC1 inactivation in melanoma. J Invest Dermatol 122:337–341
68. Liang Z et al (2004) Inhibition of breast cancer metastasis by selective synthetic polypeptide against CXCR4. Cancer Res 64:4302–4308
69. Scala S et al (2007) CXC chemokine receptor 4 is expressed in uveal malignant melanoma and correlates with the epithelioid-mixed cell type. Cancer Immunol Immunother. Oct; 56: 1589–1595. Epub 5 Apr 2007
70. Demicheli R et al (1996) Time distribution of the recurrence risk for breast cancer patients undergoing mastectomy: further support about the concept of tumor dormancy. Breast Cancer Res Treat 41:177–185
71. Crowley NJ, Seigler HF (1992) Relationship between disease-free interval and survival in patients with recurrent melanoma. Arch Surg 127:1303–1308
72. Yoshida BA et al (2000) Metastasis-suppressor genes: a review and perspective on an emerging field. J Natl Cancer Inst 92:1717–1730
73. Ohtaki T et al (2001) Metastasis suppressor gene KiSS-1 encodes peptide ligand of a G-protein-coupled receptor. Nature 411:613–617
74. Nash KT et al (2007) Requirement of KISS1 secretion for multiple organ metastasis suppression and maintenance of tumor dormancy. J Natl Cancer Inst 99:309–321
75. Miele ME et al (1996) Metastasis suppressed, but tumorigenicity and local invasiveness unaffected, in the human melanoma cell line MelJuSo after introduction of human chromosomes 1 or 6. Mol Carcinog 15:284–299

76. Welch DR et al (1994) Microcell-mediated transfer of chromosome 6 into metastatic human C8161 melanoma cells suppresses metastasis but does not inhibit tumorigenicity. Oncogene 9:255–262

77. Lee JH, Welch DR (1997) Suppression of metastasis in human breast carcinoma MDA-MB-435 cells after transfection with the metastasis suppressor gene, KiSS-1. Cancer Res 57: 2384–2387

78. Shirasaki F et al (2001) Loss of expression of the metastasis suppressor gene KiSS1 during melanoma progression and its association with LOH of chromosome 6q16.3-q23. Cancer Res 61:7422–7425

79. Martins CM et al (2008) Expression of the metastasis suppressor gene KISS1 in uveal melanoma. Eye 22:707–711

Index

P. Brodt (ed.), *Liver Metastasis: Biology and Clinical Management*, Cancer
Metastasis – Biology and Treatment 16, DOI 10.1007/978-94-007-0292-9,
© Springer Science+Business Media B.V. 2011

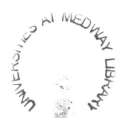